MECHANICAL VENTILATION

Second Edition

MECHANICAL VENTILATION

Neil R. MacIntyre, MD
Professor of Medicine
Medical Director of Respiratory Care
Clinical Chief of the Division of Pulmonary and Critical Care Medicine
Duke University Medical Center
Durham, North Carolina

Richard D. Branson, MSc, RRT
Associate Professor of Surgery
Adjunct Faculty
College of Pharmacy
University of Cincinnati
Cincinnati, Ohio
Adjunct Faculty
School of Aerospace Medicine
United States Air Force

with 234 illustrations

SAUNDERS
ELSEVIER

SAUNDERS
ELSEVIER

11830 Westline Industrial Drive
St. Louis, Missouri 63146

MECHANICAL VENTILATION
ISBN: 978-1-4160-3141-3

Library of Congress Control Number 2007930779

Publisher: Jeanne Wilke
Managing Editor: Billi Sharp
Senior Developmental Editor: Mindy Hutchinson
Publishing Services Manager: Pat Joiner-Myers
Senior Project Manager: Rachel E. Dowell
Design Direction: Maggie Reid

Printed in the United States of America

Last digit is the print number: 9 8 7 6 5 4 3 2 1

To my family and the Duke Respiratory Care Department for their support.

NM

I want to thank my long time colleagues in the Department of Surgery at the University of Cincinnati who have taught me so much and been good friends.

RB

Contributors

Mariam Al-Ansari, MD, FRCSI
Consultant Intensivist
Intensive Care Unit
Salmaniya Medical Complex
Manama, Kingdom of Bahrain

Shannon S. Carson, MD
Associate Professor
Pulmonary and Critical Care Medicine
University of North Carolina School of Medicine
Chapel Hill, North Carolina

Robert L. Chatburn, BS, RRT-NPS, FAARC
Clinical Research Manager
Respiratory Therapy
The Cleveland Clinic
Cleveland, Ohio

Ira M. Cheifetz, MD, FCCM, FAARC
Associate Professor of Pediatrics
Division Chief, Pediatric Critical Care Medicine
Medical Director, Pediatric ICU
Medical Director, Pediatric Respiratory Care and ECMO Programs
Duke Children's Hospital
Durham, North Carolina

Christopher E. Cox, MD, MPH
Assistant Professor of Medicine
Duke University Medical Center
Durham, North Carolina

John D. Davies, MA, RRT, FAARC
Clinical Research Coordinator
Respiratory Care Services
Duke University Medical Center
Durham, North Carolina

Henry E. Fessler, MD
Associate Professor
Pulmonary and Critical Care Medicine
Johns Hopkins Medical Institutions
Baltimore, Marlyand

Bryan A. Fisk, MD, MSc
Assistant Chief, Critical Care Medicine Service
Department of Surgery
Walter Reed Army Medical Center
Washington, D.C.

Michael A. Gentile, BS, RRT, FAARC
Associate in Research Department
Pulmonary and Critical Care Medicine
Duke University Medical Center
Durham, North Carolina

Joseph A. Govert, MD
Associate Professor of Medicine
Internal Medicine Department
Duke University Medical Center
Durham, North Carolina

David N. Hager, MD
Fellow
Pulmonary and Critical Care Medicine
Johns Hopkins School of Medicine
Baltimore, Maryland

Dean R. Hess, PhD, RRT
Associate Professor of Anesthesia
Harvard Medical School;
Assistant Director of Respiratory Care
Massachusetts General Hospital
Boston, Massachusetts

Mohammed Hijazi, MD, FCCP
Consultant Intensivist
Director, Quality Resource Management Department
Department of Medicine
King Faisal Specialist Hospital and Research Center
Riyadh, Saudi Arabia

Nicholas S. Hill, MD
Professor of Medicine
Tufts University School of Medicine;
Chief, Pulmonary and Critical Care and Sleep Division
Tufts-New England Medical Center
Boston, Massachusetts

Jay A. Johannigman, MD, FACS, FCCM
Associate Professor of Surgery
Director, Division of Trauma/Critical Care
Department of Surgery
University of Cincinnati
Cincinnati, Ohio

Lisa K. Moores, MD
Associate Professor of Medicine
Assistant Dean for Clinical Sciences
The Uniformed Services University of the Health Sciences
Bethesda, Maryland

Catherine S.H. Sassoon, MD
Professor of Medicine
Pulmonary and Critical Care Section, Department of Medicine
University of California, Irvine; VA Long Beach Health Care System
Irvine, California

John H. Sherner, MD
Staff Physician
Pulmonary, Critical Care and Sleep Medicine Service
Walter Reed Army Medical Center
Washington, D.C.

Renee D. Stapleton, MD, MSC
Acting Instructor
Medicine, Pulmonary and Critical Care Medicine
Harborview Medical Center/University of Washington School of Medicine
Seattle, Washington

Kenneth P. Steinberg, MD
Associate Professor of Medicine
Section Head, Pulmonary and Critical Care Medicine
University of Washington School of Medicine;
Director, Medical Intensive Care Unit
Harborview Medical Center
Seattle, Washington

Lawrence Tom, MD
Fellow, Pulmonary and Critical Care Medicine
Pulmonary and Critical Care Section, Department of Medicine
University of California, Irvine
Irvine, California

Reviewers

Allen W. Barbaro, MS, RRT
Clinical Coordinator
Respiratory Care Program
Labette Community College
Parsons, Kansas

Catherine A. Bitsche, MA, RRT-NPS, RCP
Program Director
Respiratory Therapy Program
Catawba Valley Community College
Hickory, North Carolina

Phillip Bushman, MS, RRT
Associate Professor
Shenandoah University
Winchester, Virginia

Christine Hamilton, MA, RRT, AE-C
Program Director, Respiratory Care
Nebraska Methodist College
Omaha, Nebraska

John Jarosz, MS, RRT
Director of Clinical Education
Nebraska Methodist College
Omaha, Nebraska

Robert L. Joyner, Jr., PhD, RRT
Associate Professor and Chair
Department of Health Sciences
Director, Respiratory Therapy Program
Salisbury University
Salisbury, Maryland

Timothy B. Op't Holt, EdD, RRT, AE-C, FAARC
Professor
Cardiorespiratory Care
College of Allied Health
University of South Alabama
Mobile, Alabama

Stanley M. Pearson, MSEd, RRT, C-CPT
Program Representative/Assistant Professor Respiratory Therapy
Southern Illinois University
College of Applied Sciences and Arts
Health Care Professions
Carbondale, Illinois

Preface

Mechanical ventilation is ubiquitous to intensive care. In fact, the modern day intensive care unit (ICU) owes its origins to the need to care for patients on ventilators in a common location. The implementation, management, and monitoring of mechanical ventilation are core competencies for physicians, respiratory therapists, and nurses in the ICU. Recent evidence demonstrates that the appropriate use of the mechanical ventilator in the patient with acute respiratory distress syndrome (ARDS) reduces morbidity and mortality. Implementation of the lung protective approach to ventilation is a paradigm shift for most critical care clinicians, and expertise in ventilator operation and patient-ventilator interaction are critical to successful use of this strategy.

Mechanical ventilation without intubation, commonly referred to as noninvasive ventilation (NIV), has also been shown to improve outcomes. Use of NIV in the patient with an exacerbation of chronic obstructive pulmonary disease (COPD) reduces the need for intubation, decreases ICU stay, and improves survival. The appropriate use of NIV requires a complete understanding of the devices and interfaces used, as well as the appropriate settings to maximize success. Nuances of NIV, including spending time to introduce the patient to therapy, noninvasive monitoring of response, and recognizing failure are all paramount to success.

Mechanical ventilator technology moves far ahead of evidence for new modes and techniques, making it difficult for even the most dedicated practitioners to remain abreast of all the changes. Microprocessors and miniaturization allow ventilator operation to be limited only by the imagination. Clinicians must understand new technology to separate the wheat from the chaff. This second edition of *Mechanical Ventilation* is intended to address these issues and many more.

The main goal has been to write a practical and useful text for clinicians and students. Each topic is covered from the clinician's perspective. We have endeavored to provide the evidence and the art of mechanical ventilation to aid the clinician in caring for the mechanically ventilated patient.

NEW TO THIS EDITION

Every chapter has been updated to include discussions of new technology and propose best practices using evidence-based medicine. Discussions of devices and techniques that have failed to meet their promise have been eliminated, and discussions of future technologies have been added.

A new chapter on "Unique Patient Populations" has been added to cover the unique features, pathophysiology, and management of patients requiring mechanical ventilation who may not be suffering from lung disease. Patient populations include those with traumatic brain injury, neuromuscular disease, lung transplantation, and burn injury, and perioperative patient populations.

In addition, more case studies have been added to the appendix. The glossary has been expanded to include more useful terms, and a new appendix has been added with answers to all of the assessment questions found within the chapters.

LEARNING AIDS

Outlines, objectives, key terms, key points, and assessment questions have been included for each chapter to make the text more useful for instructors and students. Our emphasis remains a clinically useful, comprehensive discussion of the engineering issues, physiologic principles, and patient management strategies toward improved outcomes in mechanically ventilated patients.

EVOLVE RESOURCES

Evolve is an interactive learning environment designed to work in coordination with *Mechanical Ventilation,* second edition. Instructors may use Evolve to provide an Internet-based course component that reinforces and expands the concepts presented in class. Evolve may be used to publish the class syllabus, outlines, and lecture notes; set up "virtual office hours" and e-mail communication; share important dates and information through the online class calendar; and encourage student participation through chat rooms and discussion boards. Evolve allows instructors to post exams and manage their grade books online. For more information, visit http://evolve.elsevier.com/MacIntyre/ or contact an Elsevier sales representative.

The Evolve site features a web-based Instructor's Electronic Resource, which includes a collection of all of the images from this text in both jpeg and PowerPoint formats, a test bank in ExamView, and an instructor's manual.

Contents

SECTION IV CLINICAL APPLICATIONS, 287

SECTION I TECHNICAL ASPECTS OF MECHANICAL VENTILATION

CHAPTER 1

Classification of Mechanical Ventilators

ROBERT L. CHATBURN; RICHARD D. BRANSON

OUTLINE

OBJECTIVES

- Describe a logical classification system for describing ventilator function.
- Describe the equation of motion for the respiratory system and how this equation delineates the phase variables for describing ventilator operation.
- Compare and contrast pressure and volume control ventilation.
- Describe the criteria for determining the control variable during ventilator evaluation.
- Describe the unique characteristics that describe and distinguish spontaneous and mandatory breaths.
- Define trigger, limit, and cycle variables.
- Describe ventilator modes based on the control, trigger, limit, and cycle variables and breath types.
- Compare and contrast the methods of triggering a breath.
- Compare and contrast the methods of cycling a breath.
- Compare and contrast the control and driving mechanisms used by mechanical ventilators.
- Compare and contrast the output waveforms of mechanical ventilators.
- Describe ventilator alarms with respect to ventilator function.

KEY TERMS

alarm event
closed-loop control
compressor
control circuit
control variables
cycle time
cycle variable
elastance
end-expiratory pressure
expiratory flow time
expiratory pause time
expiratory phase
expiratory time
external compressor
inspiratory flow time
inspiratory pause time
inspiratory phase
inspiratory time
internal compressors
limit
mandatory breath
open-loop control
phases
phase variables
phase variable values
resistance
spontaneous breaths
transrespiratory pressure

Ventilators have evolved into highly complex, microprocessor-controlled devices with a wide range of operating characteristics. Unfortunately, our language and conceptual models, which we use to understand how ventilators work, have not kept pace with the technologic development. Mushin's classic text,[1] based on ventilators common in the 1960s, provides a theoretical framework for understanding ventilators, but cannot adequately describe all the characteristics of current ventilators. This is not meant as criticism, but simply reflects the fact that Mushin did not anticipate these advancements in technology.

When Mushin developed his framework, the ventilator output was dictated by the mechanical driving system. For instance, a piston ventilator provided a quasisinusoidal flow waveform, whereas early pneumatic ventilators (Bird Mark 14) provided a rectangular pressure pattern. These patterns were not able to be altered without some external modification. The advent of microprocessor technology allows a single ventilator to produce any number of output waveforms, some as limitless as the operator's imagination. This chapter presents an updated classification scheme that effectively deals with new technology that has been accepted by leading members of the pulmonary medicine community[2-4] and most authors of respiratory care textbooks.

BOX 1-1 *Outline of Ventilator Classification System*

- I. Input Power
  - A. Electric
  - B. Pneumatic
- II. Control Scheme
  - A. Control Variables
    1. Pressure
    2. Volume
    3. Flow
    4. Time
  - B. Phase Variables
    1. Trigger
    2. Limit
    3. Cycle
    4. Baseline
  - C. Conditional Variables
  - D. Modes of Ventilation
  - E. Control Subsystems
    1. Control Circuit
    2. Drive Mechanism
    3. Output Control Valve
- III. Output
  - A. Waveforms
    1. Pressure
    2. Volume
    3. Flow
  - B. Displays
- IV. Alarm Systems
  - A. Input Power Systems
  - B. Control Circuit Alarms
  - C. Output Alarms

BASIC CONCEPTS

A ventilator is simply a machine—a system of related elements designed to alter, transmit, and direct applied energy in a predetermined manner to perform useful work.[5] Energy enters the ventilator in the form of electricity (energy = volts × amperes × time) or compressed gas (energy = pressure × volume). That energy is transmitted or transformed (by the ventilator's drive mechanism) in a predetermined manner (by the control circuit) to augment or replace the patient's muscles in performing the work of breathing (the desired output). Therefore to understand mechanical ventilators in general, we first must understand their basic functions of:

- Power input
- Control scheme (including power transmission or conversion)
- Output (pressure, volume, and flow waveforms)

This simple outline format can be expanded to add as much detail about a given ventilator as desired (Box 1-1).

INPUT POWER

All ventilators require a source of power that can be used to perform the work of ventilating the respiratory system. In effect, ventilators convert input power in a readily available form to a form that is more convenient for the delicate and exacting task of supporting ventilation. The most common forms of input power for ventilators are electric and pneumatic (compressed gas). Input power should not be confused with the power for the control circuit. For example, many ventilators use pneumatic input power to drive inspiration but electric power for the control circuit. As an example, compressed O_2 at 50 pounds per square inch gauge (psig) can be delivered to a ventilator that uses a solenoid valve to control respiratory frequency and inspiratory : expiratory (I : E) ratio. The compressed gas delivers the energy (input power) to ventilate the lungs, whereas the solenoid uses electric power to operate the control circuit.

Electric

Most ventilators in the United States use 110 to 115 volts of alternating current (AC) (60 Hz) from common electrical outlets to power drive mechanisms. The AC voltage also is reduced and converted to direct current (DC) to power electronic control circuits. Many ventilators, notably infant and transport ventilators, are designed to use rechargeable batteries as alternative sources of power when the usual AC current is not available. This capability makes them useful for transferring ventilator-dependent patients from one place to another within the hospital and for external transport. In the home care setting, a battery backup can be a life-saving feature in the event of a power outage. Common ventilator batteries are the lead-acid type, which supplies approximately 2.5 amp-hours of energy. This usually powers a ventilator for up to 1 hour. This type of battery normally requires 8 to 12 hours to recharge. Nickel-cadmium (NiCad) batteries can be used, but because the batteries develop memory and require complete discharge before recharging, careful monitoring must be done. More recently, lithium-ion batteries have been used for powering mechanical ventilators. The lithium-ion battery is capable of carrying a longer charge at a lower weight and faster recharge time than the NiCad batteries.

Pneumatic

Because compressed air and O_2 are in abundant supply in most hospital intensive care units, many ventilators are designed to use the energy stored in pressurized gas. Pressure is usually thought to be a force per unit area, but pressure also has the units of energy density—thus the more pressure available, the more useful work that can be generated. Besides being used to inflate the lungs, the input pressure often is used as the source of power for the control circuit, as in the case of fluidic logic circuits. Ventilators operated by pressurized gas typically have internal pressure-reducing regulators, so that the normal operating pressure is lower than the source pressure. This allows uninterrupted operation from piped gas sources in hospitals, which usually are regulated to 50 psig but are subject to periodic fluctuations. The use of compressed gas as a power source makes a ventilator useful in environments in which no electrical power is available, such as during transport, or where it is undesirable, such as near magnetic resonance imaging (MRI) equipment.

CONTROL SCHEME

To understand how a machine can be controlled to replace or augment the natural function of breathing, a basic understanding of the mechanics of breathing is required. The study of mechanics deals with forces, displacements, and the rate of change of displacement. In physiology, force is measured as pressure (pressure = force × area), displacement is measured as volume (volume = area × displacement), and the relevant rate of change is measured as flow (e.g., average flow = change in volume/change in time; instantaneous flow = dv/dt, the derivative of volume with respect to time). Specifically, we are interested in the pressure necessary to cause a flow of gas to flow through the airways and increase the volume of the lungs.

The study of respiratory mechanics is essentially the search for simple but useful models of respiratory system mechanical behavior. Conceptually the relatively complex respiratory system can be represented by a simple graphic model (e.g., a straw connected to a balloon). The simple graphic model is analogous to simple electrical circuits in which compliance is analogous to capacitance, flow resistance is analogous to electrical resistance, and pressure is analogous to a voltage source. The similarity of the physical and electrical models makes it possible to borrow mathematical models from electrical engineering, substituting pressure, volume, and flow for voltage, charge, and current, respectively (Figure 1-1). The result is known as the equation of motion for the respiratory system (a simplified version)[6,7]:

$$\text{Muscle pressure} + \text{ventilator pressure} = \text{elastance} \times \text{volume} + \text{resistance} \times \text{flow} \quad (1)$$

$$\text{Muscle pressure} + \text{ventilator pressure} = \text{elastic load} + \text{resistive load} \quad (2)$$

In this simplified form, muscle pressure is the imaginary **transrespiratory pressure** (i.e., airway pressure minus body surface pressure) generated by the ventilatory muscles to expand the thoracic cage and lungs. Muscle pressure is said to be imaginary because it is not directly measurable. Ventilator pressure is the transrespiratory pressure generated by the ventilator during inspiration. The combined muscle and ventilator pressure causes volume and flow to be delivered to the patient. In more simple terms, the patient's muscle effort increases lung volume by decreasing pressure relative to atmospheric pressure, whereas the ventilator increases lung volume by increasing pressure relative to atmospheric pressure. Total pressure results from the patient pulling gas into

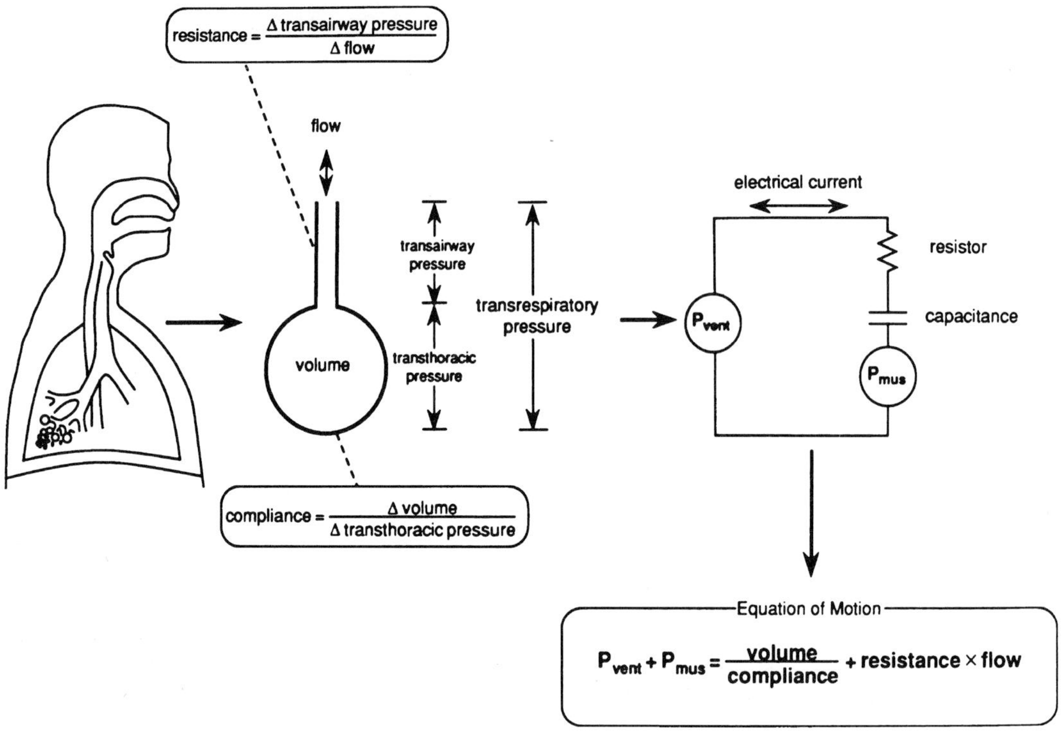

FIGURE 1-1 The study of respiratory system mechanics is based on graphic and mathematical models. The respiratory system can be modeled as a single-flow conducting tube connected to a single elastic compartment. This physical model is analogous to a simple electrical circuit consisting of a resistor and a capacitor. Two voltage sources in the circuit represent pressures generated by the muscles and the ventilator; electrical current represents airflow. The electrical circuit can be modeled by a mathematical model called the equation of motion for the respiratory system. In this model, pressure, volume, and flow are variables (i.e., functions of time), whereas resistance and compliance are constants. P_{vent}, Ventilator pressure; P_{mus}, muscle pressure.

the lung and the ventilator pushing gas into the lung. Pressure, volume, and flow change with time and hence are variables. Elastance and resistance are assumed to remain constant and are called parameters. Their combined effect constitutes the load experienced by the ventilator and ventilatory muscles. **Elastance** is defined as the ratio of pressure change to volume change (i.e., the reciprocal of compliance), and **resistance** is defined as the ratio of pressure change to flow change. The elastic load is the pressure necessary to overcome the elastance (or compliance) of the respiratory system, and the resistive load is the pressure necessary to overcome the flow resistance of the airways (including endotracheal tube) along with lung and chest wall tissue resistance. The term parameter also may refer to a particular aspect of a variable, such as the peak or mean value.

Note that pressure, volume, and flow all are measured relative to their baseline values (i.e., their values at end-expiration). This means that the pressure to cause inspiration is measured as the change in airway pressure above positive end-expiratory pressure (PEEP). This is the reason, for example, that pressure support levels are measured relative to PEEP. Thinking of ventilator pressure as simply airway pressure (i.e., pressure measured at one point in space, the airway) limits our understanding of the mechanics involved in breathing. Volume is measured as the change in lung volume above functional residual capacity, and the change in lung volume during the inspiratory period is defined as the tidal volume. Flow is measured relative to its end-expiratory value (usually zero). When pressure, volume, and flow are plotted as functions of time, characteristic waveforms

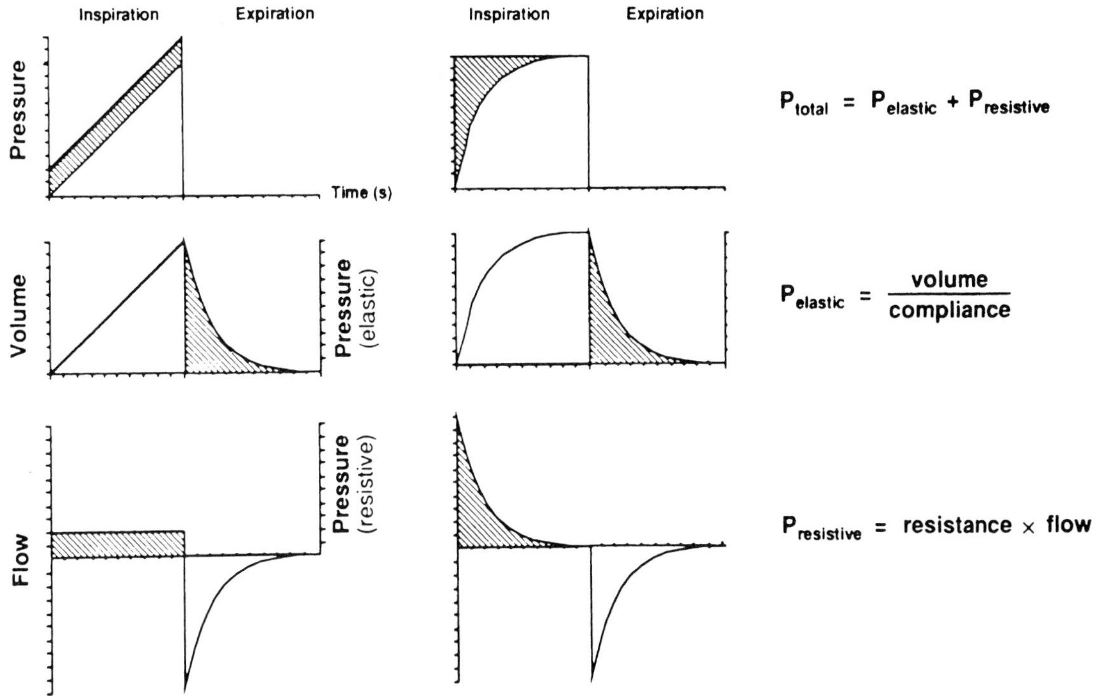

FIGURE 1-2 Some conventions for the presentation of graphic data. The theoretical output waveforms for flow-controlled inspiration with a rectangular (i.e., pulse) flow waveform on the left compared with pressure-controlled inspiration with a rectangular pressure waveform are shown. The order of presentation is pressure, volume, and flow, according to the order specified by the equation of motion. Note that the volume waveform has the same shape as the transthoracic or lung pressure waveform (i.e., pressure caused by elastic recoil). The flow waveform has the same shape as the transairway pressure waveform (i.e., pressure caused by airway resistance). If all the pressure scales are the same, then the height of the airway pressure waveform at any instant is the sum of the heights of the other two waveforms. The origin of the airway pressure waveform is the end-expiratory pressure; the origins of the volume and flow waveforms are both zero. The shaded areas represent pressures caused by flow resistance; the open areas represent pressure caused by elastic recoil.

for volume-controlled ventilation and pressure-controlled ventilation are produced (Figure 1-2).

Notice that if the patient's ventilatory muscles are not functioning, muscle pressure is zero and the ventilator must generate all of the pressure required to deliver the tidal volume and inspiratory flow. Conversely, if ventilator pressure is zero (i.e., airway pressure does not rise above baseline during inspiration) and the patient is not breathing, there is no ventilatory support. In between these two extremes, there are an infinite variety of combinations of muscle pressure (i.e., patient effort) and ventilator support that are theoretically possible for partial ventilatory support.

The concept of muscle pressure is important for another reason. There are many ventilators and bedside pulmonary function monitors that provide the clinician with estimates of respiratory system compliance and resistance based on transrespiratory system pressure (i.e., ventilator pressure), volume, and flow. All of them make calculations on the basis of this version of the equation of motion:

$$\text{Ventilator pressure} = \text{elastance} \times \text{volume} + \text{resistance} \times \text{flow} \quad (3)$$

which does not contain a term for muscle pressure. This implies that any measurement of respiratory system mechanics is valid only if the ventilatory

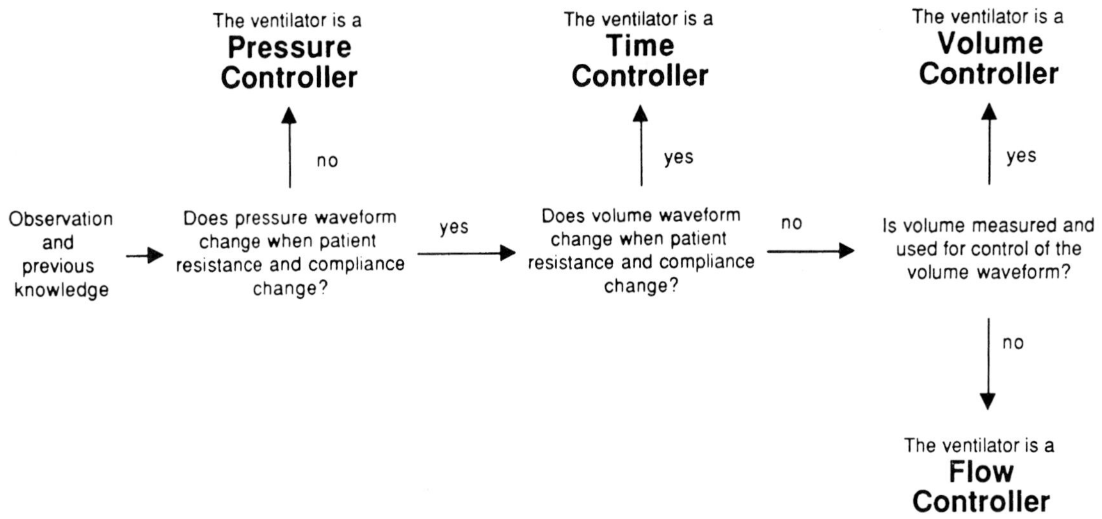

FIGURE 1-3 Criteria for determining the control variable during a ventilator-assisted inspiration.

muscles are inactive. If the patient makes an inspiratory effort during an assisted breath, he or she adds an unmeasured amount of driving pressure to that generated by the ventilator. Thus elastance and resistance based only on the ventilator's airway pressure sensor measurements underestimate the true values.

Analysis of ventilator-patient interaction on the basis of a mathematical model suggests the proper use of the word *assist,* which is another frequently confused concept. *Webster's Dictionary* defines assist as "to help; to aid; to give support." From the perspective of the equation of motion, whenever airway pressure (i.e., ventilator pressure) rises above baseline during inspiration, the ventilator does work on the patient. Thus the breath is said to be assisted, independent of other breath characteristics (i.e., whether the breath is classified as spontaneous or mandatory). Do not confuse this meaning of the word *assist* with specific names of modes of ventilation (e.g., assist/control). Ventilator manufacturers often coin terms for modes without regard to consistency or theoretical relevance.

In the equation of motion (3), the form of any one of the three variables (i.e., pressure, volume, or flow expressed as functions of time) can be predetermined, making it the independent variable and making the other two dependent variables. This is precisely analogous to the way in which ventilators operate. Thus during pressure-controlled ventilation, pressure is the independent variable, and the shape of the volume and flow waveforms depends on the shape of the pressure waveform and also on the resistance and compliance of the respiratory system. Conversely, during flow-controlled ventilation, we can specify the shape of the flow waveform. This makes flow the independent variable and the shape of the volume waveform depends on the shape of the flow waveform. The shape of the pressure waveform depends on the flow waveform and on resistance and compliance.

Thus there is a theoretical basis for classifying ventilators as pressure, volume, or flow controllers. The necessary and sufficient criteria for determining which variable is controlled (i.e., which variable is the independent variable) are illustrated in Figure 1-3. If the waveforms for all three variables are not predetermined (i.e., none of the variables can be considered independent), then the ventilator is considered to control only the timing of the inspiratory and **expiratory phase** and is called a time controller. From a practical standpoint, the only time controllers are some types of high-frequency ventilators.

This theoretical framework is more than just an intellectual exercise. It is essential for the understanding and interpretation of bedside pulmonary mechanics values (e.g., resistance, compliance, time constant, and the like) calculated by many ventilators. It is the basis of a new mode of ventilatory support known as "proportional assist."[8] The idea of this mode of ventilation is to allow the clinician to support—and essentially cancel—the specific effects of pulmonary pathology. Thus the ventilator can be set to support either the extra elastance or the extra resistance caused by lung disease, or both. To understand this, we start with the equation describing spontaneous breathing:

$$\text{Muscle pressure} = \text{normal elastance} \times \text{volume} + \text{normal resistance} \times \text{flow} \quad (4)$$

When pathology increases elastance and/or resistance, we have:

$$\text{Muscle pressure} = (\text{normal elastance} + \text{abnormal elastance}) \times \text{volume} + (\text{normal resistance} + \text{abnormal resistance}) \times \text{flow} \quad (5)$$

Equation 5 can be rearranged to show the normal and abnormal loads. Recall that load, in this context, is the pressure to overcome either elastance or resistance (i.e., elastance × volume = pressure; resistance × flow = pressure).

$$\text{Muscle pressure} = (\text{normal elastance} \times \text{volume}) + (\text{normal resistance} \times \text{flow}) + (\text{abnormal elastance} \times \text{volume}) + (\text{abnormal resistance} \times \text{flow}) \quad (6a)$$

$$\text{Muscle pressure} = (\text{normal elastance} \times \text{volume}) + (\text{normal resistance} \times \text{flow}) + \text{abnormal load} \quad (6b)$$

Because both the abnormal elastic load and the abnormal resistive load have units of pressure, they can be added together. This shows that in the presence of increased load, the muscle pressure must increase to provide the same (i.e., normal) tidal volume and flow. If we want to mechanically support the abnormal load(s) and allow muscle pressure to return to normal levels, all we have to do is set the ventilator to generate a sufficiently large inspiratory pressure. This can be seen by equating load to ventilator pressure and adding it to the left side of Equation 6b:

$$\text{Muscle pressure} + \text{ventilator pressure} = (\text{normal elastance} \times \text{volume}) + (\text{normal resistance} \times \text{flow}) + \text{abnormal load} \quad (7)$$

In this case, the muscle pressure generates the force to overcome normal elastance and resistance whereas the ventilator pressure generates the force to overcome abnormal elastance and resistance so that normal tidal volume and inspiratory flow result. This analysis shows that proportional assist is a form of pressure control ventilation. Furthermore, we can see that it differs from the pressure support mode because the ventilator pressure does not necessarily generate a rectangular pressure waveform. On the contrary, the ventilator pressure varies continuously throughout inspiration.

To understand how this works, look at Equations 6 and 7. We see that ventilator pressure has two components. One is elastance × volume and the other is resistance × flow. Elastance and resistance are assumed to be constant throughout inspiration, whereas volume and flow change with the continuously varying muscle pressure. Because of the requirement for muscle pressure, proportional assist works only with spontaneous breaths. Ventilator pressure is proportional to the volume and flow signals (hence the name *proportional assist*) where the constants of proportionality are the abnormal elastance and resistance. In engineering terms, these constants are gain (or amplification) factors set on the volume and flow signals. The ventilator measures airway pressure and flow. The flow signal is integrated to get a volume signal. The flow and volume signals are fed through two amplifiers, through a mixer (that combines the amplified signals). The mixed signal is fed to a pressure generator (e.g., a piston) connected to the patient's airway.

The ventilator's control circuit is programmed with the equation of motion so that each moment, airway pressure is controlled to be equal to the amplified volume signal plus the amplified flow signal. The gain of the flow amplifier is set to the abnormal resistance, and the gain of the volume amplifier is set to the abnormal elastance, assuming these values have been measured or estimated. Thus the specific mechanical abnormality of the patient is supported. In effect, the abnormal load is eliminated and the patient perceives only normal ventilatory load. It is analogous to power steering on an automobile, making driving easier while maintaining complete responsiveness to the operator's motions. No ventilator power is wasted, forcing the patient to breathe in an unnatural pattern, as can happen with pressure support. This makes proportional assist potentially the most comfortable mode of ventilation yet designed. Of course, there are some practical problems, such as how to continually monitor and reset the abnormal elastance and resistance levels, but these issues should be resolved soon.

The most significant revelation provided by the equation of motion, however, is that any conceivable ventilator can directly control only one variable at a time: pressure, volume, or flow. Therefore we can think of a ventilator as simply a machine that controls either the airway pressure waveform, the inspired volume waveform, or the inspiratory flow waveform. Thus pressure, volume, and flow are referred to in this context as **control variables.** Time is a variable that is implicit in the equation of motion. As shown in the following examples, in some cases time is viewed as a control variable. This concept allows us to understand any mode, no matter how complex, by simply observing how control switches from one variable to the next.

The use of the term control presents a problem for many clinicians. In many instances the clinician says "control" to mean that the ventilator does not respond to patient effort. As previously mentioned, often "control" means a breath that is part of a mode, such as assist control. In this classification system, "control" refers to the variable that the ventilator maintains constant regardless of changes in elastance or resistance. This historical basis for nomenclature causes many authors to mix and match the term control, leading to confusion. For the remaining chapters of the text, control will be as defined for describing ventilator operation. However, in some cases the reader may find the term "targeted" to mean the same as control.

Knowing what is controlled will help understand how it is controlled. In discussing respiratory mechanics, the term *system* is used without definition. Formally, a system is defined as a collection of elements that interact according to some particular process or function. A model is a simplified version of a real world system used to help us understand the relationships among system elements (e.g., the equation of motion is a model of the respiratory system). Specifically, we are interested in understanding the relationship between the input and the output of the system (e.g., we need to create a model). This understanding then may help us to control the system behavior.

A system can be controlled in two different ways to achieve the desired output[9]:

1. Select an input and wait for an output with no interference during the waiting period.
2. Select an input, observe the trend in the output, and modify the input accordingly to get as close as possible to the desired output.

For example, when a helmsman steers a boat toward the dock, he may do it in one of the two ways described previously:

1. Point the boat in the direction of the dock and retire to his cabin.
2. Continuously steer the boat toward the dock, by observing the direction of the dock, observing the direction the boat is moving, and making adjustments as necessary.

In this example, the system is the boat (motor, propeller, steering mechanism, etc.), the input is the position of the boat's steering wheel, and the output is the direction of the boat's motion. In both cases a change in the input causes a change in the output. However, in the first case, there is no flow of information from the output to generate a new input to *close the loop*. Hence, this type of control scheme is called **open-loop control.** In the second case, the helmsman uses information about the output to modify the input, which in turn improves the output. This control scheme is called **closed-loop control** or feedback control. Feedback control is also called servo control. Figure 1-4 illustrates block diagrams (i.e., models) of open- and closed-loop control systems.

To perform closed-loop control, the output must be measured and compared with a reference value. In the aforementioned example, a human performed the measuring and comparing functions. But in ventilators, pressure and flow transducers and electronic circuitry are necessary to perform automatic closed-loop control. Closed-loop control provides the advantage of a more consistent output in the presence of unanticipated disturbances. In the previous example, disturbances that affect the direction of the boat might include wind and water currents. In the case of ventilators, disturbances that might affect the delivery of pressure, volume, and flow include pooled condensation or leaks in the patient circuit, endotracheal tube obstructions, and changes in respiratory system resistance and compliance.

Ventilators use closed-loop control to maintain consistent inspiratory pressure, volume, or flow waveforms in the presence of changing loads. The load presented by the respiratory system changes frequently as a result of lung pathology. Ventilator design has evolved from simple open-loop control of pressure to closed-loop control of pressure, volume, and flow within a breath, to the current double-closed-loop or dual control. This scheme was developed to obtain the advantages of both pressure-controlled and volume-controlled ventilation while avoiding each of their disadvantages. Dual control provides the advantage of pressure control (i.e., limiting peak inspiratory pressure, at least within a given range, to prevent overdistending the lungs) while maintaining the advantage of volume control (i.e., delivering a constant, minute ventilation even if lung mechanics change).

There are currently two basic approaches to dual control. The first method is to adjust the pressure waveform between breaths. This scheme was introduced by Siemens with the volume support mode on the Siemens Servo 300. Inspiration is pressure controlled within a breath, but the pressure **limit** is automatically adjusted up or down to achieve a preset

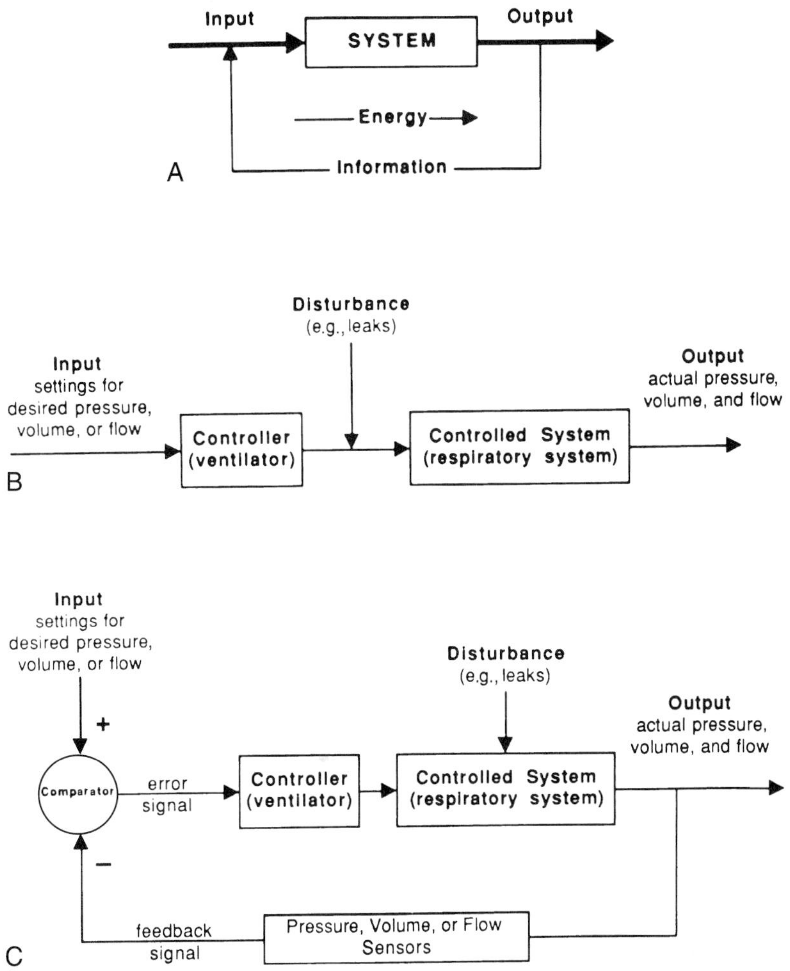

FIGURE 1-4 A, A simple block diagram of an unspecified system having one input and one output. Energy flows from input to output, and information flows from output to input. **B,** Block diagram for a ventilator using open-loop control. For example, the Newport Breeze ventilator controls airway pressure using open-loop control. **C,** Block diagram for a ventilator using closed-loop control. This is also called feedback or servo control. For example, the Infant Star ventilator uses closed-loop control of airway pressure.

target tidal volume (Figure 1-5, *top*). The initial pressure limit (i.e., change in airway pressure above PEEP) is set automatically based on the calculated value for respiratory system compliance (also automatically derived from a test breath):

initial pressure limit = set tidal volume/compliance

If the actual tidal volume based on the initial pressure limit is different from the set tidal volume, the pressure limit is adjusted up or down (no more than 3 cm H_2O per breath) to get closer to the set tidal volume. This process is repeated over several breaths until the delivered tidal volume equals the set tidal volume. A similar approach is used in the pressure-regulated volume control mode on the Siemens 300, in the autoflow mode on the Drager Evita 4, and in the adaptive pressure ventilation mode on the Hamilton Galileo.

The other basic approach is to make adjustments within a breath to achieve the target volume. This is demonstrated in the pressure augment mode on the Bear 1000 (Bear, Riverside, Calif.) and the volume assured pressure support (VAPS) mode on the Bird 8400 Sti or Tbird. Here, the ventilator may switch between pressure control and flow control within a breath depending on whether a preset tidal volume

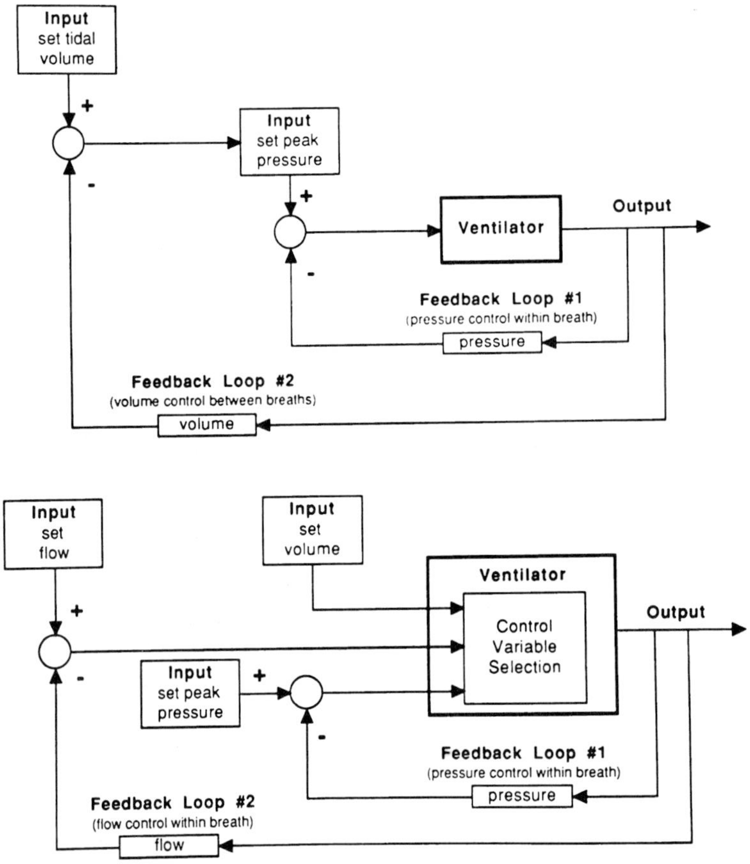

FIGURE 1-5 Double-loop or dual control. *Top,* dual control between breaths. The ventilator controls pressure during inspiration and then looks at the resultant tidal volume. The initial pressure limit is based on the set tidal volume and the value for respiratory system compliance the ventilator has calculated from a test breath (e.g., volume support on the Siemens 300). If the volume delivered with the initial pressure limit is different from the preset target value, the pressure waveform is changed for the next breath (either higher pressure limit or longer inspiratory flow time). *Bottom,* dual control within a breath. The ventilator starts inspiration in the pressure-controlled mode. If the set target volume has not been delivered by the time inspiratory flow has decayed to the preset inspiratory flow, the ventilator switches to flow control.

has been met (see Figure 1-5, *bottom*). Typical pressure and flow waveforms with this form of dual control are illustrated in Figure 1-6. Another variation of this theme is illustrated by the P_{max} feature on the Drager Evita 4, in which the ventilator begins inspiration in flow control at the set flow limit. When airway pressure reaches the set P_{max} value, the ventilator switches to pressure control at the set pressure limit while tidal volume is monitored. The ventilator attempts to increase the **inspiratory flow time** (i.e., the period from the beginning of inspiratory flow to the end of inspiratory flow) until the set tidal volume is delivered, provided that the set inspiratory time (i.e., the period from the beginning of inspiratory flow to the beginning of expiratory flow) is long enough. If the set tidal volume is not delivered in the set inspiratory time, an alarm is activated.

Control Variables

A ventilator may be classified as a pressure, volume, or flow controller. In some cases, it is logical to classify a ventilator as a time controller (i.e., it controls only inspiratory and expiratory times).

Ventilators can combine control schemes to create complex modes. For example, the NPB 7200a ventilator can mix flow-controlled breaths with pressure-

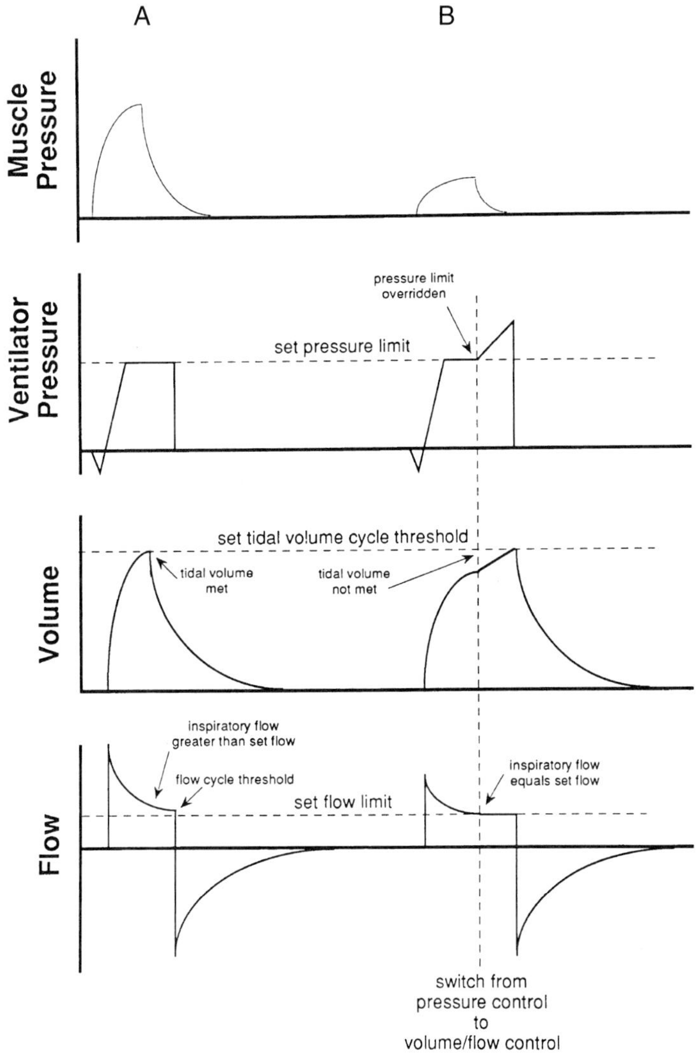

FIGURE 1-6 Pressure and flow waveforms showing the effects of dual control within breaths. **A,** Pressure-controlled breath with large patient effort (muscle pressure). The set tidal volume has been reached before flow has decayed to the set flow limit so the breath continues in pressure control until the flow cycle threshold value is reached. This value may be an arbitrary percentage of the peak value for the pressure-controlled portion of the breath (e.g., pressure augment in the Bear 1000) or the set flow rate (e.g., VAPS in the Bird 8400ST). The breath is essentially a pressure support breath. **B,** Switch from pressure control to flow control because flow decayed to the set flow before the set tidal volume was reached. This was due to a smaller patient inspiratory effort. Inspiration continues at the set flow and pressure rises as expected for a volume/flow-controlled breath.

controlled breaths in the SIMV+pressure support mode. The Bear 1000 can mix pressure control with flow control within a single breath in its pressure augment mode. The Siemens Servo 300 can adjust the level of pressure control automatically to achieve a preset target volume. The Hamilton Galileo can automatically adjust the number of mandatory breaths and the pressure limit on both mandatory and spontaneous breaths along with manipulating inspiratory and expiratory times based on the measurement of expiratory time constants. The great flexibility of current ventilators is achieved at the expense of added complexity. Thus when evaluating ventilator performance, simple and unambiguous criteria must be used for deciding which control variables are operational.

Pressure

The equation of motion tells us that if the ventilator is an ideal pressure controller, then the left side of the equation (i.e., ventilator pressure as a function of time) is determined by the ventilator settings and is unaffected by changes in parameter values on the right side (i.e., compliance and resistance).

If the control variable is pressure, then the ventilator can control either the airway pressure (causing it to rise above body surface pressure for inspiration) or the pressure on the body surface (causing it to fall below airway opening pressure for inspiration). This is the basis for classifying ventilators as being either positive or negative pressure types. For example, the Newport Wave ventilator would be classified as a positive-pressure controller that generates a rectangular pressure waveform, and the Emerson Iron Lung is a negative-pressure controller that produces a quasisinusoidal pressure waveform.

Volume

If the pressure waveform varies as the load imposed by the patient's respiratory system changes, the volume waveform is examined. However, the observation that the volume waveform remains unchanged is a necessary but insufficient condition to warrant the classification of volume controller because the same holds true for a flow controller. The reason is that once the volume waveform is specified, the flow waveform is determined because they are inverse functions of each other (i.e., volume is the integral of flow and flow is the derivative of volume). Therefore, if changes in compliance and resistance do not change the volume waveform, they will not affect the flow waveform, and vice versa.

To qualify as a volume controller, a ventilator must (1) maintain a consistent volume waveform in the presence of a varying load and (2) measure volume and use the signal to control the volume waveform. Volume can be measured directly only by the displacement of a piston or bellows or similar device. With a piston or bellows, controlling the excursion of the device automatically controls the volume waveform. Alternatively, a volume signal could be derived by integrating a flow signal. Note that although some ventilators—such as the Siemens Servo 900C, the NPB 7200, the Bear 5, and the Hamilton Veolar—display volume readings, they all actually measure and control flow and calculate volume for displays. Thus they all are flow controllers unless they are operated in a pressure-controlled mode (e.g., during pressure support ventilation). An examination of a ventilator's schematic diagrams and an operator's manual should provide the information necessary to decide whether volume or flow is being measured. This distinction is important in the engineering evaluation of a ventilator and in understanding ventilator performance. However, at the bedside, the difference between flow and volume control is not necessarily important. Although not correct in the engineering sense, referring to a flow-controlled breath as a volume-controlled breath is considered clinically acceptable. Similarly, this technique can be called volume targeted.

Flow

If the volume change (i.e., tidal volume) remains consistent when compliance and resistance are varied and if volume change is not measured and used for control, the ventilator is classified as a flow controller. The simplest example of open-loop flow control in a ventilator consists of a pressure regulator supplying gas to a flowmeter, such as found in infant ventilators. An infant ventilator becomes a flow controller rather than a pressure controller if the airway pressure does not reach the set pressure limit.[10] (However, the flowmeter is usually not back-pressure compensated and will vary its output slightly in the presence of a changing load.) In contrast, the Siemens Servo 900C (so-called because it uses servo control) measures flow and adjusts the output control valve (i.e., the inspiratory scissors valve) accordingly. It can maintain a more consistent inspiratory flow waveform as the load changes.

Time

Suppose that both pressure and volume are affected substantially by changes in lung mechanics. Then the only form of control is that of defining the ventilatory cycle, or alternating between inspiration and expiration. Therefore the only variables being controlled are the **inspiratory** and **expiratory times.** This situation arises in some forms of high-frequency ventilation, when even the designation of an inspiratory and expiratory phase becomes somewhat obscure.

Phase Variables

Once the control variables and the associated waveforms are identified, more detail can be obtained by examining the events that take place during a ventilatory cycle (i.e., the period of time between the begin-

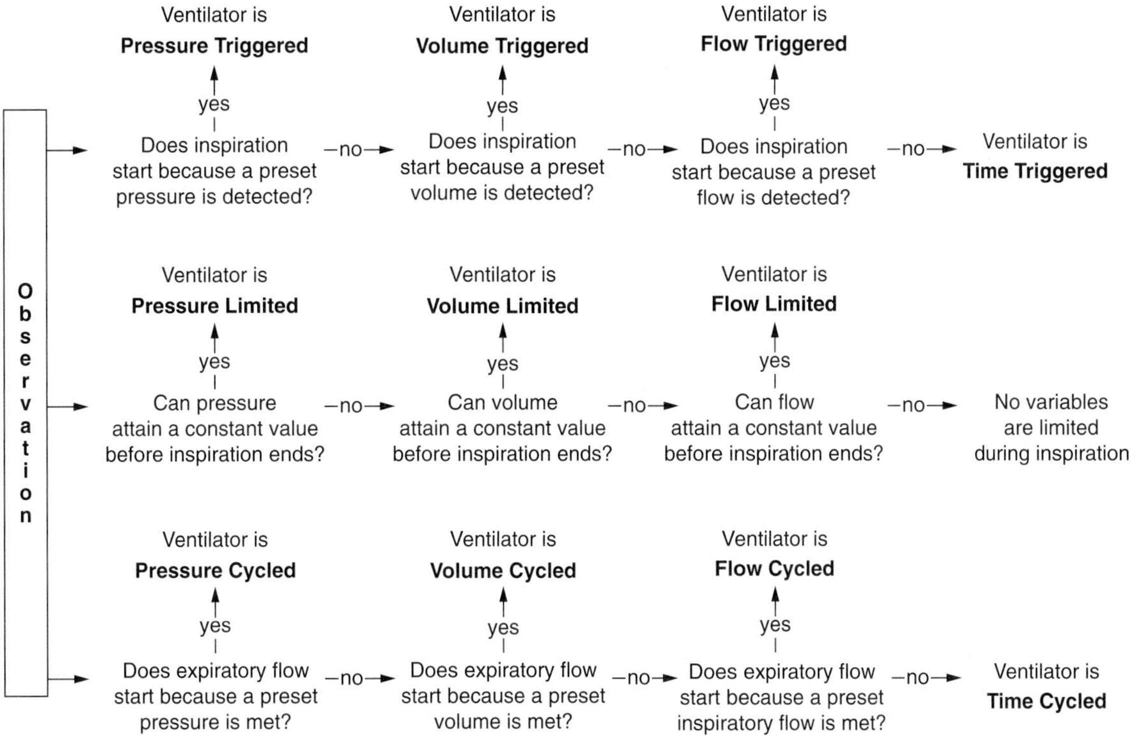

FIGURE 1-7 Criteria for determining the phase variables during a ventilator-assisted breath.

ning of one breath and the beginning of the next). Mushin and colleagues[1] proposed that this time span be divided into four **phases:** (1) the change from expiration to inspiration, (2) inspiration, (3) the change from inspiration to expiration, and (4) expiration. This convention is useful for examining how a ventilator starts, sustains, and stops an inspiration and what it does between inspirations. In each phase, a particular variable is measured and used to start, sustain, and end the phase. In this context, pressure, volume, flow, and time are referred to as **phase variables.**[11] The criteria for determining phase variables are defined in Figure 1-7.

Trigger

All ventilators measure one or more of the variables associated with the equation of motion (i.e., pressure, volume, flow, or time). Inspiration is started when one of these variables reaches a preset value. Thus the variable of interest is considered an initiating or trigger variable. The most common trigger variables are time (the ventilator initiates a breath according to a set frequency, independent of the patient's spontaneous efforts), pressure (the ventilator senses the patient's inspiratory effort in the form of a decrease in baseline pressure and starts inspiration independent of the set frequency), and flow (the ventilator senses the patient's inspiratory effort as a decrease in the baseline flow through the patient circuit or senses inspiratory flow directly with a sensor at the patient's airway opening). Any variable that can be measured can potentially be used to trigger inspiration. For example, the Star Sync module allows triggering of the Infant Star ventilator by chest wall movement, and the Sechrist SAVI system senses inspiration as a change in chest impedance. Of course, it is relatively simple to manually trigger inspiration.

Triggering based on a change in flow has been shown to reduce the work the patient must perform to trigger inspiration.[12] This is because work is proportional to the volume the patient inspires times the change in baseline pressure necessary to trigger. Pressure triggering requires some pressure change and hence an irreducible amount of work to trigger. But with flow or volume triggering, baseline pressure need not change, and theoretically, the patient need do no work on the ventilator to trigger. At least one ventilator, the Drager Babylog, may be volume triggered. The possible advantage of volume triggering over flow triggering is that when flow signal is integrated to get volume, much of the noise in the signal (e.g., from condensate in the patient circuit) is removed and the chance of false triggering is reduced. A possible disadvantage of this is the increased delay from signal processing and the phase lag between flow and volume signals.

The patient effort required to trigger inspiration is determined by the ventilator's sensitivity. Sensitivity generally is defined as the ratio of output signal amplitude to input signal amplitude. In the case of a ventilator, the output is the triggering of inspiration and the input is the change in the trigger signal required to trigger. The smaller the change in trigger signal (e.g., pressure change below baseline) required to trigger, the larger the mathematical ratio and the greater the sensitivity. Many ventilators indicate sensitivity adjustments qualitatively ("min" or "max"). Alternatively, a ventilator may specify a trigger threshold quantitatively (e.g., so many cm H_2O below baseline). For example, to make a pressure-triggered ventilator more sensitive, the trigger threshold might be adjusted from 5 to 1 cm H_2O below the baseline pressure. Sometimes the ventilator has a readout called "sensitivity" with units of pressure or flow. This confuses the issue because the readout is only half of the sensitivity ratio and a higher number in the readout is really a lower sensitivity. In such a case, the label should be "trigger threshold."

Triggering the ventilator has been studied intensively. Because the ability of the ventilator to sense patient effort and respond quickly and with sufficient flow to meet patient demands is so crucial to patient/ventilator synchrony, a technical review is in order. Time and manual triggering of the ventilator do not depend on patient effort and as such are not described in the same detail.

Manual Triggering. A breath can be triggered by activating the manual breath control on the ventilator. This is usually accomplished by means of a push button or membrane keypad. Manual triggering generally takes one of two forms. The first uses electronic control of the breath, and when the function is activated, a breath at the set tidal volume or pressure is delivered at the set inspiratory flow or time. The second type is often a mechanical control, and when the function is activated, inspiration continues until the operator disengages from the control. The flow is typically controlled using this method, and the high-pressure relief valve remains activated. In some instances, a maximum inspiratory time of three seconds automatically ends the manual breath even if the operator fails to disengage the function.

Time Triggering. A breath is time triggered when the set respiratory rate on the ventilator requires that a breath be delivered.

Pressure Triggering. Pressure triggering is the oldest and simplest technique for detecting patient effort. The sensitivity or trigger threshold is set in centimeters of H_2O relative to the baseline pressure. As an example, if baseline pressure is 5 cm H_2O and the trigger threshold is 2 cm H_2O, then when patient effort causes pressure in the circuit to fall to 3 cm H_2O, the breath is triggered. If the baseline pressure is changed—for instance, to 10 cm H_2O—and the trigger threshold remains the same (2 cm H_2O), the ventilator is triggered when circuit pressure decreases to less than 8 cm H_2O. The ability to maintain the trigger threshold constant regardless of alterations in baseline pressure is frequently referred to as "PEEP (positive end-expiratory pressure) compensation." Modern intensive care unit (ICU) ventilators all have this ability, but in many simpler devices such as transport ventilators, PEEP compensation may not be available. In this instance, the trigger threshold is referenced to atmosphere. If baseline pressure is 5 cm H_2O and trigger threshold is 2 cm H_2O, then triggering will not occur until circuit pressure is −2 cm H_2O (2 cm H_2O below atmospheric pressure). This requires that the patient create a pressure change in the circuit of 7 cm H_2O (5 cm H_2O baseline pressure + 2 cm H_2O trigger threshold) to trigger inspiration. Figure 1-8 illustrates these pressure relationships.

Pressure triggering performance of a ventilator also can be influenced by accuracy and speed of the pressure transducer.[12-14] Factors leading to delay include errors due to the speed of the pressure signal propagation through sensor tubing, errors due to the polling interval of the pressure transducer, errors in the pressure transducer, errors due to differences in set and actual PEEP, errors due to circuit noise, and position of the pressure transducer in the ventilator circuit. This initial delay is typically less than 150 msec and represents only a small amount of the work of breathing imposed during triggering.

Position of the pressure transducer in the circuit may also affect triggering (Figure 1-9). Ventilators sense pressure in the inspiratory portion of the ventilator, at the proximal airway, and in the expiratory side of the ventilator. Transducers in the inspiratory limb are adversely affected by the presence of any source of resistance between the patient and the transducer. This includes the ventilator circuit, filters, and humidifiers. Expiratory limb placement avoids the humidifier, but still must contend with filters and circuit resistance. Proximal pressure monitoring at

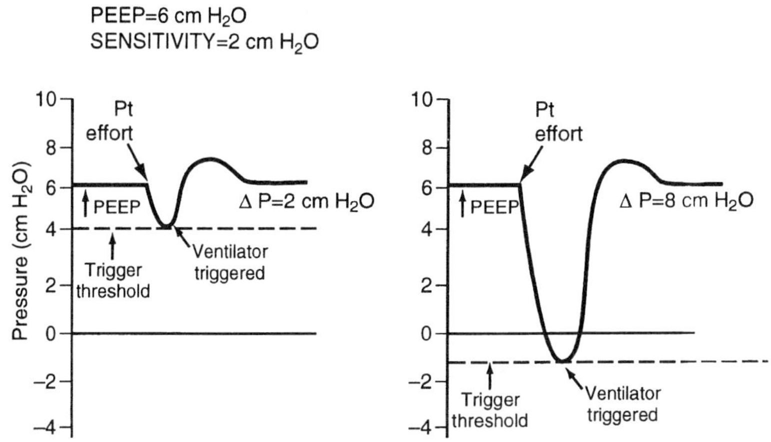

FIGURE 1-8 Demonstration of pressure triggering. On the left, pressure triggering is compensated by positive end-expiratory pressure (PEEP). On the right, pressure triggering is not PEEP compensated.

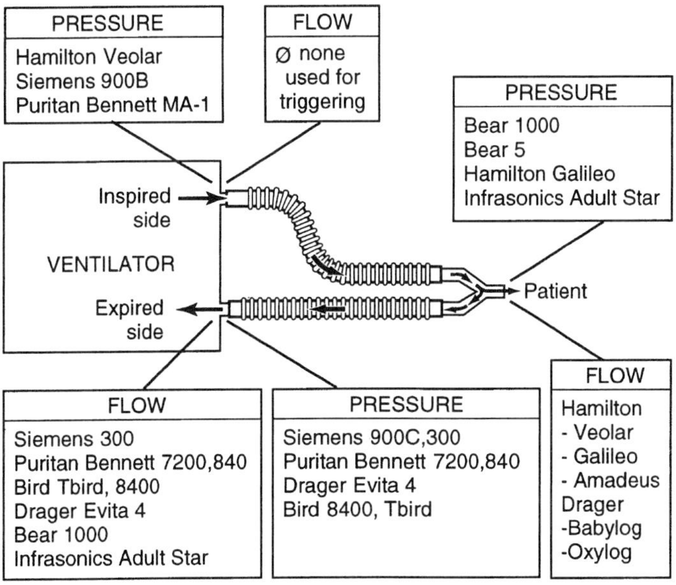

FIGURE 1-9 Position of flow ($\dot{V}$) and pressure (P) sensors used for triggering in current ventilators.

the Y-piece of the ventilator eliminates most circuit issues except the use of filters and passive humidifiers connected to the endotracheal tube. The endotracheal tube is typically the greatest source of resistance in the patient ventilator system, and several authors have suggested placement of the pressure transducer at the distal tip of the tube.[15,16] This eliminates the additional work needed to overcome endotracheal tube resistance. Unfortunately, this also places the transducer in a humid, contaminated environment in which secretions may create new problems. As of this writing, use of pressure triggering at the distal tip of the endotracheal tube has not been commercialized.

Flow Triggering. Flow triggering was introduced by Engstrom in the early 1980s, but did not become popular until it was reintroduced by Puritan Bennett in 1988. Since then, flow triggering has become standard on current ventilators. Like so much of ventilator technology, the methods of flow triggering vary from manufacturer to manufacturer. Flow-triggering systems vary in placement of the flow transducer, presence or absence of a continuous (bias) flow, and the ability to adjust bias flow and flow sensitivity.[17,18]

Generically, flow triggering occurs when a flow transducer in the patient/ventilator system detects a change in flow (i.e., flow moves into the airway opening). This is similar to the pressure-triggering concept. The implementation of flow triggering, however, has taken on several versions. Flow triggering is implemented using one of three methods. The first simply measures a change in flow caused by the patient's inspiratory effort. There is no continuous flow in the circuit, and at end-expiration flow is zero. The second provides a preset, nonadjustable level of continuous flow in the circuit, from which a change in flow (the flow sensitivity) is detected. The third allows the clinician to set the continuous flow and the flow sensitivity. In this case, a change in flow through the circuit caused by the patient's inspiratory effort reduces the flow below the flow trigger threshold setting and a breath is triggered. In the presence of a leak, this system can be tailored to overcome the leak while maintaining appropriate triggering.

As an example, the Puritan Bennett 7200ae uses a flow-triggering system known as FlowBy. The clinician selects a level of continuous flow, called the "base flow," between 5 and 20 L/min. This flow traverses the inspiratory and expiratory flow transducers, and the two values are compared every 20 msec. The clinician then sets the flow sensitivity between 1 and 10 L/min. With the 7200ae, the flow sensitivity cannot exceed one half the continuous flow. Using this system at a continuous flow of 5 L/min and flow sensitivity of 2 L/min, when the patient's inspiratory effort causes flow traversing the expiratory flow transducer to fall to 3 L/min, a breath is triggered. Continuing to use the 7200ae as an example, once a spontaneous breath is triggered, flow up to 180 L/min is available. The limit and cycle variables with flow triggering are different from pressure triggering for a spontaneous breath. Once the flow-triggered breath is initiated, the ventilator attempts to maintain airway pressure at 1 cm H_2O above the end-expiratory pressure, and the breath is cycled when flow through the expiratory flow transducer is 2 L/min greater than the set continuous flow. As mentioned in the section on pressure triggering, this demonstrates that the operation of the 7200ae is quite different for pressure- and flow-triggered spontaneous breaths.

Another example of differences between a ventilator's pressure-triggering and flow-triggering system can be seen in the Hamilton Veolar ventilator. With this system, the limit and cycle variables for the two triggering methods are identical. However, during pressure triggering, the site of pressure measurement is inside the inspiratory side of the ventilator. As such, any resistance in the ventilator circuit (heated humidifiers, artificial noses, and so on) represents an imposed workload to triggering. In the flow-triggering mode, the ventilator is triggered from a variable orifice flow transducer placed at the Y-piece of the ventilator circuit. In this instance, the reduction in the work of breathing with flow triggering results from improved sensor placement.[19] The Veolar allows the clinician to set the flow sensitivity (2 to 10 L/min) and the continuous flow is automatically twice that value, with a minimum continuous flow of 4 L/min.

The Siemens 300 ventilator uses a combination of flow and pressure triggering, with flow triggering selected by decreasing the pressure sensitivity control into an uncalibrated range on the dial. The Siemens 300 uses set continuous flows of 2 L/min, 1 L/min, and 0.5 L/min during flow triggering during adult, pediatric, and neonatal operation, respectively. Because the sensitivity dial is uncalibrated, the actual flow sensitivity setting is unknown. The site of pressure and flow measurement is located on the expiratory side of the ventilator, and the limit and cycle variables are indent.

The Bird ventilators (8400 Sti and Tbird) use a nonadjustable continuous flow of 10 L/min and allow flow sensitivity to be set from 1 to 9 L/min. Flow is measured by the expiratory flow transducer, and when the flow sensitivity threshold is exceeded, a breath is triggered. The breath then is pressure-limited and flow-cycled (when flow through the expiratory flow transducer is greater than 10 L/min). A comparison of flow-triggering systems is shown in Table 1-1. Schematic examples of the types of flow triggering are shown in Figure 1-10.

In some instances, manufacturers have provided a combination of continuous flow and pressure triggering. Conceptually, the continuous flow meets the patient's initial demand for flow, and when circuit pressure is reduced, the breath is triggered. This system has not been shown to have advantages compared with traditional flow or pressure triggering. Only the Newport ventilators continue to use this technique.

Potential problems with flow triggering include auto-triggering resulting from system leaks or the presence of condensate in the ventilator circuit.

TABLE 1-1 *Comparison of Pressure- and Flow-Triggering Systems for Certain Ventilators*

VENTILATOR	TRIGGER	SENSITIVITY	CONTINUOUS FLOW	LIMIT	CYCLE	SENSOR LOCATION
Puritan Bennett 7200ae	Pressure	0.5-20 cm H_2O	NA	PEEP sensitivity	1 cm H_2O above PEEP	Expiratory side
	Flow	1-10 L/min	5-20 L/min	PEEP + 1 cm H_2O	Expiratory flow 2 L/min > inspiratory flow	Expiratory side
Hamilton Veolar	Pressure	0.5-10 cm H_2O	NA	PEEP + 1.5 cm H_2O	37% of initial peak flow	Inspiratory side
	Flow	3-15 L/min	6-30 L/min (twice the sensitivity)	PEEP + 1.5 cm H_2O	37% of initial peak flow	Proximal airway
Siemens 300	Pressure	0-17 cm H_2O	Adults: 2 L/min Children: 1 L/min Neonates 0.5 L/min	PEEP + 3 cm H_2O	5% of initial peak flow	Expiratory side
	Flow	Uncalibrated	Adults: 2 L/min Children: 1 L/min Neonates: 0.5 L/min	PEEP + 3 cm H_2O	5% of initial peak flow	Expiratory side
Bird 8400 Sti	Pressure	1-20 cm H_2O	NA	PEEP	PEEP + 1.0 cm H_2O	Expiratory side
	Flow	1-9 L/min	10 L/min	PEEP	Flow returns to 10 L/min	Expiratory side

PEEP, Positive end-expiratory pressure.

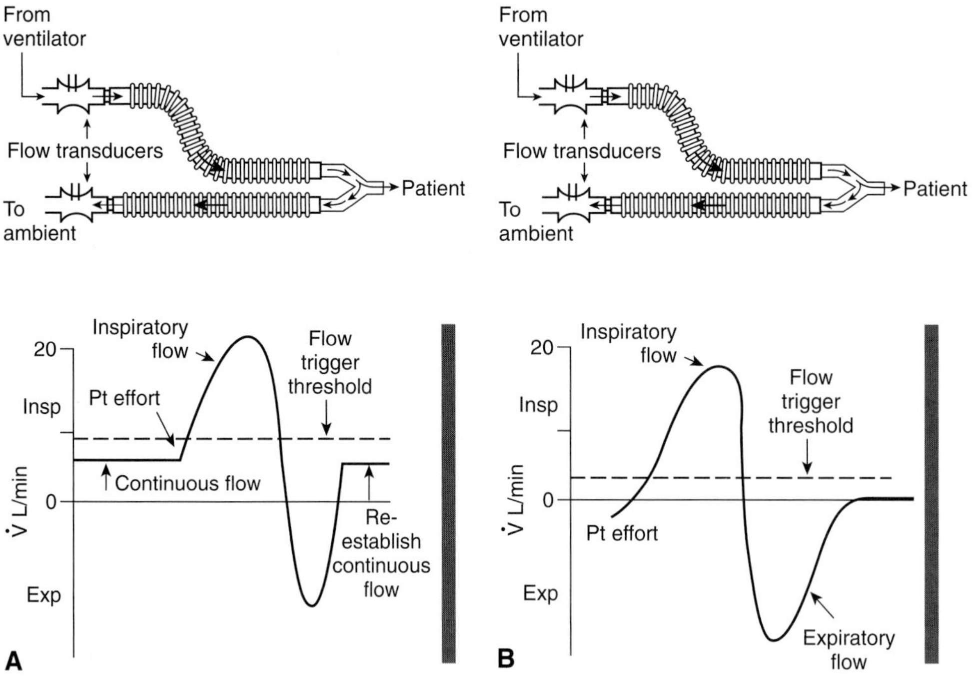

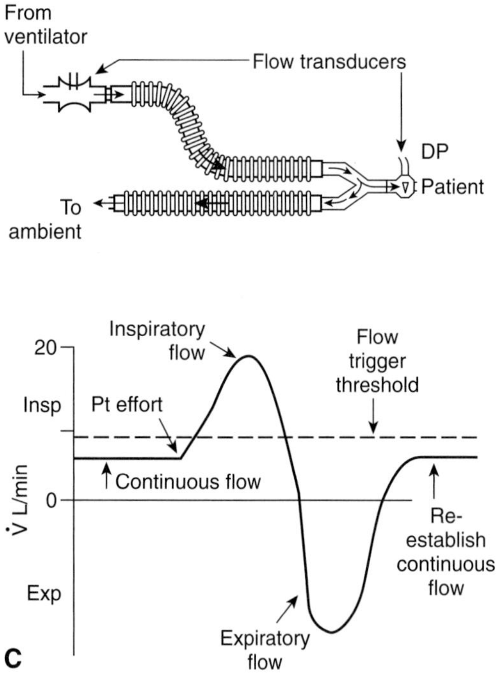

FIGURE 1-10 Three flow triggering systems. **A,** Flow triggering using inspiratory and expiratory flow sensors (e.g., 7200ae). **B,** Flow triggering using the expiratory sensor and no continuous flow (e.g., Bird Tbird). **C,** Flow triggering using a flow sensor at the proximal airway and an adjustable continuous flow (e.g., Hamilton Galileo).

Devices that measure flow at the airway opening reduce problems associated with circuit condensate. Flow-triggering systems with an adjustable continuous flow can be used to compensate for leaks. In systems with a constant continuous flow, particularly at low levels, leaks may preclude the system from triggering appropriately.

Volume Triggering. Volume triggering has been used infrequently in adults. However, the Drager Babylog ventilator uses a hot wire anemometer at the proximal airway to volume-trigger breaths. This device is also capable of calculating leaks around the uncuffed endotracheal tube. The use of volume as a trigger signal has not been studied. Conceptually,

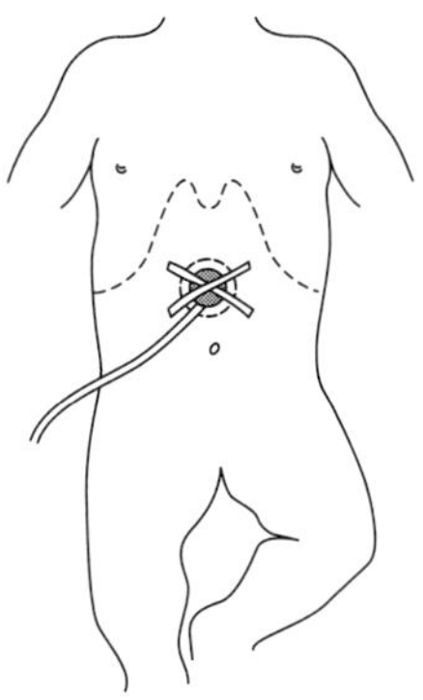

FIGURE 1-11 Placement of the abdominal sensor on infant's abdomen for motion triggering (Infrasonics Star-Sync).

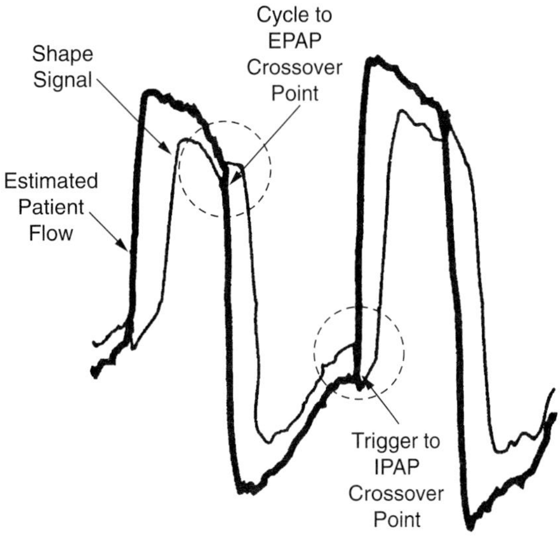

FIGURE 1-12 Flow waveform triggering. *EPAP,* Expiratory positive airway pressure; *IPAP,* inspiratory positive airway pressure.

by integrating measured flow to calculate volume, signal noise is reduced. Evaluations of this technique need to be accomplished.

Impedance Triggering. Because of the difficulties associated with measuring respiratory efforts in neonates and the small endotracheal tubes required, several investigators have searched for alternate trigger signals to initiate patient effort. The first of these introduced is chest wall impedance triggering. This technique was introduced by Sechrist and is known as the SAVI system.[20] Standard electrocardiogram (ECG) electrodes are used, and as the chest wall expands, the change in impedance initiates inspiration. Using this technique, the control of the ventilator limit and the cycling variable returns to airway pressure—once inspiratory effort is detected.

Motion Triggering. The Infrasonics Infant Star ventilator has introduced a motion sensor for triggering the neonatal ventilator. This device (Star Sync) uses an abdominal sensor to detect inspiration. The sensor is a small, air-filled flexible capsule. This device is taped to the infant's abdomen (Figure 1-11) midway between the umbilicus and the xiphisternum. As the abdomen rises, the capsule is compressed, generating a small pressure signal that is transmitted to the device and that generates an electrical signal that triggers the ventilator. Pressure in the sensor is sampled eight times every 5 msec and the response time from the onset of patient effort to breath delivery is 47 msec. From a technical standpoint, this is pressure-triggered ventilation. This may require improved definitions of triggering. Pressure triggering might be considered airway pressure triggered (citing the pressure measurement site) or abdominal pressure triggered. We prefer to refer to this method as motion triggered because although pressure is the measured signal, abdominal motion is the cause of the pressure change.

Flow Waveform Triggering. A unique type of triggering is used by the Respironics devices for noninvasive ventilation (BiPAP, BiPAP Vision), which the manufacturer terms "AutoTrak Sensitivity." This method of triggering has been investigated by Prinianakis and colleagues.[21,22] This group has termed this technique flow waveform triggering. Flow waveform triggering incorporates several possible triggers, including waveform and volume triggering (Figure 1-12). During flow waveform triggering the ventilator's algorithm creates a flow shape signal, which is an offset of the actual flow signal. This can be thought of as a shadow of the actual flow signal. This new signal is offset by 0.25 L/s (15 L/min) and delayed by 300 msec. This intentional delay causes the new flow signal to lag behind and shadow the actual flow signal. When the patient creates an inspiratory effort, the actual flow signal crosses the shadow flow signal and a breath is triggered. This same method can be used for cycling the breath. If the actual signal does not cross the shadow signal, the accumulation of 6 ml of volume above the baseline flow will also trigger the breath. Prinianakis et al found that this method reduced the number of missed triggers in a lung model study, suggesting it was more sensitive than a traditional flow triggering system. However, they also showed that auto-triggering (breaths initiated by the

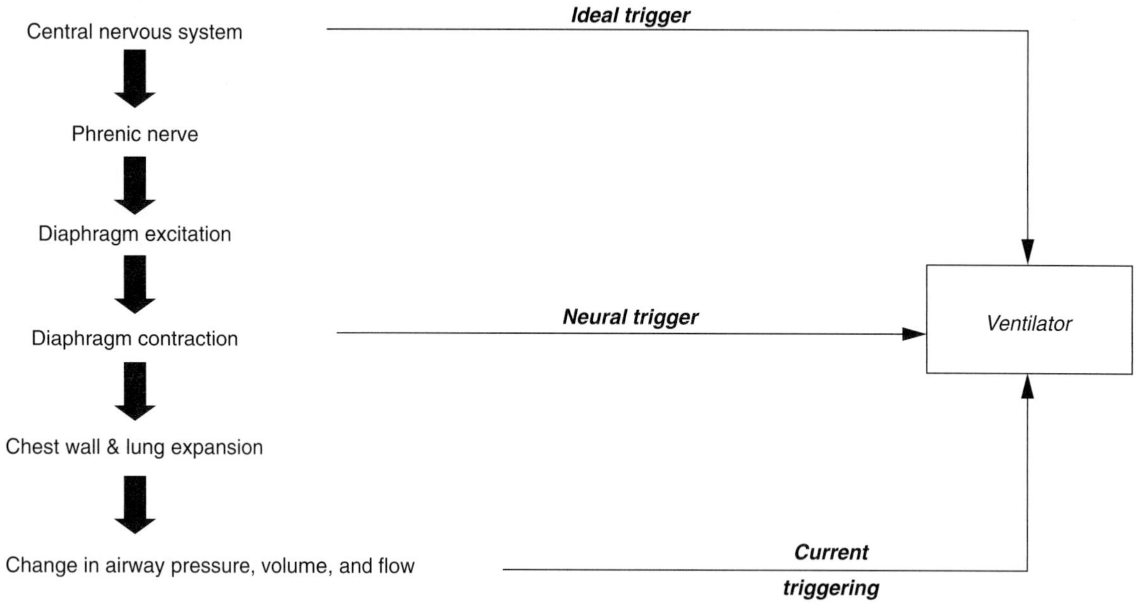

FIGURE 1-13 Schematic demonstrating the transmission of the signal to initiate a breath through the components of the respiratory system and the site of traditional airway triggers and the proposed EMG triggering (NAVA).

ventilator without a patient effort) were also more frequent with the flow waveform method of triggering.

Alternate Triggers. As the description of triggering until now implies, nearly any signal that is measurable and processed to create digital information can trigger the ventilator. Theoretically, if we could harness the electrical signal from the respiratory control center, we could trigger the ventilator to coincide directly with the neural control of breathing. Recently, Sinderby et al have described a triggering technique that uses diaphragmatic electromyography (EMG) to trigger the ventilator.[22,23] This technique uses an esophageal catheter containing an array of electrodes. The electrodes detect the diaphragmatic contraction and allow ventilator triggering upstream of the traditional airway pressure or flow signals (Figure 1-13). This technique has promise for overcoming difficulties in triggering due to intrinsic positive end-expiratory pressure and difficulties caused by leaks during mask ventilation. The key to the EMG triggering is filtering of the cardiac signal (by far the prominent electrical signal in the chest) and development of redundant systems in the airway to distinguish diaphragmatic contraction due to breathing from other functions. At the time of this writing, there are no commercially available EMG triggers. This proposed system is called neural triggering or neurally adjusted ventilatory assist (NAVA), yet another name in the ventilator lexicon that is not founded on the principle of operation.[23]

Limit

During the inspiratory phase, pressure, volume, and flow increase above their end-expiratory values. The **inspiratory phase** is quantitated by specifying the inspiratory time, defined as the time interval from the start of inspiratory flow to the start of expiratory flow. Note that any inspiratory hold (or pause) time is included in the inspiratory time. It is sometimes helpful to distinguish inspiratory flow time as the interval from the start of inspiratory flow to the end of inspiratory flow and the **inspiratory pause time** as the interval from the end of inspiratory flow to the start of expiratory flow. This distinction is useful because there is no standardized way to set these intervals on ventilators and the terminology that manufacturers use may be confusing. For example, on one ventilator, inspiratory flow time may be set indirectly by setting tidal volume and flow, whereas pause time may be set directly (in seconds), thus indirectly increasing inspiratory time. On another ventilator, inspiratory time may be set directly with no provision for directly setting inspiratory pause time. On yet another ventilator, inspiratory time may be set using the rate and "% cycle time" controls and then changing inspiratory flow time by changing a

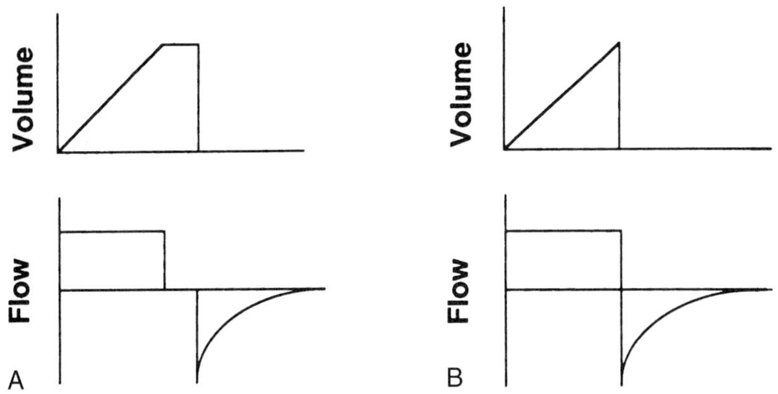

FIGURE 1-14 The importance of distinguishing between the terms limit and cycle is shown. In **(A)** both volume and flow are limited (because they reach preset values before end inspiration), and inspiration is time cycled (after the preset inspiratory pause time). In **(B)** flow is limited, but volume is not and inspiration is volume cycled.

"% inspiration" control. Finally, inspiratory flow time must be distinguished from inspiratory time to understand the way that P_{max} works on the Evita 4 ventilator (see previous description of dual control between breaths).

Cycle time (or total cycle time) is another name for ventilatory period, the reciprocal of ventilatory frequency (i.e., 60 seconds per minute/number of breaths per minute). The percent cycle time is the ratio of inspiratory time to total cycle time expressed as a percentage. The percent inspiratory time is the inspiratory flow time expressed as a percentage of total cycle time. The percent pause time is the pause time expressed as a percentage of total cycle time. An inspiratory pause is important in estimating lung pressures and calculating respiratory system mechanics.

If one (or more) of the inspiratory variables rises no higher than some preset value, we refer to the variable as a limit variable. But we must distinguish the limit variable from the variable that is used to end inspiration (called a cycle variable). Therefore we impose the additional criterion that inspiration is not terminated because a variable has met its preset limit value. In other words, a variable is "limited" if it increases to a preset value before inspiration ends. These criteria are illustrated in Figure 1-14.

Clinicians commonly misuse the terms limit and cycle by using them interchangeably. This is encouraged by some ventilator manufacturers who use the term limit to describe what happens when a pressure alarm threshold is met (i.e., inspiration is terminated and an alarm is activated). The term cycle is more appropriate in this situation.

Another potentially confusing issue is that, by convention, peak inspiratory pressure (PIP) and baseline pressure are measured relative to atmospheric pressure, whereas the pressure limit sometimes is measured relative to baseline pressure (e.g., Siemens Servo 900C) and sometimes relative to atmospheric pressure (e.g., Bird V.I.P.). On the Bird V.I.P., the high pressure limit control sets the PIP limit (above ambient pressure) during pressure-controlled ventilation but cycles the breath off and activates a high-pressure alarm during volume-controlled ventilation. Hence the term *pressure limit,* in common usage, can indicate several different clinically significant situations depending on both the mode of ventilation and the manufacturer. Thus the lack of standardization among ventilator manufacturers makes it especially important that clinicians use terminology properly.

Cycle

Inspiration always ends (i.e., is cycled off) because some variable has reached a preset value. The variable that is measured and used to terminate inspiratory time and begin expiratory time is called the **cycle variable.** Deciding which variable is used to cycle off inspiration for a given ventilator can be confusing. For a variable to be used as a feedback signal (in this case, a cycling signal), it first must be measured. Most current-generation adult ventilators allow the operator to set a tidal volume and inspiratory flow, which would lead one to believe that the ventilator could be volume cycled. However, closer inspection reveals that these ventilators do not measure volume (which is consistent with the fact that all current-generation ventilators are flow controllers). Rather, they set the inspiratory time necessary to achieve the set tidal volume with the set inspiratory flow rate, making them time cycled. The tidal volume dial can be thought of as an inspiratory time dial calibrated in units of volume rather than time.

As mentioned earlier, the term *limit* often is substituted incorrectly for cycle in common usage. But the distinction also is ignored by ventilator designers. An example of the difficulty created by improper terminology is illustrated by the Bear Cub 750vs. This ventilator is designed to be used primarily as a pressure controller for infants. The operator typically sets both inspiratory time and inspiratory pressure limit (the knob is labeled "Inspiratory Pressure" and the ventilator is designed to maintain the pressure until the cycle mechanism is activated). Inspiration is normally time cycled. However, there is a control knob that is labeled "Volume Limit," so it would seem that inspiration could be both pressure and volume limited at the same time. However, this is not true. First, the equation of motion shows that it cannot control both volume and pressure to some preset value at the same time. This is not an example of dual control (which does not control two things at the same time but rather switches back and forth). If the clinician tries to set a pressure limit, the delivered volume will depend on lung mechanics, and if the clinician tries to set a volume limit, the pressure will vary with lung mechanics. Second, the operator's manual says that "When the set threshold is reached, the ventilator will cycle into expiration." Thus the ventilator does one thing when the pressure limit is met (namely, stay at that level until inspiration ends) and it does another thing when the volume "limit" is met (terminate inspiration). The "volume limit" is really a "volume cycle threshold." Calling both functions by the same name is confusing and may obscure one's understanding of the ventilator's unique ability to volume cycle in a pressure-controlled mode.

Some investigators think that a ventilator can have "mixed" cycling, which is contrary to the idea presented here that a ventilator can control only one variable at a time. The most common example given by these authors is a ventilator drive mechanism composed of a piston connected to a rod and a rotating crank. It is argued that one cannot distinguish time (i.e., inspiratory time set by the frequency at which the crank rotates) or volume (i.e., the stroke volume of the piston) as the cycling variable. However, if the inspiratory time is set low enough and the volume and patient load are high enough, a point can be reached when a piston-driven ventilator "sacrifices" (i.e., extends) the set inspiratory time as the motor struggles against the load to deliver the volume. This unmasks its true volume-cycled nature.

Baseline

The variable that is controlled during the expiratory time is the baseline variable. Expiratory time is defined as the time interval from the start of expiratory flow to the start of inspiratory flow. As with inspiratory time, it is helpful to distinguish the components of expiratory time: **expiratory flow time,** defined as the interval from the start of expiratory flow to the end of expiratory flow, and **expiratory pause time,** defined as the interval from the end of expiratory flow to the start of inspiratory flow. Expiratory pause time often is initiated to measure auto-PEEP.

Note that in the equation of motion, pressure, volume, and flow are measured relative to end-expiratory or baseline values and are thus initially all zero. Although the baseline value of any of these variables theoretically could be controlled, pressure control is the most practical and is implemented by all commonly used ventilators.

Conditional Variables

Figure 1-15 illustrates that, for each breath, the ventilator creates a specific pattern of control and phase variables. The ventilator either may keep this pattern constant for each breath or it may introduce other patterns (e.g., one for mandatory and one for spontaneous breaths). In essence, the ventilator must decide which pattern of control and which phase variables to implement before each breath, depending on the value of some preset conditional variables. Conditional variables can be thought of as initiating conditional logic in the form of "if-then" statements. That is, if the value of a conditional variable reaches some preset threshold, some action occurs to change the ventilatory pattern.

A simple example would be the NPB MA-1 in the control mode. Each breath is time triggered, flow limited, and volume cycled. The trigger, limit, and cycle variables have preset values (e.g., trigger at frequency = 20 cycles/min, limit inspiratory flow at 60 L/min, and cycle at tidal volume = 750 ml). However, every few minutes a sigh breath is introduced that has a different set of **phase variable values** (e.g., trigger at frequency = 2 sighs every 15 minutes; cycle at tidal volume = 1500 ml). How did the ventilator know to do this? Conceptually, the ventilator examines the value of some conditional variable to see whether it has reached a preset thresh-

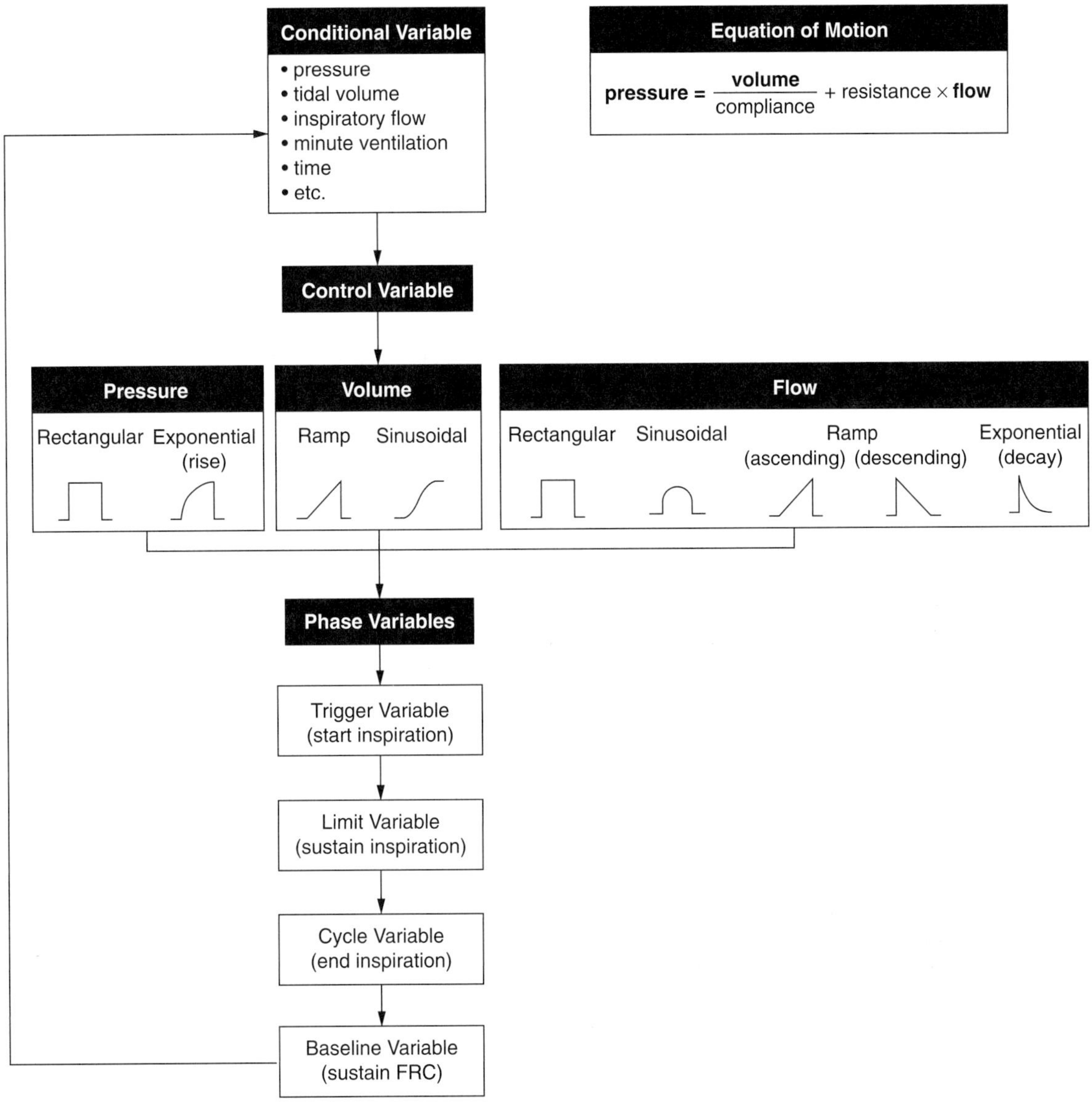

FIGURE 1-15 A ventilator classification scheme based on a mathematical model known as the "equation of motion" for the respiratory system is shown. This model indicates that during inspiration, the ventilator is able to directly control one and only one variable at a time (i.e., pressure, volume, or flow). Some common waveforms provided by current ventilators are shown for each control variable. Pressure, volume, flow, and time are also used as phase variables that determine the parameters of each ventilatory cycle (e.g., trigger sensitivity, peak inspiratory flow rate or pressure, inspiratory time, and baseline pressure). *FRC,* Functional residual capacity.

old value before each breath pattern is selected. If the threshold value has been met, then one pattern is selected; if not, another pattern is selected. In the case of the NPB MA-1, the conditional variable was time: if a preset time interval has elapsed (i.e., the sigh interval), then the ventilator switches to the sigh pattern. Other examples include switching from patient-triggered to machine-triggered breaths in the SIMV and mandatory minute ventilation (MMV) modes.

So far in this discussion, the terms mandatory and spontaneous have been used without explanation.

TABLE 1-2 *Comparison of Breath Types*

TYPE OF BREATH	TRIGGER	LIMIT	CYCLE
Mandatory	Ventilator (time)	Ventilator (pressure or flow)	Ventilator (time, flow, volume)
Assisted	Patient (pressure, flow, volume, impedance, motion)	Ventilator (pressure or flow)	Ventilator (time, flow, volume)
Spontaneous	Patient (pressure, flow, volume, impedance, motion)	Ventilator (pressure or flow) Inspiratory pressure=Baseline pressure	Patient
Supported	Patient (pressure, flow, volume, impedance, motion)	Ventilator (pressure or flow) Inspiratory pressure>Baseline pressure	Patient

Clinicians have an intuitive understanding of the meanings of these terms. But because they play a central role in defining and understanding modes of ventilation, formal definitions must be provided. **Spontaneous breaths** are those that are both initiated and terminated by the patient. That is, the patient triggers the breath and participates in cycling of the breath. A **mandatory breath** is defined as one in which the ventilator determines either the start or end of inspiration. A breath that is time triggered always is considered a mandatory breath. A breath that is patient triggered, but time- or volume-cycled (i.e., the patient does not play a role in the cycle criteria) is also a mandatory breath.

The naming of breath types is crucial to understanding ventilator modes, but is also an area of confusion and disagreement. The current classification system requires that breaths simply be distinguished only as *mandatory* or *spontaneous*. A consensus conference of experts (which did not exactly achieve consensus) thought that four breath types were necessary to describe the types of breaths. The consensus group added the terms *assisted* breath and *supported* breath. An *assisted breath* is a *mandatory breath* that is patient triggered. A *supported breath* is a *spontaneous breath* that has an inspiratory pressure greater than baseline pressure. We prefer to think of assisted breath as a type of mandatory breath and supported as a type of spontaneous breath. Table 1-2 describes the differences between these breaths. Although the two new breath types are certainly different in clinical application and clinical effect, from an engineering perspective they are not different. This is the origin of the lack of consensus. From a clinical perspective, a breath that is time-triggered is significantly different from one that is patient-triggered. Issues related to measurement of pressures, flow demand, and the work of breathing are all different in the triggered breath. However, to the ventilator, the breath was just initiated for a different reason. It is problematic when we attempt to incorporate the patient into the equation. Ventilator classification is a study of the ventilator, not the patient.

Figure 1-16 illustrates these definitions with an algorithm. Note that if the ventilator either time or volume cycles an inspiration, the breath is considered mandatory because it is terminated by the ventilator. If, however, the ventilator flow cycles after being patient triggered, as in the pressure support mode, the breath is considered to be (supported) spontaneous. The rate of decay of inspiratory flow is determined by the patient's lung mechanics and ventilatory muscle activity. Hence, during the pressure support mode, pressure-limiting inspiration does not constrain inspiratory flow rate, and flow cycling does not necessarily dictate either the inspiratory time or the tidal volume if the ventilatory muscles are active. In other words, the ventilator attempts to match the patient's inspiratory demand and it is really the patient who terminates the breath. If the ventilator is pressure cycled (usually an alarm condition) after being patient triggered, the breath is also spontaneous. Again, the patient's lung mechanics or ventilatory muscle activity has caused airway pressure to go above the preset threshold (in the absence of ventilator malfunction).

Modes of Ventilation

There are two general approaches to supporting the patient's inspiration: volume/flow control and pressure control. Figure 1-17 is a simplified influence diagram[24-27] that illustrates the important variables for ventilators that are either volume or flow controllers. Figure 1-18 is the influence diagram for ventilators that are pressure controllers. The equations relating these variables[24] are given in Table 1-3. For pressure-controlled ventilation, with a rectangular pressure

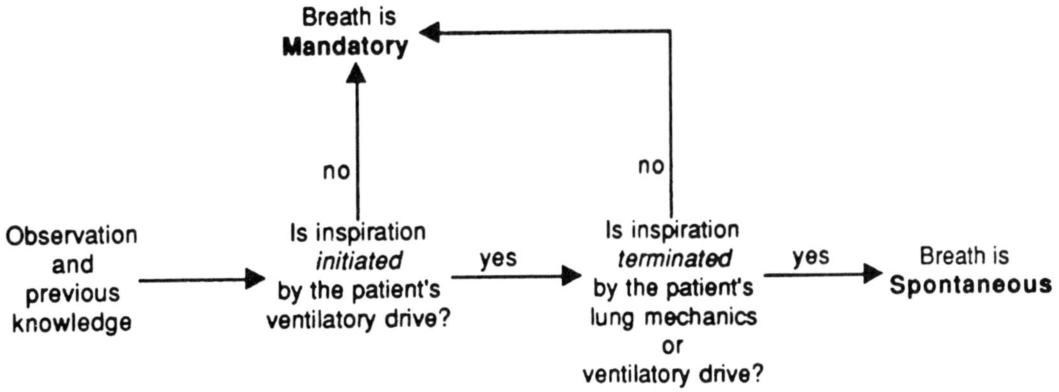

FIGURE 1-16 Algorithm defining spontaneous and mandatory breaths. In terms of current technology, if the breath is triggered according to a preset frequency or minimum minute ventilation or cycled according to a preset frequency or tidal volume, the breath is mandatory. A patient-triggered mandatory breath is an assisted breath. Spontaneous breaths are patient triggered and cycled. A spontaneous breath with an inspiratory pressure greater than expiratory pressure is a supported breath.

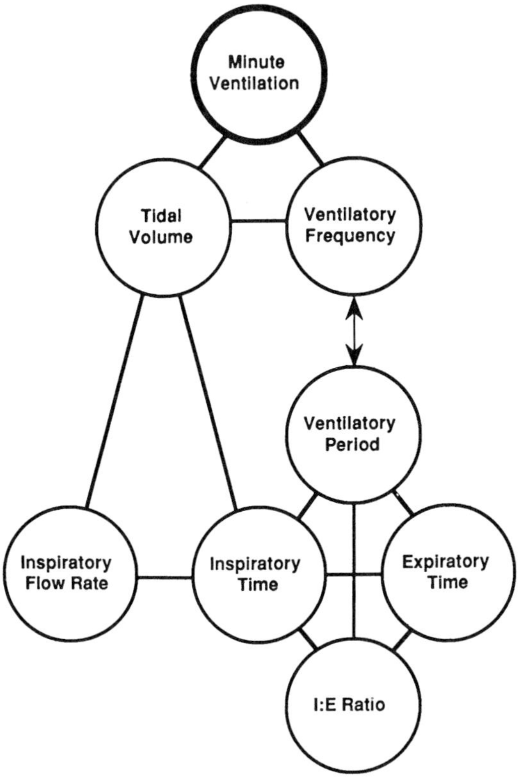

FIGURE 1-17 Influence diagram for volume-controlled ventilation. Variables are connected by straight lines so that if any two are known, the third can be calculated using standard equations (see Table 1-3). The double arrow indicates that ventilatory period is the reciprocal of ventilatory frequency.

waveform, peak inspiratory flow is equal to the set pressure difference (inspiratory pressure limit – PEEP) divided by the respiratory system resistance. Many ventilators (especially infant ventilators) provide the user with a control knob labeled "flow" (e.g., Bear Cub, Nellcor Puritan Bennett Infant Star). The meaning of this flow can be confusing. If flow is set relatively low, the set pressure limit is never reached. In this case, the set flow is the peak inspiratory flow. However, if flow is set relatively high, the pressure limit is reached almost immediately. Then peak inspiratory flow is determined by the pressure difference and resistance, as explained previously. If an intermediate flow is set, it has the effect of shaping the airway pressure waveform and generally decreasing the peak inspiratory flow. Compare the figures for rectangular and exponential pressure waveforms in the following section describing ventilator output.

Beyond these two general approaches to ventilatory support, it is possible to create a variety of breathing patterns or "modes" of ventilation. A mode of ventilation represents a set of breath characteristics that are important to the clinician. Specifically, a mode of ventilation is defined as a particular set of control variables, phase variables, and conditional variables.

Classification of Ventilation Modes

The task of understanding mechanical ventilators has become increasingly difficult in the past few years.

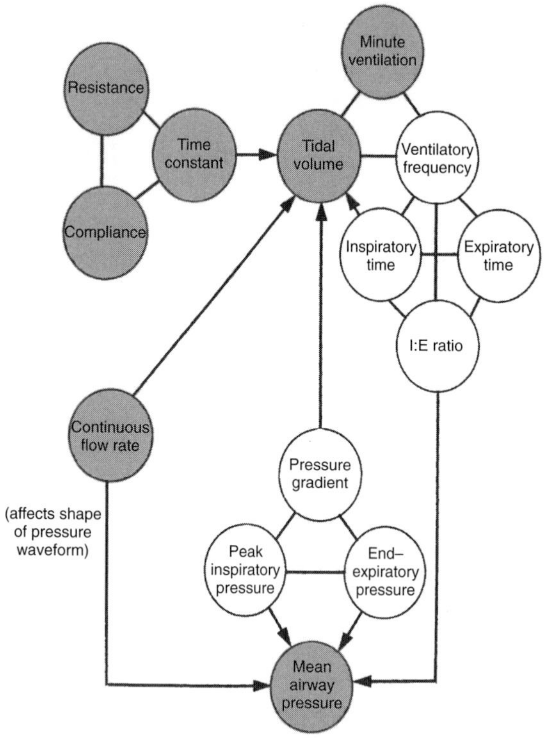

FIGURE 1-18 **Influence diagram for pressure-controlled ventilation. Variables are connected by straight lines so that if any two are known, the third can be calculated using standard equations (see Table 1-3). Arrows represent relations that are either more complex or less predictable. Open circles represent variables that can be controlled directly by the ventilator; shaded circles are controlled indirectly.** (Modified from Chatburn RL, Lough MD: Mechanical ventilation. In: Lough MD, Doershuk CF, Stern RC, editors: Pediatric respiratory therapy, Chicago, 1985, Year Book Medical Publishers.)

Manufacturers try to achieve product differential by creating new and different names for ventilator features that may be fundamentally the same. However, as discussed, the same word may be used for fundamentally different features. Goals in clarifying terminology should be to:

- Avoid promotion of new terms that do not add to the ability to understand ventilator operating fundamentals.
- Use words and concepts, when possible, that are widely used and presumably understood.
- Maintain logical consistency among terms and, when possible, link to an underlying theoretical structure consistent with classical physiology.
- Create simple terms that can be combined to create varying degrees of complexity, such as using letters of the alphabet to create words and sentences rather than separate icons for each idea. This promotes the concept that it is easier to memorize a small number of terms and the rules for combining them (governed by the profession) rather than a never-ending list of unrelated jargon (generated by marketing interests). Manufacturers cannot be compelled to adopt a consistent classification scheme, but practitioners can develop one that clearly explains what ventilators do, independent of what the manufacturers call it. The alternative is to memorize the manufacturers' descriptions for all the different ventilators in use and try to ignore the contradictions.

The first step in creating a unified and consistent mode classification scheme is to set up some definitions. The following terms represent a minimum set of concepts needed to construct a convenient lexicon of mechanical ventilation modes:

- Mandatory breath: inspiration is machine triggered and/or machine cycled.
- Spontaneous breath: inspiration is patient triggered and patient cycled.
- CMV: continuous mandatory ventilation—every breath is mandatory.
- IMV: intermittent (machine-triggered) mandatory ventilation (breaths) with spontaneous breaths allowed in between.
- SIMV: synchronized intermittent (patient or machine triggered) mandatory ventilation (breaths) with spontaneous breaths allowed in between.
- CSV (commonly called pressure support ventilation or PSV): continuous spontaneous ventilation—every breath is spontaneous.
- Pressure control: the ventilator attempts to maintain a preset airway pressure waveform during inspiration.
- Volume/flow control: the ventilator attempts to maintain a preset volume or flow waveform during inspiration; direct control of flow implies indirect control of volume and vice versa.
- Dual control: two variables are controlled by independent but synergistic feedback loops. Current examples are: (1) inspiration is pressure controlled within breaths, but the pressure limit is adjusted automatically between breaths to achieve a target tidal volume; and (2) inspiration switches between pressure control and flow control within a breath depending on the level of patient effort relative to machine settings.

TABLE 1-3 *Pressure, Volume, and Flow Functions of Time During Mechanical Ventilation*

	PRESSURE CONTROL	VOLUME/FLOW CONTROL
INSPIRATION		
Pressure	$\Delta P_{AW} = PIP - PEEP$	$P_{AW} = \left(\frac{V_T}{C}\right) + (R)(\dot{V})$
	$\bar{P}_{AW} \approx (PIP - PEEP)\left(\frac{I}{I+E}\right) + PEEP$	$\bar{P}_{AW} \approx (0.5)(PIP - PEEP)\left(\frac{I}{I+E}\right) + PEEP$
	$P_A \approx (\Delta P_{AW})(1 - e^{-t/\tau})$	$P_A = \left(\frac{V_T}{C}\right)$
Volume	$V_T = (\Delta P_{AW})(C)\ (1 - e^{-t/\tau})$	$V_T = \int_{t=0}^{t=T_I} \dot{V}dt$ (any flow waveform)
		$V_T = (\dot{V})(T_I)$ (constant flow)
Flow	$\dot{V} = \left(\frac{\Delta P}{R}\right)(e^{-t/\tau})$	$\dot{V}$ = constant
EXPIRATION		
Pressure	$P_A = \left(\frac{V_T}{C}\right)(e^{-t/\tau})$	$P_A = \left(\frac{V_T}{C}\right)(e^{-t/\tau})$
Volume	$V_A = (V_T)\ (e^{-t/\tau})$	$V_A = (V_T)\ (e^{-t/\tau})$
Flow	$\dot{V} = -\left(\frac{P_A}{R}\right)(e^{-t/\tau})$	$\dot{V} = -\left(\frac{P_A}{R}\right)(e^{-t/\tau})$
GENERAL EQUATIONS APPLICABLE TO ANY MODE OF VENTILATION		
$\dot{V}_E = (f)\ (V_T)$	$T_I = \frac{(I)(60)}{(I+E)(f)}$	$T_E = \frac{(E)(60)}{(I+E)(f)}$
$I{:}E = \frac{T_I}{T_E}$	$f = \frac{(I)(60)}{(I+E)(T_I)} = \frac{(E)(60)}{(I+E)(T_E)}$	$\text{period} = \frac{f}{60} = T_I + T_E$

From Chatburn RL: Classification of mechanical ventilators. Respir Care 37:1009-1025, 1992.
P_{AW}, Airway pressure; *$\bar{P}_{AW}$,* mean airway pressure; *P_A,* alveolar pressure; *V_T,* tidal volume; *$\dot{V}$,* flow; *$\dot{V}_E$,* minute ventilation; *R,* respiratory system resistance; *C,* respiratory system compliance; *t,* time from beginning of inspiration; *τ,* respiratory system time constant; *f,* ventilatory frequency (cycles/min); *T_I,* inspiratory time; *T_E,* expiratory time; *I,* numerator of I:E; *E,* denominator of I:E; *e,* base of natural logarithm≈2.72; *PIP,* peak inspiratory pressure; *PEEP,* positive end-expiratory pressure; *ΔP,* pressure gradient.

- Assist, assisted inspiration: inspiratory flow associated with a rise in transrespiratory pressure above baseline caused by an external agent (e.g., a ventilator assists the patient in breathing).

The next step in classifying modes is to realize that simple deductive reasoning, from general to specific, can be applied to the characteristics of mandatory and spontaneous breaths. This order is analogous to the taxonomy applied in biology, in which family, genus, and species characteristics take on a hierarchical order of increasing detail. Figure 1-19 illustrates this concept. It shows that at the "family" level, we have the categories of mandatory and spontaneous breaths. At the "genus" level, detail is added by describing the possible control variables. Finally, at the "species" level is the smallest group to which distinctive characteristics (i.e., phase variables) can be assigned.

General Modes of Ventilation

There are many reasons that we need to describe ventilator function. Sometimes we need only to convey the most general information. At other times, we need to be quite specific about the nature of the ventilator-patient interaction. Our classification system should provide this flexibility as a logical progression of detail. One practical way to do this is to base the classification system on the pattern of mandatory breaths. The format is to specify the following characteristics:

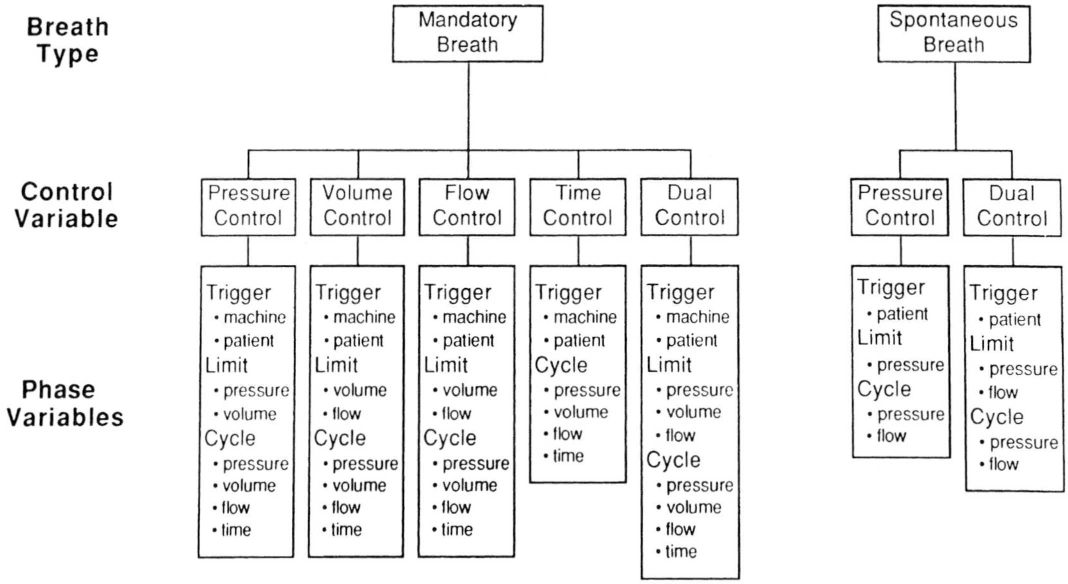

FIGURE 1-19 A hierarchical order of characteristics applied to mandatory and spontaneous breath. Once the clinician understands the way that breath types are described, he or she can combine breath types to describe modes of ventilation.

1. The control variable (i.e., pressure, volume, or dual control)
2. The pattern of mandatory versus spontaneous breaths (i.e., CMV, SIMV, and CSV)
3. The phase variables for mandatory breaths, in particular the trigger and cycle variables
4. Whether spontaneous breaths are assisted
5. Conditional variables; modes are discussed in detail in Chapter 2

At this point something should be said about the potential conflict between the concepts described previously and the terms and concepts in common usage. Much common terminology is driven by manufacturers. They, in turn, are driven by manufacturing standards. For example, the American Society for Testing and Materials (ASTM) published *Standard Specifications for Ventilators Intended for Use in Critical Care* (designation: F 1100-90) in 1990. There is a section on ventilator classification that references Mushin and co-workers' text,[1] which was published in 1980. Thus ideas that were relevant almost 20 years ago, but which are largely irrelevant today, still are influencing the understanding of current clinicians. The aforementioned ASTM standard states that there are four types of ventilators:

- Controller: a device or mode of operation of a device that inflates the lungs independently of the patient's inspiratory effort.
- Assister: a device designed to augment the patient's breathing synchronously with his or her inspiratory effort.
- Assister/controller: an apparatus that is designed to function as an assister, or in the absence of the patient's inspiratory effort, a controller.
- Assister/controller/spontaneous breathing: those devices that incorporate various modes of operation that allow the patient to breathe spontaneously at or above ambient pressure levels or with or without supplemental mandatory positive pressure breaths.

The deficiencies in this classification system should be clear, despite its widespread use. The term "control," although not defined explicitly, centers on whether the mode responds to the patient's inspiratory effort. It implies that the machine is controlling the ventilatory rate. However, when the ventilator triggers in response to the patient's effort, it is called an "assister." That was a big deal 20 years ago, but currently the ability to respond to patient effort is only one of many features that shape a breathing pattern. It seems relatively insignificant compared with the complexity of, for example, dual-control pressure and flow patterns. The term "control" is much more useful when it is broadened to its true engineering meaning, in the sense of feedback control, as described previously. In the same way, the term "assist" should not be limited to the patient-triggering feature but should be seen in the broader sense of adding force to the patient's inspiratory effort throughout inspiration (e.g., see the description of the "proportional assist" mode). Thus inspiratory assistance can be achieved by controlling the pressure, volume, or flow pattern generated by the ventilator. Another problem is that the terms "mandatory" and "spontaneous" are not defined. The reader evidently is supposed to "intuit" the meaning. However, if the terms are not defined explicitly, as explained earlier, much contradiction and confusion result when the detailed workings of modern ventilators are examined.

Once the system is understood, the meaning of the jargon can easily be grasped on the job. For example, if the concept of volume-controlled CMV is understood, it can be seen that it is what many call "assist/control" or "A/C." But it can also be seen that assist/control implies only that there is both patient and machine triggering of breaths, whereas VC-CMV conveys more information. It tells about the control variable (volume) and the phase variables (patient or machine triggered, flow limited, machine cycled, due to the fact that each breath is mandatory).

The most general way of describing a mode is to state the control variable and the pattern, as in pressure-controlled intermittent mandatory ventilation (PC-IMV). This indicates that both mandatory and spontaneous breaths are allowed and that pressure, rather than volume or flow, is predetermined for mandatory breaths. If more detail is needed, it can be said that mandatory breaths are either patient or time triggered or time cycled. Further detail can include the fact that spontaneous breaths are pressure supported. Finally, we can add that conditional variables determine that spontaneous inspiratory efforts can only trigger a mandatory breath within a particular trigger window as determined by the set mandatory breath frequency.

This system can be applied to even the most complex ventilator control schemes. For example, on the Siemens Servo 300, there is a mode called "volume support." This term must be memorized, regardless of how any other mode on the machine works (e.g., pressure support) and independent of how other ventilators work. Translated, this mode becomes dual-controlled continuous spontaneous ventilation. Every breath is pressure or flow triggered, pressure limited, and flow cycled and that conditional logic adjusts the pressure limit between breaths in an attempt to achieve a preset tidal volume.

Consider another example: Using the terminology of the Bear 1000 ventilator, there is a mode called "Assist CMV plus Pressure Augment." Translated, this would be dual-control SIMV. Each breath begins as patient triggered and pressure limited. If the conditional logic detects that the tidal volume has been delivered by the time flow decays to 30% of the peak flow, the breath is flow cycled (and therefore classified as spontaneous or supported). If, however, this condition is not met, then the breath switches to flow limited (i.e., volume controlled) and volume cycled (and therefore classified as a mandatory or assisted breath). Because a breath can be either mandatory or spontaneous depending on the relative value of patient effort and ventilator settings, the mode is a form of IMV rather than CMV or CSV.

By now, the reader should be able to discern three things: (1) there is a logical way to explain ventilator performance and with increasing detail to meet any communication need; (2) there are a great number of possible "modes"; and (3) it is essential to have a good theoretical understanding of ventilators independent of their terminology or the operator's manuals may cause confusion, especially if several brands of ventilators are used.

Perhaps the most compelling reason to use the general mode classification scheme presented in this chapter is the increasing use of computerized hospital information systems to automate physician orders and patient notes. For example, at University Hospitals of Cleveland, a system was recently needed that allowed computer entry of orders for specific modes of ventilation. The basic software allowed selection of various menu items presented on different screens. The problem was that the same system would be used in seven different intensive care units (ICUs) spanning neonatal, pediatric, and adult practices plus a variety of acute care divisions that might use home care ventilators. In addition to the wide range of possible modes for ventilation, the capabilities of more than half a dozen different ventilator brands had to be accommodated. In addition, there were the following goals:

- Orders could be written at various levels of detail.
- The most commonly changed parameters should appear in earlier screens to save time looking for them.
- Higher level-of-order detail means longer chain-of-order screens, encouraging brief orders that rely on external care paths and practice guidelines.

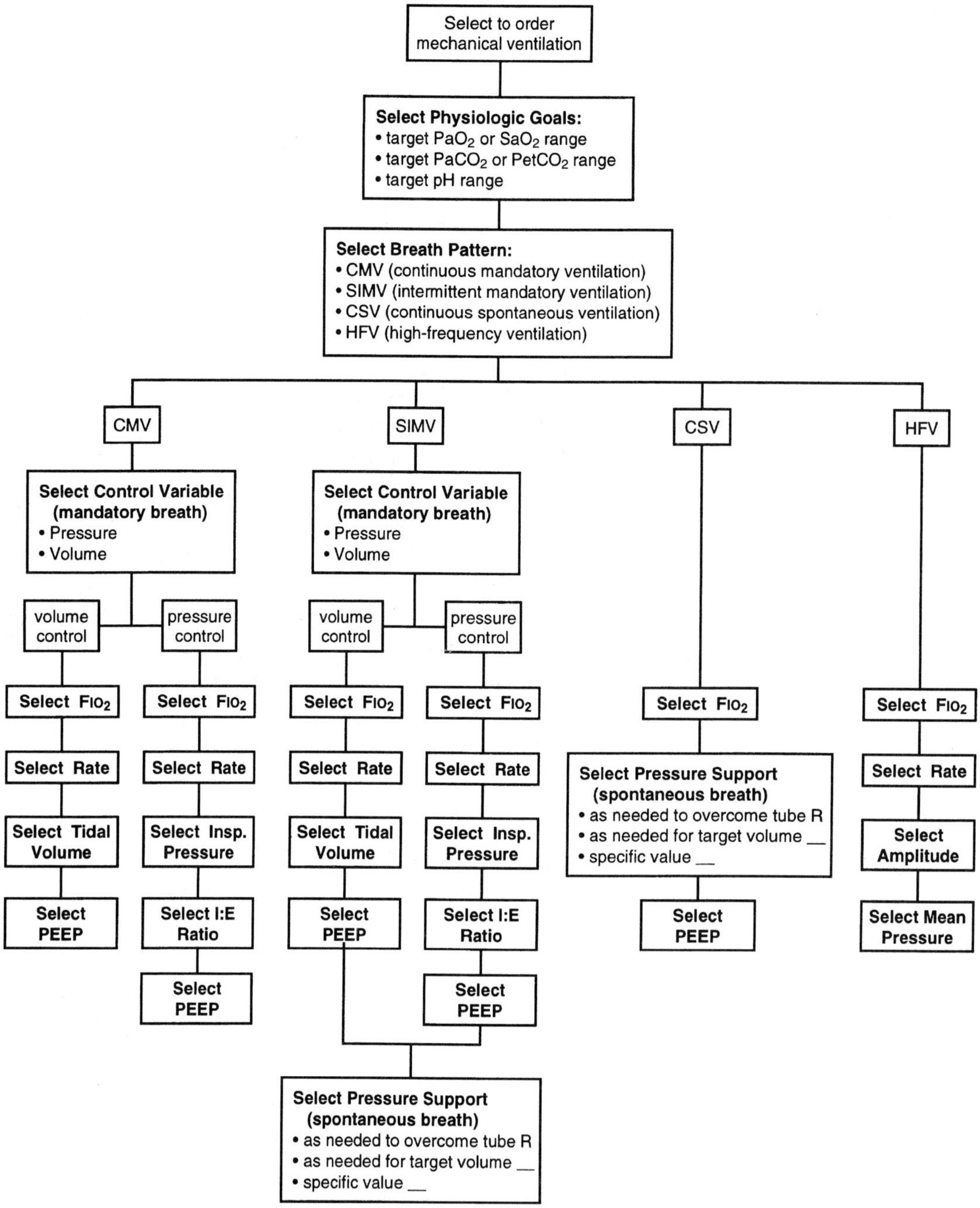

FIGURE 1-20 Schematic diagram of computerized physician order entry screens for mechanical ventilation on a hospitalwide information system.

- The user could not exit until a minimum set of order details was entered.
- Consistency should be maintained between neonatal, pediatric, and adult areas.

By applying the general mode classification system in this chapter, a logical system of entry screens, as illustrated in Figure 1-20, was created. The general flow of information is to first select the breath pattern (CMV, SIMV, CSV, or HFV [high-frequency ventilation]), then select the control variable (for mandatory breaths), the phase variables (for mandatory breaths), and lastly the pressure support level (for spontaneous breaths). It would be easy to modify this system to include dual control.

Control Subsystems

Control Circuit

The **control circuit** is the subsystem responsible for controlling the drive mechanism and/or the output control valve. A ventilator may have more than one control circuit and more than one type.

Mechanical. Mechanical control circuits use levers, pulleys, cams, and so on. These types of circuits were used in the early manually operated ventilators illustrated in history books.[28]

Pneumatic. Pneumatic control circuits use gas pressure to operate diaphragms, jet entrainment devices, pistons, and so on. The original Bird and Bennett PR series ventilators used pneumatic control. A simple ventilator can be constructed with just two poppet valves and three flow resistors (Figure 1-21).

Fluidic. Fluidic circuits are analogs of electronic logic circuits (Figure 1-22).[29] They use minute gas flows to generate signals that operate timing systems and pressure switches. This makes them immune to failure from electromagnetic interference (such as around MRI equipment). Fluidic circuits can be constructed with discrete components, such as comparators and flip-flops, or they can be combined in the form of integrated circuits, analogous to electronic integrated circuits. Examples of ventilators using fluidic logic control circuits are the Sechrist IV-100B and the Bio-Med IC-2A. A simple fluidic ventilator is shown in Figure 1-23.

Electric. Electric control circuits use only simple switches, rheostats (or potentiometers), and magnets to control ventilator operation. An example of a completely electrically controlled ventilator is the Emerson Iron Lung.

Electronic. Electronic control circuits use devices such as resistors, capacitors, diodes, and transistors and combinations of these components in the form of integrated circuits. Integrated circuits can range in complexity from simple logic gates and operational amplifiers to microprocessors.

Drive Mechanism

The power transmission and conversion system, sometimes referred to as the *drive mechanism,* generates the force necessary to deliver gas to the patient. In general terms, this system is composed of either a compressor external to the ventilator in conjunction with a regulator inside the ventilator or an internal compressor linked to a motor. A complete description of all possible systems is beyond the scope of this chapter but may be found elsewhere.[30]

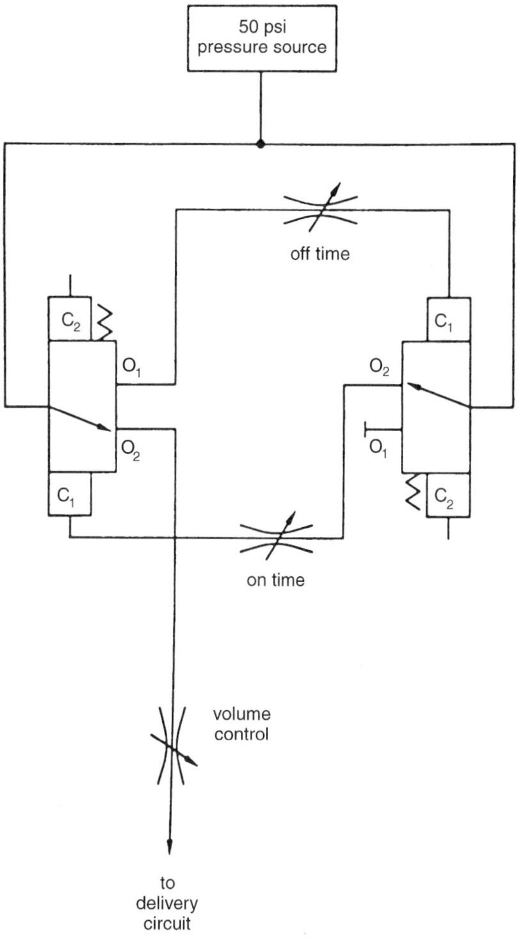

FIGURE 1-21 A simple ventilator control circuit composed of pneumatic components. Two poppet valves are connected to form a simple oscillator circuit. The on and off times (i.e., inspiratory and expiratory times) are controlled by two flow resistors. O_1 and O_2 are pneumatic signal outputs. C_1 ports are pneumatic signal inputs. The C_2 ports are spring loaded.

Compressor. A **compressor** is a device whose internal volume can be changed to increase the pressure of the gas it contains. Large, water-cooled, piston-type compressors often are used to supply gas under pressure to outlets near patient beds in hospitals. When a ventilator uses compressed gas from wall outlets as its only source of power to drive inspiration, the ventilator is considered to have an **external compressor.** Alternatively, a small compressor designed for use with a single ventilator may be employed. There are three types of compressors commonly used inside ventilators:

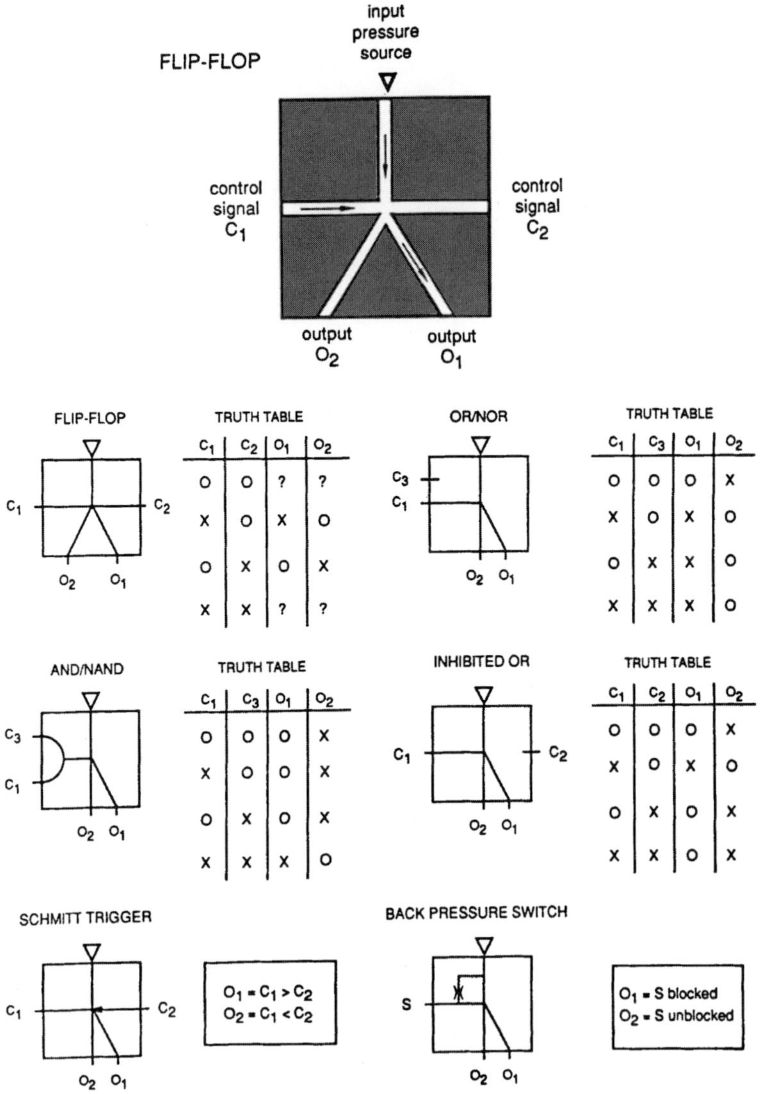

FIGURE 1-22 Basic fluidic components along with their associated input-output relations in the form of "truth tables."

- Piston and cylinder (e.g., Emerson IMV)
- Bellows (e.g., Siemens Servo 900C)
- Turbine (e.g., Pulmonetics LTV-1000)

Motor and Linkage. A motor is anything that produces motion. In a mechanical ventilator, the motor is the device used to drive the compressor. For ventilators with **internal compressors,** the characteristics of interest are the type of motor and the linkage between the compressor and motor because these influence the waveforms that the ventilator can produce.

Electric Motor/Rotating Crank and Piston Rod. This sometimes is referred to as an "eccentric wheel" (Figure 1-24). It produces a quasisinusoidal motion at the distal end of the piston rod (e.g., Emerson IMV). A true sinusoidal is generated only by a rotating crank in combination with a Scotch yoke.[31]

Electric Motor/Rack and Pinion. This produces a linear motion of the rack, driving the piston forward at either a constant (e.g., Bourns LS 104-150) or variable rate, depending on the control circuit (Figure 1-25).

Electric Motor/Direct. This can produce either a rotary motion of the output shaft, such as on a rotating vane air compressor (e.g., Bear 2), or a

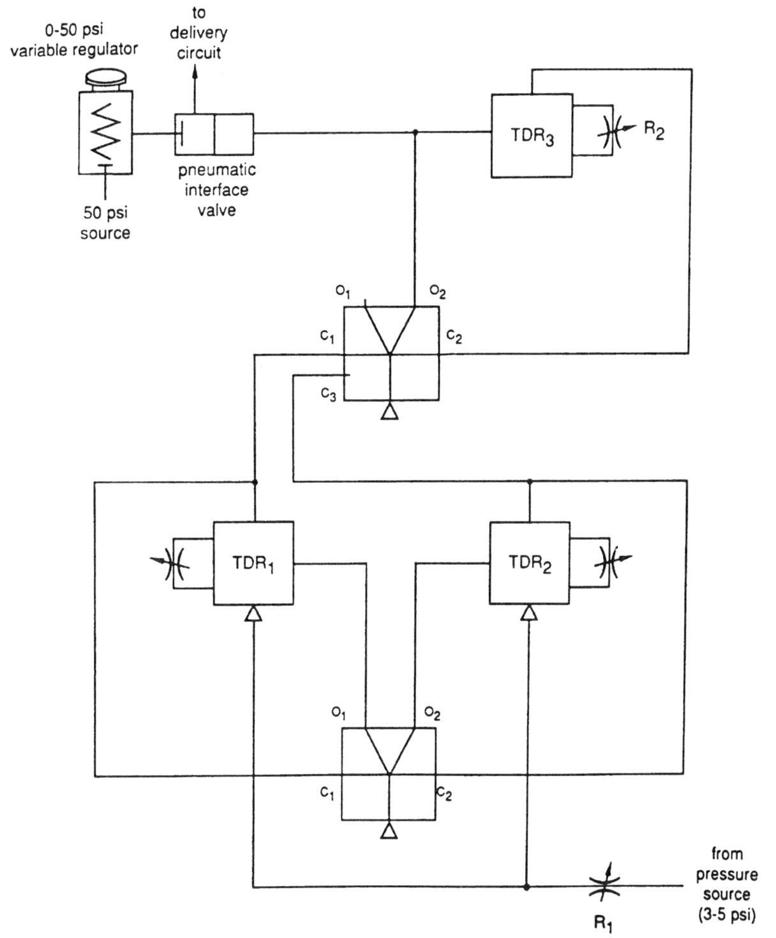

FIGURE 1-23 A simple ventilator control circuit composed of fluidic logic components. *TDR,* Time delay relay.

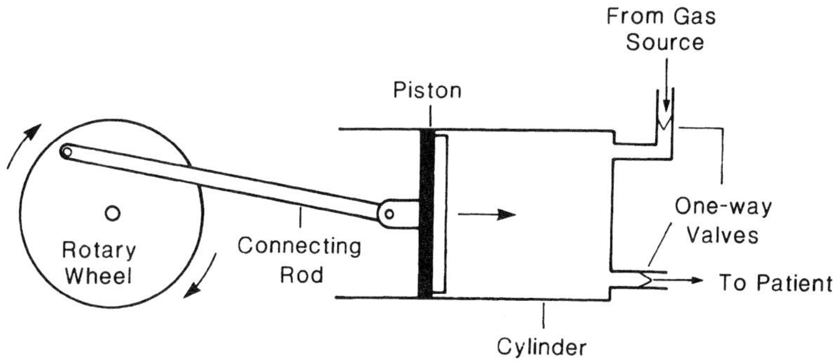

FIGURE 1-24 Drive mechanism consisting of eccentric wheel, piston rod, and piston.

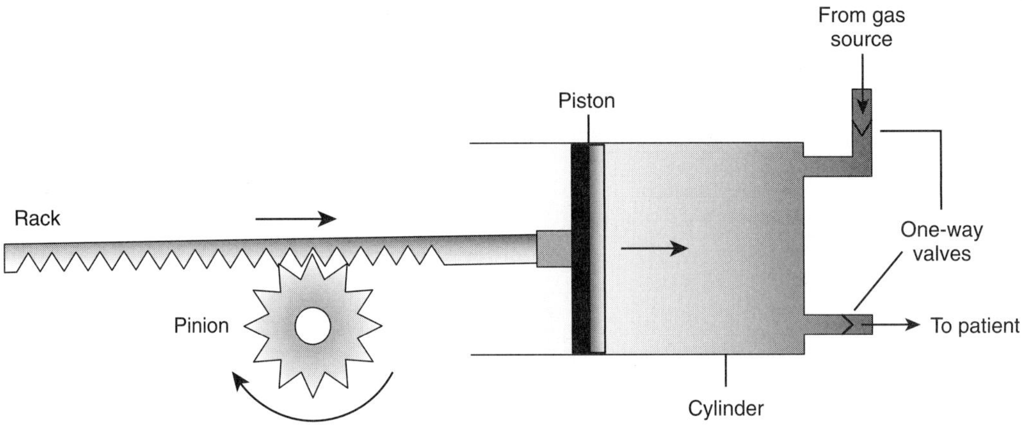

FIGURE 1-25 Drive mechanism consisting of a rack and pinion, piston rod, and piston.

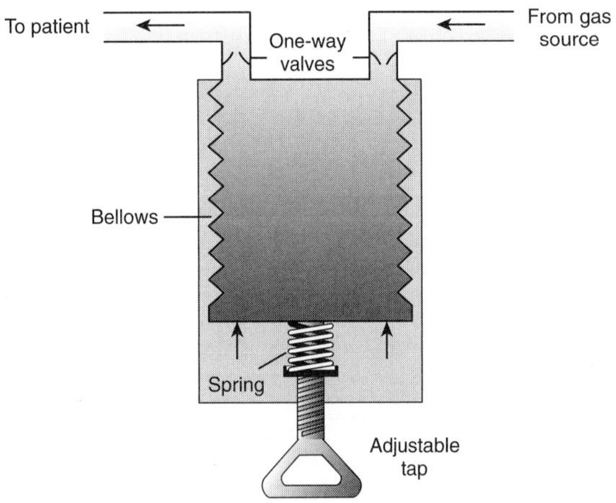

FIGURE 1-26 Drive mechanism consisting of a bellows under spring tension.

linear motion, as in the case of a linear drive motor. The linear drive motor is particularly versatile because it can produce a wide variety of easily controllable output waveforms.

Compressed Gas Regulator/Direct. When compressed gas is used as the motor, its force often is adjusted by a pressure regulator (pressure reducing valve). The compressed gas either directly inflates the lungs (e.g., Bennett 7200) or stores energy in a spring (e.g., Siemens Servo 900C) mechanism, shown in Figure 1-26.

Output Control Valve

This valve is used to regulate the flow of gas to the patient. It may be a simple on/off valve (also called an *exhalation valve*), as in the NPB MA-1, or it may be used to shape the output waveform, as in the Siemens Servo 900C. Discussions of the most commonly used types follow.

Electromagnetic Poppet Valve. This type of device (also called a solenoid valve) uses magnetic force caused by an electric current to allow a small voltage to control a large pneumatic pressure in an on/off manner. Examples include the electronic interface valve (e.g., Infant Star, which uses a set of valves to approximate various pressure or flow waveforms), the plunger (e.g., Bear Cub), and the pinch valve (e.g., Bunnell Life Pulse Jet Ventilator).

Pneumatic Poppet Valve. This type of valve is similar to a solenoid valve except that it uses a small pneumatic pressure (e.g., a fluidic signal) to control a larger pneumatic pressure. These valves are particularly useful when electronic signals are inconvenient or hazardous.

Proportional Valve. Also known in industrial settings as a mass flow control valve, this device is similar to the solenoid valve because it is operated by an electromagnet, perhaps in the form of a stepper motor (i.e., an electric motor whose rotation can be controlled in discrete arcs or "steps"). The major difference is that rather than simply turning flow on and off, this type of valve can shape the flow waveform during inspiration by changing the diameter of its outflow port and can be used to create a variety of waveforms. Proportional valves are used in the Bennett 7200 and the Hamilton Veolar ventilators and in the form of scissors valves in the Siemens Servo 900C or stepper motors in the Bear 5.

Pneumatic Diaphragm. Usually an on/off type of valve, this device uses a flexible diaphragm or membrane (e.g., a "mushroom" valve) to divert gas

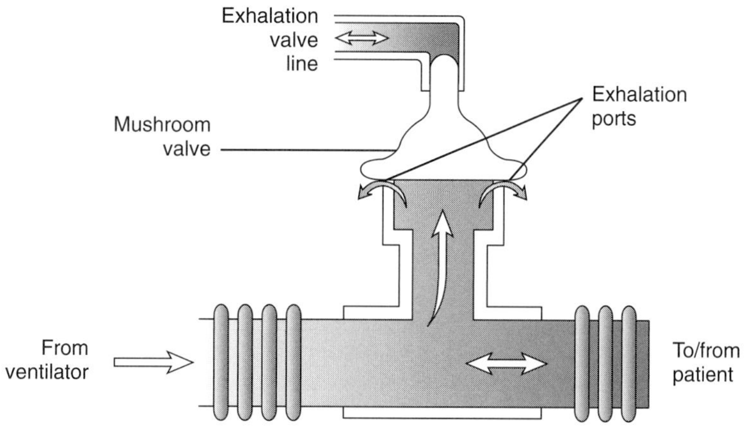

FIGURE 1-27 Balloon or mushroom style exhalation valve often used to direct inspiratory gases to the patient.

from one pathway to another (Figure 1-27). These are commonly referred to as "exhalation valves," which is a misnomer because they are primarily responsible for diverting gas into the patient's lungs during inspiration. However, they are also responsible for slowing exhalation ("expiratory retard") and maintaining PEEP. Pneumatic diaphragms are commonly used, such as in the Newport ventilators.

Many ventilators use more than one output control valve. In particular, one valve often is used to direct flow into the patient's airway (e.g., a mushroom valve) whereas another may be used to shape the waveform (e.g., a proportional valve).

Output Waveforms

Just as the study of heart physiology involves the use of ECGs and blood pressure waveforms, the study of ventilator operation requires the examination of output waveforms. The waveforms of interest, of course, are the pressure, volume, and flow waveforms we have used throughout this discussion.

For each control variable, there are a limited number of waveforms that commonly are used by current ventilators. These waveforms can be idealized and have been grouped into four basic categories: rectangular (pulse), exponential, ramp, and sinusoidal. (Note that a rectangular volume waveform is theoretically impossible because volume cannot change instantaneously from zero to some preset value as pressure and flow can.)

Output waveforms are graphed in groups of three (Figure 1-28). The horizontal axes of all graphs are the same and have the units of time. The vertical axes are in units of the measured variables (e.g., cm H_2O for pressure). For the purpose of identifying waveforms, the specific baseline values of each variable are irrelevant. Therefore the origin of the vertical axis is labeled zero. The relative magnitude of each of the variables and how the value of one affects or is affected by the value of the others are important.

Characteristic ventilator output waveforms are shown in Figures 1-29 through 1-35. They are idealized (i.e., they are defined precisely by mathematical equations and are meant to characterize the operation of the ventilator's control system). As such, they do not show the minor deviations or "noise" often seen in waveforms recorded during actual ventilator use. These waveform imperfections can be caused by a variety of extraneous variables, such as vibration and turbulence, and the appearance of the waveform is affected by the scaling of the time axis. The waveforms also do not show the effects of the resistance of the expiratory side of the patient circuit because this varies depending on the ventilator and type of circuit.

No ventilator is an ideal controller, and ventilators are designed only to approximate a particular waveform. Idealized or standard waveforms are nevertheless helpful because they are common in other fields (e.g., electrical engineering), which makes it possible to use mathematical procedures and terminology that already have been developed. For example, a standard mathematical equation is used to describe the most common waveforms for each control variable. This known equation may be substituted into the equation of motion, which then is solved to get the equations of the other two variables. Once the equations for pressure, volume, and flow are known, they are

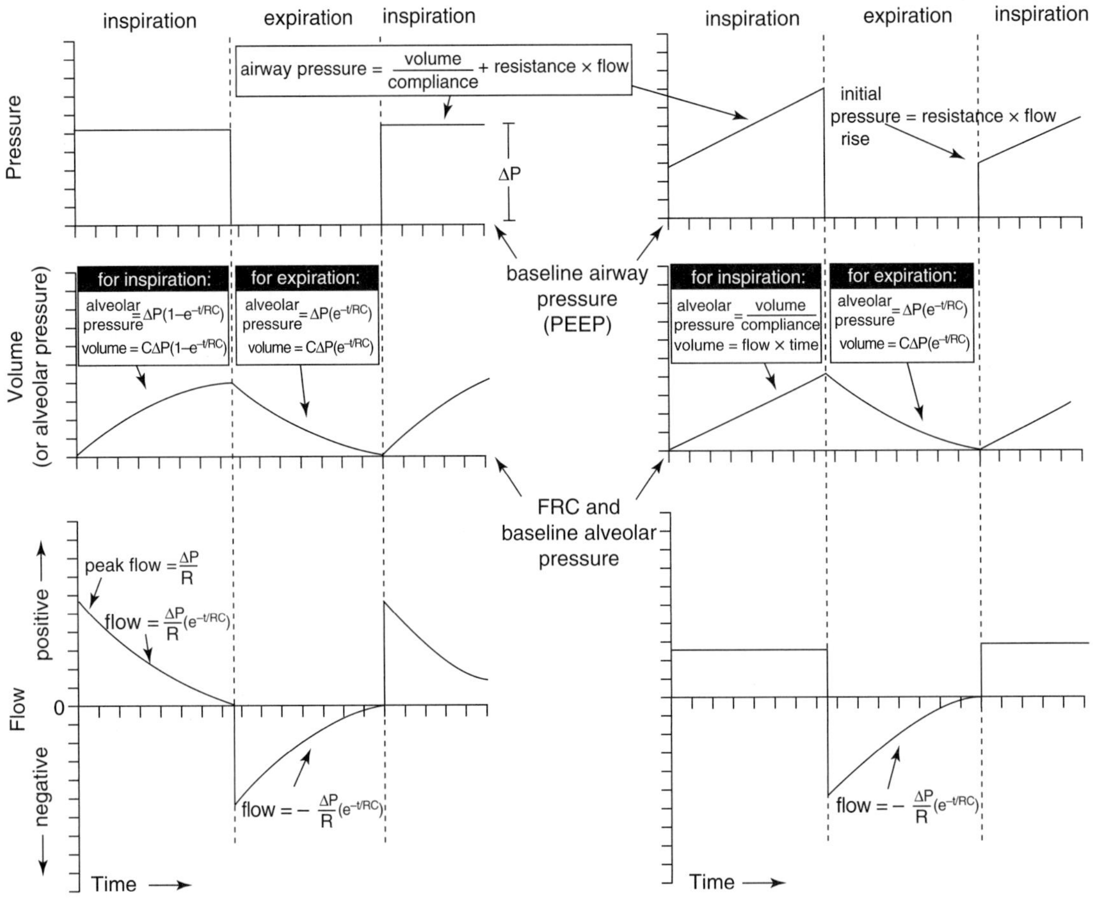

FIGURE 1-28 Typical pressure, volume, and flow waveforms for pressure-controlled (rectangular pressure waveform) and volume-controlled (rectangular flow waveform) ventilation. The curves show pressure, volume, and flow as functions of time in accordance with the equation of motion (where muscle pressure = 0). Note that all variables are measured relative to their baseline, or end-expiratory, values. *ΔP,* Change in airway pressure; *R,* resistance; *C,* compliance; *t,* time; *e,* base of natural logarithm (less than 2.72); *FRC,* functional residual (lung) capacity.

graphed easily. This is the process used to generate the graphs in Figures 1-29 through 1-35.

As mentioned previously, most ventilator waveforms can be classified as one of four general types: rectangular, exponential, ramp, or sinusoidal (including sigmoidal and oscillating). Although many subtypes are possible, only the most common are described. Waveforms are listed according to the shape of the control variable waveform. Any new waveforms produced by future ventilators can be accommodated easily by this system.

Pressure

Rectangular. Mathematically, a rectangular waveform is referred to as a step or instantaneous change in transrespiratory pressure from one constant value to another (see Figure 1-29). In response, volume rises exponentially from zero to a steady-state value equal to compliance times the change in airway pressure (i.e., PIP – PEEP). Inspiratory flow falls exponentially from a peak value (at the start of inspiration) equal to (PIP – PEEP) times resistance.

Exponential. Exponential pressure waveforms are used most commonly during neonatal ventilation (see Figure 1-30). Ventilators such as the Bear Cub are designed to deliver a modified rectangular waveform that typically results in a gradual rather than an instantaneous change in pressure at the start of inspiration. Depending on the specific ventilator settings (e.g., short inspiratory time, low flow rate, and high

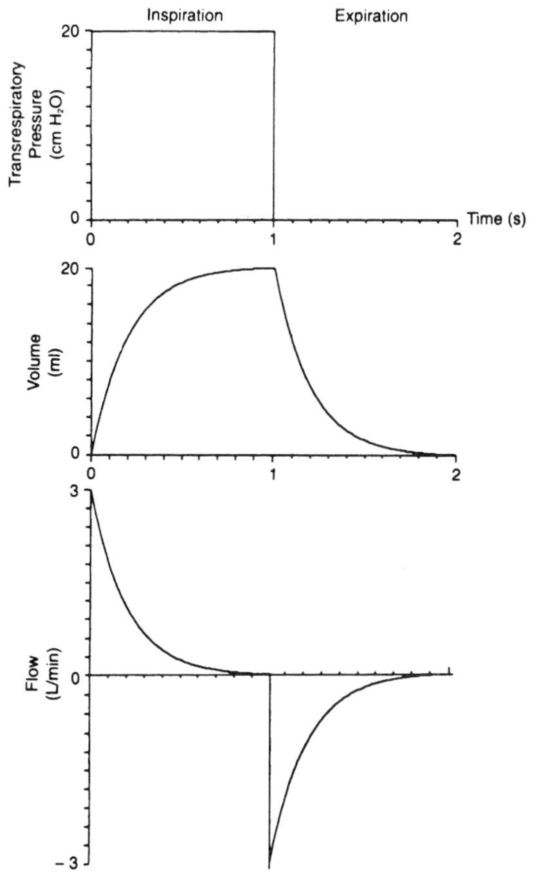

FIGURE 1-29 Characteristic waveforms for pressure-controlled ventilation with a rectangular pressure waveform. C = 0.001 L/cm H_2O; R = 200 cm H_2O/L/s.

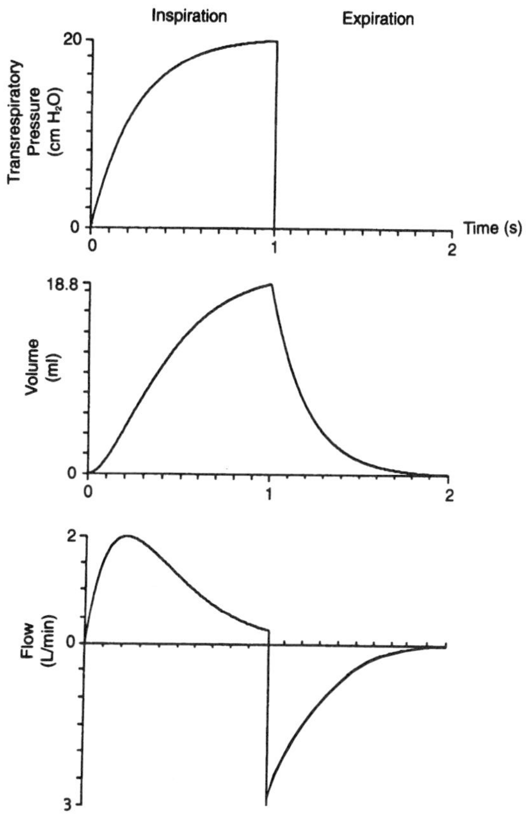

FIGURE 1-30 Characteristic waveforms for pressure-controlled ventilation with an exponential pressure waveform. C = 0.001 L/cm H_2O; R = 200 cm H_2O/L/s.

PIP), the pressure waveform may never attain a constant value and may resemble an exponential curve instead. In response, the volume and flow waveforms are also exponential, but their peak values are less than with a rectangular pressure waveform. Newer ventilators sometimes have a "slope" control that adjusts the rate of airway pressure rise (e.g., Drager Evita 4).

Sinusoidal. A sinusoidal pressure waveform can be created by attaching a piston either to a rotating crank or to a linear drive motor driven by an oscillating signal generator (see Figure 1-31). In response, the volume and flow waveforms are also sinusoidal, but they attain their peak values at different times (i.e., they are out of phase with each other).

Oscillating. Oscillating pressure waveforms can take on a variety of shapes from sinusoidal to ramp (e.g., SensorMedics 3100 oscillator) to roughly triangular (e.g., Nellcor Puritan Bennett Adult Star 1010 high-frequency jet ventilator). The distinguishing feature of a ventilator classified as an oscillator is that it can generate negative transrespiratory pressure. Thus, if the mean airway pressure is set equal to atmospheric pressure, then the airway pressure waveform oscillates above and below zero. If the pressure waveform is sinusoidal, volume and flow will also be sinusoidal, but will be out of phase with each other. Other waveforms produce more complex volume and flow waveforms.

Volume

Ramp. Volume controllers that produce an ascending ramp waveform (e.g., the Bennett MA-1) produce a linear rise in volume from zero at the start of inspiration to the peak value (i.e., the set tidal volume) at end inspiration (see Figure 1-32). In response, the flow waveform is rectangular. The pressure waveform rises instantaneously from zero to a value equal to resistance times flow at the start of inspiration. From here, it rises linearly to its peak

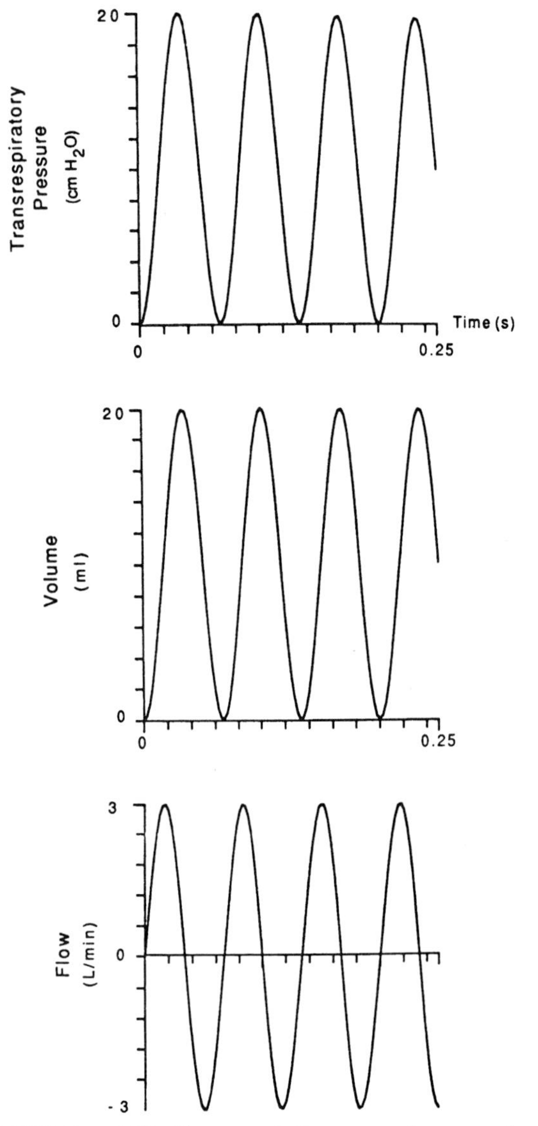

FIGURE 1-31 Characteristic waveforms for pressure-controlled ventilation with a sinusoidal pressure waveform. C = 0.001 L/cm H_2O; R = 200 cm H_2O/L/s.

value (PIP) equal to (tidal volume/compliance) + (flow × resistance).

Sinusoidal. This waveform is produced most often by ventilators whose drive mechanism is a piston attached to a rotating crank (e.g., Emerson ventilators). The output waveform of this type of ventilator can be approximated by the first half of a cosine curve, whose shape in this case is sometimes referred to as a sigmoidal curve (see Figure 1-33). Because volume is sinusoidal during inspiration, pressure and flow are also sinusoidal.

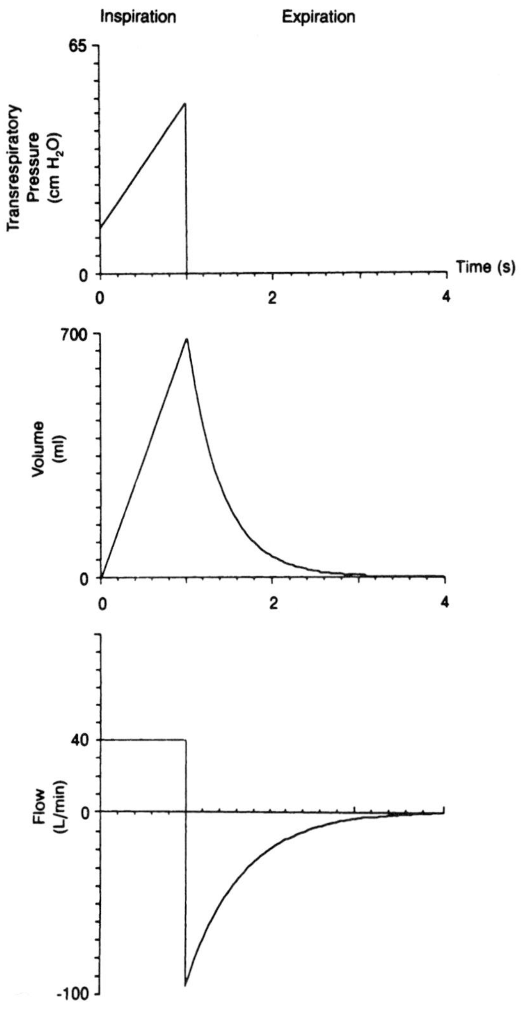

FIGURE 1-32 Characteristic waveforms for volume-controlled ventilation with an ascending ramp volume waveform. Identical to flow-controlled ventilation with a rectangular flow waveform. C = 0.02 L/cm H_2O; R = 20 cm H_2O/L/s.

Flow

Rectangular. A rectangular flow waveform is perhaps the most common output (see Figure 1-32). When the flow waveform is rectangular, volume is a ramp waveform and pressure is a step followed by a ramp, as described for the ramp volume waveform.

Ramp. The ramp waveform is what many respiratory care practitioners (and ventilator manufacturers) call an "accelerating" or "decelerating" flow waveform. The term ramp is borrowed from electronic engineering and is preferred for three reasons. First, the name "ramp" gives a more obvious visual image of actual shape of the waveform. Second, the

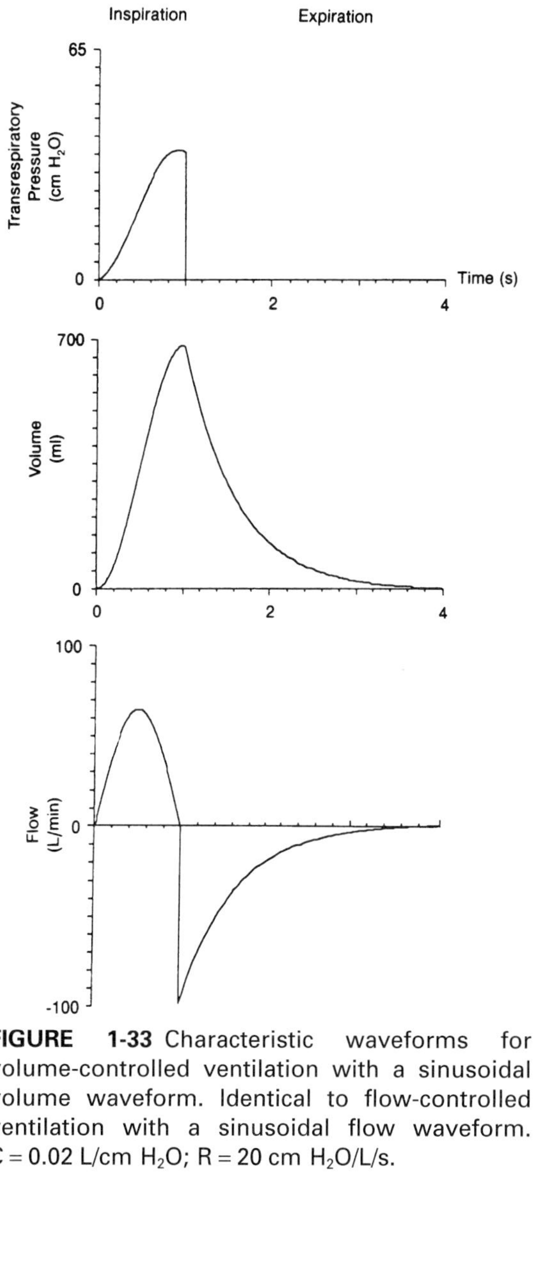

FIGURE 1-33 Characteristic waveforms for volume-controlled ventilation with a sinusoidal volume waveform. Identical to flow-controlled ventilation with a sinusoidal flow waveform. $C = 0.02$ L/cm H_2O; $R = 20$ cm H_2O/L/s.

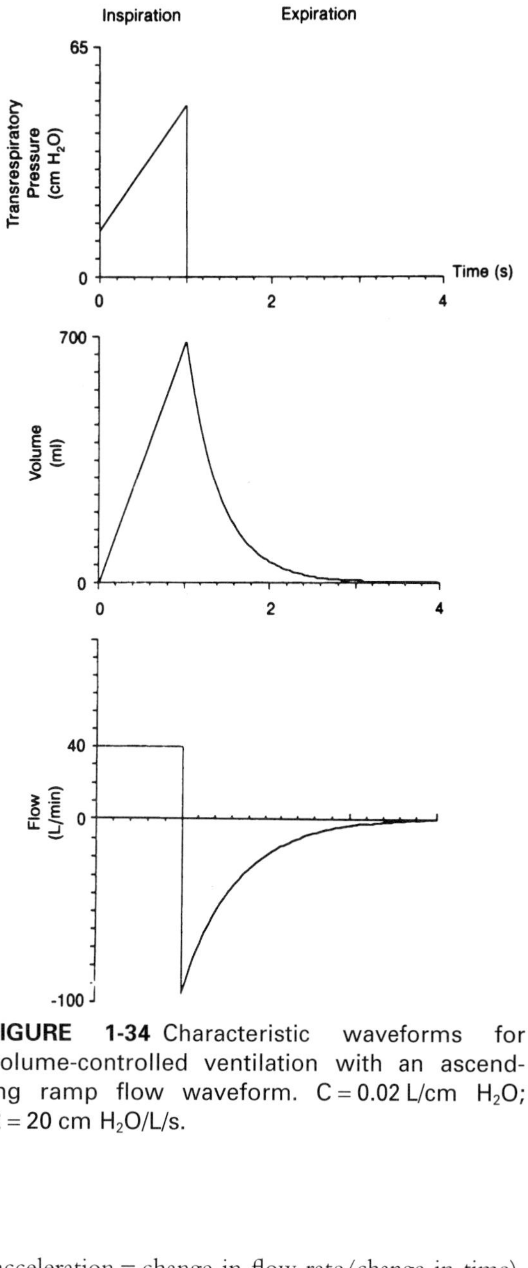

FIGURE 1-34 Characteristic waveforms for volume-controlled ventilation with an ascending ramp flow waveform. $C = 0.02$ L/cm H_2O; $R = 20$ cm H_2O/L/s.

term ramp has been described mathematically and used universally for much longer than mechanical ventilators have been in existence. Third, the analogy of something accelerating or decelerating is misapplied. For example, when a car is moving, we say it has a certain speed (speed = change in distance/change in time). If the speed increases with time, we say that the car accelerates (acceleration = change in speed/change in time), not that the speed accelerates. The speed of moving gas is expressed as a flow rate (flow rate = area of tube × change in distance/change in time). If the flow rate increases, we would properly say that the gas accelerates (acceleration = change in flow rate/change in time), not that the flow accelerates. In scientific terms, the acceleration of a particle is the rate of change of its velocity with time.[32]

Ascending Ramp. A true ascending ramp waveform starts at zero and increases linearly to the peak value (see Figure 1-34). Ventilator flow waveforms sometimes are truncated; inspiration starts with an initial instantaneous flow (e.g., the Bear 5 ventilator starts inspiration at 50% of the set peak flow). Flow then increases linearly to the set peak flow rate. In response to an ascending ramp flow waveform, the pressure and volume waveforms are exponential with a concave upward shape.

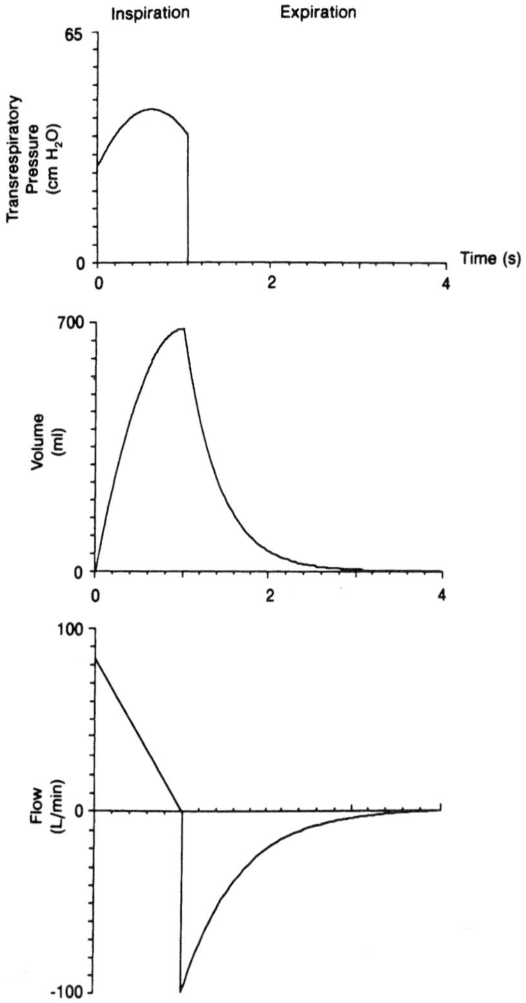

FIGURE 1-35 Characteristic waveforms for volume-controlled ventilation with a descending ramp flow waveform. C = 0.02 L/cm H_2O; R = 20 cm H_2O/L/s.

Descending Ramp. A true descending ramp waveform starts at the peak value and decreases linearly to zero (see Figure 1-35). Ventilator flow waveforms sometimes are truncated; inspiratory flow rate decreases linearly from the set peak flow until it reaches some arbitrary threshold at which flow drops immediately to zero (e.g., the Bennett 7200a ends inspiration when the flow rate drops to 5 L/min). In response to a descending ramp flow waveform, the pressure and volume waveforms are exponential with a concave downward shape. Like many other topics we discuss, manufacturers may give the same technique different names, occasionally using a different technique and the same terminology. The descending ramp waveform is a good example of this problem. Depending on the manufacturer, the descending ramp may begin at a maximum flow and decelerate to 0 L/min or to a percentage of the initial flow. This is illustrated in Figure 1-36.

Sinusoidal. Some ventilators offer a mode in which the inspiratory flow waveform approximates the shape of the first half of a sine wave (see Figure 1-33). As with the ramp waveform, ventilators often truncate the sine waveform by starting and ending flow at some percentage of the set peak flow rather than start and end at zero flow. In response to a sinusoidal flow waveform, the pressure and volume waveforms also will be sinusoidal but out of phase with each other.

Effects of the Patient Circuit

Thus far, we have implied that what comes out of the ventilator is the same as what goes into the patient. However, pressure, volume, and flow measured inside the ventilator are never the same as pressure, volume, and flow measured at the patient's airway opening. This is because the patient circuit has its own compliance (actually, the compliance of the tubing material plus the compressibility of the inspired gas) and resistance. Therefore the pressure measured inside the ventilator on the inspiratory side (e.g., on a NPB MA-1) is always higher than the pressure at the airway opening because of the elastic and flow-resistive pressure decreases created by the patient circuit. Volume and flow coming out of the ventilator are always more than those delivered to the patient because of the effective compliance of the patient circuit. Patient circuit compliance includes not only the compliance of the material from which the circuit is made but also the compressibility of the gas within the circuit. This compliance effect absorbs both volume and flow.

It can be shown by analogy to electrical circuits that the compliance of the delivery circuit is connected in parallel with the compliance of the respiratory system (i.e., both elements share the same driving pressure). Pneumatic compliance is analogous to electrical capacitance, and pneumatic resistance is analogous to electrical resistance.[7] Therefore the total compliance of the ventilator-patient system is simply the sum of the two compliances. In a similar manner, the resistance of the delivery circuit is shown to be connected in series with the respiratory system resistance (i.e., both elements share the same flow) so that the total resistance is the sum of the two. From these assumptions, it can be shown that the relationship between the volume input to the patient (at the point of connection to the patient's airway opening) and

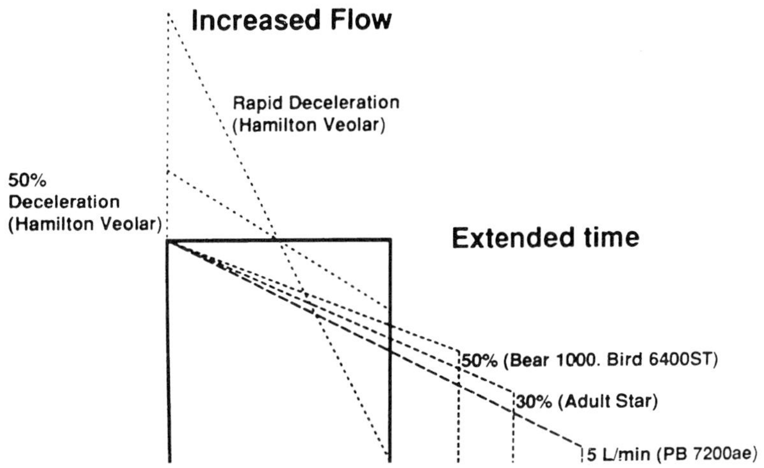

FIGURE 1-36 Differences in the flow profiles provided by different ventilators delivering the same tidal volume. The solid line represents the initial rectangular flow waveform. The Hamilton Veolar increases peak flow and decreases to 50% or 0% of the peak flow. Other ventilators maintain peak flow and decrease to 50% of peak flow to 5 L/min. In these ventilators, inspiratory time is extended and expiratory time is shortened. (From Nahum A, Shapiro R: Adjuncts to mechanical ventilation, Clin Chest Med 17:491-511, 1996.)

the volume output from the ventilator (at the point of connection to the patient circuit) is described by:

$$\text{Volume input to patient} = [1/(1 + C_{PC}/C_{RS})] \times \text{volume output from ventilator} \quad (8)$$

where C_{PC} is the compliance of the patient circuit and C_{RS} is the total compliance of the patient's respiratory system. The equation shows that the larger the patient circuit compliance, compared with the patient's respiratory system, the larger the denominator on the right-hand side of the equation. Hence, the smaller the delivered tidal volume is compared with the volume coming out of the ventilator's drive mechanism.

Assuming that the volume exiting the ventilator is the set tidal volume, the patient circuit compliance is calculated as:

$$C_{PC} = \text{set tidal volume}/(\text{Pplt} - \text{PEEP}) \quad (9)$$

where Pplt is the pressure measured during an inspiratory hold maneuver with the Y-adapter of the patient circuit occluded (patient is not connected) and PEEP is end-expiratory pressure (i.e., baseline pressure). Most authors recommend the use of peak inspiratory pressure (PIP) for Pplt in the aforementioned equation. This is acceptable, but it may lead to a slight underestimation of patient circuit compliance. Pplt is slightly lower than PIP because of the flow-resistive pressure drop of the patient circuit if pressure is not measured at the Y-adapter. This difference is greatest in small-bore, corrugated patient circuit tubing but is probably insignificant.

The effects of patient circuit compliance are most troublesome during volume-controlled ventilation. For example, when ventilating neonates, the patient circuit compliance can be as much as three times that of the respiratory system, even with small-bore tubing and a small-volume humidifier. Thus when trying to deliver a preset tidal volume, the volume delivered to the patient may be as little as 25% of that coming from the ventilator, whereas 75% is compressed in the patient circuit. An example using adult values is shown in Figure 1-37.

Another area in which patient circuit compliance causes trouble is in the determination of auto-PEEP. Auto-PEEP is pressure in the lung at end-expiration caused by either insufficient expiratory time or early closure of small airways secondary to lung disease. The result is unintended positive pressure, which can result in a number of clinical problems. The patient's airway opening is occluded at end-expiration until static conditions prevail throughout the lungs. The pressure at this time is auto-PEEP ($PEEP_A$) and is an index of the volume of gas trapped in the lungs:

$$\text{True } PEEP_A = V_{RS}/C_{RS} \quad (10)$$

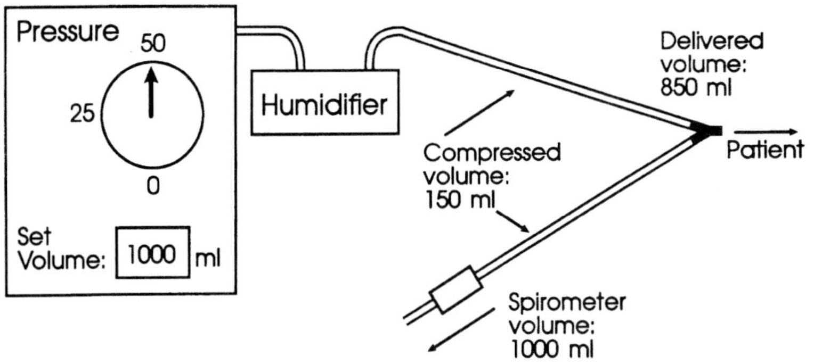

FIGURE 1-37 The concept of compressible volume is illustrated. The ventilator is set to deliver 1000 ml to the patient. If the tubing compliance is 3 ml/cm H_2O and plateau pressure is 50 cm H_2O, then compressible volume is (3 ml/cm H_2O) × 50 cm H_2O = 150 ml. Actual volume delivered to the patient is 1000 ml − 150 ml = 850 ml. If the ventilator measures volume distal to the exhalation valve, tidal volume equals set volume but does not reflect the actual tidal volume delivered to the patient.

where V_{RS} is the volume of the respiratory system at end-expiration and C_{RS} is respiratory system compliance.

Many ventilators allow the clinician to perform the maneuver without disconnecting the patient from the ventilator. In this case, however, the end-expiratory respiratory system volume is distributed between the lungs and the patient circuit. Thus the auto-PEEP measured under these conditions underestimates the true auto-PEEP because the patient circuit compliance is added in parallel with the compliance of the respiratory system:

$$\text{Estimated PEEP}_A = V_{RS}/(C_{RS} + C_{PC}) \quad (11)$$

The relationship between true and estimated auto-PEEP is derived by solving Equation 4 for volume and substituting it into Equation 3:

$$\text{True PEEP}_A = [(C_{RS} + C_{PC})/C_{RS}] \times \text{Estimated PEEP}_A \quad (12)$$

Thus true auto-PEEP may be calculated from the estimated auto-PEEP by multiplying by an error factor that is a function of the patient circuit compliance. This error can be substantial for small patients with stiff lungs.

The patient circuit has the same magnitude of effect on mean inspiratory flow rate by dividing both sides of Equation 8 by inspiratory time. The discrepancy between the set and delivered tidal volume and flow must be taken into account when using most ventilators. However, some ventilators, such as the NPB 7200 series, automatically make the appropriate calculations and adjustments.

During pressure-controlled ventilation, the compliance of the patient circuit has the effect of rounding the leading edge of a rectangular pressure waveform, which could reduce the volume delivered to the patient. This effect is avoided if the pressure limit is maintained for at least five time constants (of the respiratory system). The time constant is a measure of the time required for the passive respiratory system to respond to abrupt changes in ventilatory pressure. It has units of time (usually seconds) and is calculated as resistance times compliance.[7]

For both pressure- and volume-controlled ventilation, the patient circuit compliance and resistance, along with the resistance of the exhalation valve (in series with the patient circuit and respiratory system resistance) increase the expiratory time constant. Thus a large circuit compliance coupled with a short expiratory time can lead to inadvertent **end-expiratory pressure.**

In summary, the "set" values for pressure, volumes, and flow may be different from the "output (from ventilator)" values because of calibration errors and different from the "input (to the patient)" because of the effects of the patient circuit. Thus there are two general sources of error that cause discrepancies between the desired and actual patient values.

VENTILATOR ALARM SYSTEMS

The ventilator classification scheme described previously centers on the basic functions of input, control, and output. If any of these functions fails, a life-threatening situation may result. Thus ventilators are equipped with various types of alarms, which may be classified in the same manner as the other major ventilator characteristics.

Day and MacIntyre[33,34] have stressed that the goal of ventilator alarms is to warn of events. They define an "event" as any condition or occurrence that requires clinician awareness or action. Technical events are those involving an inadvertent change in the ventilator's performance; patient events are those involving a change in the patient's clinical status that can be detected by the ventilator.[30] A ventilator may be equipped with any conceivable vital sign monitor, but we limit the scope here to include the ventilator's mechanical/electronic operation and those variables associated with the mechanics of breathing (i.e., pressure, volume, flow, and time). Because the ventilator is in intimate contact with exhaled gas, we also include the analysis of exhaled O_2 and CO_2 concentrations as possible variables to monitor.

Alarms may be audible, visual, or both, depending on the seriousness of the alarm condition. Visual alarms may be as simple as colored lights or may be as complex as alphanumeric messages to the operator indicating the exact nature of the fault condition. Specifications for an **alarm event** should include: (1) conditions that trigger the alarm, (2) the alarm response in the form of audible and/or visual messages, (3) any associated ventilator response, such as termination of inspiration or failure to operate, and (4) whether the alarm must be manually reset or whether it resets itself when the alarm condition is rectified. Table 1-4 outlines the various levels of alarm priority along with alarm characteristics and appropriate alarm categories. Alarm categories are based on the ventilator classification scheme and are detailed in the following sections.

Input Power Alarms

Loss of Electric Power

Most ventilators have some sort of battery backup in case of electrical power failure, even if the batteries only power alarms. Ventilators typically have alarms that are activated if the electrical power is cut off while the machine still is switched on (e.g., if the power cord is accidentally pulled out of the wall socket).

If the ventilator is designed to operate on battery power (e.g., transport ventilators), there is usually an alarm to warn of a low-battery condition.

Loss of Pneumatic Power

Ventilators that use pneumatic power have alarms that are activated if either the O_2 or air supply is cut off or reduced below some specified driving pressure. In some cases, the alarm is activated by an electronic pressure switch (e.g., NPB 7200), but in others the alarm is operated pneumatically as part of the blender (e.g., Siemens Servo 900C).

Control Circuit Alarms

Control circuit alarms are those that either warn the operator that the set control variable parameters are incompatible (e.g., inverse I:E ratio) or indicate that some aspect of a ventilator self-test has failed. In the latter case, there may be something wrong with the ventilator control circuitry itself (e.g., a microprocessor failure) and the ventilator generally responds with a generic message such as "Ventilator Inoperative."

Output Alarms

Output alarms are those that are activated by an unacceptable state of the ventilator's output. More specifically, an output alarm is activated when the value of a control variable (pressure, volume, flow, or time) falls outside an expected range. Some possibilities include the following.

Pressure

Pressure alarms may be available for the following conditions:

High and Low Peak Airway Pressure. These alarms occur when there is a possible endotracheal tube obstruction or leak in the patient circuit, respectively.

High and Low Mean Airway Pressure. These alarms indicate a possible leak in the patient circuit or a change in ventilatory pattern that might lead to a change in the patient's oxygenation status (i.e., within reasonable limits, oxygenation is roughly proportional to mean airway pressure).

High and Low Baseline Pressure. These alarms indicate a possible patient circuit or exhalation manifold obstruction (or inadvertent PEEP) and disconnection of the patient from the patient circuit, respectively.

Failure to Return to Baseline Pressure. Failure of airway pressure to return to baseline within a specified period indicates a possible patient circuit obstruction or exhalation manifold malfunction.

Volume

High and Low Expired Volume. These alarms indicate changes in respiratory system time constant during pressure-controlled ventilation, leaks around the endotracheal tube or from the lungs, or

TABLE 1-4 *Classification of Ventilator Alarms*

	PRIORITY			
	LEVEL 1	LEVEL 2	LEVEL 3	LEVEL 4
EVENT	*Critical ventilator malfunction*[a]	*Noncritical ventilator malfunction*[b]	*Patient status change*[c]	*Operator alert*[d]
ALARM CHARACTERISTICS				
Mandatory	Yes	Yes	No	Yes
Redundant[e]	Yes	No	No	No
Noncancelling[f]	Yes	No	No	Yes
Audible	Yes	Yes	Yes	No
Visual	Yes	Yes	Yes	Yes
Automatic Backup Response	Yes	No	No	No
AUTOMATIC RESET				
Audible	Yes	Yes	Yes	—
Visual	No	Yes	Yes	Yes
APPLICABLE ALARM CATEGORIES				
Input				
Electric power	Yes	No	No	No
Pneumatic power	Yes	No	No	No
Control Circuit				
Inverse I:E	Yes	Yes	No	Yes
Incompatible settings	No	No	No	Yes
Mechanical/electronic fault	Yes	No	No	No
Output				
Pressure[g]	Yes	Yes	Yes	Yes
Volume[h]	Yes	Yes	Yes	Yes
Flow[i]	Yes	Yes	Yes	Yes
Minute ventilation	Yes	Yes	Yes	Yes
Time[j]	Yes	Yes	Yes	Yes
Inspired gas (F_{IO_2}, temp)[k]	Yes	Yes	No	Yes
Expired gas (F_{EO_2})[k]	No	No	Yes	No

[a]Immediately life threatening.
[b]Not immediately life threatening.
[c]Change in neurologic ventilatory drive, respiratory system mechanics, hemodynamic, or metabolic status.
[d]Ventilator warns of potential danger (e.g., control variable settings high or low, alarms inappropriately set).
Specific alarm mechanisms designed in duplicate or backed up by related alarm mechanisms.
[e]Operator cannot reset alarm until the alarm condition has been corrected.
[f]Backup ventilator mode or patient ventilator circuit opens to atmosphere.
[g]High/low peak, mean, and baseline pressure.
[h]High/low inhaled and exhaled tidal volume. May also include alarms for leaks.
[i]Alarm triggered if expiratory flow does not fall below a threshold. Warns of gas trapping.
[j]Warns that inspiratory or expiratory times are too long/short.
[k]Analysis of inspired and expired gas may include other tracer gases for measurement of functional residual capacity.

possible disconnection of the patient from the patient circuit.

Flow

High and Low Expired Minute Ventilation. These alarms indicate hyperventilation (or possible machine self-triggering) and possible apnea or disconnection of the patient from the patient circuit, respectively.

Time

High or Low Ventilatory Frequency. When these alarms occur, hyperventilation (or possible machine self-triggering) and possible apnea, respectively, may be occurring.

Inappropriate Inspiratory Time. Inspiratory time that is too long indicates a possible patient circuit obstruction or exhalation manifold malfunction. Inspiratory time that is too short indicates that adequate tidal volume may not be delivered (in a pressure-controlled mode) or that gas distribution in the lungs may not be optimal.

Inappropriate Expiratory Time. Expiratory time that is too long may indicate apnea. Expiratory time that is too short may warn of alveolar gas trapping (i.e., expiratory time should be greater than or equal to five time constants of the respiratory system).

Inspired Gas

Inspired gas conditions have been standard alarm parameters for some time.

- High/low inspired gas temperature
- High/low FIO_2

Expired Gas

Because ventilators are designed to control the mechanical results of exhalation, they may be adapted easily to the analysis of exhaled gas composition, and alarms may be set for specific parameters.

Exhaled CO_2 Tension. End-tidal CO_2 monitoring may reflect arterial CO_2 tension and thus indicate the level of ventilation. Calculation of mean expired CO_2 tension along with minute ventilation measurements could provide information about CO_2 production and contribute to the calculation of the respiratory exchange ratio and the tidal volume/dead space ratio.[35]

Exhaled O_2 Tension. Analysis of end-tidal and mean expired O_2 tension may provide information about gas exchange and could be used along with CO_2 data to calculate the respiratory exchange ratio.

KEY POINT SUMMARY

- All ventilators require an input power to deliver positive pressure breaths.
- Ventilators may use gas pressure (pneumatic) or electric power inputs or both.
- The equation of motion for the respiratory system describes the relationships between the pressure required to deliver mechanical ventilation and patient variables (elastance × tidal volume and resistance × flow).
- Within the equation of motion, the pressure to deliver ventilation can be created by the ventilator alone, the patient alone, or a combination of the two.
- Open loop control uses a set point with no feedback signal to assure that the set point is achieved.
- Closed loop control uses a set point and a feedback signal to modify the output to achieve the desired set point.
- The control variable is the variable that remains constant during ventilation regardless of changes in elastance or resistance.
- A ventilator may control time, pressure, flow, or volume, but may only control one at a time.
- There are four phases of a respiratory cycle: (1) the change from expiration to inspiration, (2) inspiration, (3) the change from inspiration to expiration, and (4) expiration.
- The change from expiration to inspiration is known as triggering and initiates a breath.
- The change from inspiration to expiration is known as cycling and ends a breath.
- Conditional variables alter ventilator output based on logic.
- A ventilator may deliver four types of breaths: mandatory, assisted, supported, and spontaneous.
- A mode of ventilation is defined as a particular set of control variables, phase variables, and conditional variables.
- Pressure control and volume control refer to the specific characteristics of individual breaths; pressure control and volume control are not modes.
- The driving mechanism of a ventilator is the particular system that transforms electric or pneumatic energy into useful energy for ventilation. Good examples are pistons or turbines.
- An output waveform describes the shape of pressure or flow delivery to the patient. The output waveform may affect important variables, such as peak airway pressure and mean airway pressure.
- Compressible volume refers to the loss of delivered tidal volume into the ventilator circuit as it is expanded with pressure.
- Alarms alert the user to violations of predetermined safety variables.
- Alarms should be both audible and visual to alert the user.

ASSESSMENT QUESTIONS

1. Input power for a mechanical ventilator includes all of the following:
   - I. Mechanical
   - II. Pneumatic
   - III. Electronic
   - IV. Microprocessor
     - A. I and II
     - B. II and III
     - C. II, III, and IV
     - D. All of the above
2. The equation of motion for the respiratory system includes the following variables:
   - I. Ventilator pressure
   - II. Muscle pressure
   - III. Flow × resistance
   - IV. Volume × elastance
     - A. I and II
     - B. I, III, and IV
     - C. II, III, and IV
     - D. All of the above
3. True or False. The difference between open and closed loop control schemes is that closed loop control uses measurement of the desired set point to alter output.
4. True or False. Dual control of a breath describes a technique where both volume and pressure are controlled simultaneously.
5. When elastance and resistance are changed in a model system and pressure remains constant as volume and flow vary, this is an example of what kind of control?
   - I. Time control
   - II. Flow control
   - III. Volume control
   - IV. Pressure control
     - A. I
     - B. II and III
     - C. IV
     - D. All of the above
6. The phase variables include
   - I. Pressure
   - II. Volume
   - III. Time
   - IV. Flow
     - A. I and II
     - B. III
     - C. I, II, and IV
     - D. All of the above
7. The four phases include all but which of the following:
   - A. The change from expiration to inspiration
   - B. Inspiration
   - C. The change from inspiration to expiration
   - D. The change from spontaneous to mandatory breaths
8. True or False. The cycle refers to the variable that both initiates and ends inspiration.
9. A breath may be triggered by which of the following:
   - I. Time
   - II. Flow
   - III. Pressure
   - IV. Volume
     - A. I
     - B. I, II, and III
     - C. II, III, and IV
     - D. All of the above
10. True or False. An assisted breath is a type of spontaneous breath triggered and cycled by the ventilator?
11. The four breath types include:
    - A. Spontaneous, assisted, mandatory, and supported
    - B. Spontaneous, assisted, mechanical, and supported
    - C. Spontaneous, assisted, mandatory, and limited
    - D. Spurious, assisted, mandatory, and supported
12. A conditional variable may be:
    - I. Any of the phase variables
    - II. Pressure and flow only
    - III. Spontaneous or assisted
    - IV. An if/then statement that alters ventilatory pattern based on a measured variable
      - A. I
      - B. I and IV
      - C. IV
      - D. All of the above
13. A fluidic control circuit operates using:
    - A. Gas movement
    - B. Microprocessors
    - C. Electric circuits
    - D. Liquid circuits

ASSESSMENT QUESTIONS—cont'd

14. The drive mechanism generates the power to cause ventilation and may include:
- **I.** Compressors
- **II.** Turbines
- **III.** Pistons
- **IV.** Spring-loaded bellows
  - **A.** I and II
  - **B.** I, II, and III
  - **C.** I, II, and IV
  - **D.** All of the above

15. Ventilator output waveforms include the following:
- **A.** Rectangular, exponential, ramp, or aggressive
- **B.** Rectangular, exponential, ramp, or sinusoidal
- **C.** Rectangular, inverse, ramp, or sinusoidal
- **D.** Rectangular, exponential, modified, or sinusoidal

16. A rectangular pressure waveform and a ramp flow waveform are indicative of what kind of breath?
- **A.** Volume control
- **B.** Time control
- **C.** Pressure control
- **D.** Flow control

17. Compressible volume in the ventilator circuit causes:
- **A.** An increase in delivered tidal volume compared with set tidal volume
- **B.** A decrease in delivered tidal volume compared with set tidal volume
- **C.** An increase in dead space
- **D.** A decrease in dead space

18. Ventilator alarms warn the clinician of:
- **A.** Changes in patient condition
- **B.** Ventilator malfunction
- **C.** Both A and B
- **D.** B only

REFERENCES

1. Mushin M, Rendell-Baker W, Thompson PW et al: Automatic ventilation of the lungs, Oxford, 1980, Blackwell Scientific Publications.
2. Consensus statement on the essentials of mechanical ventilators-1992, Respir Care 37:1000-1008, 1992.
3. Chatburn RL: Classification of mechanical ventilators, Respir Care 37:1009-1025, 1992.
4. Branson RD, Chatburn RL: Technical description and classification of modes of ventilator operation, Respir Care 37:1026-1044, 1992.
5. Morris W: The American heritage dictionary of the English language, Boston, 1975, American Heritage Publishing and Houghton Mifflin.
6. Otis AB, McKerrow CB, Bartlett RA et al: Mechanical factors in distribution of pulmonary ventilation, J Appl Physiol 2:427-443, 1956.
7. Chatburn RL, Primiano FP Jr: Mathematical models of respiratory mechanics. In: Chatburn RL, Craig KC, editors: Fundamentals of respiratory care research, Norwalk, Conn, 1988, Appleton & Lange.
8. Younes M: Proportional assist ventilation: a new approach to ventilatory support, Am Rev Respir Dis 45:114-120, 1992.
9. Rubinstein MF: Patterns of problem solving, Englewood Cliffs, NJ, 1975, Prentice-Hall.
10. Hess D, Lind L: Nomograms for the application of the Bourns Model BP200 as a volume-constant ventilator, Respir Care 25:248-250, 1980.
11. Desautels DA: Ventilator performance evaluation. In: Kirby RR, Smith RA, Desautels DA, editors: Mechanical ventilation, New York, 1985, Churchill Livingstone.
12. Sassoon CSH, Giron AE, Ely EA et al: Inspiratory work of breathing on flow-by and demand-flow continuous positive airway pressure, Crit Care Med 17:1108-1114, 1989.
13. Sassoon CSH, Gruer SE: Characteristics of the ventilator pressure and flow trigger variables, Intensive Care Med 21:159-168, 1995.
14. Sassoon CSH, Light RW, Lodia R et al: Pressure-time product during continuous positive airway pressure, pressure support ventilation, and T-piece during weaning from mechanical ventilation, Am Rev Respir Dis 143:469-475, 1991.
15. Messinger G, Banner MJ, Blanch PB et al: Using tracheal pressure to trigger the ventilator and control airway pressure during continuous positive airway pressure decreases the work of breathing, Chest 108:509-514, 1995.
16. Messinger G, Banner MJ: Tracheal pressure triggering a demand flow continuous positive airway pressure system decreases patient work of breathing, Crit Care Med 24:1829-1834, 1996.
17. Branson RD: Flow triggering systems, Respir Care 39:892-896, 1994.
18. Sassoon CSH, Del Rosario N, Fei R et al: Influence of pressure and flow triggered synchronous intermittent mandatory ventilation on inspiratory muscle work, Crit Care Med 22:1933-1941, 1994.
19. Branson RD, Campbell RS, Davis K Jr et al: Comparison of pressure and flow triggering systems during continuous positive airway pressure, Chest 106:540-544, 1994.
20. Nikischin W, Gerhardt T, Everett R et al: Patient triggered ventilation: a comparison of tidal volume and

chest wall and abdominal motion as trigger signals, Pediatr Pulmonol 22:28-34, 1996.
21. Prinianakis G, Kondili E, Georgopoulos D: Effects of flow waveform method of triggering and cycling on patient ventilator interaction during pressure support, Intens Care Med 29:1950-1959, 2003.
22. Kondili E, Prinianakis G, Georgopoulos D: Patient ventilator interaction, Br J Anaesth 91:106-119, 2003.
23. Sinderby C, Navalesi P, Beck J et al: Neural control of mechanical ventilation in respiratory failure, Nature Med 12:1433-1438, 1999.
24. Shachter RD: Evaluating influence diagrams, Operations Res 34:871-882, 1986.
25. Seiver A, Holtzman S: Decision analysis: a framework for critical care decision assistance, Int J Clin Monit Comput 6:137-156, 1989.
26. Chatburn RL, Lough MD, Primiano FP Jr: Mechanical ventilation. In: Chatburn RL, Lough MD, editors: Handbook of respiratory care, ed 2, Chicago, 1990, Year Book Medical Publishers, pp 159-223.
27. Perry DG: A simplified diagram for understanding the operation of volume-preset ventilators, Respir Care 22:42-49, 1977.
28. Morch ET: History of mechanical ventilation. In: Kirby RR, Smith RA, Desautels DA, editors: Mechanical ventilation. New York, 1985, Churchill Livingstone, pp 1-58.
29. Russell DF, Ross DG, Manson HJ: Fluidic cycling devices for inspiratory and expiratory timing in automatic ventilators, J Biomed Eng 5:227-234, 1983.
30. Dupuis YG: Ventilators: theory and application, St Louis, 1986, CV Mosby.
31. Beckwith TG, Buck NL, Marangoni RD: Mechanical measurements, ed 3, Reading, Mass, 1982, Addison-Wesley.
32. Halliday D, Resnick R: Fundamentals of physics, ed 2, New York, 1981, John Wiley.
33. Day S, Maclntyre NR: Ventilator alarm systems, Prob Respir Care 4:118-126, 1991.
34. MacIntyre NR, Day S: Essentials for ventilator-alarm systems, Respir Care 37:1108-1112, 1992.
35. Weingarten M: Respiratory monitoring of carbon dioxide and oxygen: a ten-year perspective, J Clin Monit 6:217-225, 1990.

CHAPTER

2

Modes of Ventilator Operation

Richard D. Branson

OUTLINE

OBJECTIVES

- Compare and contrast pressure and volume targeted breaths.
- Describe the modes of ventilation.
- Evaluate dual control with pressure and volume targeted ventilation.
- Describe the operation and principle of:
  - proportional assist ventilation
  - adaptive support ventilation
  - SmartCare
  - automatic tube compensation
- Explain the effects of changing rise time on pressure support breaths.
- Explain the effects of changing flow termination on pressure support breaths.

KEY TERMS

adaptive support ventilation (ASV)
adaptive tidal volume support (AVtS)
airway pressure release ventilation (APRV)
assist-control ventilation (A-C)
assisted mechanical ventilation (AMV)
automatic tube compensation
continuous mandatory ventilation (CMV)
continuous positive airway pressure (CPAP)
dual control
intermittent mandatory ventilation (IMV)
mandatory minute ventilation (MMV)
positive end-expiratory pressure (PEEP)
pressure control
pressure control inverse ratio ventilation (PCIRV)
pressure support ventilation (PSV)
proportional assist ventilation (PAV)
SmartCarePS
synchronized intermittent mandatory ventilation (SIMV)
volume-assured pressure support (VAPS)
volume control

According to the framework presented in Chapter 1, a mode is a specific combination of control, phase, and conditional variables defined for both mandatory and spontaneous breaths.[1] More simply, a mode describes whether the breaths are volume constant (volume controlled) or pressure constant (pressure controlled); whether breaths are mandatory, spontaneous, or a combination of the two; and which conditional variables determine a change in ventilator function. There are numerous names for any given mode, despite similar function. This chapter attempts to group these together whenever possible.

Unfortunately, the "names" of modes frequently are the result of a whim of the designer or are concocted by the marketing group of a manufacturer. Understanding the ventilator's function during a given mode is crucial to applying the appropriate ventilatory care to the patient. Each mode has its staunch supporters and equally determined detractors. No group seems to understand the approach of another, and most fail to realize that experience and skill with a specific mode are probably the greatest determinants of success. In subsequent chapters, when application of the modes is discussed, it should become evident that mode selection should be based on patient need, not clinician preference.

In this chapter, the modes of mechanical ventilation are described and the plethora of names for each one are listed. Important concepts related to setting ventilatory variables are included. Clinical application of these techniques, however, is not described in this chapter.

PRESSURE CONTROL VERSUS VOLUME CONTROL

Pressure Target Versus Volume Target

As described in Chapter 1, the ventilator is capable of controlling breath delivery with any one of the variables in the equation of motion. From a practical standpoint, conventional modes of mechanical ventilation control either pressure or volume. Newer modes are capable of switching from pressure to volume or vice versa and are called **dual control** modes. Pressure control and volume control are not modes; they indicate which variable is constant during breath delivery regardless of changes in lung mechanics. **Pressure control** simply means the breaths are pressure constant and volume variable. **Volume control** simply means that the breaths are volume constant and pressure variable. Once this distinction is made, the ventilator's response to patient effort determines the mode.

This can be the source of some confusion. Often, pressure control is thought to mean pressure-limited, time-cycled ventilation in the control (continuous mandatory ventilation [CMV]) mode. This may be true for a given ventilator (e.g., the 900C, Siemens, Danvers, Mass.); however, pressure control breaths can be delivered in the intermittent mandatory ventilation (IMV) mode and the CMV mode. Again, pressure control and volume control only describe the variable in the equation of motion that the ventilator is maintaining constant during breath delivery.

Throughout this text, the terms pressure control and volume control may be used interchangeably with the terms *pressure targeted* and *volume targeted*. This is done for two reasons. First, the word control often causes the clinician to think of "controlled" ventilation in which the patient is paralyzed and prevented from interacting with the ventilator. Secondly, control is often used as part of the mode CMV, again leading people to confuse what is being controlled. One of the most difficult aspects of understanding ventilators is realizing that when describing how a machine works, the patient is secondary. A perfect example occurs when comparing a volume targeted breath, which is triggered by the patient, to one that is time triggered based on the set respiratory rate. Clearly, to the clinician and the patient these two breaths are different with respect to patient work of breathing, timing, and required pressure. However, to the ventilator, the breath is the same.

The breath delivery technique (pressure, volume, or dual control) should be used as a prefix for each "mode" of ventilation—for example, volume control IMV or pressure control IMV. Volume targeted IMV or pressure targeted IMV may be used for consistency. In these two examples, the mode is the same. That is, a certain number of ventilator (mandatory) breaths are delivered per minute while the patient breathes spontaneously in between ventilator breaths. Pressure control IMV implies that the ventilator (mandatory) breaths are at a constant pressure, whereas volume control implies that the ventilator breaths are at a constant volume.

The practical aspects of pressure and volume breath delivery should be mentioned. During volume control, the clinician must set tidal volume, inspiratory flow or inspiratory time, inspiratory flow pattern, and respiratory frequency. During a volume control breath, the tidal volume, flow, and flow pattern remain constant regardless of patient effort or respira-

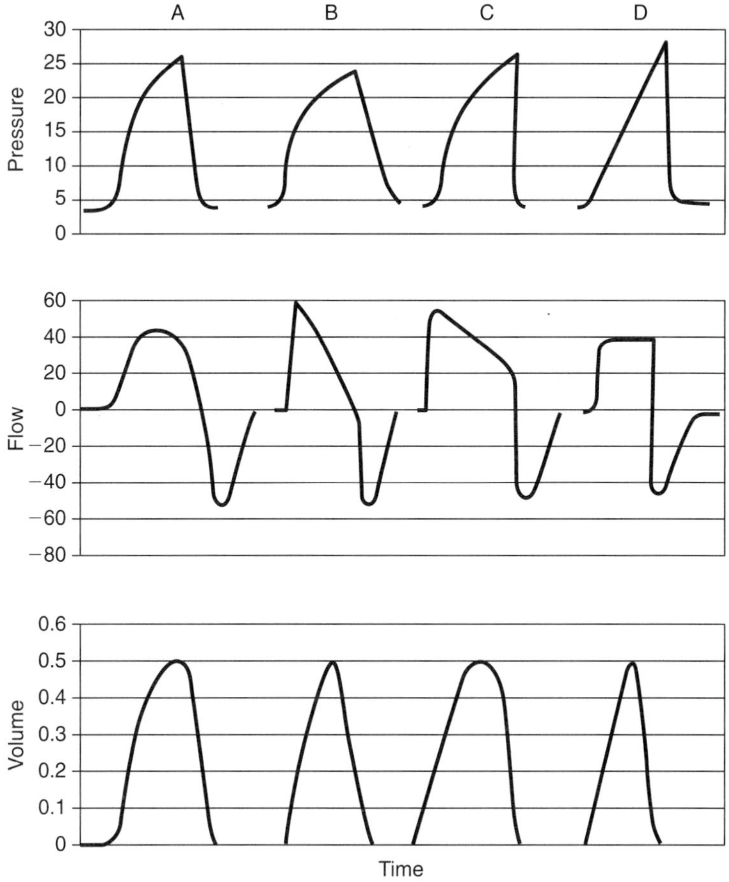

FIGURE 2-1 The effects of changing inspiratory flow pattern during volume control ventilation on pressure waveform. Breath A shows a volume control breath using a sine wave flow pattern. Breath B shows a volume control breath using a full decelerating flow pattern. Breath C shows a volume control breath using a 50% decelerating flow pattern. Breath D shows a volume control breath using a constant (square) flow waveform.

tory system impedance. The clinician may select the flow pattern during a volume control breath. Figure 2-1 demonstrates the effects of changing flow patterns during volume control ventilation on appearance of the pressure and volume waveforms.

During a pressure control breath, the clinician must set the peak inspiratory pressure, inspiratory time, and respiratory frequency. During a pressure control breath, the peak inspiratory pressure and inspiratory time remain constant. Flow during a pressure control breath is variable, depending on patient effort and respiratory system impedance. Flow during a pressure control breath always takes the shape of a decelerating waveform. This is necessary to allow the set pressure to be reached early during the breath and remain constant throughout the inspiratory time. The speed at which the flow decelerates during a pressure control breath, and hence the appearance, changes with changes in respiratory system impedance. Table 2-1 compares the characteristics of pressure and volume control breaths. Figure 2-2 demonstrates pressure, volume, and flow waveforms against time for both kinds of breaths and depicts the changes caused by respiratory system impedance changes.

MODES

Continuous Mandatory Ventilation

Descriptive Definition

Continuous mandatory ventilation (CMV) is a mode of ventilator operation in which all breaths are mandatory and are delivered by the ventilator at a preset frequency (f), volume or pressure, and

TABLE 2-1 *Comparison of Pressure Control and Volume Control Breaths*

VARIABLE	VOLUME CONTROL BREATH	PRESSURE CONTROL BREATH
Tidal volume	Set by clinician; remains constant	Variable with changes in patient effort and respiratory system impedance
Peak inspiratory pressure	Variable with changes in patient effort and respiratory system impedance	Set by clinician; remains constant
Inspiratory time	Set directly or as a function of respiratory frequency and inspiratory flow settings	Set by clinician; remains constant
Inspiratory flow	Set directly or as a function of respiratory frequency and inspiratory flow settings	Variable with changes in patient effort and respiratory system impedance
Inspiratory flow waveform	Set by clinician; remains constant; can use constant, sine, or decelerating flow waveform	Variable with changes in patient effort and respiratory system impedance; flow waveform always is decelerating

inspiratory time. In the proposed list of modes, CMV encompasses all modes that deliver only mandatory or a combination of mandatory and assisted breaths. The only difference between an assisted breath and a control breath is that the patient triggers the assisted breath, whereas the ventilator triggers the mandatory breath.

Other Terms

The term CMV is listed in the literature as:

- continuous mechanical ventilation.
- continuous mandatory ventilation.
- controlled mechanical ventilation.
- controlled mandatory ventilation.[2-5]

Interestingly, many authors preserve the CMV acronym while choosing its meaning haphazardly. CMV also frequently is called volume-controlled ventilation (VCV) or just simply control mode.[2,3]

Manufacturer Terms

Currently available mechanical ventilators refer to CMV as CMV assist control, control, volume control, and a host of others. In some cases, this mode strictly adheres to the aforementioned definition, but in others the patient is allowed to trigger mandatory breaths by exceeding the sensitivity setting. This mode often is called assist-control. On many ventilators, CMV and assist-control are the same, the only difference being the sensitivity setting. For instance, on the Hamilton Veolar (Hamilton Medical, Reno, Nev.), if desired, the sensitivity setting is dialed to its least sensitive position (−20 cm H_2O).[6] Otherwise, patient triggering is possible. It would be wise to sedate and paralyze the patient in this situation.

Classification

CMV is classified as volume or pressure controlled; time or patient triggered; volume, pressure, or flow limited; and volume, pressure, flow, or time cycled. All breaths are mandatory breaths. Figure 2-3 demonstrates volume-controlled CMV and Figure 2-4 demonstrates pressure-controlled CMV. In these examples, the modes are volume control CMV (all breaths are volume constant, and each breath is triggered by the ventilator) and pressure control CMV (all breaths are pressure constant, and each breath is time triggered by the ventilator).

Simplifying this by substituting the more generic terms, CMV is pressure or volume controlled; machine triggered; and machine cycled (Table 2-2). It should be understood that simply conveying the message that the patient is "on CMV" hardly describes the mode of operation. Depending on the ventilator used and local practice, CMV could mean that mandatory breaths are pressure or volume controlled; patient (using any of the possible variables) and/or machine triggered; pressure, volume, or flow limited; and time, flow, volume, or pressure cycled. This requires that the mode be referred to as volume control CMV or pressure control CMV.

Assist-Control Ventilation

Descriptive Definition

Assist-control ventilation (A-C) is a mode of ventilator operation in which mandatory breaths are delivered at a set frequency, pressure or volume, and inspiratory flow. Between machine-initiated breaths, the patient can trigger the ventilator and receive an

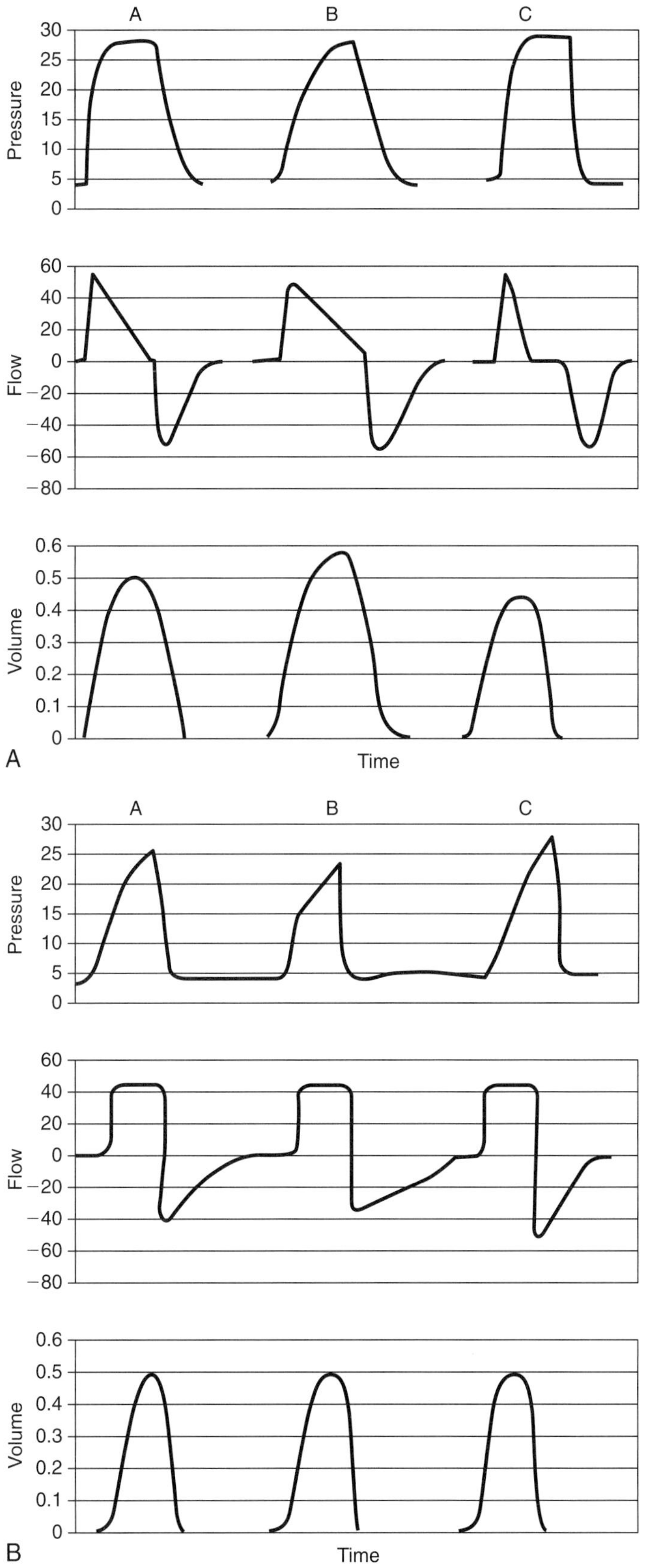

FIGURE 2-2 A, Comparison of pressure control ventilation at a normal lung compliance (Breath A) to elevated compliance (Breath B) and reduced compliance (Breath C). **B,** Comparison of a volume control breath at normal lung compliance (Breath A) to elevated compliance (Breath B) and reduced (Breath C) lung compliance.

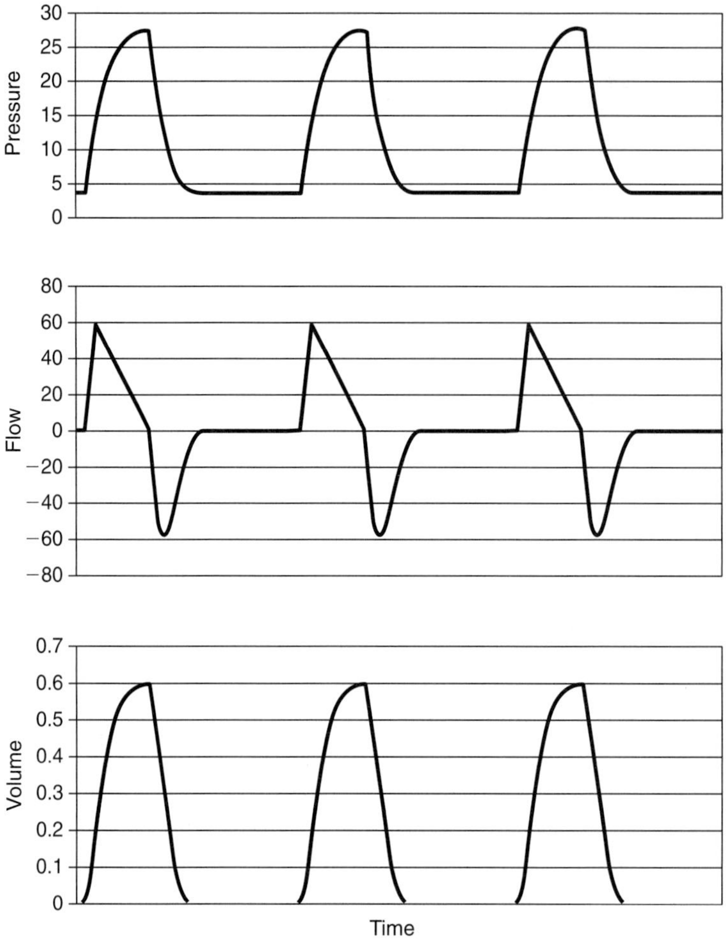

FIGURE 2-3 Pressure, flow, and volume versus time during volume control-continuous mechanical ventilation (VC-CMV) with a decelerating flow pattern.

assisted breath at the volume or pressure set on the ventilator.[2-5] Machine- and patient-triggered breaths are delivered using the same limit and cycle variables. Technically speaking, the only difference between CMV and A-C ventilation is that during A-C ventilation, the patient also can trigger a breath. From a ventilator classification standpoint, this is a subtle difference. In fact, A-C ventilation could be considered "patient- and time-triggered CMV." However, the clinical implications of patient triggering and active respiratory muscles are clinically important. Distinguishing between breaths that are time triggered and those that are patient triggered is important to monitoring and manipulating the ventilator.

Other Terms

A-C ventilation has been described in the literature as:

- assisted mechanical ventilation (AMV).
- assisted ventilation.
- CMV with assist.

Manufacturer Terms

Many ventilators use the term CMV to describe assist-control, the only difference being the position of the sensitivity setting. Other terms include assist-control and volume control.

Classification

Regardless of the terminology used, A-C can be described as pressure or volume controlled; time, pressure, flow, or volume triggered; pressure, flow, or volume limited; and flow, volume, pressure, or time cycled (see Table 2-2). Again, it is quite obvious that although a group of similarly trained clinicians understand what the term A-C indicates, the term is

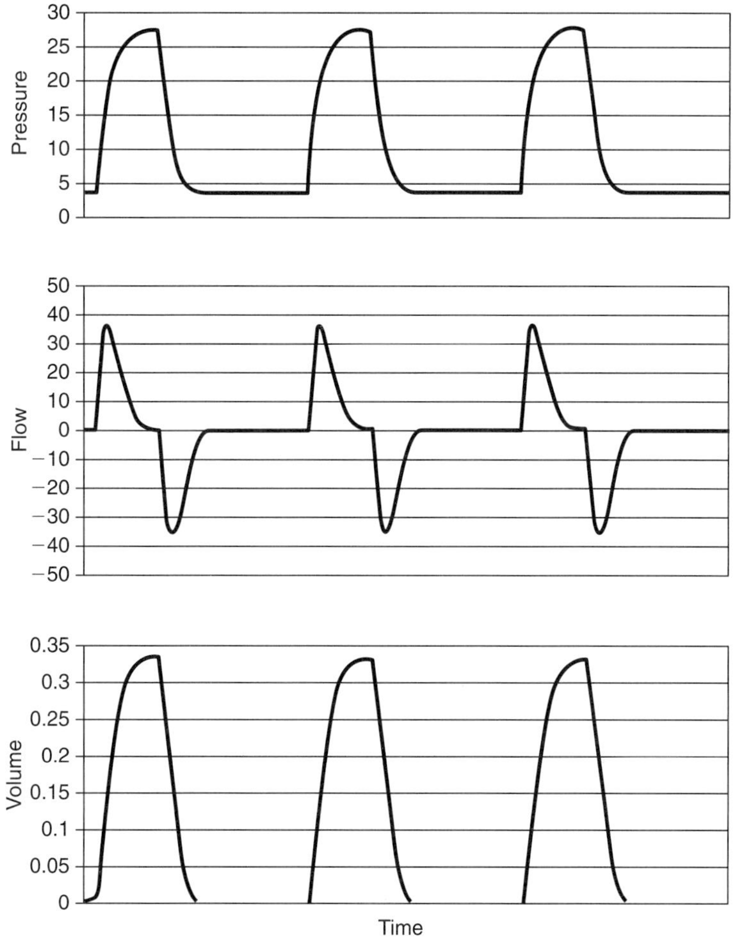

FIGURE 2-4 Pressure, flow, and volume versus time during pressure control-continuous mechanical ventilation (PC-CMV).

too imprecise to allow real understanding. Using the simplified version, A-C ventilation can be described as pressure or volume controlled; machine and patient triggered; and machine cycled. Breaths would be either time triggered (based on the set rate) or patient triggered (based on patient effort and sensitivity). Thus, A-C ventilation combines mandatory and assisted breaths that can be either volume controlled (Figure 2-5) or pressure controlled (Figure 2-6).

Assisted Mechanical Ventilation

Descriptive Definition

Assisted mechanical ventilation (AMV) is a proposed version of A-C ventilation in which there is no set frequency.[2-5] In this case, all breaths are patient triggered and delivered at the ventilator's set tidal volume or pressure. This means that all breaths are assisted breaths.

Other Terms

The pure form of AMV, without a set backup rate, is not often discussed. The term assisted ventilation has been used but frequently alludes to A-C ventilation. In subsequent chapters, this mode may be called *pressure assist* when the breaths are pressure controlled and *volume assist* when breaths are volume constant.

Manufacturer Terms

At this time, no manufacturer labels a mode of operation as only assist. AMV can be produced by placing the patient in the CMV or A-C mode and turning the rate control to "0 breaths/min."

Classification

Assist mode ventilation is classified as volume or pressure controlled; pressure, flow, or volume triggered; flow, volume, or pressure limited; and time, flow,

TABLE 2-2 *Breath Types for the Modes of Ventilator Operations*

	MANDATORY			ASSISTED		
MODE (COMMON NAMES)	TRIGGER	LIMIT	CYCLE	TRIGGER	LIMIT	CYCLE
VC-CMV	Time	Flow	Volume or time	—	—	—
VC-A-C	Time	Flow	Volume or time	Patient	Flow	Volume or time
VC-IMV	Time	Flow	Volume or time	—	—	—
VC-SIMV	Time	Flow	Volume or time	—	—	—
PC-CMV	Time	Pressure	Time	—	—	—
PC-A-C	Time	Pressure	Time	Patient	Pressure	Time
PC-IMV	Time	Pressure	Time	—	—	—
PC-SIMV	Time	Pressure	Time	—	—	—
PSV	—	—	—	—	—	—
CPAP	—	—	—	—	—	—
APRV	Time	Pressure	Time	—	—	—
PAV	—	—	—	—	—	—
DC within a breath VAPS	Time	Pressure or flow	Flow or volume	Patient	Pressure or flow	Flow or volume
If V_T<set V_T=volume cycled breath						
DC breath to breath volume support	—	—	—	—	—	—
DC breath to breath AutoFlow	Time	Pressure	Time	Patient	Pressure	Time
ATC	—	—	—	—	—	—
ASV	Time	Pressure	Time	—	—	—

APRV, Airway pressure release ventilation; *ASV,* adaptive support ventilation; *ATC,* automatic tube compensation; *CPAP,* continuous positive airway pressure; *DC,* dual control; I:E, inspiratory:expiratory ratio; *PAV,* proportional assist ventilation; *PC-A-C,* pressure control-assist-control (ventilation); *PC-CMV,* pressure control-continuous mandatory ventilation; *PC-IMV,* pressure control-intermittent mandatory ventilation; *PC-SIMV,* pressure control-synchronized IMV; *PSV,* pressure support ventilation; *VAPS,* volume-assured pressure support; *VC-A-C,* volume control-assist-control (ventilation); *VC-CMV,* volume control-continuous mandatory ventilation; *VC-IMV,* volume control-intermittent mandatory ventilation; *VC-SIMV,* volume control-synchronized IMV; V_T, tidal volume.

SUPPORTED			SPONTANEOUS				
TRIGGER	LIMIT	CYCLE	TRIGGER	LIMIT	CYCLE	CONDITIONAL VARIABLE	ACTION
—	—	—	—	—	—	—	—
—	—	—	—	—	—	Patient effort and time	Mandatory or assisted breath
—	—	—	Patient	Pressure	Pressure or flow	—	—
—	—	—	Patient	Pressure	Pressure or flow	Patient effort and time	Mandatory or assisted breath
—	—	—	—	—	—	—	—
—	—	—	—	—	—	Patient effort and time	Mandatory or assisted breath
—	—	—	Patient	Pressure	Pressure or flow	—	—
—	—	—	Patient	Pressure	Pressure or flow	Patient effort and time	Mandatory or assisted breath
Patient	Pressure	Flow	—	—	—	—	—
—	—	—	Patient	Pressure	Pressure or flow	—	—
—	—	—	Patient	Pressure	Flow or pressure		
Patient	Pressure	Flow	—	—	—	Patient effort, elastance, and resistance	Increase or decrease pressure to overcome resistive and elastic work
Patient	Pressure or flow	Flow or volume	—	—	—	Delivered volume vs. set tidal volume	If V_T>set=PSV breath
Patient	Pressure	Flow	—	—	—	Tidal volume	Increase or decrease pressure limit to keep V_T constant
—	—	—	—	—	—	Tidal volume	Increase or decrease pressure limit to keep V_T constant
Patient	Pressure	Flow	—	—	—	Patient flow demand	Pressure increases or decreases to overcome a known resistance
Patient	Pressure	Flow	—	—	—	Patient effort changes in impedance	Deliver mandatory or supported breaths Increase or decrease pressure limit to adjust V_T Change I:E to prevent air trapping

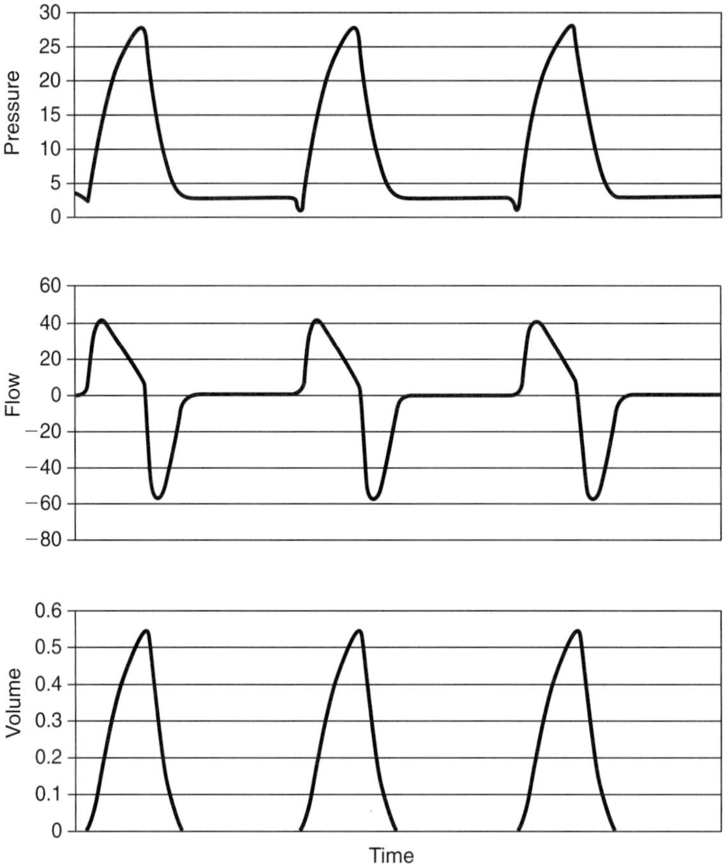

FIGURE 2-5 Pressure, flow, and volume versus time during volume control-assist-control ventilation (VC-A-C).

volume, or pressure cycled. The simpler classification system (see Table 2-2) classifies this mode as volume or pressure controlled; patient triggered; and machine cycled. Volume controlled AMV and pressure controlled AMV appear the same as Figures 2-5 and 2-6, except that every breath is patient triggered.

Intermittent Mandatory Ventilation

Descriptive Definition

Intermittent mandatory ventilation (IMV) is a mode of ventilator operation in which mandatory (machine) breaths are delivered at a set frequency and volume or pressure. Between machine breaths, the patient can breathe spontaneously from either a continuous flow of gas or demand system.[2-5,7-12]

Other Terms

For the most part, IMV has survived the interchangeable name calling if not the derogatory name calling. At one time, IMV was frequently referred to as intermittent demand ventilation (IDV) and was occasionally called "intermittent respiratory failure" by its most ardent critics.[13]

Manufacturer Terms

The terms IMV or synchronized IMV (SIMV, discussed subsequently) are used to identify this mode by most manufacturers. The term IMV sometimes is linked with continuous positive airway pressure (CPAP) on the mode selection switch, dial, or keypad. CPAP is discussed later in this chapter.

Classification

As a mode, IMV presents the new problem of classifying both mandatory and spontaneous breaths. According to our classification system, mandatory breaths during IMV are volume or pressure controlled; time triggered; pressure, volume, or flow limited; and pressure, volume, flow, or time cycled. Spontaneous breaths are not controlled and therefore have no trigger, limit, or cycle variable if a continu-

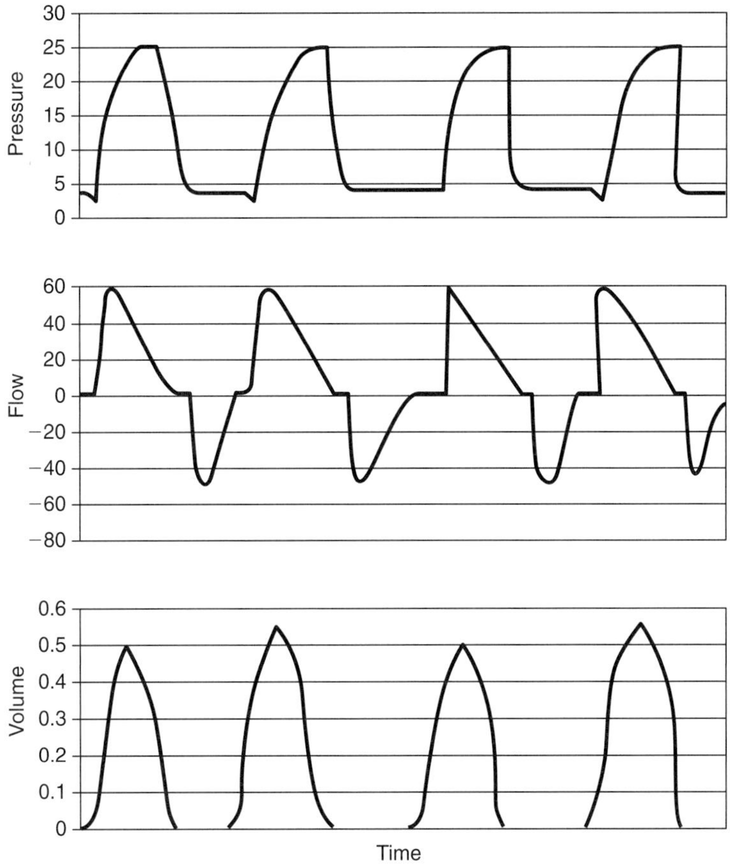

FIGURE 2-6 Pressure, flow, and volume versus time during pressure control-assist-control ventilation (PC-A-C).

ous flow of gas is used. Demand systems (i.e., a system that responds to the patient's inspiratory effort by varying gas delivery) allow spontaneous breaths to be classified. During IMV, spontaneous breaths are pressure controlled; pressure, volume, or flow triggered; pressure limited; and pressure or flow cycled (see Table 2-2). Using the simpler system allows a more succinct description. Mandatory breaths are pressure or volume controlled; machine or patient triggered; and machine cycled. Spontaneous breaths are pressure controlled, patient triggered, and patient cycled. Figure 2-7 demonstrates pressure, volume, and flow waveforms for pressure control IMV.

Synchronized Intermittent Mandatory Ventilation

Descriptive Definition

Synchronized intermittent mandatory ventilation (SIMV) is a version of IMV in which the ventilator creates a timing window around the scheduled delivery of the mandatory breath and attempts to deliver the breath in concert with the patient's inspiratory effort.[2-5,13,14] This mode uses a conditional variable to determine which type of breath to deliver. If no inspiratory effort occurs during this time, the ventilator delivers the mandatory breath at the scheduled time (time triggered). If the patient initiates an inspiration, the mandatory breath is synchronized with the patient's effort. In practical terms, the "S" in SIMV can probably be assumed. All modern microprocessor ventilators provide SIMV. Only in neonatal ventilators is traditional IMV still found.

Other Terms

The term SIMV appears to be accepted universally, although the first description of this mode named it intermittent demand ventilation (IDV).[13]

Manufacturer Terms

All manufacturers who offer SIMV refer to it as such.

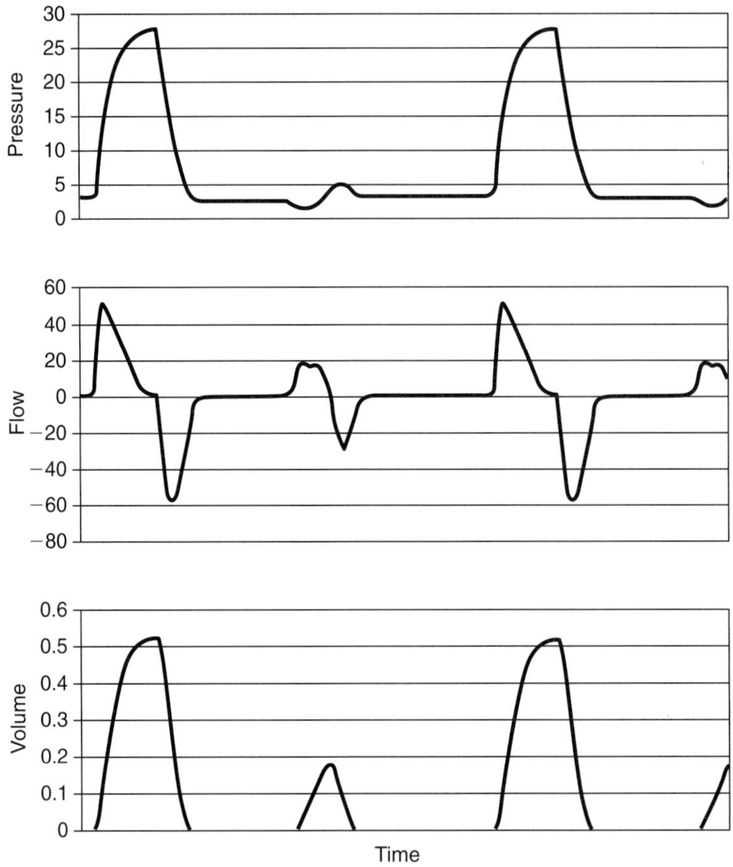

FIGURE 2-7 Pressure, flow, and volume versus time during pressure control-intermittent mandatory ventilation (PC-IMV).

Classification

Classification of SIMV is identical to that of IMV, except that mandatory breaths can be machine or patient triggered. During SIMV, mandatory breaths are pressure or volume/flow controlled; time, pressure, flow, or volume triggered; pressure, volume, or flow limited; and pressure, volume, flow, or time cycled. Spontaneous breaths are pressure controlled; pressure, volume, or flow triggered; pressure limited; and pressure or flow cycled. The simpler classification describes mandatory breaths during SIMV as pressure or volume controlled; machine or patient triggered; and machine cycled. Spontaneous breaths are classified as pressure controlled, patient triggered, and patient cycled. Because of the synchronization process, SIMV is not possible with only a continuous flow source. Some authors describe demand flow IMV and continuous flow IMV as different modes, which clearly is not the case. Although the implications to the respiratory care practitioner are quite different, the fundamental operation is the same. Figure 2-8 demonstrates the SIMV "window" concept, which allows synchronization of the mandatory breath with patient effort. Figure 2-9 demonstrates pressure control SIMV.

Pressure Support Ventilation

Descriptive Definition

Pressure support ventilation (PSV) is a mode of ventilator operation in which the patient's inspiratory effort is assisted by the ventilator up to a preset level of inspiratory pressure. Inspiration is terminated when peak inspiratory flow rate reaches a minimum level or a percentage of initial inspiratory flow. Quite simply, PSV is patient triggered, pressure limited, and flow cycled. This allows patients to determine their own frequency, inspiratory time, and tidal volume.[2-3,15-17]

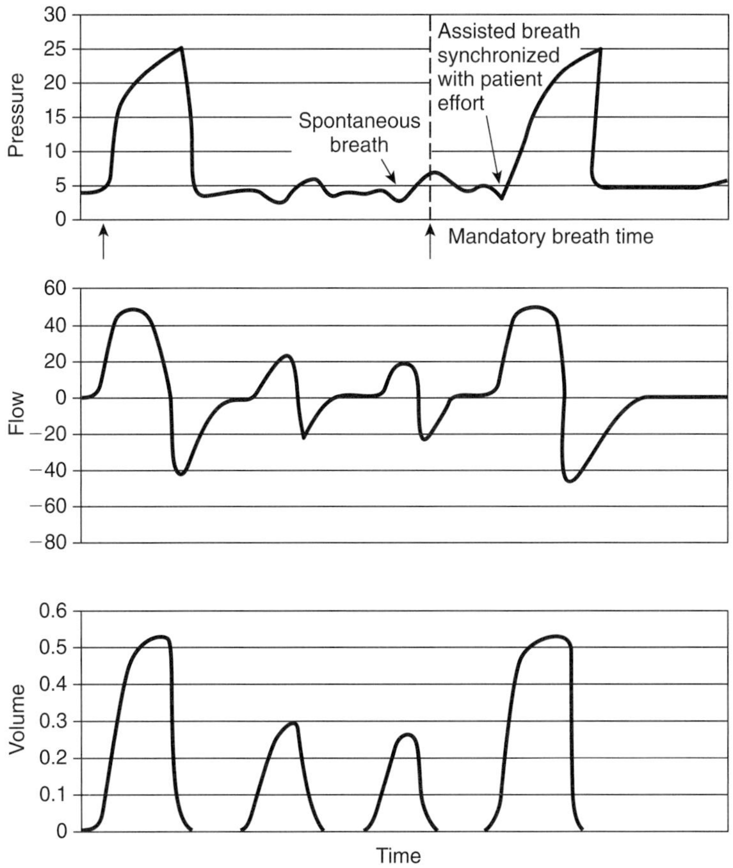

FIGURE 2-8 Pressure, volume, and flow waveforms demonstrating the "window" concept for synchronizing mandatory breaths during synchronized intermittent mandatory ventilation (SIMV) with patient effort. The bottom arrows demonstrate the clock time where a mandatory breath is due based on set respiratory frequency. The first breath is a mandatory (time-triggered) breath. At the second arrow, the patient is exhaling a spontaneous breath. The ventilatory algorithm allows exhalation and synchronizes the mandatory (assisted) breath with patient effort.

Other Terms

PSV has suffered a fate similar to CPAP in the variations of its name. The literature refers to PSV as:

- inspiratory assist (IA).
- inspiratory pressure support (IPS).
- spontaneous pressure support (SPS).
- inspiratory flow assist (IFA).

Ventilators used for noninvasive ventilation via a mask often are thought of as bilevel, but typically provide pressure support.

Manufacturer Terms

All manufacturers have different algorithms for the provision of pressure support, but all label it PSV. Unfortunately, the PSV mode often is invoked through the spontaneous mode control, leading some to believe that the ventilator is not providing positive pressure ventilation.

Classification

According to the definitions of spontaneous and mandatory breaths, all PSV breaths are spontaneous. However, because the inspiratory pressure is greater than the baseline pressure, breaths are considered *supported.* The difference between a spontaneous breath and a supported breath is that in the former, inspiratory pressure equals baseline pressure, and in the latter, inspiratory pressure is greater than baseline pressure. Therefore, PSV can be classified as pressure controlled (pressure is constant); pressure, flow, or volume triggered; pressure limited; and flow cycled.

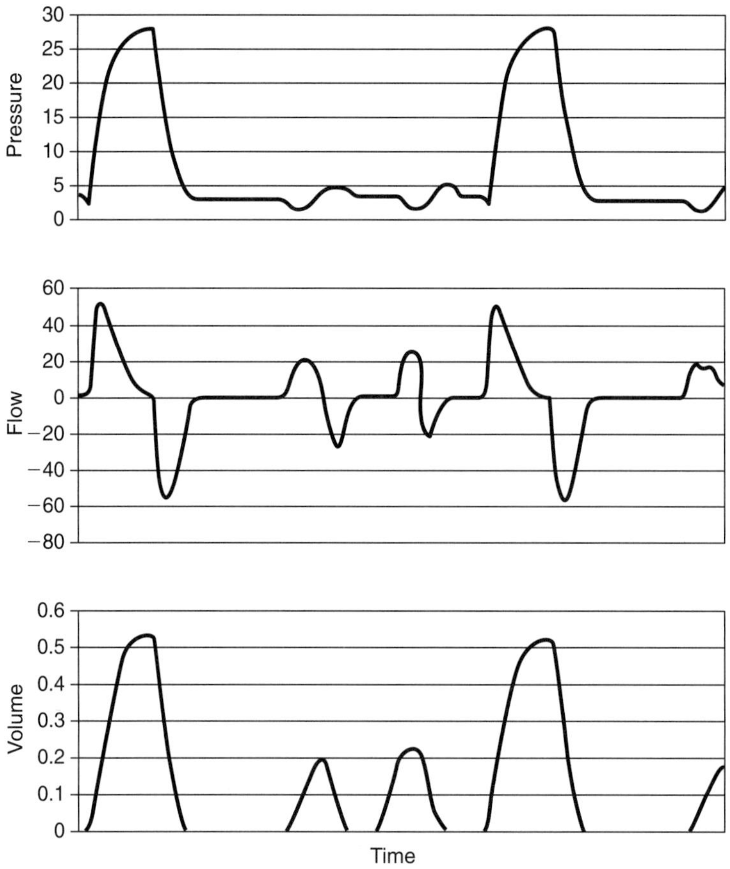

FIGURE 2-9 Pressure, flow, and volume versus time during pressure control-intermittent mandatory ventilation (PC-SIMV).

The simpler classification is pressure-controlled, patient-triggered, pressure-limited, patient-cycled ventilation. Figure 2-10 depicts pressure, flow, and volume waveforms seen during pressure support ventilation.

Algorithms for delivering pressure support vary between manufacturers. The important components of the pressure support breath include the trigger, the rise time to pressure, the limit, and the cycle variable. Triggering can be accomplished by ventilator detection of a change in pressure, flow, or other input. The speed at which the breath reaches the set pressure is referred to as the rise time. In many ventilators, this is preset and nonadjustable. Other ventilators use a clinician-set control to adjust the speed (faster or slower) at which the ventilator attempts to reach the pressure limit. If the speed is too fast, "overshoot" of the pressure limit can occur and premature cycling may result. If the speed is too slow, the patient's work of breathing increases. The limit variable demonstrates the ability of the ventilator to maintain a constant pressure.

The cycle variable of a pressure support breath typically is flow. Two schemes are commonly used, a percentage of the initial peak flow or a set terminal flow. However, there are other cycle variables implemented for safety. These typically include time and pressure. During a pressure support breath, the longest allowed inspiratory time is usually 3 seconds. This prevents prolonged inspiratory times when a low cycle flow criterion is used (i.e., 5 L/min) in the presence of an air leak. Cycling of the PSV breath also can occur if the pressure exceeds the set pressure by a set value (1.5 cm H_2O) or the pressure alarm setting is reached. In most ventilators, these cycle variables are buried in the software. Many ventilators (Puritan Bennett 840, Carlsbad, Calif.; Viasys Avea, Yorba Linda, Calif.; Newport E500, Newport Beach, Calif.; and Hamilton Galileo, Hamilton Medical, Reno, Nev.) allow the flow cycle variable to be set

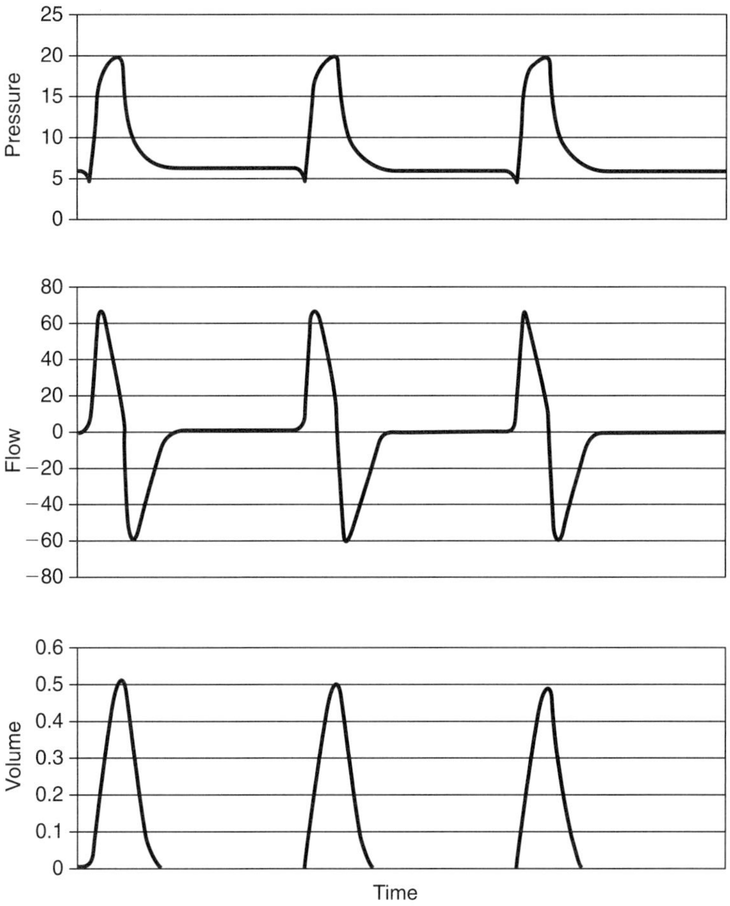

FIGURE 2-10 Pressure, flow, and volume versus time during pressure support ventilation (PSV).

at a percentage of the initial flow. Figure 2-11 depicts the important components of a pressure support breath. Table 2-3 compares the capabilities of currently available ventilators in the pressure support mode.

Simplicity always has been a hallmark of the pressure support mode. However, these changes can allow the more sophisticated clinician to tailor the mode to the patient's needs. As examples, looking at the Puritan Bennett 7200ae (Puritan Bennett Corp., Carlsbad, Calif.) and Hamilton Galileo may provide some clarity.

The 7200ae uses pressure or flow triggering, has a set rise time, and cycles when flow reaches a set flow of 5 L/min. Secondary cycle variables include an inspiratory time greater than 3 seconds and a pressure 1.5 cm H_2O greater than the set pressure limit. In this case, it is not unusual to see pressure support breaths become pressure cycled, when the patient wants to exhale before the ventilator reaches the 5 L/min flow criteria (Figure 2-12).

The Galileo can be pressure or flow triggered, the rise time is adjustable between 50 and 200 msec, and the flow cycle variable is adjustable from 10% to 40% of the initial peak flow. Secondary cycle criteria include an inspiratory time greater than 3 seconds and a pressure exceeding the high pressure alarm setting. Figure 2-13 depicts a normal pressure support breath, with additional breaths demonstrating the effects of altering rise time and expiratory termination (cycle) criteria.

The Newport E500 uses an automated system to control the flow termination based on the measurement of time constants. When the lung compliance is low and airway resistance is normal as with a patient with acute lung injury (short time constant), the ventilator chooses a flow termination of 5% to 25% of initial peak flow. This results in a longer inspiratory

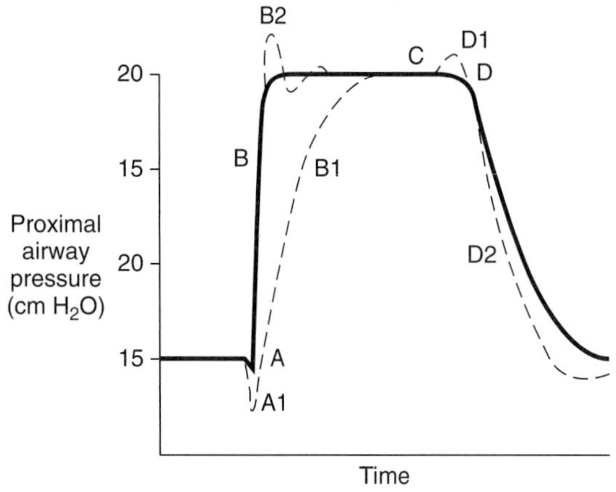

FIGURE 2-11 Important components of a pressure support breath. **A,** Trigger; **B,** rise time; **C,** pressure limit (plateau); **D,** cycle. Under ideal conditions, the PSV breath appears as the solid line. Alterations in patient effort and ventilator algorithm can cause the pressure waveform to appear different. **A1,** Inappropriate sensitivity setting or slow response time; **B1,** slow rise time relative to patient demand, which can result in an increased work of breathing; **B2,** rise time too fast, causing overshoot and contributing to premature cycling; **D1,** inspiratory time too long (caused by late-cycle criteria), causing the patient to exhale, creating a pressure spike; **D2,** breath cycles too early because of B2 or early cycle criteria.

time and larger tidal volume. If lung compliance is normal and resistance is high, as seen in COPD, the time constant will be long. In this instance, the ventilator will choose a flow termination of 40% to 55% of peak flow. This results in a smaller tidal volume, shorter inspiratory time, and better matching of patient and ventilator timing. The earlier flow termination also helps to prevent air-trapping and missed triggers due to intrinsic PEEP.

Continuous Positive Airway Pressure

Descriptive Definition

Continuous positive airway pressure (CPAP) is a mode of ventilator operation in which a clinician-set level of pressure is maintained constant while the patient is allowed to breathe spontaneously.[2-5,18]

Other Terms

Few processes have garnered the virtual avalanche of acronyms heaped on CPAP. Although differences do exist, the following all have been used to describe or have been used interchangeably with CPAP:

- **Positive end-expiratory pressure** (PEEP).
- End-expiratory pressure (EEP).
- Inspiratory positive airway pressure (IPAP).
- Expiratory positive airway pressure (EPAP).
- Continuous distending pressure (CDP).
- Continuous positive pressure breathing (CPPB).

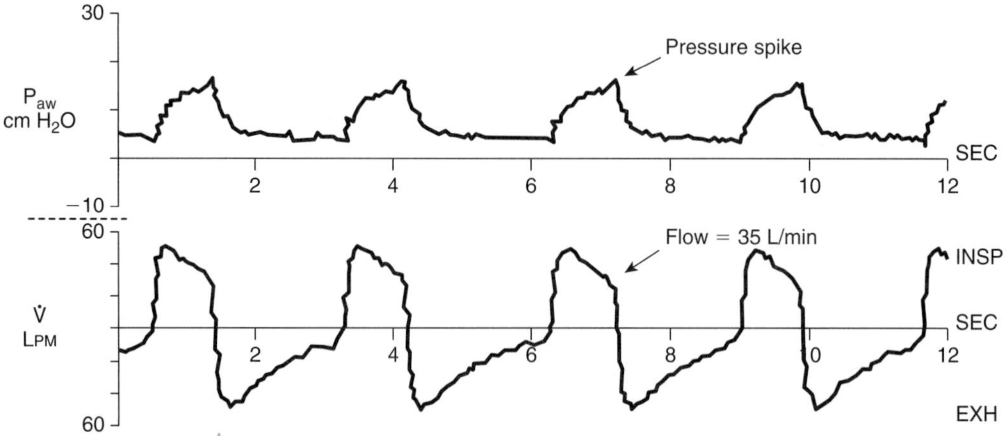

FIGURE 2-12 Pressure and flow waveforms demonstrating pressure cycling of a pressure support breath. The flow cycle criterion is 5 L/min. However, because the patient exhales before flow decelerating to this value, the breath is cycled by pressure (1.5 cm H_2O above set pressure limit). The inspiratory flow at the time the breath is terminated is 35 L/min.

TABLE 2-3 *Comparison of the Pressure Support Mode Operation of Different Ventilators*

			CYCLE VARIABLE			
VENTILATOR	**TRIGGER**	**RISE TIME**	**FLOW**	**PRESSURE**	**TIME**	**FLOW CYCLE (FIXED OR ADJUSTABLE)**
Viasys Avea (Yorba, Linda, Calif.)	Flow or pressure	Adjustable	5%-45%	High pressure alarm	0.2-5 sec adjustable	Adjustable
Newport E500	Flow or pressure	Adjustable	5%-50%	High pressure alarm	3 sec	Adjustable–uses an automated algorithm
Newport HT-50 (Newport Beach, Calif.)	Pressure	Fixed	25%	High pressure alarm	3 sec	Fixed
Drager E4 (Drager, Telford, Pa.)	Flow or pressure	Adjustable	25% adult 6% pediatric	High pressure alarm	4 sec adult 1.5 sec pediatric	Fixed
Hamilton Galileo (Hamilton Medical, Reno, Nev.)	Flow or pressure	Adjustable	25%	High pressure alarm	25%	Adjustable 10%-50%
Puritan Bennett 7200 (Mallinckrodt, Carlsbad, Calif.)	Flow or pressure	Fixed	5 L/min	1.5 cm above set	3 sec	Fixed
Puritan Bennett 840 (Mallinckrodt, Carlsbad, Calif.)	Flow or pressure	Adjustable	1%-80%	2 cm H_2O above set	2 sec	Adjustable 1%-80%
Puritan Bennett 740 (Mallinckrodt, Carlsbad, Calif.)	Flow or pressure	Fixed	25%	2 cm H_2O above set	2 sec	Fixed
Pulmonetics LTV 1000 (Pulmonetic Systems, Inc., Colton, Calif.)	Flow	Adjustable	10%-40%	High pressure alarm	3 sec	Adjustable Flow 10%-40% Time 0.5-3 sec
Siemens 900C (Siemens, Danvers, Mass.)	Pressure	Fixed	25%	High pressure alarm	3 sec	Fixed
Siemens 300 (Siemens, Danvers, Mass.)	Flow or pressure	Adjustable	5%	High pressure alarm	80% of total cycle time	Fixed
Servo *i* (Maquette, Danvers, Mass.)	Flow or pressure	Adjustable	1%-40%	High pressure alarm	2.5 sec or less	Adjustable

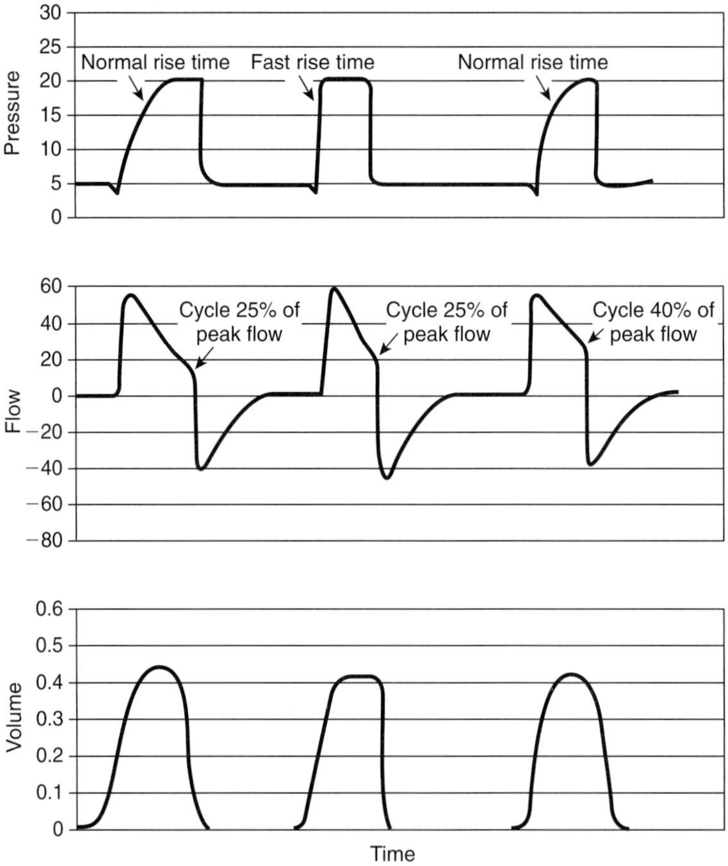

FIGURE 2-13 A pressure support breath *(left)* and the effects of increasing the rise time *(middle)* and decreasing the cycle criteria *(right).* As rise time increases, flow and volume increase whereas inspiratory time tends to decrease. When rise time is constant and the cycle criteria change from 25% to 40% of peak flow, inspiratory time is shortened and tidal volume tends to diminish.

The most common explanation of the difference between PEEP and CPAP is that PEEP is elevated baseline pressure during mechanical ventilation, whereas CPAP is elevated baseline pressure during spontaneous breathing. This explanation falls short when IMV is used because an elevated baseline pressure is used after both spontaneous and mandatory breaths. Perhaps the best way to differentiate the two is that CPAP is, as we are discussing, a mode of ventilator operation, whereas PEEP is simply control of baseline pressure during use of a separate mode of ventilation. On some occasions, CPAP has been described as IMV with a frequency of zero.

Manufacturer Terms

The term CPAP is used by all manufacturers to describe this mode. In some instances, there is a control labeled CPAP, and in others the mode is accessed via the "spontaneous" mode. In both cases, the level of end-expiratory pressure is selected using a baseline or PEEP/CPAP control.

Classification

Because CPAP is devoid of mandatory breaths, only the spontaneous breaths need to be considered. Spontaneous breaths are pressure controlled; pressure, flow, or volume triggered; pressure limited; and pressure or flow cycled. More simply, CPAP is pressure-controlled, patient-triggered, patient-cycled, unsupported spontaneous breathing. Figure 2-14 depicts spontaneous breathing during CPAP.

Airway Pressure Release Ventilation

Descriptive Definition

Airway pressure release ventilation (APRV) often is described as two levels of CPAP that are

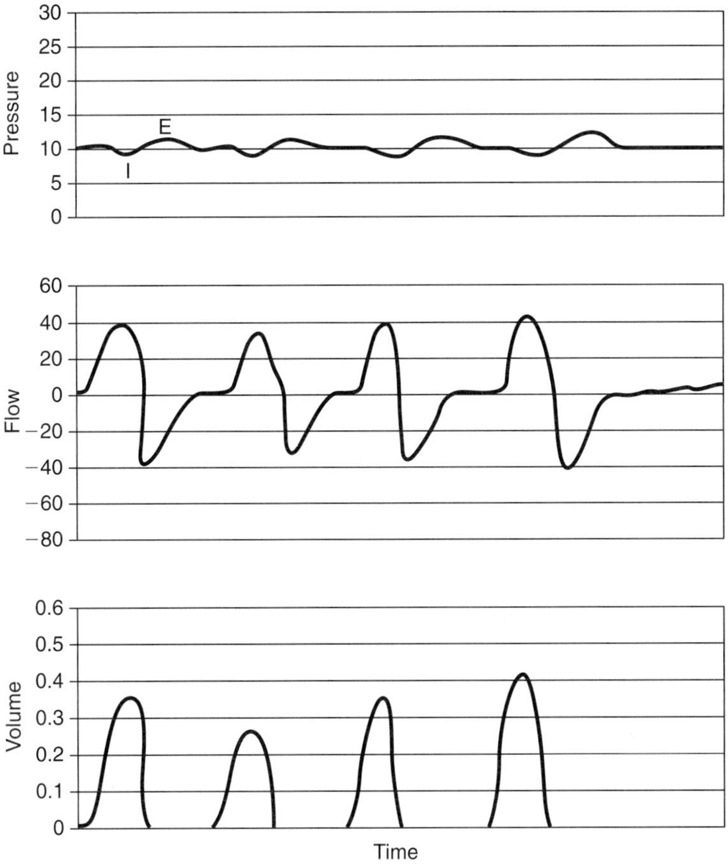

FIGURE 2-14 Pressure, flow, and volume versus time during continuous positive airway pressure (CPAP). *I,* Inspiration; *E,* expiration.

applied for set periods of time, allowing spontaneous breathing to occur at both levels. This mode is said to allow the clinician to set the two CPAP levels (known as CPAP or pressure high and release pressure or pressure low) and the time spent at each level (time high or inspiratory time and time low or expiratory time).[2-5,19-23]

Other Terms

APRV has been referred to as:

- bilevel airway pressure (BiPAP).
- variable positive airway pressure (VPAP).
- intermittent CPAP.
- CPAP with release.

Manufacturer Terms

The Drager Dura and Evita 4 (Drager Inc., Telford, Pa.) offer APRV and use that terminology. The Puritan Bennett 840 provides APRV and calls the mode bilevel. The Hamilton Galileo provides APRV as Duo-PAP. The Viasys Avea provides ARPV/ Biphasic.

Classification

Scrutiny of the APRV pressure, volume, and flow waveforms demonstrates its similarity to pressure control inverse ratio ventilation (PCIRV) (discussed below). In fact, if spontaneous breathing is absent, the two modes are indistinguishable. Mandatory breaths, which occur when the pressure increases from low pressure to higher pressure, are pressure controlled, time triggered, pressure limited, and time cycled. Spontaneous breaths are pressure controlled, pressure triggered, pressure limited, and pressure cycled during APRV (Figure 2-15). In the original description by Downs and Stock,[19] a continuous flow of gas was used; therefore, spontaneous breaths were not controlled. This mode demonstrates the strength of this classification system. Whereas proponents

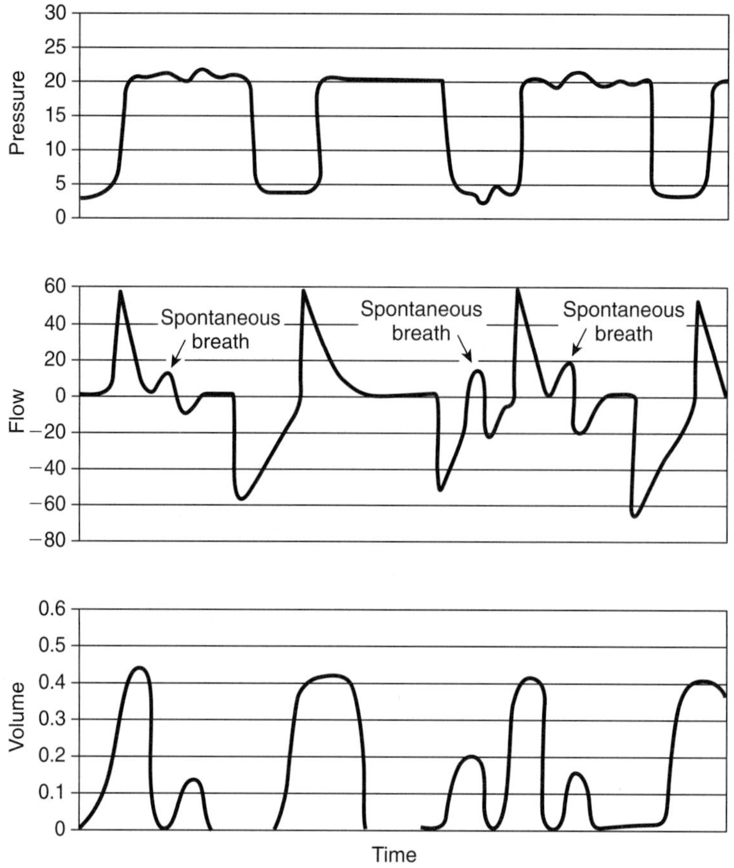

FIGURE 2-15 Pressure, flow, and volume versus time during airway pressure release ventilation (APRV).

of APRV talk about bilevel CPAP, dropping from CPAP to release pressure, applying the classification principles unmasks the black box. Certainly, every neonatal ventilator performs what has been described as APRV and has done so for more than 20 years.

The uniqueness of APRV rests in how it is applied, not in the specific ventilator function. In a patient who is paralyzed, APRV is simply pressure control, time-triggered, pressure-limited, time-cycled ventilation. However, when the patient is breathing spontaneously, the transition of pressure from higher to lower results in tidal movement of gas and subsequent CO_2 elimination. The short expiratory time (time at the low pressure) prevents complete exhalation and maintains alveolar distention. The ability of APRV to allow the patient to breathe spontaneously during any phase of the ventilator's mechanical cycle makes it a viable alternative as a partial support mode.

Pressure Control Inverse Ratio Ventilation

Descriptive Definition

Pressure control inverse ratio ventilation (PCIRV) is a particular version of pressure control-CMV (PC-CMV) in which all breaths are pressure limited and time cycled and the patient cannot initiate an inspiration.[2-5,24-29] Additionally, as the name implies, inspiration is longer than expiration.

Other Terms

PCIRV sometimes is shortened simply to IRV; otherwise, it has few aliases.

Manufacturer Terms

No manufacturer has labeled a mode as PCIRV. In most instances, PCIRV is initiated by selecting the PCV mode and adjusting parameters to provide the desired inspiratory : expiratory (I : E) ratio.

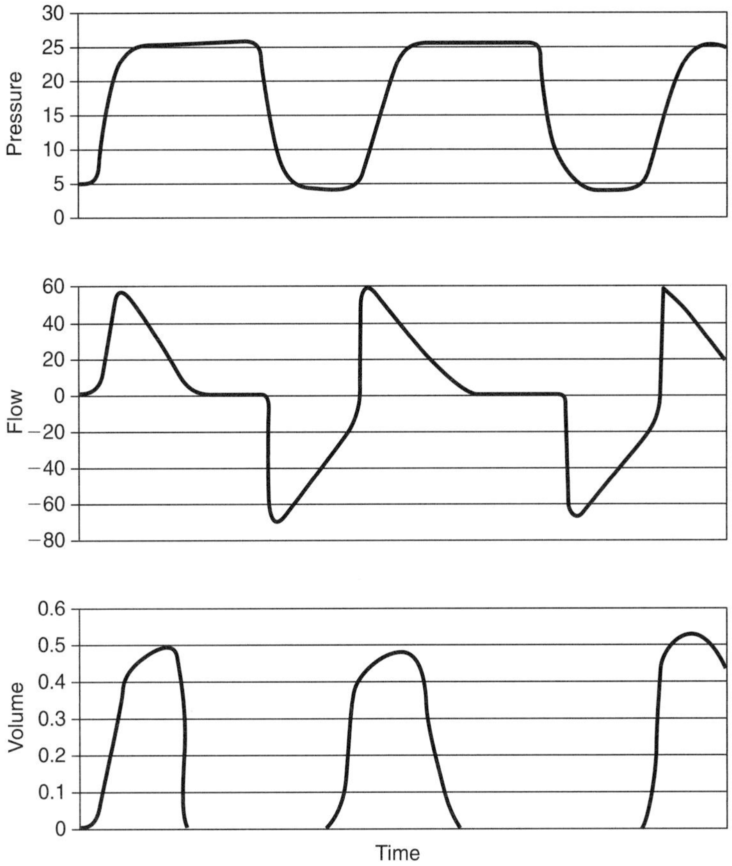

FIGURE 2-16 Pressure, flow, and volume versus time during pressure control-continuous mandatory ventilation (PC-CMV) using an inspiratory time greater than the expiratory time.

Classification

PCIRV can be classified as pressure controlled, time triggered, pressure limited, and time cycled. All breaths are mandatory. The simpler classification refers to PCIRV as pressure controlled, machine triggered, pressure limited, and machine cycled (Figure 2-16). These descriptions should lead the reader to question why PCIRV is considered a separate mode because the only difference between it and PCV is the I:E ratio. Volume-oriented modes are not classified separately with respect to I:E ratio, although VCV certainly can be delivered using a prolonged inspiratory time (Figure 2-17). This technique is not a new mode but rather is pressure control CMV in which the inspiratory time is longer than the expiratory time.

Mandatory Minute Ventilation

Descriptive Definition

Mandatory minute ventilation (MMV) is a mode of ventilator operation that allows the patient to breathe spontaneously yet ensures that a minimum level of minute ventilation (V_E), set by the clinician, always is achieved.[4,5,30-32] This can be accomplished by the use of increasing levels of PSV (Hamilton Veolar)[6] or by delivery of mandatory breaths (Bear 5,[33] Drager E4[34]).

Other Terms

MMV has been called:

- minimum minute volume.
- augmented minute volume (AMV).
- extended mandatory minute ventilation (EMMV).

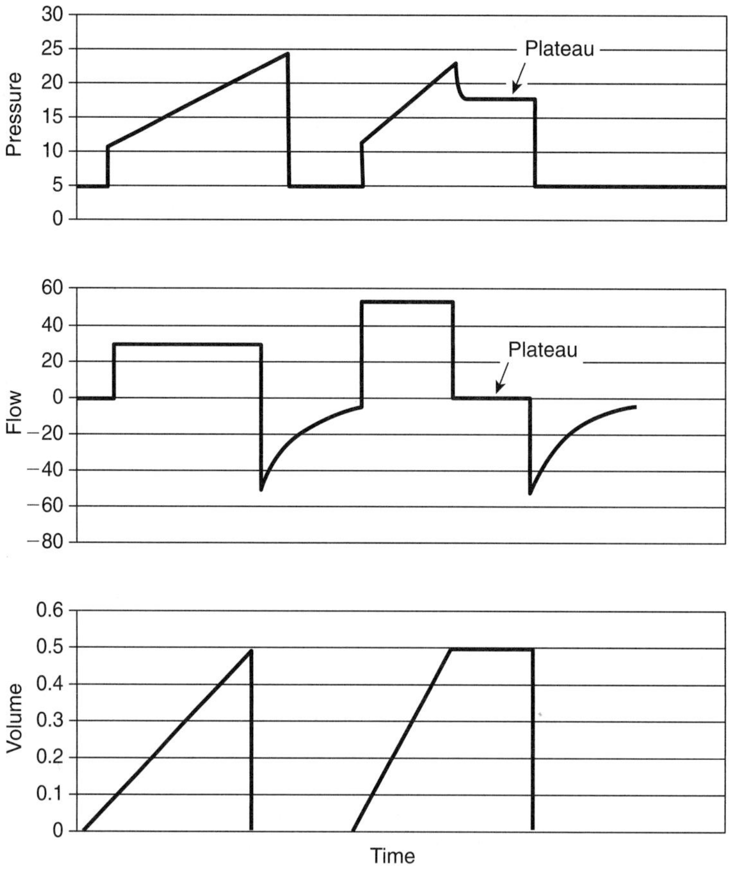

FIGURE 2-17 Pressure, flow, and volume versus time during volume control-continuous mandatory ventilation (VC-CMV) using an inspiratory time greater than the expiratory time. On the left, this is accomplished by a low inspiratory flow, and on the right, by using normal flows with an inspiratory pause.

Manufacturer Terms

The initial description of MMV was termed mandatory minute volume, and ventilators use all the terms listed previously (EMMV, MMV, AMV).

Classification

MMV is one of the modes in which the conditional variable (in this case, V_E) is critically important to classification. In fact, MMV is the first of the modes that can be considered closed loop modes. Closed loop simply means that the ventilator changes its output based on a measured input variable. If spontaneous breathing is used, breaths are pressure controlled, patient triggered, pressure limited, and flow cycled. Essentially, the patient is receiving pressure support ventilation with a varying pressure support level. As long as the conditional variable is met, this system does not change the output (in this instance pressure of preceding breaths). If V_E decreases below the minimum, classification depends on the ventilator used. With the Hamilton Veolar, breaths are supported with increasing levels of PSV. In this instance, there are still no mandatory breaths. Therefore, MMV is pressure controlled, patient triggered, pressure limited, and flow cycled. The simpler classification is pressure-controlled, patient-triggered, pressure-limited, patient-cycled ventilation. If the conditional variable is not met with the other ventilators, mandatory breaths are delivered. In this case, the ventilator anticipates the minute volume based on the minute volume occurring in the past 30 seconds. If the predicted minute volume is lower than the set minute volume, mandatory breaths at the volume set on the ventilator are delivered to make up the difference. This creates an IMV-like situation in which both spontaneous and mandatory breaths must be described. Spontaneous breaths are classified identically to CPAP or PSV depending on the clinician's setting of parameters, and mandatory breaths are volume/flow controlled, time triggered, flow or volume limited, and time or flow cycled. More simply, mandatory breaths are volume controlled, machine initiated, and machine cycled.

COMBINING MODES

Modes of ventilator operation do not have to be used in isolation. Although certain modes have to stand alone based on their function, others can be combined. The combination of IMV and CPAP was previously discussed. Essentially, any mode that has both spontaneous breathing and mandatory breaths can be combined. For instance, PSV can be combined with IMV, but not with CMV. In these cases, creation of a new term to describe the combined modes is undesirable. It is simpler and more descriptive to acknowledge the contributions of each mode (i.e., IMV + PSV, IMV + CPAP).

DUAL CONTROL MODES

Dual control modes are capable of controlling either pressure or volume based on a measured input variable. They cannot control both at the same time, but rather one or the other. There are currently two techniques for performing dual control. We prefer to think of these techniques as *dual control within a breath* and *dual control from breath-to-breath*. The former uses a measured input to switch from pressure control to volume control in the middle of the breath. The latter simply uses a measured input to manipulate the pressure level of a pressure-limited breath (either a pressure control mandatory breath or a pressure support breath).

Dual Control Within a Breath

Descriptive Definition

These modes allow the ventilator to deliver a pressure support breath (pressure control) or switch from a pressure support breath to a volume-controlled breath within the breath. As such, two types of breaths can be delivered during **volume-assured pressure support (VAPS).** The first is a pressure-controlled, patient- or time-triggered, pressure-limited, and flow-cycled breath. The second is a volume-controlled, patient- or time-triggered, flow-limited, volume-cycled breath.

Other Terms

VAPS sometimes is known as volume-assisted pressure support. Currently, no other ventilators use this mode or another name.

Manufacturer Terms

VAPS (Bird 8400ST and Tbird, Bird Corp., Palm Springs, Calif.; Avea, Viasys, Yorba Linda, Calif.) and pressure augmentation (PA) (Bear 1000, Bear Medical, Riverside, Calif.) are common terms. Although each manufacturer uses a different mode name, operation is the same.

Classification

Both of these techniques can operate during mandatory breaths or pressure-supported breaths. Conceptually, VAPS and PA are meant to combine the high variable flow of a pressure-limited breath with the constant volume delivery of a volume-limited breath. The initial description of VAPS by Amato and associates[35] described volume-*assisted* pressure support. This initial report clearly considers VAPS a technique to be used instead of volume control-continuous mandatory ventilation (VC-CMV). During pressure support, VAPS and PA can be considered a safety net that always supplies a minimum tidal volume.

During VAPS and PA, the clinician must set the respiratory frequency, peak flow, PEEP, inspired oxygen concentration, trigger sensitivity, and minimum desired tidal volume. During VAPS or PA, the ventilator's inspiratory flow waveform is constant (square). Additionally, the pressure support setting must be set. The pressure support control is nonfunctional during VC-CMV unless the VAPS or PA mode is activated. Selecting the appropriate pressure support setting is difficult, and no studies have been accomplished that identify the best setting. Our practice has been to set the pressure support setting at a level equivalent to the plateau pressure obtained during a volume control breath at the desired tidal volume. The peak flow setting is also important during VAPS and PA. Peak flow should be adjusted to allow for the appropriate inspiratory time and I:E ratio required by the patient.[36-38]

A VAPS or PA breath may be initiated by the patient or may be time triggered. Once the breath is triggered, the ventilator attempts to reach the pressure support setting as quickly as possible. This portion of the breath is the pressure control portion and is associated with a rapid variable flow, which

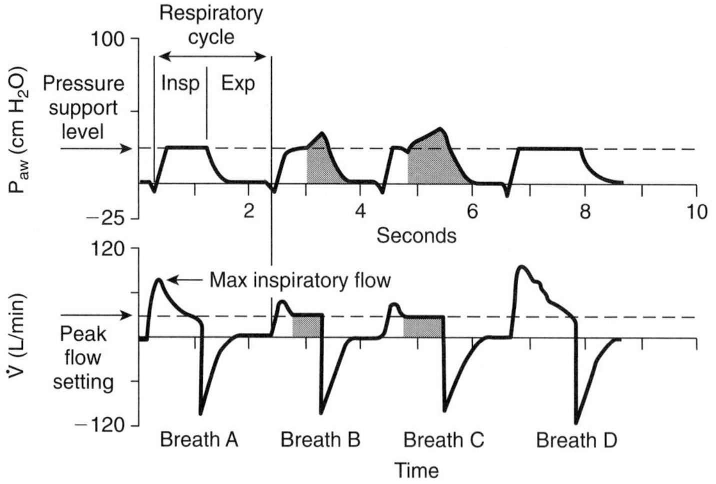

FIGURE 2-18 The possible breath delivery characteristics occurring during the use of volume-assured pressure support. See text for details. (From Branson RD: Volume assured pressure support ventilation: a clinical manual. Bird Products Corp., Palm Springs, Calif, 1996.)

may reduce the work of breathing. As this pressure level is reached, the ventilator's microprocessor determines the volume that has been delivered from the machine (note that this is not exhaled tidal volume), compares this measurement with the desired tidal volume, and determines whether the minimum desired tidal volume will be reached.

There are several differences in ventilator output based on the relationship between delivered and set tidal volume. These are shown in Figure 2-18. If the delivered tidal volume and set tidal volume are equivalent, the breath is a pressure support breath. That is, the breath is pressure limited at the pressure support setting and flow cycled—in this instance, at 25% of the initial peak flow. This type of breath occurring during VAPS is shown in Figure 2-18, breath A.

If the patient's inspiratory effort is diminished, the ventilator delivers a smaller volume, and when delivered and set volume are compared, the microprocessor determines that the minimum set tidal volume will not be delivered. As the flow decelerates and reaches the set peak flow, the breath changes from a pressure-limited to a volume-limited breath. The flow remains constant, increasing the inspiratory time, until the volume has been delivered. Again, remember that the volume is volume exiting the ventilator, not exhaled tidal volume. During this time, the pressure increases above the set pressure support setting. Setting the high pressure alarm remains important during VAPS. If pressure increases abruptly, the high pressure alarm setting is reached and the breath is pressure cycled. This type of breath is shown in Figure 2-18, breath B.

A similar condition can occur if there is an acute decrease in lung compliance or an increase in airways resistance. This is shown in Figure 2-18, breath C. The same sequence of events occurs as described for breath B. However, this breath demonstrates the possibility of prolonging inspiratory time during a VAPS breath. There are secondary cycle characteristics for these breaths, and an inspiratory time lasting longer than 3 seconds automatically is time cycled. This finding suggests that when used for patients with airflow obstruction, intrusions of the constant flow on the patient's I:E ratio should be monitored.

Lastly, and perhaps most importantly, the VAPS breath can allow the patient a tidal volume larger than the set volume. Because the pressure limit remains the same, this breath is also a pressure support breath (i.e., it is pressure limited and flow cycled). Figure 2-18, breath D demonstrates the effect of an increase in patient effort. This system allows for normal variations in patient tidal volume and sighing and increased volumes during times of hyperpnea.

VAPS then is patient or machine triggered, pressure or flow limited (depending on the relationship of set and actual tidal volume), and flow or volume cycled.

Dual Control Breath-to-Breath—Pressure-Limited, Flow-Cycled Ventilation

Descriptive Definition

Dual control breath-to-breath in the pressure support mode quite simply is closed loop pressure support ventilation, with tidal volume as the input variable.

Other Terms

No other terms are used.

Manufacturer Terms

Volume support (Siemens 300, Servo*i* Maquette, Danvers, Mass.) is the current term.

Classification

Dual control breath-to-breath during the pressure support mode was introduced on the Siemens 300 ventilator. Volume support is pressure support ventilation that uses tidal volume as a feedback control for continuously adjusting the pressure support level.[39,40] All breaths are patient triggered, pressure limited, and flow cycled. Volume support is selected with the mode selector switch, and the desired tidal volume is set. The ventilator initiates volume support by delivering a "test breath" with a peak pressure of 5 cm H_2O when a patient effort is sensed. The delivered tidal volume (again, this is not exhaled tidal volume, but volume exiting the ventilator) is measured, and total system compliance is calculated. The following three breaths are delivered at a peak inspiratory pressure of 75% of the pressure calculated to deliver the minimum tidal volume. Each subsequent breath uses the previous calculation of system compliance to manipulate peak pressure to achieve the desired tidal volume. From breath-to-breath, the maximum pressure change is less than 3 cm H_2O and can range from 0 cm H_2O above PEEP to 5 cm H_2O below the high-pressure alarm setting. Because all breaths are pressure support breaths, cycling normally occurs at 5% of the initial peak flow. A secondary cycling mechanism is activated if inspiratory time exceeds 80% of the set total cycle time. There is also a relationship between the set ventilator frequency and tidal volume. If the desired tidal volume is 500 ml and the respiratory frequency is set at 15 breaths per minute, the minute volume setting is 7.5 L/min. If the patient's respiratory frequency decreases below 15 breaths per minute, the tidal volume target automatically is increased by the ventilator up to 150% of the initial value (in this example, 750 ml). This is done in an effort to maintain the minute volume constant. Figure 2-19 depicts the volume support mode response to a decrease in lung compliance. If lung compliance increases, the opposite response (decreasing pressure support and constant tidal volume) occurs.

Dual Control Breath-to-Breath–Pressure-Limited, Time-Cycled Ventilation

Descriptive Definition

Dual control in the pressure control mode, like volume support, is simply closed loop pressure-controlled, patient- or time-triggered, pressure-limited, time-cycled ventilation with tidal volume as the input variable.

Other Terms

No other terms are used.

Manufacturer Terms

Pressure-regulated volume control (PRVC) (Siemens 300 and Servo*i* and Viasys Avea), Adaptive pressure ventilation (APV) (Hamilton Galileo), Auto-flow (Evita 4), Volume Control + (Puritan Bennet 840) and variable pressure control (Venturi) are commonly used terms.

Classification

All these techniques are forms of pressure-limited, time-cycled ventilation that use tidal volume as a feedback control for continuously adjusting the pressure limit. As such, these modes are patient or machine triggered, pressure limited, and time cycled, with tidal volume as the conditional variable used to change the pressure limit.[41] As in previous examples, the volume signal used for ventilator feedback is not exhaled tidal volume, but volume exiting the ventilator. This prevents a kind of runaway effect that could occur if a leak in the circuit prevented accurate measurement of exhaled tidal volume.

Despite the fact that each technique has a different name, operation is fairly consistent between devices. All breaths in these modes are time or patient triggered, pressure limited, and time cycled. One difference between devices is that the Siemens 300 only allows PRVC in the CMV mode. The other ventilators allow dual control breath-to-breath using CMV or SIMV. During SIMV, the mandatory breaths are the dual control breaths.

Volume measurement for the feedback signal is also different between ventilators. The Siemens 300 uses the volume leaving the inspiratory flow sensor.

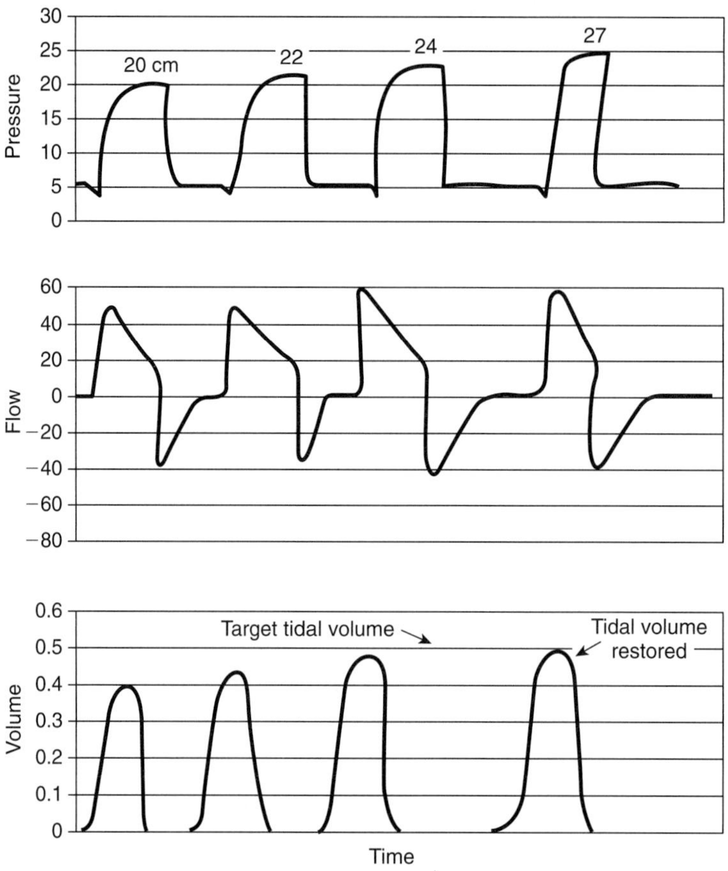

FIGURE 2-19 The effect of decreased compliance on dual control breath-to-breath (pressure support). The target tidal volume is 500 ml. When compliance decreases, pressure increases gradually until tidal volume is restored

The Hamilton Galileo uses the flow sensor at the airway and the inspiratory flow sensor to determine an average volume. This latter technique eliminates compressible volume, can detect the presence of leaks, and may be the preferred method of volume monitoring in dual control.

PRVC is selected on the mode selector switch, and the desired tidal volume is set. Like volume support, a "test breath" is delivered, and total system compliance is calculated. The next three breaths are delivered at a pressure limit 75% of that necessary to achieve the desired tidal volume based on the compliance calculation. The ensuing breaths increase or decrease the pressure limit at less than 3 cm H_2O per breath in an attempt to deliver the desired tidal volume. The pressure limit fluctuates between 0 cm H_2O above the PEEP level and 5 cm H_2O below the upper-pressure alarm setting. The ventilator sounds an alarm if the tidal volume and maximum pressure limit settings are incompatible.

Like volume support, the proposed advantage of PRVC or other dual control breath-to-breath modes is maintaining the minimum peak pressure, which provides a constant set tidal volume and automatic weaning of the pressure as the patient improves. Likewise, during periods of limited staffing, these modes maintain a more consistent tidal volume as compliance decreases or increases. Figure 2-20 depicts the effects of increasing compliance on the ventilator response during dual control breath to breath.

AUTOMODE

Descriptive Definition

AutoMode combines dual control breath-to-breath time-cycled breaths with dual control breath-to-breath flow-cycled breaths. AutoMode allows the ventilator to alternate between these two modes based on another input. In this instance, patient effort

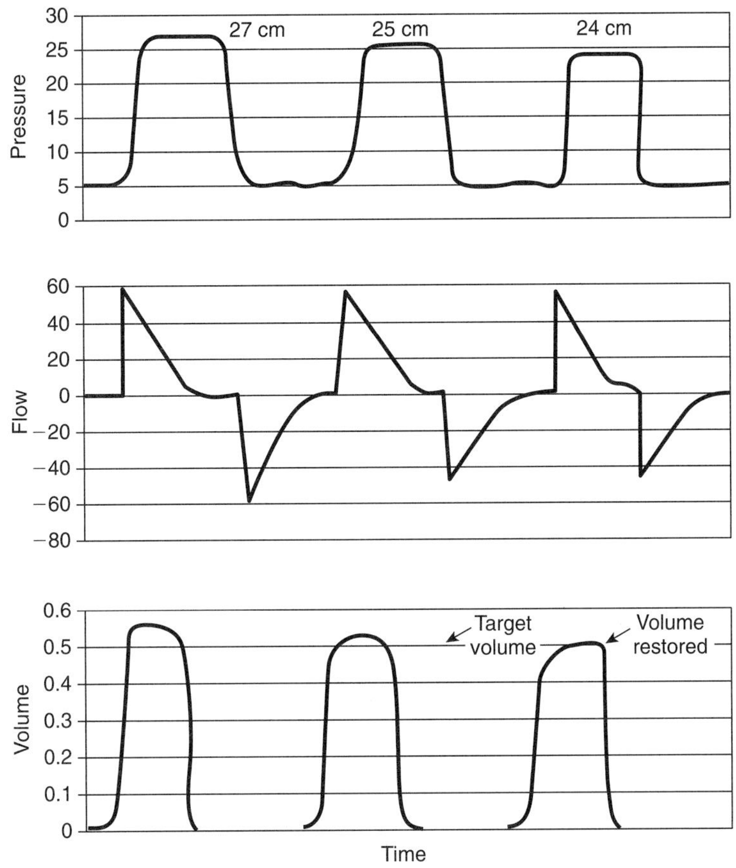

FIGURE 2-20 The effects of an improvement in compliance on dual control breath-to-breath (pressure control). The target tidal volume is 500 ml. As compliance improves, tidal volume exceeds the target. Pressure is decreased by 1- to 3-cm H_2O increments on a breath-to-breath basis until the tidal volume target is achieved.

or the lack of patient effort determines whether the breaths are time cycled or flow cycled.[42,43]

Other Terms

No other terms are used.

Manufacturer Terms

AutoMode is a mode available on the Siemens 300A ventilator.

Classification

AutoMode combines volume support and PRVC in a single mode. If the patient is paralyzed, the ventilator provides PRVC. All breaths are mandatory breaths that are time triggered, pressure limited, and time cycled. The pressure limit increases or decreases to maintain the desired tidal volume set by the clinician. If the patient breathes spontaneously for two consecutive breaths, the ventilator switches to volume support. In this case, all breaths are supported breaths that are patient triggered, pressure limited, and flow cycled. If the patient becomes apneic for 12 seconds in the adult setting, 8 seconds in the pediatric setting, or 5 seconds in the neonatal setting, the ventilator switches back to the PRVC mode. The change from PRVC to volume support is accomplished at equivalent peak pressures. This mode is simply the combination of two existing modes using the conditional variable of patient effort to decide whether the next breath is time cycled or flow cycled.

AutoMode also switches between pressure control and pressure support or volume control to volume support. In the volume control to volume support switch, the volume support pressure limit is equivalent to the pause pressure during volume control. If an inspiratory plateau is not available, the pressure level is calculated as:

$$(\text{Peak pressure} - \text{PEEP}) \times 50\% + \text{PEEP}$$

AutoMode only recently has been introduced. One concern is that during the switch from time-cycled to flow-cycled ventilation, mean airway pressure will decrease. This may result in hypoxemia in the patient with acute lung injury. The ventilator's algorithm is fairly simple, and the patient is either assisting all the breaths or none of the breaths.

ADAPTIVE SUPPORT VENTILATION

Descriptive Definition

Adaptive support ventilation (ASV) is a mode that combines the dual control breath to breath time-cycled and flow-cycled breaths and allows the ventilator to choose the initial ventilator settings based on the clinician input of ideal body weight and percent minute volume. This is the most sophisticated of closed loop techniques, allowing the ventilator to choose set respiratory frequency, tidal volume, pressure limit of mandatory and spontaneous breaths, inspiratory time of mandatory breaths, and, when spontaneous breathing is absent, I:E ratio.

Other Terms

No other terms are used.

Manufacturer Terms

Adaptive support ventilation (ASV) (Hamilton Galileo) is used.

Classification

ASV is based on the minimal work of breathing concept developed by Arthur B. Otis, which was published in 1950.[44] This concept suggests that the patient breathes at a tidal volume and respiratory frequency that minimizes the elastic and resistive loads while maintaining oxygenation and acid-base balance. Otis and colleagues[44] developed an equation that describes the minimal work concept shown below:

$$f = \sqrt{\frac{1 + 4\pi^2 RCe \times \dfrac{MV - f \times VD}{VD} - 1}{2\pi^2 RCe}}$$

The ASV algorithm uses this formula along with patient weight (which determines dead space) to adjust a number of ventilator variables. The clinician inputs the patient's ideal body weight; sets the high pressure alarm, PEEP, and inspired oxygen concentration; and adjusts the rise time and flow cycle variable for pressure support breaths from 10% to 40% of initial peak flow. The ventilator attempts to deliver 100 ml/min/kg of minute ventilation for an adult and 200 ml/min/kg for children. This can be adjusted by a setting known as the percent minute volume control. This control can be set from 20% to 200%. In the latter case, 200%, a minute volume of 200 ml/min/kg would be delivered to an adult patient. This setting allows the clinician to provide full ventilatory support or encourage spontaneous breathing and facilitate weaning.

When connected to the patient, the ventilator delivers a series of test breaths and measures system compliance, airway resistance, and intrinsic PEEP (PEEPi) using a least squares, fitting technique.[45,46] This measurement system is important for accurate measurement of variables used in the minimal work equation. The input of body weight allows the ventilator algorithm to choose a required minute volume. The ventilator then uses the clinician input and measured respiratory mechanics to select a respiratory frequency, inspiratory time, I:E ratio, and pressure limit for mandatory and spontaneous breaths. These variables are measured on a breath-to-breath basis and are altered by the ventilator's algorithm to meet the desired targets. If the patient breathes spontaneously, the ventilator pressure supports breaths and encourages spontaneous breathing. However, spontaneous and mandatory breaths can be combined to meet the minute ventilation target. The pressure limit of both the mandatory and spontaneous breaths is always being adjusted. This means that ASV continuously is employing dual control breath-to-breath of mandatory and spontaneous breaths.

ASV uses the input from the clinician and the patient's respiratory mechanics to determine the target breath rate and tidal volume. A "safety box" will be constructed according to the ASV rules base. Table 2-4 lists lung protective ASV rules, which determine the minimum and maximum values for each control parameter. Figure 2-21 shows the limits imposed by ASV rules. The patient will be guided to the target point (respiratory frequency [f], tidal volume, minute ventilation [V_E]) through manipulation of mandatory breath rate and inspiratory pressure according to the algorithm depicted in Figure 2-22. In quadrant I, the tidal volume exceeds the target and the respiratory rate is below the target. ASV will respond by decreasing the inspiratory pressure and

TABLE 2-4 *Minimum and Maximum Values for All Control Parameters Determined by the ASV Lung Protective Rules Base*

PARAMETER	MINIMUM	MAXIMUM
Inspiratory pressure (cm H_2O)	5 above baseline airway pressure (PEEP/CPAP)	10 below P_{MAX} alarm setting
Tidal volume (ml)	4.4•IBW	15.4•IBW or V_E/5, whichever is lower *May be limited by P_{MAX} alarm
Target respiratory rate (b/min)	5 bpm	22 bpm•% Min Vol/100 (if IBW greater than 15 kg) 45 bpm•% Min Vol/100 (if IBW less than 15 kg)
Mandatory breath rate (b/min)	5 bpm	60 bpm
Inspiratory time (seconds)	0.5 sec or 1•RCe, whichever is longer	2 sec
Expiratory time (seconds)	3•RCe	15 sec
I:E ratio range (seconds)	1:4	1:1

PEEP, Positive end-expiratory pressure; *CPAP,* continuous positive airway pressure; P_{MAX}, maximum inspiratory pressure; *IBW,* ideal body weight; *RCe,* expiratory time constant; V_E, minute ventilation.

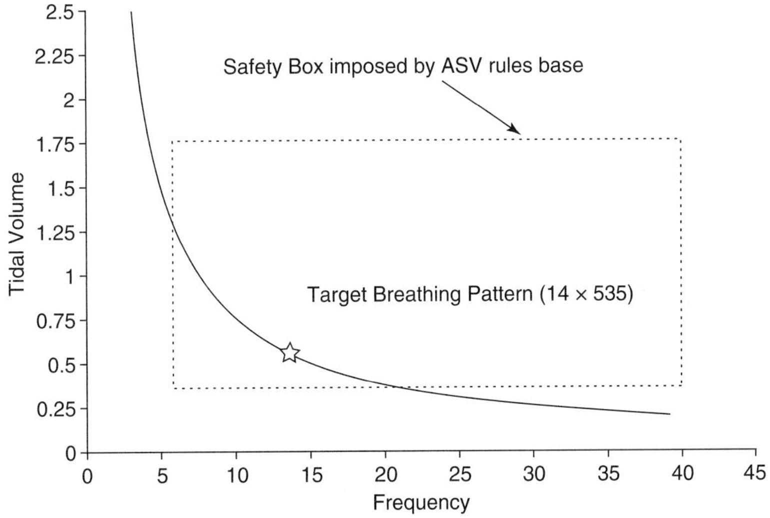

FIGURE 2-21 ASV selection of the target frequency and tidal volume using the equation of Otis in a 70 kg patient. The safety box displays the limits for respiratory rate (high and low) and the limits for tidal volume (high and low).

increasing the mandatory breath rate. In quadrant II, the tidal volume exceeds the target while the respiratory rate is above the target. ASV response includes reducing both inspiratory pressure and mandatory breath rate. In quadrant III, tidal volume is lower than the target value and respiratory rate exceeds the target. In this case, ASV will increase the inspiratory pressure while decreasing the mandatory breath rate. Finally, in quadrant IV, both the tidal volume and respiratory rate are below the target values and ASV responds by increasing the inspiratory pressure and mandatory breath rate. Clinical interpretation of these findings and the rationale for changes are shown in Table 2-5.

The ventilator also can adjust the I:E ratio and inspiratory time of mandatory breaths to prevent air trapping and PEEPi. This is done by calculation of the expiratory time constant (compliance × resistance) and maintenance of sufficient expiratory time.

If the patient is paralyzed, the ventilator determines the respiratory frequency, tidal volume, pressure limit required to deliver that tidal volume, inspiratory time, and I:E ratio. As the patient begins to breathe spontaneously, the number of mandatory breaths decreases and the ventilator chooses a pressure support level that maintains a tidal volume sufficient to ensure alveolar ventilation, based on a dead space calculation of 2.2 ml/kg.

As a synopsis, ASV can provide pressure-limited, time-cycled ventilation; add dual control of those breaths on a breath-to-breath basis; allow for mandatory breaths and spontaneous breaths (a kind of dual control PC-SIMV + pressure support); and eventually switch to pressure support with dual control breath-to-breath (variable pressure with each pressure support breath). During mandatory breath delivery, the ventilator can set inspiratory time and I : E ratio.[47-57]

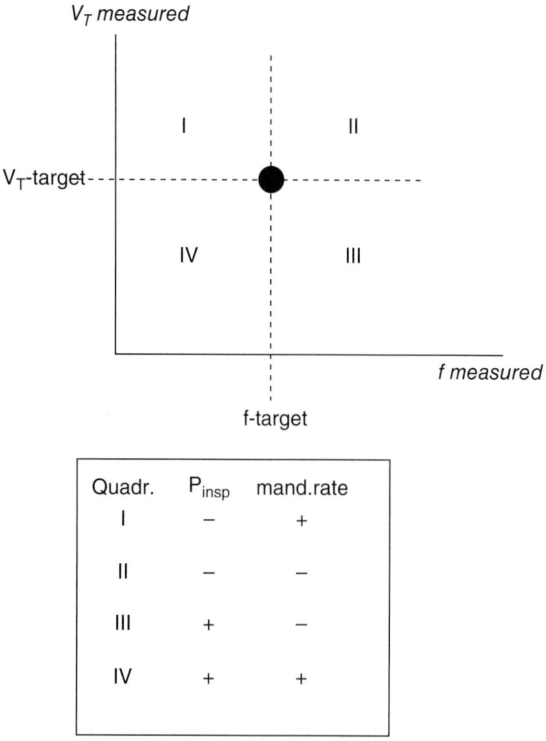

FIGURE 2-22 Guidance of frequency and tidal volume to the ASV selected targets through manipulation of airway pressure and ventilator frequency.

ADAPTIVE TIDAL VOLUME SUPPORT

Descriptive Definition

Adaptive tidal volume support (AVtS) is a mode that combines the dual control breath-to-breath time-cycled and flow-cycled breaths and allows the ventilator to choose the initial ventilator settings based on the clinician input of ideal body weight, percent minute volume, inspiratory time, and target tidal volume.

Other Terms

No other terms are used.

Manufacturer Terms

Adaptive tidal volume support (AVtS) (Hamilton Galileo) is used.

Classification

AVtS is a form of ASV where the clinician inputs the patient's ideal body weight and then sets the tidal volume target in ml/kg, high-pressure limit, and inspiratory time. AVtS operates in the same manner as ASV, the only difference being greater clinician control over selected variables.

TABLE 2-5 *Clinical Interpretation of Breath Pattern During ASV and the Changes Implemented by the ASV Algorithm*

QUADRANT	MEANING	CLINICAL CONTEXT	ACTION
1	Low tidal volume in spite of high inspiratory activity	High respiratory system impedance	Increase pressure support
2	High inspiratory activity in spite of high tidal volume	Low efficiency of CO_2 elimination Increased metabolic demand Metabolic acidosis Central neurologic disorders	Increase pressure support
3	Lack of adequate inspiratory activity in spite of low tidal volume	Anesthesia Fatigue Neuromuscular disease	Increase pressure support
4	High tidal volume at low inspiratory activity	Excess of pressure support	Decrease pressure support

AUTOMATIC TUBE COMPENSATION

Descriptive Definition

Automatic tube compensation (ATC) is a technique of ventilator operation that uses the known resistive characteristics of artificial airways to overcome the imposed work of breathing caused by those airways.[58,59] Automatic tube compensation is not a mode of ventilation, but rather an addition to other modes aimed at eliminating the resistive characteristics of the artificial airway (endotracheal tube or tracheostomy tube).

Other Terms

No other terms are used.

Manufacturer Terms

Automatic tube compensation (Evita 4, Drager Inc., Telford, Pa.; Viasys Avea), tube compensation (Puritan Bennett 840), and tube resistance compensation (Hamilton Galileo and Raphael, Reno, Nev.) are the common terms.

Classification

ATC is pressure controlled, patient triggered, pressure limited, and flow cycled. The pressure delivered is a consequence of the known resistive characteristics of the airway and the flow demand of the patient. As the airway diameter decreases, the pressure applied for any given flow increases. As the flow demand increases, the pressure increases for any given airway caliber.

According to Poiseuille's law, pressure decrease across the endotracheal tube is inversely proportional to the radius to the fourth power and is directly proportional to the length. Increasing flow through the same size endotracheal tube results in a curvilinear increase in resistance. Several investigators have advocated using pressure support ventilation to overcome the imposed work presented by the endotracheal tube.[60-63] This method requires increasing pressure support levels as endotracheal tube diameter diminishes and inspiratory flow increases. Under static conditions, pressure support can effectively eliminate endotracheal tube resistance. However, variable inspiratory flow and changing demands of the patient cannot be met by a single level of pressure support (Figure 2-23). During periods of tachypnea, the previously chosen level of pressure support no longer eliminates work imposed by the endotracheal tube.

Additionally, the resistance of the endotracheal tube creates a condition early in the breath in which ventilator flow is high, tracheal pressure remains low, and undercompensation for imposed work occurs. Late in the breath, when pressure begins to equilibrate during the pressure plateau, pressure support tends to overcompensate, prolong inspiration, and exacerbate overinflation.

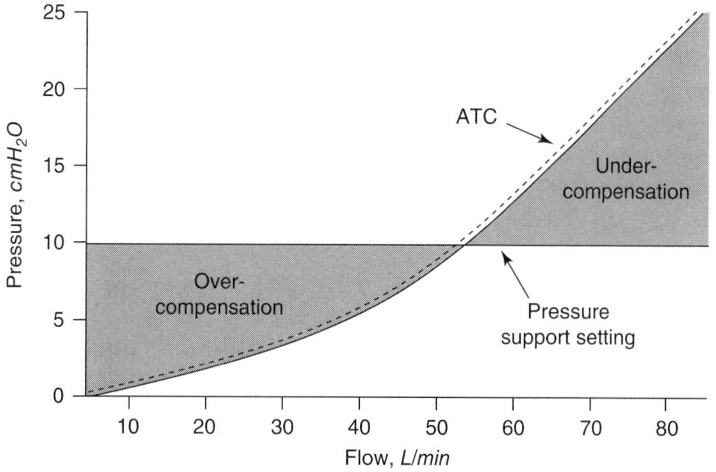

FIGURE 2-23 The capabilities of pressure support and automatic tube compensation (ATC) on overcoming the work of breathing caused by the artificial airway. Pressure support only eliminates the work precisely at a given flow. Above and below that flow, pressure support undercompensates or overcompensates for resistance. ATC compensation can overcome resistance regardless of patient flow demand.

In 1993, Guttmann and associates described a technique for continuously calculating tracheal pressure in intubated, mechanically ventilated patients.[61] This system uses the known resistive component of the endotracheal tube and the measurement of flow to calculate tracheal pressure. These authors successfully validated their system in a group of mechanically ventilated patients, finding favorable comparisons between calculated and measured tracheal pressure.

This work led to the introduction of ATC on the Drager Evita 4.[34] ATC attempts to compensate for endotracheal tube resistance via closed loop control of *calculated* tracheal pressure. This system uses the known resistive coefficients of the tracheal tube (tracheostomy or endotracheal) and measurement of instantaneous flow to apply pressure proportional to resistance throughout the total respiratory cycle. The equation for calculating tracheal pressure is:

$$\text{Tracheal pressure (cm } H_2O) = \text{Proximal airway pressure (cm } H_2O) - \text{tube coefficient (cm } H_2O/L/s) \times \text{flow}^2 \text{ (L/min)}$$

The operator inputs the type of tube, endotracheal or tracheostomy, and the percentage of compensation desired (10% to 100%). Most of the interest in ATC revolves around eliminating the imposed work of breathing during inspiration. However, during expiration there is also a flow-dependent pressure decrease across the tube. ATC also compensates for this flow-resistive component and may reduce expiratory resistance and unintentional hyperinflation. During expiration, the calculated tracheal pressure is greater than airway pressure. Under ideal conditions, a negative pressure at the airway may help reduce expiratory resistance. Because this is not always desirable or possible, ATC can reduce PEEP to 0 cm H_2O during expiration to facilitate compensation of expiratory resistance posed by the endotracheal tube.[64-72]

PROPORTIONAL ASSIST VENTILATION

Descriptive Definition

Proportional assist ventilation (PAV) is a mode of mechanical ventilation based on the equation of motion.[73-77] This concept was presented in Chapter 1 and is reviewed briefly.

The equation of motion for the respiratory system states:

$$P_{AW} + P_{MUS} = \text{Volume} \times \text{elastance} + \text{Flow} \times \text{resistance}$$

where P_{AW} is pressure created by the ventilator and P_{MUS} is pressure created by the respiratory muscles. The larger the volume and greater the elastance, the more pressure required (either greater driving pressure by the ventilator or greater respiratory muscle effort by the patient). Similarly, as resistance or flow increases, the pressure provided by the ventilator or pressure created by the respiratory muscles must increase. This proportionality is the hallmark of PAV. Regardless of changes in patient effort, the ventilator continues to do the same percentage of work.

The design of PAV allows the ventilator to change the pressure output (pressure control) to always perform work proportionally to patient effort. Because the left side of the equation includes both ventilator pressure and patient muscle pressure, the ventilator can determine its output based on the online measurement of elastance (the reciprocal of compliance) and resistance. PAV requires only the traditional values of PEEP and inspired oxygen concentration (FIO_2) to be set. The other settings are the percent volume assist (to overcome elastance) and percent flow assist (to overcome resistance). The interface for PAV remains a challenge. Another method might be to set percent work, which would control both the volume and flow assist. PAV is still new enough that we do not know whether there ever is any reason to set the assist settings at any value other than 80%.

Other Terms

Proportional assist ventilation was named by the designer, Magdy Younes. To date, no new terms for PAV have been introduced.

Manufacturer Terms

At present three manufacturers have PAV modes. The Drager Evita 4 uses proportional pressure support, while the Puritan Bennett 840 and the Respironics Vision both use the term proportional assist ventilation.

Classification

PAV uses the measurement of elastance and resistance to determine ventilator output. PAV is pressure controlled, patient triggered, pressure limited, and flow cycled. The pressure delivered is not a set value, as in pressure support, but changes as a multiple of the sum of the volume and flow signals. Safety settings for high pressure and high tidal volume also can be set and cause the breaths to be pressure or volume limited (cycled if this is set as the alarm threshold). The pressure delivered changes from breath-to-breath depending on elastance, resistance, and flow demand.

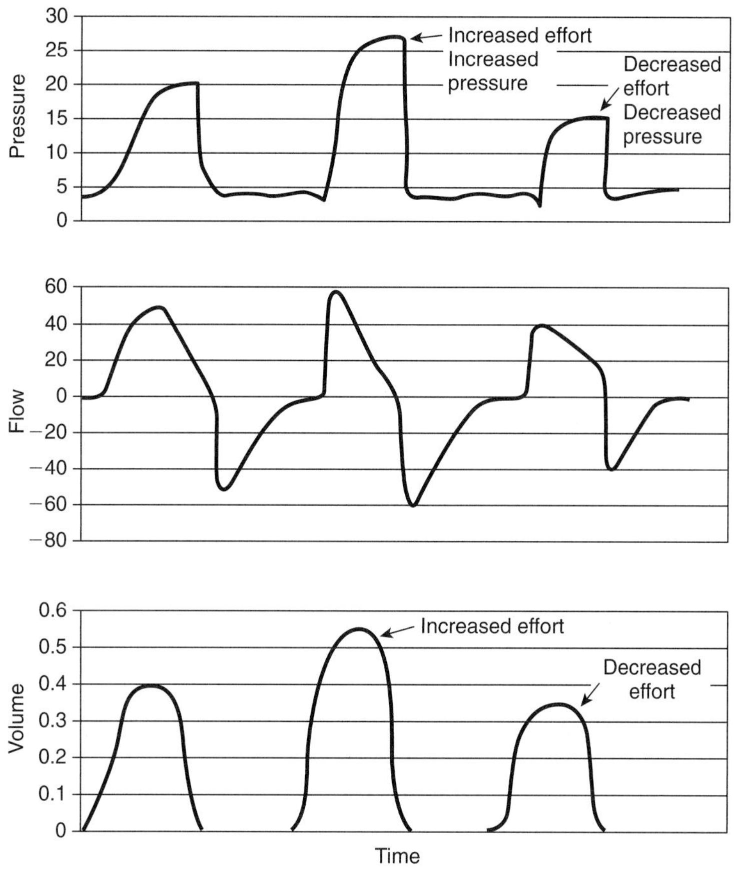

FIGURE 2-24 Pressure volume and flow waveforms during proportional assist ventilation (PAV). Note that as patient effort and volume increase, pressure applied by the ventilator increases.

Typically, PAV is set to overcome 80% of the elastic and resistive loads. If elastance is measured at 40 cm H_2O/L, the ventilator provides a pressure for that breath that overcomes 80% of that elastance value. In this example, the pressure required to overcome 80% of the work of breathing for a 1 L tidal volume is 32 cm H_2O.

PAV can be thought of as similar to cruise control on a car. When the cruise control is set, the accelerator changes position to maintain a constant speed regardless of terrain (uphill or downhill). With PAV, if the volume and flow assist are set at 80% (overcome 80% of the elastic and resistive load), as the patient's tidal volume increases, the pressure applied by the ventilator increases. This is shown in Figure 2-24. The percentage of patient work stays the same, regardless of the volume. In the original piston device described by Younes, as the patient demand or volume increased, the forward movement of the piston increased (larger volume delivered). If the volume remains constant but inspiratory flow increases, the ventilator increases pressure to overcome the increased resistive load. In the piston device, the stroke of the piston would be quicker, whereas the piston displacement remained constant. In essence, the ventilator attempts to maintain the percentage of work the patient performs per breath, regardless of the volume of the breath or inspiratory flow of the breath. The successful introduction of PAV requires that elastance and resistance be measured instantaneously breath-to-breath.

The major impediments to implementing PAV include the accurate breath-to-breath measurement of elastance and resistance, the confounding effects of endotracheal tube resistance and auto-PEEP, the problem of the nonlinearity of elastance and resistance, and the effect termed "runaway." Runaway is a form of overassist that occurs when the elastance improves dramatically or is measured inaccurately and the ventilator continues to provide volume after the patient has terminated inspiration. This could lead to overdistention, worsening of air trapping, and, potentially, barotrauma. This requires that high pressure and high tidal volume alarms be set appropriately. Additionally, because PAV always is patient triggered, a backup mode is necessary to take over in the event of apnea.

Recent research has found that PAV is both better than or equivalent to PSV.[78-93] Many of the issues complicating PAV continue to improve as the ability to monitor elastance and resistance on the fly improves. Recent introduction of an improved interface with PAV on the Puritan Bennett 840 may also lead to simplifying set up and implementation. This interface uses a sliding bar to allow the operator to select the percentage of work the ventilator performs per breath.

SMARTCAREPS

Descriptive Definition

SmartCarePS is patient-triggered, pressure-limited, flow-cycled ventilation. More simply, SmartCarePS is pressure support ventilation. The unique aspect of SmartCarePS is that the level of pressure support is automatically adjusted by the ventilator to maintain a series of variables (tidal volume, end tidal CO_2 ($ETCO_2$), and respiratory rate) within a range of normal limits.

Other Terms

SmartCarePS was initially designed by Dojat et al and known as NeoGanesh.[94-96] Ganesh being the Hindu God with an elephant head and multiple arms, "Ga" symbolizes Buddhi (intellect) and "Na" symbolizes Vidnyana (wisdom). Ganesh is thus considered the master of intellect and wisdom.

Manufacturer Terms

SmartCarePS is marketed under that trademark by Drager.

Classification

SmartCarePS is a pressure targeted, patient triggered, pressure limited, flow cycled mode of ventilation. All breaths are spontaneous. There is no set rate.

SmartCare attempts to maintain the patient's respiratory pattern in a "comfort zone." This is defined by predetermined values for respiratory frequency, tidal volume, and $ETCO_2$. The comfort zone is defined as a respiratory rate between 15 and 30 breaths per minute, a tidal volume greater than 300 ml (250 ml if body weight is less than 55 kg) and $ETCO_2$ less than 55 mm Hg (less than 65 mm Hg for patients with COPD). The pressure support level is increased or decreased in 2 to 4 cm H_2O increments based on these variables along with the patient's breathing pattern history. The system is an automated weaning technique and the ventilator is always trying

BOX 2-1 *Changes in Pressure Support Associated with Changes in the Physiologic Endpoints Using SmartCare*

Comfort Zone- *f* 15-20 breaths per minute, tidal volume greater than 300 ml, $ETCO_2$ less than 55 mm Hg. SmartCare attempts to maintain this breathing pattern with the lowest possible pressure support. Instability of 2-4 min is tolerated to prevent frequent changes.

Changes based on current physiology

If f is 28-35 b/min and $ETCO_2$ and V_T are normal – Increase PS by 2 cm H_2O.

If f is greater than 35 b/min – Increase PS by 4 cm H_2O.

If f is less than 15 b/min – Decrease PS by 4 cm H_2O.

If V_T is less than 300 ml – Increase PS by 2 cm H_2O. If $ETCO_2$ is greater than 55 mm Hg (65 mm Hg in COPD) – Increase PS by 2 cm H_2O.

If apnea lasts greater than 30 sec – ventilation is provided in CMV with an alarm to alert the caregiver.

Changes based on current physiology and breathing pattern history

If PS is less than 15 cm H_2O for 30 min – Decrease PS by 2 cm H_2O.

If PS is greater than 15 cm H_2O for 60 min – Decrease PS by 4 cm H_2O.

If f is greater than 35 b/min – Increase PS by 4 cm H_2O. (PS greater than 15 cm H_2O) Increase PS by 2 (PS less than 15 cm H_2O).

If PS is increased by 4 cm H_2O – 4 min are allowed before further changes can be made.

If 3 changes in PS are made consecutively and the breathing pattern does not change, an alarm sounds.

When PS is less than 9 cm H_2O (endotracheal tube) or less than 5 cm H_2O (tracheostomy tube), a message suggesting ventilator disconnection is displayed.

to wean the pressure support level to a minimum of 9 cm H_2O. When this is reached, the system displays a message to consider removal of the patient from the ventilator. In this way the system terminates in a spontaneous breathing trial. An early paper suggests that this technique can reduce ventilation times compared with traditional weaning.[97] Box 2-1 depicts changes in the pressure support level associated with alterations in respiratory frequency, tidal volume, and $ETCO_2$.

KEY POINTS

- Volume control ventilation delivers a constant tidal volume at a set flow and flow waveform.
- Pressure control ventilation delivers a constant airway pressure with a variable flow and flow waveform.
- During a volume breath, the peak inspiratory pressure varies with patient effort, lung compliance, and airways resistance.
- During a pressure breath, the tidal volume varies with patient effort, lung compliance, and airways resistance.
- During CMV, if the patient's respiratory rate increases, the expiratory time is shortened.
- During CMV, an increase in respiratory rate can lead to air-trapping.
- During SIMV, the patient can breathe spontaneously or breaths can be pressure supported.
- Spontaneous breathing is associated with improved ventilation–perfusion matching.
- Airway pressure release ventilation uses a release time typically less than 1.5 seconds to prevent de-recruitment.
- Adaptive support ventilation controls respiratory frequency, inspiratory time, peak inspiratory pressure, and I:E ratio when the patient is passive.
- Adaptive support ventilation controls only the pressure support level when the patient is active.
- SmartCare uses measurements of the patient's respiratory frequency, tidal volume, and $ETCO_2$ to control the level of pressure support.
- Proportional assist attempts to perform the same percentage of work per breath; as such the pressure of each breath is variable.
- Dual control breath-to-breath describes a breath that is pressure controlled, but the pressure varies from one breath to the next to achieve a volume target.

ASSESSMENT QUESTIONS

1. Volume targeted breaths require that the clinician set which of the following variables?

I. Tidal volume
II. Inspiratory flow
III. Peak airway pressure
IV. Flow pattern

A. I, II, and IV
B. II and III
C. II, III, and IV
D. All of the above

2. Pressure targeted breaths require that the clinician set which of the following variables?

I. Tidal volume
II. Inspiratory time
III. Flow pattern
IV. Inspiratory flow

A. I, III, and IV
B. II, III, and IV
C. I and II
D. All of the above

3. True or False. Pressure control and pressure target refer to the same description of a breath type.

4. True or False. During pressure support ventilation, the inspiratory flow is controlled by the clinician.

5. During pressure support ventilation, a breath can be terminated by which of the following variables?

I. Time
II. Flow
III. Volume
IV. Pressure

A. II and III
B. I only
C. I, II, and IV
D. All of the above

Continued

ASSESSMENT QUESTIONS—cont'd

6. Adjustment of the flow termination criteria during pressure support from 25% to 50% results in what changes in the following variables?
   I. Larger tidal volume
   II. Smaller tidal volume
   III. Longer inspiratory time
   IV. Shorter inspiratory time
   - A. I and III
   - B. I, II, and IV
   - C. I and II
   - D. II and IV
7. Adjusting rise time during pressure support has the following effect:
   - A. Reduced work of breathing
   - B. Increased work of breathing
   - C. Longer inspiratory time
   - D. No changes
8. True or False. Proportional assist ventilation is based on the minimal work of breathing concept developed by Otis.
9. Adaptive support ventilation uses which of the following inputs to control the ventilation pattern?
   I. Expiratory time constant
   II. Ideal body weight
   III. Patient respiratory effort
   IV. Equation of motion
   - A. II, III, and IV
   - B. I only
   - C. All of the above
   - D. I, II, and III
10. True or False. Proportional assist ventilation results in the ventilator performing the same percentage of work for each breath regardless of the tidal volume.
11. Which of the following variables are used by automatic tube compensation?
    - A. Known resistance of the endotracheal tube, flow, and proximal airway pressure
    - B. Known resistance of the endotracheal tube, flow, and tracheal pressure
    - C. Known resistance of the endotracheal tube and airway pressure
    - D. Tracheal pressure, flow, and airway pressure
12. Dual control, breath-to-breath describes a technique that automatically adjusts ___ to keep ___ at a minimum value.
    - A. volume, pressure
    - B. pressure, volume
    - C. pressure, minute volume
    - D. pressure, inspiratory time
13. During dual control breath-to-breath, if the depth of patient effort increases, then
    - A. airway pressure is automatically reduced.
    - B. airway pressure is automatically increased.
    - C. airway pressure remains the same.
    - D. None of the above
14. During application of SmartCare, the ventilator uses what in-out variables to control the pressure support level?
    I. Elastance and resistance
    II. Pa_{CO_2}, respiratory frequency, and tidal volume
    III. $ETCO_2$, respiratory frequency, and tidal volume
    IV. Pa_{O_2}, respiratory frequency, and tidal volume
    - A. I only
    - B. III only
    - C. I and II
    - D. I and III
15. Airway pressure release ventilation requires the following variables to be set:
    - A. High pressure, low pressure, high time, low time
    - B. High pressure, low pressure, high tidal volume, low tidal volume
    - C. High pressure, low pressure, flow
    - D. High pressure, high time, I:E
16. During ASV, if the patient breathes spontaneously greater than 10 breaths per minute, what variable(s) does the ventilator control?
    - A. Tidal volume
    - B. I:E
    - C. Pressure
    - D. Flow

ASSESSMENT QUESTIONS—cont'd

17. Pressure control inverse ratio ventilation and APRV are similar except that:
  A. No difference
  B. APRV allows spontaneous breathing, PCIRV does not.
  C. PCIRV is more comfortable for the patient.
  D. APRV maintains a constant tidal volume.

18. During volume targeted ventilation, an increase in patient effort results in:
  I. an increase in delivered tidal volume compared to set tidal volume.
  II. a constant tidal volume and lower peak airway pressure.
  III. an increase in the patient work of breathing.
  IV. an increase in dead space.
  V. a decrease in delivered tidal volume.
    A. III and V
    B. Both I and III
    C. II only
    D. Both II and III

19. During pressure targeted ventilation, an increase in patient effort results in:
  I. an increase in delivered tidal volume.
  II. a constant tidal volume and lower peak airway pressure.
  III. longer inspiratory time.
  IV. an increase in dead space.
  V. a decrease in delivered tidal volume.
    A. I only
    B. Both I and III
    C. II only
    D. Both II and III

20. During dual control ventilation, an increase in patient effort results in:
  I. an increase in delivered tidal volume.
  II. a constant tidal volume and lower peak airway pressure.
  III. an increase in the patient work of breathing.
  IV. an increase in dead space.
  V. a decrease in delivered tidal volume.
    A. III and V
    B. Both I and III
    C. II only
    D. Both II and III

CASE STUDIES

For additional practice, refer to Case Studies 7-9 and 11-13 in the appendix at the back of this book.

REFERENCES

1. Chatburn RL: A new system for understanding mechanical ventilators, Respir Care 36:1123-1155, 1992.
2. Sassoon CSH, Mahutte CK, Light RW: Ventilator modes old and new, Crit Care Clin 6:605-634, 1990.
3. Sassoon CSH: Positive pressure ventilation: alternate modes, Chest 100:1421-1429, 1991.
4. Hotchkiss RS, Wilson RS: Mechanical ventilatory support, Surg Clin North Am 63:417-438, 1983.
5. DuPuis YG: Ventilators: theory and clinical application, St Louis, CV Mosby, 1986.
6. Hamilton Veolar: Operators manual, Reno, Nev, Hamilton Medical, 1990.
7. Luce JM, Pierson DJ, Hudson LD: Intermittent mandatory ventilation, Chest 79:678-685, 1981.
8. Weisman IM, Rinaldo JE, Rogers RM et al: Intermittent mandatory ventilation, Am Rev Respir Dis 127:641-647, 1983.
9. Downs JB, Stock MC, Tabeling B: Intermittent mandatory ventilation (IMV): a primary ventilatory support mode, Ann Chir Gynaecol 196(suppl):57-63, 1982.
10. Downs JB, Block AJ, Venum KB: Intermittent mandatory ventilation in the treatment of patients with chronic obstructive pulmonary disease, Anesth Analg 55:437-443, 1974.
11. Downs JB, Douglas ME, Sanfelippo PM et al: Ventilatory pattern, intrapleural pressure, and cardiac output, Anesth Analg 56:88-96, 1977.
12. Downs JB, Klein EF, Desautels D et al: Intermittent mandatory ventilation: a new approach to weaning patients from mechanical ventilators, Chest 64:331-335, 1973.
13. Shapiro BA, Harrison RA, Walton JR et al: Intermittent demand ventilation: a new technique for supporting ventilation in critically ill patients, Respir Care 21:521-525, 1976.
14. Heenan TJ, Downs JB, Douglas ME et al: Intermittent mandatory ventilation: is synchronization important? Chest 77:598-602, 1980.
15. MacIntyre NR: Respiratory function during pressure support ventilation, Chest 89:677-683, 1986.
16. Murphy DF, Dobb GD: Effect of pressure support of spontaneous breathing during intermittent mandatory ventilation, Crit Care Med 15:612-613, 1987.

17. MacIntyre NR: Weaning from mechanical ventilatory support: volume-assisting intermittent breaths versus pressure-assisting every breath, Respir Care 33:121-125, 1988.
18. Gregory GA, Kitterman JA, Phibbs RH et al: Treatment of the idiopathic respiratory distress syndrome with continuous positive airway pressure, N Engl J Med 284:1333-1340, 1971.
19. Stock MC, Downs JB: Airway pressure release ventilation: a new approach to ventilation support during acute lung injury, Respir Care 32:517-524, 1987.
20. Stock MC, Downs JB, Frolicher DA: Airway pressure release ventilation, Crit Care Med 15:462-466, 1987.
21. Downs JB, Stock MC: Airway pressure release ventilation: a new concept in ventilatory support, Crit Care Med 15:459-461, 1987.
22. Rasanen J, Downs JB, Stock MC: Cardiovascular effect of conventional positive pressure ventilation and airway pressure release ventilation, Chest 93:911-915, 1988.
23. Garner W, Downs JB, Stock MC et al: Airway pressure release ventilation (APRV): a human trial, Chest 94:779-781, 1988.
24. Abraham E, Yoshihara G: Cardiorespiratory effects of pressure control ventilation in severe respiratory failure, Chest 98:1445-1449, 1990.
25. Gurevitch MJ, Van Dyke J, Young ES et al: Improved oxygenation and lower peak airway pressure in severe adult respiratory distress syndrome: treatment with inverse ratio ventilation, Chest 89:211-213, 1986.
26. Abraham E, Yoshihara G: Cardiorespiratory effects of pressure controlled inverse ratio ventilation in severe respiratory failure, Chest 96:1356-1359, 1989.
27. Lain DC, DiBenedetto R, Morris SL et al: Pressure control inverse ratio ventilation as a method to reduce peak inspiratory pressure and provide adequate ventilation and oxygenation, Chest 95:1081-1088, 1989.
28. Marini JJ, Crooke PS III, Truwit JD: Determinants and limits of pressure-preset ventilation: a mathematical model of pressure control, J Appl Physiol 67:1081-1092, 1989.
29. Tharratt RS, Allen RP, Albertson TE: Pressure controlled inverse ratio ventilation in severe adult respiratory failure, Chest 94:755-762, 1988.
30. Hewlett AM, Platt AS, Terry VG: Mandatory minute volume, Anesth 32:163-169, 1977.
31. East TD, Elkhuizan PHM, Pace CL: Pressure support in mandatory minute ventilation supplied by the Ohmeda CPU-1 prevents alveolar hypoventilation due to respiratory depression in a canine model, Respir Care 34:795-800, 1989.
32. Ravenscroft PS: Simple mandatory minute volume, Anesth 33:246-249, 1978.
33. Operators Manual Bear 5, Riverside, Calif, Bear Medical, 1990.
34. Operators Manual Drager E4, Telford, Pa: Drager Inc. 1997.
35. Amato MBP, Barbos CSV, Bonassa J et al: Volume assisted pressure support ventilation (VAPSV): a new approach for reducing muscle workload during acute respiratory failure, Chest 102:1225-1234, 1992.
36. Haas CF, Branson RD, Folk LM et al: Patient determined inspiratory flow during assisted mechanical ventilation, Respir Care 40:716-721, 1995.
37. MacIntyre NR, Gropper C, Westfall T: Combining pressure limiting and volume cycling features in a patient-interactive mechanical ventilation, Crit Care Med 22:353-357, 1994.
38. Branson RD, MacIntyre NR: Dual control modes of mechanical ventilation, Respir Care 41:294-305, 1996.
39. Piotrowski A, Sobala W, Kawczynski P: Patient initiated, pressure regulated, volume controlled ventilation compared with intermittent mandatory ventilation in neonates: a prospective, randomized study, Intensive Care Med 23:975-981, 1997.
40. Alvarez A, Subirana M, Benito S: Decelerating flow ventilation effects in acute respiratory failure, J Crit Care 13:7-12, 1998.
41. Raneri VM: Optimization of patient ventilator interactions: closed loop technology, Intensive Care Med 23:936-939, 1997.
42. Roth H, Luecke T, Lansche G et al: Effects of patient triggered automatic switching between mandatory and supported ventilation in the postoperative weaning period, Intensive Care Med 2001;27:47-51.
43. Holt RJ, Sanders RC, Thurman TL et al: An evaluation of automode, a computer-controlled ventilator mode, with the Siemens Servo 300A ventilator, using a porcine model, Respir Care 2001;46:26-36.
44. Otis AB, Fenn WO, Rahn H: Mechanics of breathing in man, J Appl Physiol 2:592-607, 1950.
45. Brunner JX, Laubscher TP, Banner MJ et al: A simple method to measure total expiratory time constant based on the passive expiratory flow-volume curve, Crit Care Med 23:1117-1122, 1995.
46. Iotti GA, Braschi A, Brunner J et al: Respiratory mechanics by least squares fitting in mechanically ventilated patients: applications during paralysis and during pressure support ventilation, Intensive Care Med 21:406-413, 1995.
47. Weiler N, Henrichs W, Kebler W: The AVL mode: a safe closed loop algorithm for ventilation during total intravenous anesthesia, Int J Clin Monit Comput 11:85-88, 1994.
48. Laubscher TP, Frutiger A, Fanconi S et al: Automatic selection of tidal volume, respiratory frequency and minute volume in intubated ICU patients as startup procedure for closed-loop controlled ventilation, Int J Clin Monit Comput 11:19-30, 1994.
49. Laubscher TP, Frutiger A, Fanconi S: The automatic selection of ventilation parameters during the initial phase of mechanical ventilation, Intensive Care Med 22:199-207, 1996.
50. Linton DM, Potgieter PD, Davis S et al: Automatic weaning from mechanical ventilation using an adaptive lung controller, Chest 106:1843-1850, 1994.
51. Weiler N, Eberle B, Latorre F et al: Adaptive lung ventilation, Anaesthesia 45:950-956, 1996.
52. Campbell RS, Sinamban RP, Johannigman JA et al: Clinical evaluation of a new closed loop ventilation mode: adaptive support ventilation, Respir Care 43:856, 1998 (abstract).

53. Bersten AD, Rutten AJ, Vedig AE et al: Additional work of breathing imposed by endotracheal tubes, breathing circuits, and intensive care ventilators, Crit Care Med 17:671-680, 1989.
54. Sulzer CF, Chiolero R, Chassot PG et al: Adaptive support ventilation for fast tracheal extubation after cardiac surgery: a randomized controlled study, Anesthesiology 95:1339-1345, 2001.
55. Tassaux D, Dalmas E, Gratadour P et al: Patient-ventilator interactions during partial ventilatory support: a preliminary study comparing the effects of adaptive support ventilation with synchronized intermittent mandatory ventilation plus inspiratory pres-sure support, Crit Care Med 30:801-807, 2002.
56. Cassina T, Chiolero R, Mauri R et al: Clinical experience with adaptive support ventilation for fast-track cardiac surgery, J Cardiothorac Vasc Anesth 17:571-575, 2003.
57. Petter AH, Chiolero RL, Cassina T et al: Automatic "respirator/weaning" with adaptive support ventilation: the effect on duration of endotracheal intubation and patient management, Anesth Analg 97:1743-1750, 2003.
58. Shapiro M, Wilson RK, Casar G et al: Work of breathing through different sized endotracheal tubes, Crit Care Med 14:1028-1031, 1986.
59. Bersten AD, Rutten AJ, Vedig AE: Efficacy of pressure support in compensating for apparatus work, Anaesth Intensive Care 21:67-71, 1993.
60. Brochard L, Rua F, Lorini H et al: Inspiratory pressure support compensates for the additional work of breathing caused by the endotracheal tube, Anesthesiology 75:739-745, 1991.
61. Guttmann J, Eberhard L, Fabry B et al: Continuous calculation of intratracheal pressure in tracheally intubated patients, Anesthesiology 79:503-513, 1993.
62. Fiastro JF, Habib MP, Quan SF: Pressure support compensation for inspiratory work due to endotracheal tubes and demand continuous positive airway pressure, Chest 93:499-505, 1988.
63. Stocker R, Fabry B, Haberthur C: New modes of ventilatory support in spontaneously breathing intubated patients. In: Vincent JL, editor: Yearbook of intensive care and emergency medicine, vol 12, Berlin, Springer-Verlag, 1997, pp 514-533.
64. Fabry B, Guttman J, Eberhard L et al: Automatic compensation of endotracheal tube resistance in spontaneous breathing patients, Technol Health Care 1:281-291, 1994.
65. Guttmann J, Bernhard H, Mols G et al: Respiratory comfort of automatic tube compensation and inspiratory pressure support in conscious humans, Intensive Care Med 23:1119-1124, 1997.
66. Fabry B, Zappe D, Guttman J et al: Breathing pattern and additional work of breathing in spontaneously breathing patients with different ventilatory demand during inspiratory pressure support and automatic tube compensation, Intensive Care Med 23:545-552, 1997.
67. Wrigge H, Zinserling J, Hering R et al: Cardiorespiratory effects of automatic tube compensation during airway pressure release ventilation in patients with acute lung injury, Anesthesiology 95(2):382-389, 2001.
68. Haberthur C, Mols G, Elsasser S et al: Extubation after breathing trials with automatic tube compensation, T-tube, or pressure support ventilation, Acta Anaesthesiol Scand 46:973-979, 2002.
69. Oczenski W, Kepka A, Krenn H et al: Automatic tube compensation in patients after cardiac surgery: effects on oxygen consumption and breathing pattern, Crit Care Med 30(7):1467-1471, 2002.
70. Cohen JD, Shapiro M, Grozovski E et al: Automatic tube compensation-assisted respiratory rate to tidal volume ratio improves the prediction of weaning outcome, Chest 122(3):980-984, 2002.
71. Fujino Y, Uchiyama A, Mashimo T et al: Spontaneously breathing lung model comparison of work of breathing between automatic tube compensation and pressure support, Respir Care 48(1):38-45, 2003.
72. Kuhlen R, Max M, Dembinski R et al: Breathing pattern and workload during automatic tube compensation, pressure support and T-piece trials in weaning patients, Eur J Anaesthesiology 20(1):10-16, 2003.
73. Ranieri VM, Grasso S, Mascia L et al: Effects of proportional assist ventilation on inspiratory muscle effort in patients with chronic obstructive pulmonary disease and acute respiratory failure, Anesthesiology 86:79-81, 1997.
74. Younes M, Puddy A, Robert D et al: Proportional assist ventilation: results of an initial clinical trial, Am Rev Respir Dis 145:121-129, 1992.
75. Younes M: Proportional assist ventilation, a new approach to ventilatory support, Am Rev Respir Dis 145:114-120, 1992.
76. Bigatello LM, Nishimura M, Imanaka H et al: Unloading of the work of breathing by proportional assist ventilation in a lung model, Crit Care Med 25:267-272, 1997.
77. Navalesi P, Hernandez P, Wongsa A et al: Proportional assist ventilation in acute respiratory failure: effects of breathing pattern and inspiratory effort, Am J Respir Crit Care Med 154:1330-1338, 1996.
78. Grasso S, Puntillo F, Mascia L et al: Compensation for increase in respiratory workload during mechanical ventilation. Pressure-support versus proportional-assist ventilation, Am J Respir Crit Care Med 161(3 Pt 1):819-826, 2000.
79. Vitacca M, Clini E, Pagani M et al: Physiologic effects of early administered mask proportional assist ventilation in patients with chronic obstructive pulmonary disease and acute respiratory failure, Crit Care Med 28(6):1791-1797, 2000.
80. Mols G, von Ungern-Sternberg B, Rohr E et al: Respiratory comfort and breathing pattern during volume proportional assist ventilation and pressure support ventilation: a study on volunteers with artificially reduced compliance, Crit Care Med 28(6):1940-1946, 2000.
81. Polese G, Vitacca M, Bianchi L et al: Nasal proportional assist ventilation unloads the inspiratory muscles of stable patients with hypercapnia due to COPD, Eur Respir J 16(3):491-498, 2000.

82. Musante G, Schulze A, Gerhardt T et al: Proportional assist ventilation decreases thoracoabdominal asynchrony and chest wall distortion in preterm infants, Pediatr Res 49(2):175-180, 2001.
83. Hernandez P, Maltais F, Gursahaney A et al: Proportional assist ventilation may improve exercise performance in severe chronic obstructive pulmonary disease, J Cardiopulm Rehabil 21(3):135-142, 2001.
84. Gay PC, Hess DR, Hill NS: Noninvasive proportional assist ventilation for acute respiratory insufficiency. Comparison with pressure support ventilation, Am J Respir Crit Care Med 164(9):1606-1611, 2001.
85. Serra A, Polese G, Braggion C et al: Non-invasive proportional assist and pressure support ventilation in patients with cystic fibrosis and chronic respiratory failure, Thorax 57(1):50-54, 2002.
86. Wysocki M, Richard JC, Meshaka P: Noninvasive proportional assist ventilation compared with noninvasive pressure support ventilation in hypercapnic acute respiratory failure, Crit Care Med 30(2):323-329, 2002.
87. Porta R, Appendini L, Vitacca M et al: Mask proportional assist vs. pressure support ventilation in patients in clinically stable condition with chronic ventilatory failure, Chest 122(2):479-484, 2002.
88. Hawkins P, Johnson LC, Nikoletou D et al: Proportional assist ventilation as an aid to exercise training in severe chronic obstructive pulmonary disease, Thorax 57(10):853-859, 2002.
89. Hart N, Hunt A, Polkey MI et al: Comparison of proportional assist ventilation and pressure support ventilation in chronic respiratory failure due to neuromuscular and chest wall deformity, Thorax 57(11):979-981, 2002.
90. Delaere S, Roeseler J, D'hoore W et al: Respiratory muscle workload in intubated, spontaneously breathing patients without COPD: pressure support vs. proportional assist ventilation, Intensive Care Med 29(6):949-954, 2003.
91. Fernandez-Vivas M, Caturla-Such J, Gonzalez de la Rosa J et al: Noninvasive pressure support versus proportional assist ventilation in acute respiratory failure, Intensive Care Med 29(7):1126-1133, 2003.
92. Passam F, Hoing S, Prinianakis G et al: Effect of different levels of pressure support and proportional assist ventilation on breathing pattern, work of breathing and gas exchange in mechanically ventilated hypercapnic COPD patients with acute respiratory failure, Respiration 70(4):355-361, 2003.
93. Wysocki M, Meshaka P, Richard JC et al: Proportional-assist ventilation compared with pressure-support ventilation during exercise in volunteers with external thoracic restriction, Crit Care Med 32(2):409-414, 2004.
94. Dojat M, Brochard L, Lemaire F et al: A knowledge based system for assisted ventilation of patients in intensive care units, Int J Clin Monit Comput 9:239-250, 1992.
95. Dojat M, Harf A, Touchard D et al: Evaluation of a knowledge based system providing ventilatory management and decision for extubation, Am J Respir Crit Care Med 153:997-1004, 1996.
96. Dojat M, Harf A, Touchard D et al: Clinical evaluation of a computer controlled pressure support mode, Am J Respir Crit Care Med 161:1161-1166, 2000.
97. Lellouche F, Mancebo J, Jolliet P et al: A multicenter randomized trial of computer driven protocolized weaning from mechanical ventilation, Am J Respir Crit Care Med 174:894-900, 2006.

CHAPTER

3

The Patient-Ventilator Interface: Ventilator Circuit, Airway Care, and Suctioning

Richard D. Branson

OUTLINE

OBJECTIVES

- Understand the components that determine the compressible volume of the ventilator circuit.
- Understand the effects of compressible volume on tidal volume delivered to the patient and measurements of compliance, resistance, and auto-PEEP.
- Explain how the resistance of the expiratory valve may affect the inspiratory work of breathing.
- Describe the function of the active exhalation valve.
- Compare and contrast flow and threshold resistors.
- Compare and contrast the methods for determining proper placement of the endotracheal tube.
- Describe the technique for cuff pressure measurement.
- Identify the safe pressure for the endotracheal tube cuff.
- Compare and contrast the minimal seal and minimal leak techniques for setting cuff pressure.
- Describe the potential advantages of a silver-coated or silver-impregnated endotracheal tube.
- Describe the function of an endotracheal tube designed for subglottic secretion drainage.
- Compare and contrast open and closed circuit suctioning.
- List the goals of oral care in the mechanically ventilated patient.
- List the potential complications of airway suctioning and methods to prevent each.
- Describe the use of saline instillation to facilitate suctioning and list the pros and cons.

KEY TERMS

closed circuit suction catheters
colorimetric CO_2 detector
compressible volume
cuff pressure
end-expiratory valves
endotracheal tube (ETT)
esophageal detector devices (EDDs)

minimal leak technique
minimal occlusion technique
minimal seal technique
suction catheters
silver-coated/silver-impregnated tube
subglottic suction tube
ventilator associated pneumonia (VAP)
ventilator circuit

Care of the mechanically ventilated patient includes airway maintenance, secretion clearance, proper positioning, and provision of ancillary equipment. Because many of these subjects are intertwined in the fabric of other chapters, this chapter concentrates on technical and device-related issues.

THE VENTILATOR CIRCUIT

The **ventilator circuit** is approximately 60 inches of plastic tubing that connects the mechanical ventilator to an artificial airway or mask. Circuits for adults traditionally use 22-mm tubing, whereas pediatric circuits range from 9 to 13 mm in diameter. The ventilator circuit may contain filters, humidifiers, water traps, heated wires, artificial noses, closed **suction catheters,** and devices for aerosol administration. Issues related to humidification and aerosol therapy are covered elsewhere.

Ventilator circuits are associated with certain characteristics, including compliance, resistance, and dead space. Each of these characteristics can affect the efficiency of ventilation. Ventilator circuits often are associated with the potential for nosocomial infection, and the frequency of ventilator circuit changes has recently been the subject of several investigations.[1-9] These topics are discussed relative to the pertinent literature and the effects on the mechanically ventilated patient.

Ventilation

The length, diameter, and materials used to construct a ventilator circuit all affect the circuit compliance. Typical disposable adult ventilator circuits possess a compliance of 2 to 3 ml/cm H_2O. This typically is known as the **compressible volume** of the circuit. Nondisposable circuits generally have a lower compliance because of the more rigid materials used in manufacturing (1.5 to 2 ml/cm H_2O). The initial cost of a nondisposable circuit is approximately $300. These circuits tend to improve ventilator performance because they are leak free, frequently have a smooth internal bore, and are relatively unaffected by prolonged use.[10] The cost of a disposable circuit is approximately $9.00 with water traps and $19.00 with heated wires. The cost of cleaning (washing and sterilizing) nondisposable circuits is quite high and possibly the most important reason that disposable circuits remain popular.

Compressible volume usually plays a small part in the discrepancy between actual tidal volume delivered to the patient and tidal volume measured by the ventilator. If compressible volume of the circuit is known, measurement of distending pressure (peak inspiratory pressure [PIP] – positive end-expiratory pressure [PEEP]) allows the volume trapped in the tubing to be determined.

If tidal volume is 600 ml, PIP is 40 cm H_2O, PEEP is 8 cm H_2O, and compressible volume is 3 ml/cm H_2O, then:

$$(40 \text{ cm } H_2O - 8 \text{ cm } H_2O) \times 3 \text{ ml/cm } H_2O = \text{compressible volume}$$

$$32 \text{ cm } H_2O \times 3 \text{ ml/cm } H_2O = 96 \text{ ml}$$

$$600 \text{ ml} - 96 \text{ ml} = 504 \text{ ml actual tidal volume}$$

The issue of compressible volume is handled in various ways by different ventilator manufacturers. In many ventilators (Siemens 900C [Siemens, Danvers, Mass.]; Bear 1, 2, and 3 [Bear Medical Systems, Viasys HealthCare, Riverside, Calif.]), the set tidal volume is delivered into the circuit, and the expiratory flow sensor measures the actual exhaled tidal volume plus the compressible volume. Using the aforementioned example, the ventilator is set at 600 ml, the patient receives 504 ml, and the exhaled tidal volume displays 600 ml. This represents an error in tidal volume measurement of 16%, which would invalidate measurements of compliance and resistance made using this value for tidal volume.

Many ventilators (Puritan Bennett 7200ae, 840 [Puritan Bennett, Carlsbad, Calif.]) measure compressible volume of the circuit during setup and "compensate" for compressible volume. Using our example, the ventilator would deliver 696 ml (set tidal volume + calculated compressible volume), actual tidal volume would be 600 ml, and measured tidal volume would read 600 ml (measured exhaled tidal volume – calculated compressible volume). In this case, PIP would increase based on the required volume increase and patient impedance (in the example above, 6 cm H_2O).

Several ventilators (Hamilton Veolar [Hamilton Medical, Reno, Nev]; Raphael, Galileo, Pulmonetic Systems LTV [Pulmonetic Systems Inc., Colton, Calif.]; Drager Babylog [Drager, Telford, Pa.]; and Viasys Avea [Viasys Healthcare, Yorba Linda, Calif.]) use a flow sensor positioned between the circuit and **endotracheal tube (ETT).** In this case, tidal volume delivered into the circuit would be 600 ml, measured actual tidal volume would be 504 ml, and the presence of compressible volume would be unmasked. The clinician then could increase the set tidal volume until measured exhaled tidal volume was 600 ml, if desired.

Compressible volume can also result in the underestimation of autoPEEP when using the expiratory hold maneuver. When both inspiratory and expiratory valves are closed, the volume trapped in the lung can redistribute throughout the entire patient-ventilator system. As the volume of the system increases, the pressure decreases. The underestimation of autoPEEP in this situation is typically quite small.

The compliance of the circuit can also complicate evaluation of pressure and flow tracings. The circuit "exhales" the compressible volume more quickly than the patient, particularly the patient with dynamic hyperinflation. This gives the expiratory flow signal an initial steep deceleration followed by a gradual slope toward zero. Clinicians should be aware of the effects of the circuit on graphics (Figure 3-1).

Resistance of the ventilator circuit is not typically a problem during mechanical ventilation. Compared with the resistance of the ETT, circuit resistance is minute. Resistance is greatest at the Y-piece and elbow. Occasionally, these areas can interfere with proximal pressure and flow measurements.[11] These components should be inspected for excessive resistance before use.

Exhalation Valves

Exhalation valves can be a considerable source of resistance in the patient circuit, increasing the work of breathing and retarding expiratory flow.[12] Most

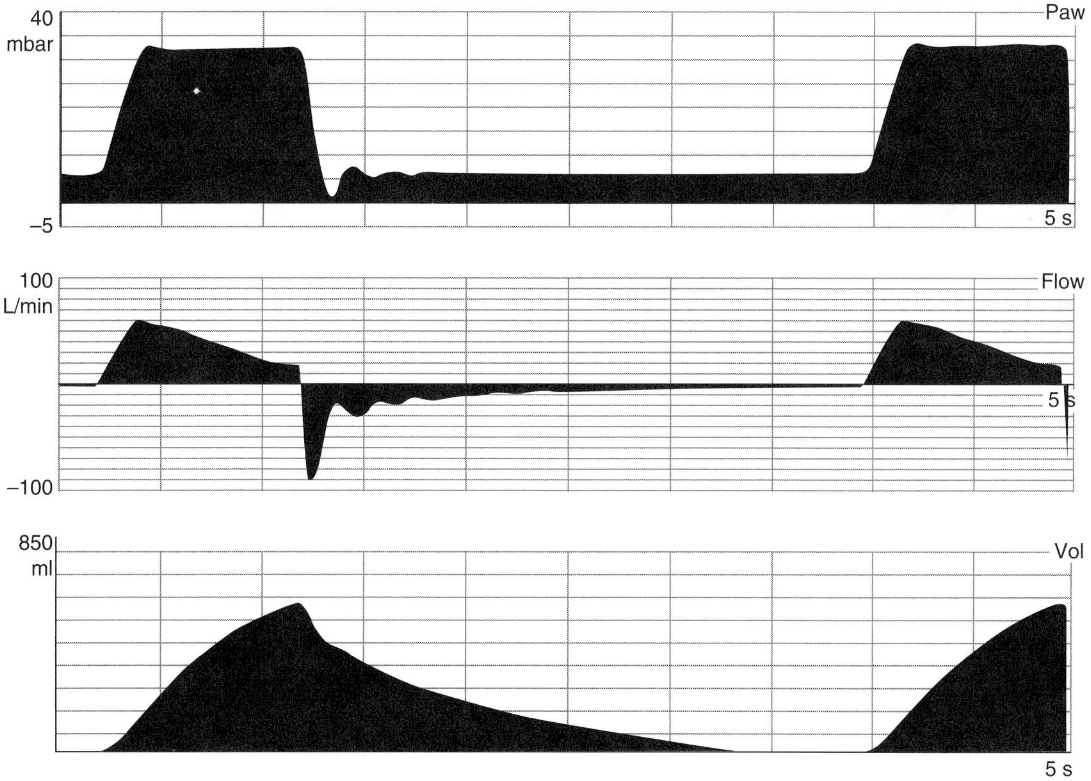

FIGURE 3-1 The effects of compressible volume on the flow time curve during mechanical ventilation. The patient is being ventilated in the pressure control mode. This is a patient with COPD; note the prolonged expiratory flow. The initial flow spike represents the volume of gas trapped in the tubing being released.

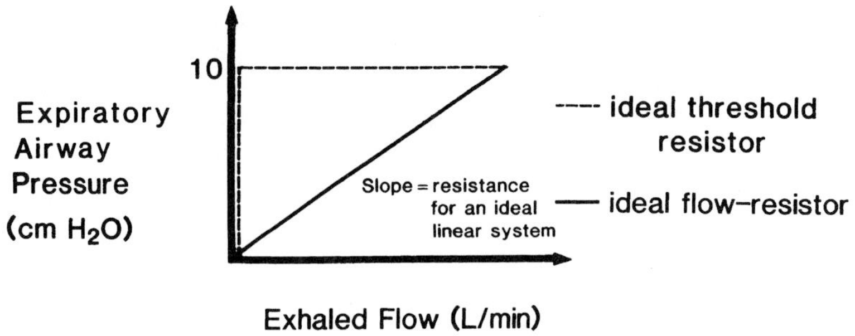

FIGURE 3-2 **The effects of increasing flow on the pressure provided by flow-resistive and threshold expiratory valve devices.** (From Banner MJ: Expiratory positive pressure valves and work of breathing. Respir Care 32:431-436, 1987.)

current-generation ventilators have internal exhalation valves, eliminating this circuit component as a point of concern. However, in many home care and transport ventilators, disposable exhalation valves remain in use.

The exhalation valve can result in an increased work of breathing because of resistance and the requirement that the valve functionally close for pressure in the circuit to fall. This is important during pressure triggering, a common triggering method in ventilators that use disposable exhalation valves. For patient effort to result in a negative pressure in the circuit, the exhalation valve must come to rest against the gas outflow port. The time required for the exhalation valve to move from an open to a closed position is a measurable delay in response time of the ventilator. The resistance to gas flow of the exhalation valve also contributes to the work of breathing as a consequence of the increased work to close the valve.

In recent years, exhalation valve systems known as "active exhalation valves" have been introduced. This is an unfortunate term as all exhalation valves are active. A traditional active exhalation valve closes during the inspiratory time. If the patient attempts to inhale or exhale, the valve remains closed and airway pressure may fall or rise. In the case of a forceful exhalation, such as a cough, the exhalation valve remains closed until airway pressure exceeds the high pressure alarm setting. The active exhalation system allows the patient to inhale or exhale while maintaining the inspiratory pressure constant. In this way, the exhalation valve is "active," allowing inspiratory and expiratory flow through the valve during the mechanical inspiration. An important note is that when an active exhalation valve is used, the clinician loses control of the delivered tidal volume. There are no studies that evaluate the potential beneficial effects of the active exhalation valve, but in the authors' experience, these systems seem to improve patient comfort and synchrony.

End-expiratory valves or PEEP valves commonly are used with home care and transport ventilators. These devices have been classified as flow resistors or threshold resistors on the basis of performance.[12-16] A flow resistor requires a constant flow to maintain a constant pressure. A decrease in flow results in a pressure lower than desired, and an increase in flow results in a pressure greater than desired (Figure 3-2). Threshold resistors maintain a constant or nearly constant pressure regardless of gas flow. Threshold resistors are preferred to flow resistors. Examples of a flow resistor and a threshold resistor are shown in Figures 3-3 and 3-4.

CARE OF THE ARTIFICIAL AIRWAY

Mechanical ventilation is most often accomplished with the use of an artificial airway. The advent of noninvasive ventilation has changed this paradigm and required re-evaluation of preconceptions. Masks and other devices are discussed in the chapter on noninvasive ventilation. Caring for the artificial airway includes ensuring proper tube placement, securing the tube, maintaining appropriate **cuff pressure,** and suctioning secretions. Following is a discussion of each of these.

Tube Placement

Ensuring appropriate airway position after placement and during prolonged use is essential for safe mechanical ventilation. Proper placement should, of course, be verified visually, during intubation. However, because even in experienced hands esophageal intubation can occur, several techniques have been devised to detect esophageal placement of an artificial airway.[17-19]

Carbon dioxide (CO_2) monitoring generally is considered the gold standard for determining esophageal intubation.[20,21] A tube inserted into the esophagus and connected to the ventilator or manual resuscitator does not have CO_2 in the expired gas. The measurement of expired CO_2 can be accomplished quantitatively through use of a capnometer (Figure 3-5) or qualitatively through use of a detector. In the former, expired CO_2 is measured in percent or millimeters of mercury (mm Hg). In the latter, the presence of CO_2 is displayed by a color change.

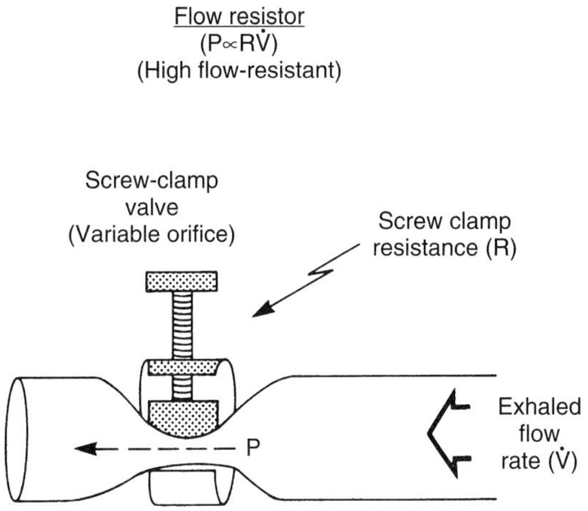

FIGURE 3-3 A flow resistor for providing PEEP. (From Banner MJ et al. Flow resistance of expiratory positive pressure valve systems. Chest 90:212-217, 1986. From Banner MJ, Lampotang S: Expiratory pressure valves. In: Branson RD, Hess D, Chatburn RL, editors: Respiratory care equipment, ed 2. Philadelphia, 1999, Lippincott.)

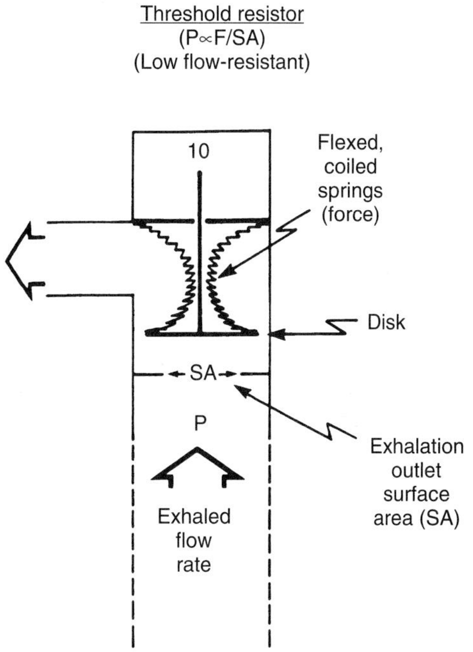

FIGURE 3-4 A threshold resistor for providing PEEP. (From Banner MJ, Lampotang S: Expiratory pressure valves. In: Branson RD, Hess D, Chatburn RL, editors: Respiratory care equipment, ed 2. Philadelphia, 1999, Lippincott.)

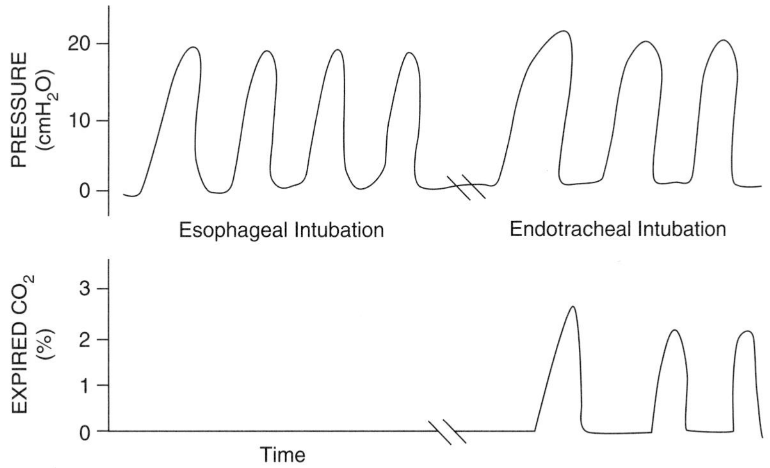

FIGURE 3-5 The response of a capnograph to esophageal intubation followed by correct placement of the ETT into the trachea.

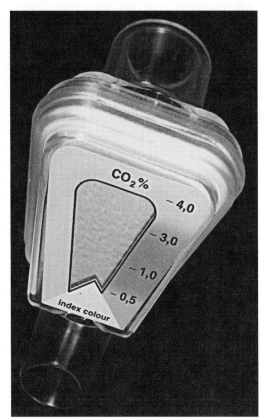

FIGURE 3-6 A colorimetric device for detecting the presence of CO_2 in expired gas.

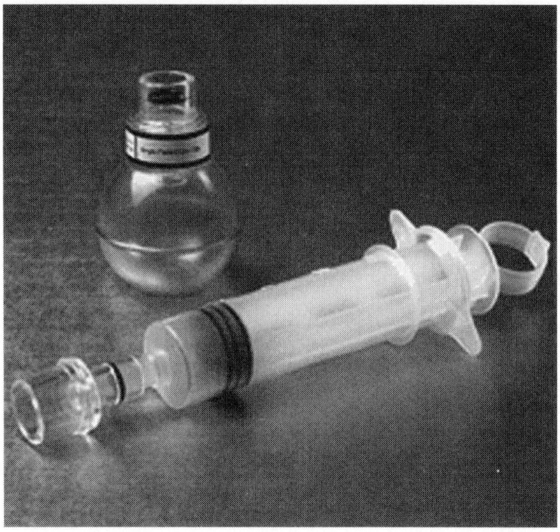

FIGURE 3-7 Two types of esophageal detector devices. The squeeze bulb *(top)* and the syringe type *(bottom).*

The **colorimetric CO_2 detector** technique uses a pH-sensitive chemical, bonded to a paper element (Figure 3-6). In the presence of CO_2, the paper changes color.[20-26] As the patient is ventilated, the detector changes color with inspiration (absence of CO_2) and expiration (presence of CO_2). This color change is typically yellow to purple. Several devices are currently available to serve this purpose. Some devices simply change one color, whereas others change through a series of shades as CO_2 concentration increases. The major limitation of CO_2 detection as a method of ensuring ETT placement is seen during cardiopulmonary resuscitation. In the absence of cardiac output and hence pulmonary blood flow, CO_2 concentration may be very low or zero. This creates the unfavorable situation in which the tube may be placed correctly, but the absence of CO_2 in expired gas causes the clinician to remove the tube.[23-30] In these instances, the clinician should use clinical judgment along with other observations (e.g., breath sounds) before removing the tube.

Another method of determining proper tube placement involves the use of negative pressure applied to the airway. These devices are collectively known as **esophageal detection devices (EDDs).** The principle of operation resides in the fact that the lungs are full of air, while under normal conditions the esophagus is collapsed. The EDD is either a syringe or squeeze bulb connected to the ETT (Figure 3-7). If the tube is in the trachea, the syringe fills easily or the bulb inflates quickly. If the tube is in the esophagus, the negative pressure further collapses the esophagus, and the syringe does not fill or the bulb stays flat. One caveat of these systems occurs after manual ventilation with a face mask. In these situations, if the stomach has been filled with air, the EDD may suggest endotracheal intubation, even though the tube is in the esophagus.[31]

Several investigators have shown that clinicians can use the EDD in determining appropriate tube placement.[31-38] Like the CO_2 monitor, the EDD also occasionally predicts esophageal tube placement, even though the tube is in the trachea. This may result from reduced lung volume, airway secretions, airway obstruction, or bronchospasm.

Chest radiographs also can be used to determine tube placement. The chest radiograph is reliable but requires considerably more time to check placement than the other devices. Auscultation of the chest also remains an important adjunct to these techniques. Auscultation is simple and readily available but is subjective. However, the use of CO_2 monitoring or the EDD can be complemented by simple auscultation.

TABLE 3-1 *A Comparison of Techniques for Assessing Appropriate Endotracheal Tube Placement*

	TIME TO RESULT	COST	COMMENT
Chest radiograph	5-10 min	Moderate	• In the presence of esophageal intubation, time is excessive • Detects endobronchial intubation
EDD	Immediate	Low	• Requires some training • Effective in adults • Cannot detect endobronchial intubation • False-positive result in stomach has been insufflated during manual ventilation • Less successful in pediatrics (<20 kg)
CO_2 detector	Immediate	Low	• Presence of low expired CO_2 due to cardiac arrest suggests esophageal placement • Cannot detect endobronchial intubation
Capnometer	Immediate	Moderate	• Cannot detect endobronchial intubation • Precise measures of $ETCO_2$ • Can be used to monitor ventilation
Auscultation	Immediate	Low	• Requires training and experience • Detects endobronchial intubation • Less reliable than other methods

EDD, Esophageal detector device.

Once the tube is placed and proper position is confirmed, the position of the tube should be noted by recording the length of the tube at the teeth. This value then can be checked during subsequent ventilator checks. The tube should be secured to prevent migration.

Previous discussions have concentrated on verifying tube placement. During the course of intubation, these techniques also may be useful if the patient becomes extubated or if the tube migrates cephalad. Distal migration of the tube into the right mainstem bronchi is also of concern, requiring different detection techniques. Commonly, distal migration of the tube is detected by an increase in airway pressure during volume control ventilation, a decrease in tidal volume during pressure control ventilation, or absence of breath sounds on one side, or it is detected on routine chest radiograph.[39,40]

The appropriate depth of endotracheal tube insertion has been determined for both endotracheal and nasotracheal tubes. Eagle[41] suggests that the distance from the teeth to the midpoint of the trachea can be predicted by the height in centimeters divided by 10, plus 2. For nasotracheal tubes, the distance from the external naris to the midpoint of the trachea is the height in centimeters divided by 10, plus 8.[41] Other studies have shown that, during orotracheal intubation, placement of the tube at the gums at 23 cm for men and 21 cm for women aids in preventing endobronchial intubation.[42,43]

There are many causes of endobronchial intubation. Patient movement and position of the head cause the ETT to move distal with flexion and proximal with extension of the neck.[44] Turning of the patient by the nursing staff, transport, and position changes for procedures all play a role in tube misplacement. Patient activity and vigorous coughing also may result in tube movement.

Chest radiographs remain the gold standard for assessing ETT position. The incidence of tube malposition has been demonstrated to be between 15% and 30%.[40,45] The risk of malposition is greatest immediately after intubation and in women.[45] Endobronchial intubation, predominantly of the right mainstem bronchus, occurs in approximately 5% of cases.[45,46] Radiographic evaluation of tube placement should be accomplished with knowledge of head and neck position. Movement of the tube 2 cm either cephalad or caudad is common with flexion and extension of the head.

Current cost-cutting strategies frequently call for less frequent chest radiographs. However, in many cases, tube malposition occurs many days after the initial intubation.[45-47] In patients at risk for tube movement (frequent movement, transport) daily chest radiographs remain important for ensuring adequate position. Additional assessments, including checking position at the gums, evaluating breath sounds, and cuff palpation, may be used when chest radiographs are unavailable. Table 3-1 compares techniques for assessment of ETT placement.

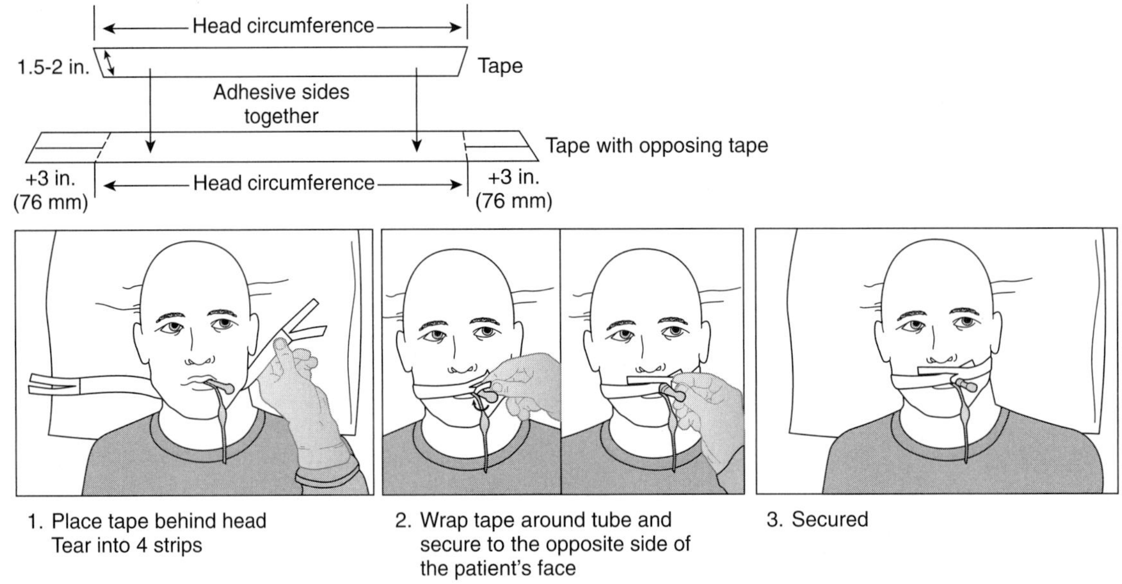

FIGURE 3-8 A method for using adhesive tape to secure an ETT.

Securing the Tube

Once tube placement has been verified, the ETT should be secured to prevent accidental extubation or migration of the tube. Unplanned extubation can result from self-extubation or accidental extubation. In the former, the patient removes the tube because of anxiety or agitation. In the latter, the tube is removed inadvertently during patient movement, transport, or positioning. The incidence of unplanned extubation ranges from 2% to 13%.[48-59] Boulain and colleagues evaluated the factors associated with unplanned extubation and found the four most frequent attributes were lack of intravenous sedation, chronic respiratory failure (prolonged intubation time), oral tube placement, and use of adhesive tape to secure the tube.[49] The use of adhesive tape also generally means that no tube-securing protocol was in place. Efforts to reduce the incidence of unplanned extubations have been instituted in the form of continuous quality improvement programs. In several cases, the use of properly controlled sedation and an ETT fixation protocol resulted in reduced rates of unplanned extubations.[49,57,59]

Methods for securing the ETT range from the very simple to application of specialty devices manufactured specifically for this purpose. Adhesive tape is a common, simple method for securing the ETT (Figure 3-8). This is best accomplished using 1-inch tape of moderate strength. A length of tape twice that necessary to encircle the patient's head is cut, and a second piece 6 to 8 inches in length is placed across the midportion in the opposite position. This second piece of tape prevents the original piece from sticking to the patient's hair and neck. This piece may be extended in patients with facial hair. Benzoin or another skin protective substance should be placed wherever the tape comes in direct contact with the patient's skin. Each end of the tape should be torn longitudinally, leaving four pieces of tape 2 to 3 inches in length. Each of these tape sections is wrapped around the ETT and resecured to the patient's face. If a bite block is used, it should be taped separately. The tape should be placed firmly around the patient's head, but binding of the skin should be prevented. The tape should be changed when soiled or aesthetically unpleasing, or when changing edema of the face results in the tape being either too loose or too tight.

Other techniques for securing the ETT include the use of cloth tape, sometimes called trach tape or twill tape. This cloth tape is wrapped around the head, looped around the tube, and tied in a bow near the patient's cheek. Other securing devices are available that use Velcro, plastic, or metal retaining devices.[60-62] These devices vary in the ability to secure the tube, prevent skin breakdown, and allow for effective mouth care. Success with any device often is predicated on clinician experience and preference.

Adequate tube fixation is crucial to prevent tube migration and unplanned extubation, facilitate mouth care, and prevent skin breakdown. Each of these should be considered when choosing a fixation device. Patient comfort also plays an important role, dictating the need for a fixation method that is as unobtrusive as possible and the judicious use of sedation in these patients.

Special Endotracheal Tubes

ETTs are designed for a number of special situations. These include wire-reinforced tubes, tubes for laser surgery, specially shaped tubes to improve the operative field, and tubes for high frequency ventilation. During mechanical ventilation in the ICU, two new types of ETTs have been introduced. These are the **silver-coated** or **silver-impregnated tube** and the **subglottic suction tube.**

Silver-Coated or Silver-Impregnated Endotracheal Tubes

Silver has long been appreciated for its bacteriostatic properties. In fact, older clinicians will remember a time when all tracheostomy tubes were silver or silver plated over stainless steel. Silver-coated or silver-impregnated urinary catheters and central venous catheters have been used for over a decade. Silver has other medically useful properties including prevention of biofilm formation, a reduction in bacterial burden, and reduction in inflammation.[63-71] To test the potential bacterial burden reduction in the respiratory tract with silver-coated ETTs, Olson et al performed an experimental study in 11 ventilated dogs.[68] They reported that silver-coated tubes reduced biofilm formation, with a significant lumen-narrowing difference between both tubes. Five of six of the noncoated tubes (83%) and none (zero) of the five coated tubes (0%) had a narrowing of greater than 50%. Coated tubes not only reduced the bacterial burden, with a statistically minor risk of colonization, but also delayed the duration of luminal side colonization from 1.8 ± 0.4 to 3.2 ± 0.8 days. This beneficial effect was correlated with a decline in the degree of histologic grade of lung parenchyma inflammation.

A prospective, randomized study has recently been completed, testing silver-coated ETTs in ICU patients. The main objective was to determine whether silver-coated ETTs reduce the incidence and/or delay the time of onset of colonization, compared to noncoated ETTs in mechanically ventilated patients. In this study the proportion of patient days with quantitative endotracheal aspirates greater than 10^5 CFU and greater than 10^6 CFU was greater among patients with uncoated ETTs. Upon removal, microbial burden was found to be 55.9×10^6 CFU/ml and 38.8×10^6 CFU/ml in control and silver-coated ETTs, respectively. In this pilot study, blood silver analysis was determined on day 1 and when the patient was extubated. No increase in blood silver or loss from the ETT was found. These data suggest that silver-coated ETTs are safe, reduce bacterial biofilm formation, can delay airway colonization, and may significantly reduce the endotracheal lumen-narrowing effect observed in patients who require long-term mechanical ventilation.

A prospective, randomized, phase II pilot study has recently been completed testing silver-coated ETTs in ICU patients.[71] The main objective was to determine whether silver-coated ETTs reduce the incidence, and/or delay the time of onset, of colonization when compared with noncoated ETTs in mechanically ventilated patients. The results of this study also demonstrate a significant reduction in microbiologic burden associated with silver-coated ETTs. The high level of bacterial concentration in the inner surface of a standard ETT can play a role in the development of late-onset VAP when biofilm fragmentation occurs. This fragmentation can be facilitated during instillation of saline and airway suctioning.

Subglottic Suction Endotracheal Tubes

Silent aspiration of oral secretions around the ETT cuff has been implicated as playing a primary role in the pathogenesis of **ventilator associated pneumonia (VAP).** Removal of secretions above the cuff has been shown to reduce the incidence of early VAP.[71-78] This procedure is typically referred to as subglottic secretion drainage (SSD) and is performed with a special ETT (Hi-Lo Evac, Mallinckrodt, Tyco Healthcare, Calif.) This special ETT has a second lumen embedded in the body of the tube that opens just above the ETT cuff on the posterior aspect (Figures 3-9 and 3-10). This lumen can be connected to continuous low wall suction (70 mm Hg) or aspirated intermittently. Studies of SSD suggest a reduction in early VAP and a potential cost savings. This is important as the cost of the Hi-Lo Evac tube is 10 to 15 times greater than that of a standard ETT.

Early practical issues with the SSD tube include placement in patients at risk and maintaining patency of the SSD lumen. At the bedside, monitoring and care of the Hi-Lo Evac tube should include:

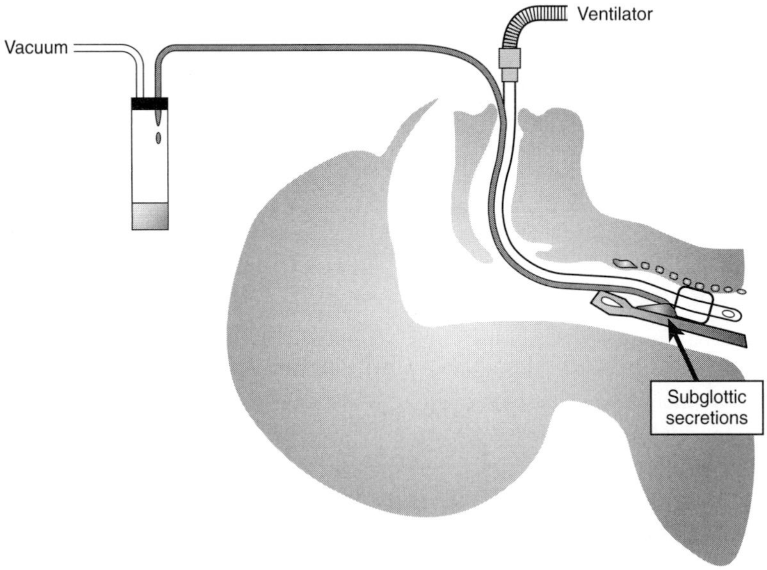

FIGURE 3-9 Placement of the Hi-Lo Evac tube for continuous subglottic secretion drainage.

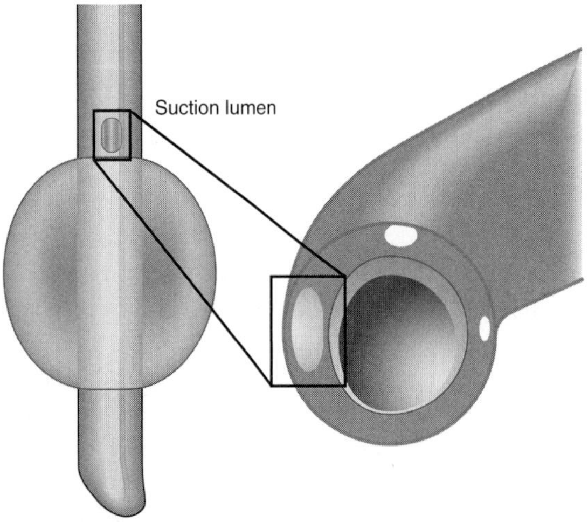

FIGURE 3-10 Position of the port for subglotic secretion drainage above the cuff and cut-away of the Hi-Lo Evac tube demonstrating the lumen for subglottic secretion drainage.

- continuous aspiration with 70 mm Hg (100 cm of water).
- monitor ETT cuff pressure every four hours to maintain 25 to 30 cm H_2O.
- check lumen patency every 4 hours by injecting 2 to 4 ml of air via syringe.
- check lumen patency if no secretions are recovered in the mucus collector.

Oral Care

The realization that early VAP results from the aspiration of oropharyngeal secretions has led a number of authors to re-evaluate the role of mouth care in reducing VAP. A number of studies using chlorhexidine, hydrogen peroxide, and other cleaners have been evaluated. The evidence remains inconclusive as to the role of effective mouth care in preventing VAP. Clearly, good oral hygiene cannot be a detriment to the patient and as such should be practiced in the ICU. More interestingly, the role of bacteria-laden dental plaque in VAP is being evaluated.[79-84]

Management of the Endotracheal Tube Cuff

The use of ETTs to facilitate mechanical ventilation is, by historical standards, a fairly modern technique. Advantages of the ETT were offset by problems associated with pressure exerted by the ETT cuff on the tracheal mucosa.[85-88] Early tubes used the so-called low-volume, high-pressure cuffs that exerted high pressures on the tracheal wall, occluding mucosal blood flow. Under normal conditions, the perfusion pressure of the tracheal mucosa (capillary pressure) is 25 to 35 mm Hg.[89] However, it should be noted that in patients with shock, sepsis, and hypotension this value may be considerably lower. Current standards suggest that the pressure in the new high-volume, low-pressure cuffs should be kept at less than

25 mm Hg to prevent mucosal damage. Lower pressures are associated with less damage but also are associated with silent aspiration around and through folds in the cuff.[68,69] This aspiration has been shown to be more prevalent at pressures less than 20 mm Hg. Aspiration of oropharyngeal secretions is responsible for nosocomial pneumonia and should be avoided. Given this small range of function, it seems prudent to maintain cuff pressures between 20 and 25 mm Hg.

Techniques for determining the adequate volume for filling the cuff include the **minimal leak** and **minimal seal techniques.**[90] The minimal seal technique also frequently is called the **minimal occlusion technique.** Both these techniques use the auscultation of air leak during inspiration around the cuff. The minimal leak technique adjusts cuff inflation volume such that at end inspiration there is a small leak of air around the cuff. This leak is sometimes audible to the naked ear but is best heard using a stethoscope placed over the trachea. Commonly, stethoscope placement for best sound detection is just above the suprasternal notch. Minimal seal or occlusion is one step past the minimal leak technique. That is, additional volume from a syringe is added to the cuff until the leak no longer can be heard. The minimal leak technique uses the lowest cuff pressure and therefore is thought to reduce tracheal damage compared with the minimal seal method. However, the minimal seal method is conceptually superior to the minimal leak method with respect to preventing silent aspiration. The minimal seal technique also facilitates mechanical ventilation, improves monitoring of respiratory mechanics, and reduces nuisance alarms. Our preference has been to use the minimal seal technique because the risk of nosocomial pneumonia from aspiration of oropharyngeal secretions is of more immediate concern than damage to the tracheal mucosa.

Monitoring Cuff Pressure

Measuring pressure within the ETT cuff is a standard of care. Cuff pressures should be monitored routinely and the results recorded on the patient's chart. The frequency of cuff pressure measurement is not well defined. Ideally, cuff pressure should be measured and recorded at least once a day. If the tube is repositioned, if a leak occurs, or if volume is added or removed from the cuff, cuff pressure should be reassessed. The measurement of cuff pressure typically is accomplished after the minimal seal technique has been used. That is, although it is desirable to maintain cuff pressure below tracheal mucosa perfusion pressure, higher pressure may be required to prevent air leaks and silent aspiration.

Measuring cuff pressure can be accomplished by a variety of means, and several commercial devices are available for this purpose. Cuff pressures typically are measured using a syringe, a three-way stopcock, and an aneroid pressure gauge. This method is easily accomplished with equipment commonly stocked in the intensive care unit. Figure 3-11 shows the system recommended for cuff pressure measurement. By using a three-way stopcock, the volume of the air in the cuff can be increased or decreased while pressure is measured continuously. Cuff pressure is affected by compliance of the cuff, volume of air inserted into the cuff, and airway pressure in the ventilator circuit. In fact, increases in airway pressure during inspiration are followed closely by increases in cuff pressure. In many circumstances, elevated cuff pressures must be tolerated to ensure adequate ventilation. Careful monitoring of the cuff pressure and using the minimum volume that maintains a seal should be accomplished frequently whenever cuff pressure exceeds 25 mm Hg.[91-93]

Cuff pressures can be elevated for many reasons. One of the most common causes of elevated cuff pressure is placement of an ETT of incorrect size. When a tube that is too small is inserted into the trachea, the cuff must be expanded to its maximum volume to form a seal. Careful choice of an appropriately sized tube is paramount in avoiding this problem. The volume of an individual tracheal tube cuff is selected to maintain pressures less than 25 mm Hg. If this volume is exceeded, cuff pressures increase rapidly. The maximum volume of a cuff is easily measured by filling the cuff with air before placement in the patient and recording the volume at which pressure less than 25 mm Hg is maintained. This is not best accomplished during an emergency intubation.

Other causes of elevated cuff pressures include malposition of the tube, overinflation of the cuff, and tracheomalacia.[93] Tube malposition, particularly migration cephalad into the larynx, requires that a greater volume be placed in the cuff to seal the larger diameter upper airway. Despite concern over cuff pressure and the production of tubes with low-pressure, high-volume cuffs, certain surgical procedures such as laser surgery require tubes with low-volume, high-pressure cuffs. Anode tubes are used during laser surgery. When these tubes are left in postoperatively, cuff pressures are high. Replacement of the tube is typically the only remedy to this problem.

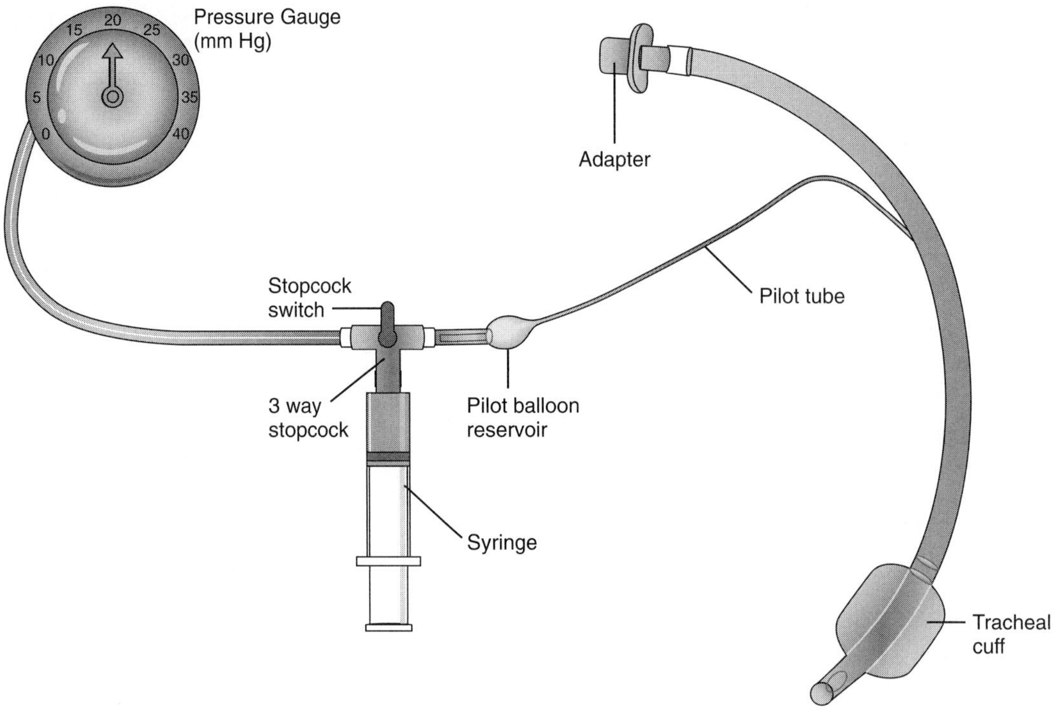

FIGURE 3-11 The system used for cuff pressure measurement.

In the course of mechanical ventilation, it is not unusual for the pilot balloon or the cuff of the tube to leak, or the pilot tube to be severed or nicked.[94] The latter commonly is caused when patients are shaved and the razor lacerates the pilot tube. Cuff leaks are less common if the tube is cared for properly. Laceration of the cuff occurs most often during nasotracheal intubation. As the tube passes through the nasal turbinates, the cuff can become ruptured. If the pilot balloon develops a leak, placing a stopcock into the port and closing it to the patient can identify this problem. If the leak persists, the problem is not in the pilot balloon. In critically ill patients, incompetent pilot balloons or leaks in the pilot tube can be overcome using a host of methods. These include severing the pilot balloon, placing a blunt needle into the pilot tube, and running a continuous flow of gas through the pilot tube to maintain the cuff inflated. This latter method requires adequate humidification of the gas to prevent drying of secretions. This method should also be considered a temporizing measure until reintubation can be accomplished safely.[95,96]

SUCTIONING

Removal of tracheobronchial and upper airway secretions to maintain airway patency and reduce the risk of silent aspiration is also a standard of care.[92] The use of routine suctioning should be avoided. Assessment of the patient, including auscultation, palpation, and visual inspection, should be used to determine the need for endotracheal suctioning. Endotracheal suctioning is associated with a litany of complications and should be undertaken only when necessary, keeping the potential complications in mind.[92]

Suction catheters vary greatly in design but have the same general characteristics (Figure 3-12). Most catheters are 56 cm in length to allow the catheter to travel into the mainstem bronchi. The distal tip of the catheter has several openings for secretion removal, and the proximal portion contains a thumb port that is occluded by the practitioner to activate the suction. The distal tip of the catheter should be blunt to avoid trauma to the mucosa and possible perforation of the tracheobronchial tree. The side holes in the distal tip of the catheter also serve to limit local tissue damage. If the catheter had a single

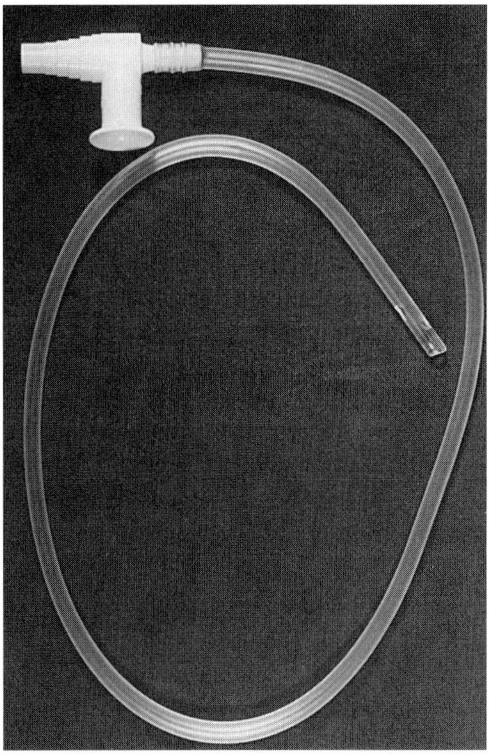

FIGURE 3-12 A standard suction catheter.

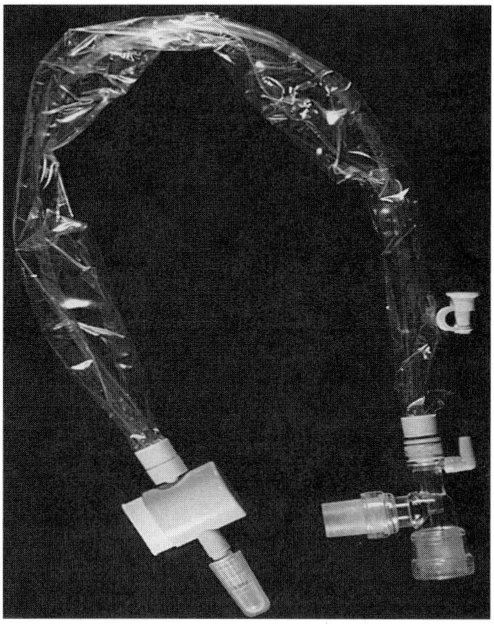

FIGURE 3-13 A closed circuit suction catheter.

opening in the distal end, the mucosa could be drawn into the catheter tip and torn during withdrawal of the catheter. The addition of side holes helps eliminate this problem. Suction catheters should be transparent to allow visual inspection of secretions, rigid enough to pass through the ETT, yet pliable enough to traverse airway structures without damaging mucosa.

In the last decade, **closed circuit suction catheters** have become popular for a number of reasons (Figure 3-13). These include prevention of problems associated with disconnecting the patient from the ventilator, reduced costs, and reduced exposure of caregivers to infectious materials. Comparisons of closed and open circuit suctioning techniques suggest that there is no difference in the ability of each device to evacuate secretions.[97-99] Because the patient does not need to be disconnected from the ventilator when closed circuit suctioning is used, several authors have suggested that this device reduces complications associated with the suctioning procedure.[100,101] These investigations have produced disparate results. Taken together, however, these authors appear to suggest that closed circuit suctioning reduces the incidence of dysrhythmias and desaturation when compared with open circuit suctioning.

Manufacturers of closed circuit suction devices have often claimed that these devices reduce patient and caregiver contamination. This contention is supported by two studies that, although not conclusive, appear to favor closed circuit suctioning for reducing caregiver exposure.[102,103] Many institutions have adopted the use of closed circuit suctioning systems for all mechanically ventilated patients. Additionally, the desire for caregivers to be protected from exposure to secretions also forces this issue.

The cost of closed circuit suction devices is considerably greater than that of open circuit devices. However, this is the out-of-box cost. Prolonged use of closed circuit catheters in patients requiring frequent suctioning attempts actually can result in cost savings. As with ventilator circuit changes, conventional wisdom and several recent studies suggest that these devices need only be changed weekly. The longer the duration of use, the more cost-effective closed circuit suctioning becomes.[104-113]

Bronchial Suctioning

During routine endotracheal suctioning, the suction catheter most likely enters the right mainstem bronchus if the catheter is advanced far enough. This is

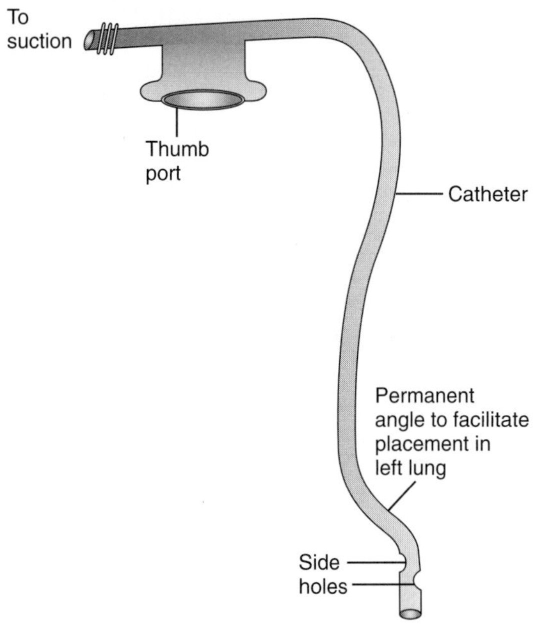

FIGURE 3-14 A catheter for selective suctioning of the left lung.

caused by the more acute angle of the left mainstem bronchus at the carina compared with the right mainstem, which is almost a direct shot. As such, the left lung is less likely to be suctioned. Attempts at suctioning the left mainstem have been described and range all the way from simple maneuvers to use of special catheters.[114-116] One simple way of suctioning the left mainstem bronchus is by turning the head to the right in an attempt to increase the likelihood of passage of the catheter into the left mainstem. The same effect may be gained by placing the patient in the left lateral position and attempting to use gravity to further the catheter's passage.

Specialized catheters using a curved tip have been shown to enter the left mainstem bronchus in up to 90% of cases (Figure 3-14). The success of bronchial suctioning can be affected by tube position, patient body and head position, and type of tube (ETT vs. tracheostomy tube). We have not found selective endobronchial suctioning to be a necessary routine technique. Frequent changes in patient body position facilitate movement of secretions to the carina, where they can be suctioned. In patients with infectious processes confined to the left lung, selective endobronchial suctioning may prove useful.

Use of Saline Instillation

During the suctioning procedure, it is common for practitioners to instill 5 to 10 ml of normal saline in an attempt to thin tracheobronchial secretions. This practice remains a point of contention, and studies have failed to show any advantage of saline instillation.[117-123] Our own studies of humidification techniques reveal that the only correlation between saline instillation and patient care is practitioner preference. That is, our research fails to show that saline instillation is used uniformly or has any benefit in terms of liquefying secretions. Saline instillation frequently does cause the patient to cough violently, which may aid in the secretion removal process. From a conceptual standpoint, this practice makes sense, but the current literature does not support the use of saline instillation. From a mucus rheology perspective, the properties of mucus are unlikely to change with the addition of water unless some physical means of mixing the two is accomplished. There appear to be no real contraindications to using saline. However, severe coughing episodes and bronchospasm occasionally may result from the instillation of saline. There is also some concern that the use of saline may dislodge bacteria-laden biofilm from the ETT, resulting in infectious consequences. Given this evidence, the use of saline to thin secretions currently is unsupported.

Complications of Suctioning

The long list of complications associated with endotracheal suctioning is frequently studied in an effort to arrive at methods that minimize patient discomfort and instability. These complications include hypoxemia, cardiac arrhythmias, trauma to the airway mucosa, and atelectasis. Contamination of the lower airway of the patient also may occur during suctioning if appropriate techniques are not used. Contamination of health care providers exposed to secretions is also of concern.[124-135]

Hypoxemia is by far the most frequent complication of endotracheal suctioning.[124-128] The causes of hypoxemia during suctioning are multifactorial. These include the obvious, such as disconnection of mechanical ventilation and the resultant loss of PEEP, decreased FIO_2, and lack of ventilator assistance. Suctioning also reduces lung volume by evacuating gas from the lung and entrains room air into the airway. The duration of suctioning is directly related to the frequency and severity of these problems. Generally speaking, the suctioning procedure should last only 10 to 15 seconds. A rule of thumb that helps limit the duration of suctioning is for the clinician to hold his or her breath during the procedure. When the clinician begins to feel air hungry, the patient certainly is, and the procedure should be ended.[129]

TABLE 3-2 *Complications of Endotracheal Suctioning Procedures and Methods to Avoid Those Complications*

COMPLICATIONS OF ENDOTRACHEAL SUCTIONING	METHODS TO AVOID COMPLICATIONS OF ENDOTRACHEAL SUCTIONING
• Hypoxemia	• Hyperoxygenation
• Airway trauma, bleeding	• Hyperinflation
• Cardiac arrhythmias	• Limit procedure to 10-15 sec
• Derecruitment, atelectasis	• Apply suction only during withdrawal
• Bronchospasm	• Limit vacuum pressure to <150 mm Hg
• Airway contamination	• Use a closed circuit suction catheter
• Elevated intracranial pressure	• Do not instill saline
• Coughing	• Use the appropriate sized suction catheter
	• Use care on insertion
	• Use a catheter with side holes

Avoiding hypoxemia during suctioning typically is accomplished by hyperoxygenation before the procedure.[124] This can be accomplished by manually ventilating the patient with an F_{IO_2} of 1.0 before the procedure, increasing the F_{IO_2} on the ventilator to 1.0 before the procedure, or using the hyperoxygenation program of the ventilator (usually a preprogrammed increase in F_{IO_2} followed by an automatic return to the previous F_{IO_2} after 2 to 3 minutes). Manual hyperinflation or sighs from the ventilator also may be used.[124-128] This type of hyperinflation therapy has fallen out of favor recently with the improved understanding of overdistention lung injury. We believe that manual ventilation is less effective and associated with more frequent complications than the use of manually triggered breaths from the ventilator. The use of manual resuscitators results in unstable tidal volume, F_{IO_2}, and minute volume. In fact, manual ventilation commonly is associated with a reduction in delivered tidal volume, rapid increase in respiratory rate, and elevated airway pressures. This combination can result in hemodynamic compromise during the manual hyperinflation procedure.

Arrhythmias commonly are seen with suctioning procedures and may be caused by hypoxemia, vagal stimulation, or both.[129-134] The use of hyperoxygenation before suctioning can help eliminate this problem. Sudden disconnection of a patient from PEEP also may cause arrhythmias because venous return is suddenly unimpeded. Closed circuit suction devices should be used when this problem is identified. Mucosal trauma from suction catheters generally results from overzealous suctioning or use of a catheter that is too rigid or has a pointed tip. As previously discussed, the use of a blunt-tipped catheter with multiple side holes reduces this problem. Proper setting of the negative pressure (less than 150 mm Hg) used for suctioning is also important.

Other complications include atelectasis, coughing, bronchospasm, and, in head-injured patients, an increase in intracranial pressure.[134-137] From the patient's side of the suction catheter, suctioning is at best uncomfortable and at worst unbearable. Irritation of the airway causes coughing, and hypoxemia can promote anxiety and dyspnea. Preoxygenation, proper suctioning technique, and careful patient monitoring are important in limiting these complications.

The issue of contamination during the suctioning procedure is often an emotional one. The procedure should be performed using the sterile technique to prevent contamination of the lower respiratory tract. Contamination of the clinician should be avoided by use of universal precautions. Despite some level of concern, contamination of caregivers during suctioning procedures has never been documented to result in illness. Table 3-2 lists complications of endotracheal suctioning and methods to avoid these complications.

PATIENT-VENTILATOR SYSTEM CHECK

Checking the ventilator has long been an important role for the respiratory care practitioner. This task or procedure recently has been redefined by the American Association for Respiratory Care (AARC) in a clinical practice guideline.[138] It should be remembered that the patient-ventilator system check need not always be recorded. Checks should be recorded on a regularly scheduled basis based on patient acuity. The guidelines suggest that in addition to regularly scheduled intervals, checks should be performed before obtaining blood gas values, before obtaining hemodynamic or respiratory mechanics data, after a change in settings (except F_{IO_2}), after an acute deterioration in patient condition, or any time the performance of the ventilator is in question. This system was adopted to allow stable patients to receive documented patient-ventilator system checks every 6 hours or more. In a critically ill patient requiring numerous manipulations and frequent blood gas determinations, patient-ventilator system checks might be done every hour. It is also crucial to remember that a patient-ventilator system check is not merely a verification of ventilator settings. It also includes documentation of patient response to ventilation and evaluation of breath sounds, tube placement, cuff pressure, and results of suctioning. The term "patient-ventilator system" emphasizes that the patient is the most important component of the system. Every patient-ventilator check should include assessment of the patient.

Akhtar et al recently reviewed documentation procedures accomplished by respiratory care departments around the United States.[139] They found significant variation of documentation with the guideline and with the current best evidence. As an example, the measurement of plateau pressure is not required and there is no mention of spontaneous breathing trials. This AARC guideline is currently under review and in the interim, documentation of the patient-ventilator system check should reflect the current best practices based on the available evidence.

KEY POINTS

- Compressible volume lost in the ventilator circuit can result in a reduction in the delivered tidal volume with respect to the set tidal volume.
- Compressible volume may be automatically compensated for with certain ventilators.
- Failure to account for compressible volume can invalidate compliance measurements.
- A high-resistance expiratory valve may increase the inspiratory work of breathing.
- The active exhalation valve allows the patient to breathe spontaneously during both the inspiratory and expiratory phases of the mandatory ventilator breath.
- The presence of an active expiratory valve prevents the clinician from limiting the delivered tidal volume.
- Following endotracheal intubation the presence of CO_2 in the exhaled breath is the standard for determining ETT placement.
- Following endotracheal intubation the clinician should use a number of methods to assure the proper placement of the tube.
- A silver-coated ETT is associated with a reduction in biofilm and tube obstructions.
- The use of a subglottic secretion drainage ETT reduces the incidence of early ventilator associated pneumonia.

ASSESSMENT QUESTIONS

1. Which of the following variables are required to calculate the compressible volume during mechanical ventilation?
   - **I.** Tidal volume
   - **II.** Ventilator circuit compliance in ml/cm H_2O
   - **III.** Peak airway pressure
   - **IV.** PEEP
   - **V.** Inspiratory time
     - **A.** I, II, and IV
     - **B.** II and III
     - **C.** II, III, and IV
     - **D.** All of the above
2. Failure to account for compressible volume results in errors in the calculation of what variables?
   - **I.** Tidal volume
   - **II.** Pulmonary compliance
   - **III.** Airway resistance
   - **IV.** Auto-PEEP
     - **A.** I, III, and IV
     - **B.** II, III, and IV
     - **C.** I and II
     - **D.** I, II, and IV
3. True or False. A ventilator that automatically compensates for compressible volume must by definition deliver a tidal volume larger than the set tidal volume.

ASSESSMENT QUESTIONS—cont'd

4. True or False. Compressible volume is not a concern during pressure control ventilation.
5. During display of the expiratory flow curve, a "spike" at the beginning of exhalation may result from?
   A. The circuit emptying the compressible volume
   B. Too large a tidal volume
   C. Too high an inspiratory flow
   D. The circuit emptying auto-PEEP
6. An active exhalation valve system has what characteristics?
   I. Allows spontaneous inspiration during the mechanical inspiratory time
   II. Maintains pressure constant
   III. Maintains tidal volume constant
   IV. Allows exhalation during the mechanical inspiratory time
   A. I and III
   B. I, II, and IV
   C. I and II
   D. II and IV
7. An exhalation valve with a high expiratory resistance can cause which of the following?
   I. Reduced work of breathing
   II. Increased work of breathing
   III. Expiratory retard
   IV. Incorrect tidal volume
   A. I and II
   B. I and III
   C. I and IV
   D. All of the above
8. True or False. The characteristics of the exhalation valve can affect the inspiratory work of breathing.
9. Which of the following methods are used to determine appropriate ETT placement?
   I. Airway pressure
   II. CO_2 detectors
   III. Chest radiograph
   IV. Capnometry
   V. Esophageal detector device
   VI. Auscultation of breath sounds
   VII. Expired O_2 concentration
   A. All of the above
   B. II, III, V, and VII only
   C. II, IV, V, and VI only
   D. II, III, IV, V, and VI only
   E. I, II, III, IV, V, and VI only
10. True or False. Instillation of saline in the ETT has been shown to improve secretion removal.
11. Closed circuit suctioning has what potential advantages?
    I. Reduction in environmental contamination
    II. Maintenance of PEEP
    III. Prevention of hypoxemia
    IV. Lower bacterial contamination
    A. I, II, and III only
    B. All of the above
    C. II and III only
    D. I and IV only
12. Which of the following are known complications of endotracheal suctioning?
    I. Bradycardia
    II. Hypoxemia
    III. Hypotension
    IV. Mucosal trauma
    A. I, II, and III only
    B. II and III only
    C. II, III, and IV only
    D. All of the above
13. Silver-coated or silver-impregnated ETTs may reduce airway colonization owing to the ___ properties of silver.
    A. Bactericidal
    B. Antibacterial
    C. Aseptic
    D. Bacteriostatic
14. Advantages of a silver-coated or silver-impregnated tube include:
    I. Reduction in secretions
    II. Reduction in bacterial colonization
    III. Reduced biofilm on the inner lumen of the tube
    IV. Prevention of VAP
    A. I, II, and III
    B. II, III, and IV
    C. I, III, and IV
    D. II and IV
15. The special ETT for removal of subglottic secretions has been proven to
    A. reduce the incidence of early VAP.
    B. reduce the incidence of late VAP.
    C. reduce the incidence of both early and late VAP.
    D. reduce ETT occlusion.

Continued

ASSESSMENT QUESTIONS—cont'd

16. The primary purpose of the patient ventilator system check is
- **A.** to verify the settings.
- **B.** to verify that the settings have not changed since the last check.
- **C.** to evaluate the patient's response to mechanical ventilation.
- **D.** to avoid lawsuits.

17. During a patient ventilator system check, which of the following should be recorded?
- **I.** Current alarm settings
- **II.** Current ventilation parameter settings (e.g., tidal volume, PEEP, etc.)
- **III.** Patient ventilator synchrony
- **IV.** Airway pressures
- **V.** Breath sounds
- **VI.** Results of suctioning procedures (volume, color, and consistency of secretions)
- **A.** I, II, III, and IV
- **B.** All of the above
- **C.** I, II, III, IV, and VI
- **D.** I, II, IV, V, and VIA, B, D, E, and F

REFERENCES

1. Hess D, Burns E, Romangnoli D et al: Weekly ventilator circuit changes, Anesthesiology 82:903-911, 1995.
2. Kollef MH, Shapiro SD, Fraser VJ et al: Mechanical ventilation with or without 7-day circuit changes, Ann Intern Med 123:168-174, 1995.
3. Dreyfuss D, Djedani K, Gros I et al: Mechanical ventilation with heated humidifiers or heat and moisture exchangers: effects on patient colonization and incidence of nosocomial pneumonia, Am J Respir Crit Care Med 151:986-992, 1995.
4. Branson RD: The ventilator circuit and ventilator associated pneumonia, Respir Care 50(6):774-785, 2005.
5. Hess DR, Kallstrom TJ, Mottram CD et al: American Association for Respiratory Care, Care of the ventilator circuit and its relation to ventilator-associated pneumonia, Respir Care 48(9):869-879, 2003.
6. Makhoul IR, Kassis I, Berant M et al: Frequency of change of ventilator circuit in premature infants: Impact on ventilator-associated pneumonia, Pediatr Crit Care Med 2(2):127-132, 2001.
7. Han JN, Liu YP, Ma S et al: Effects of decreasing the frequency of ventilator circuit changes to every 7 days on the rate of ventilator-associated pneumonia in a Beijing hospital, Respir Care 46(9):891-896, 2001.
8. Stamm AM: Ventilator-associated pneumonia and frequency of circuit changes, Am J Infect Control 26(1):71-73, 1998.
9. Boots RJ, George N, Faoagali JL et al: Double-heater-wire circuits and heat-and-moisture exchangers and the risk of ventilator-associated pneumonia, Crit Care Med 34(3):687-693, 2006.
10. Sanborn WG: Microprocessor based mechanical ventilation, Respir Care 38:72-109, 1993.
11. Branson RD, Campbell RS, Thompson D: Ventilator circuits: what you see may not be what you get, Respir Care 36:629-630, 1991.
12. Banner MJ, Lampotang S, Boysen PG et al: Flow resistance of expiratory pressure valve systems, Chest 90:212-217, 1986.
13. Banner MJ: Expiratory positive pressure valves: flow resistance and the work of breathing, Respir Care 32:431-439, 1987.
14. Marini JJ, Culver BH, Kirk W: Flow resistance of exhalation valves and positive end-expiratory pressure devices used in mechanical ventilation, Surgery 131:850-854, 1985.
15. Pinsky MR, Hrehocik D, Culpepper JA: Flow resistance of expiratory positive pressure systems, Chest 94:788-791, 1988.
16. Banner MJ, Lampotang S: End expiratory pressure valves. In: Branson RD, Hess D, Chatburn RL, editors: Respiratory care equipment, Philadelphia, JB Lippincott, 1998.
17. Birmingham PK, Cheney FW, Ward RJ: Esophageal intubation: a review of detection techniques, Anesth Analg 65:886-891, 1986.
18. Hess D: Monitoring during resuscitation, Respir Care 37:739-768, 1992.
19. Cardoso MSC, Banner MJ, Melker RJ et al: Portable devices used to detect endotracheal intubation during emergency situations: a review, Crit Care Med 26:957-964, 1998.
20. Murray IP, Modell JH: Early detection of endotracheal tube accidents by monitoring carbon dioxide concentration in respiratory gas, Anesthesiology 59:344-346, 1983.
21. Linko K, Paloheimo M, Tammisto T: Capnography for detection of accidental oesophageal intubation, Acta Anaesthesiol Scand 27:199-202, 1983.
22. Bhende MS, Thompson AE, Howland DF: Validity of a disposable end-tidal carbon dioxide detector in verifying endotracheal tube position in piglets, Crit Care Med 19:566-568, 1991.
23. Bhende MS, Thompson AE, Orr RA: Utility of an end-tidal carbon dioxide detector during stabilization and transport of critically ill children, Pediatrics 89:1042-1044, 1992.

24. Bhende MS: Colorimetric end-tidal carbon dioxide detector, Pediatr Emerg Care 11:58-61, 1995.
25. Goldberg JS, Rawle PR, Zehnder JL et al: Colorimetric end-tidal carbon dioxide monitoring for tracheal intubation, Anesth Analg 70:191-194, 1990.
26. Higgins DJ, Addy V: Efficacy of the FEF colorimetric end-tidal carbon dioxide detector in children, Anesth Analg 76:683-684, 1993.
27. Jones BR, Dorsey MJ: Sensitivity of a disposable end-tidal carbon dioxide detector, J Clin Monit 7:268-270, 1991.
28. O'Flaherty D, Adams AP: The end-tidal carbon dioxide detector: assessment of a new method to distinguish oesophageal from tracheal intubation, Anaesthesia 45:653-655, 1990.
29. Petroianu GA, Maleck WH, Bergler WF et al: Preliminary observations on the Colibri CO_2-indicator, Am J Emerg Med 16:677-680, 1998.
30. Barton C, Callaham M: Lack of correlation between end-tidal carbon dioxide concentrations and $PaCO_2$ in cardiac arrest, Crit Care Med 19:108-110, 1991.
31. Takeda T, Tanigawa K, Tanaka H et al: The assessment of three methods to verify tracheal tube placement in the emergency setting, Resuscitation Feb;56(2):153-157, 2003.
32. Kasper CL, Deem S: The self-inflating bulb to detect esophageal intubation during emergency airway management, Anesthesiology 88:898-902, 1998.
33. Ardagh M, Moodie K: The esophageal detector device can give false positives for tracheal intubation, J Emerg Med 16:747-779, 1998.
34. Zaleski L, Abello D, Gold M: The esophageal detector device: does it work? Anesthesiology 79:244-247, 1993.
35. Williams KN, Nunn JF: The oesphageal detector device: a prospective trial on 100 patients, Anaesthesia 44:412-414, 1989.
36. Wee M: The oesphageal detector device: assessment of a new method to distinguish oesphageal from tracheal intubation, Anaesthesia 43:27-29, 1988.
37. Pelucio M, Halligan L, Dhindsa H: Out-of-hospital experience with the syringe esophageal detector device, Acad Emerg Med 4:463-468, 1997.
38. Donahue PL: The esophageal detector device: an assessment of accuracy and ease of use by paramedics, Anaesthesia 49:863-865, 1994.
39. Gray P, Sullivan G, Ostryzniuk P et al: Value of postprocedural chest radiographs in the adult intensive care unit, Crit Care Med 20:1513-1518, 1992.
40. Henschke CI, Yankelevitz DF, Wand A, et al: Accuracy and efficacy of chest radiography in the intensive care unit, Intensive Care Radiol 34:21-31, 1996.
41. Eagle CCP: The relationship between a person's height and appropriate endotracheal tube length, Anaesth Intensive Care 20:156-160, 1992.
42. Owen RL, Cheney FW: Endobronchial intubation: a preventable complication, Anesthesiology 67:255-257, 1987.
43. Roberts JR, Spadafora M, Cone DC: Proper depth placement of oral endotracheal tubes in adults prior to radiographic confirmation, Acad Emerg Med 2:20-24, 1995.
44. Conrardy PA, Goodman LR, Lainge F et al: Alteration of endotracheal tube position: flexion and extension of the neck, Crit Care Med 4:8-12, 1976.
45. Kollef MH, Leagre EJ, Damiano M: Endotracheal tube misplacement: incidence, risk factors, and impact of a quality improvement program, South Med J 87:248-254, 1994.
46. Schwarts DE, Lieberman JA, Cohen NH: Women are at greater risk than men for malpositioning of the endotracheal tube after emergent intubation, Crit Care Med 22:1127-1131, 1994.
47. Brunel W, Coleman DL, Schwartz DE et al: Assessment of routine chest roentgenograms and the physical examination to confirm endotracheal tube position, Chest 96:1043-1045, 1989.
48. Tominga GT, Rudzwick H, Scannell G et al: Decreasing unplanned extubations in the intensive care unit, Am J Surg 170:586-590, 1995.
49. Boulain T: Unplanned extubations in the adult intensive care unit: a prospective multicenter study, Am J Respir Crit Care Med 157:1131-1137, 1998.
50. Listello D, Sessler CN: Unplanned extubation: clinical predictors for reintubation, Chest 105:1496-1503, 1994.
51. Christie JM, Dethlefsen M, Cane RD: Unplanned endotracheal extubation in the intensive care unit, J Clin Anesth 8:289-293, 1996.
52. Vassal T, Anh NG, Gabillet JM et al: Prospective evaluation of self-extubations in a medical intensive care unit, Intensive Care Med 19:340-342, 1993.
53. Taggart JA, Lind MA: Evaluating unplanned endotracheal intubations, Dimens Crit Care Nurse 13:114-121, 1994.
54. Whelen J, Simpson SQ, Levy H: Unplanned extubation: predictors of successful termination of mechanical ventilatory support, Chest 105:1808-1812, 1995.
55. Coppolo DP, May JJ: Self-extubations: a 12-month experience, Chest 98:165-169, 1990.
56. Atkins PM, Mion LC, Mendelson W et al: Characteristics and outcomes of patients who self-extubate from ventilatory support: a case-control study, Chest 112:1317-1323, 1997.
57. Betbase A, Perez M, Rialp G et al: A prospective study of unplanned endotracheal extubation in intensive care unit patients, Crit Care Med 26:1180-1186, 1998.
58. Chiang AA, Lee KC, Lee JC et al: Effectiveness of a continuous quality improvement program aiming to reduce unplanned extubation: a prospective study, Intensive Care Med 22:1269-1271, 1996.
59. Sessler CN: Unplanned extubations: making progress using CQI, Intensive Care Med 23:143-145, 1997.
60. Kaplow R, Bookbinder M: A comparison of four endotracheal tube holders, Heart Lung 23:59-66, 1994.
61. Levy H, Griego L: A comparative study of oral endotracheal tube securing methods, Chest 104:1537-1540, 1993.

61a. Volsko TA, Chatburn RL: Comparison of two methods for securing the endotracheal tube in neonates, Respir Care 42:288-291, 1997.
62. Clarke T, Evans S, Way P et al: A comparison of two methods of securing an endotracheal tube, Aust Crit Care 11:45-50, 1998.
63. Balazs DJ, Triandafillu K, Wood P et al: Inhibition of bacterial adhesion on PVC endotracheal tubes by RF-oxygen glow discharge, sodium hydroxide and silver nitrate treatments, Biomaterials 25(11):2139-2151, 2004.
64. Hollinger MA: Toxicological aspects of topical silver pharmaceuticals, Crit Rev Toxicol 26(2):255-260, 1996.
65. Jansen B, Kohnen W: Prevention of biofilm formation by polymer modification, J Ind Microbiol 15(4):391-396, 1995.
66. Kumon H, Hashimoto H et al: Catheter-associated urinary tract infections: impact of catheter materials on their management, Int J Antimicrob Agents 17(4):311-316, 2002.
67. Diaz E, Rodriguez AH et al: Ventilator-associated pneumonia: issues related to the artificial airway, Respir Care 50(7):900-906, 2005.
68. Olson ME, Harmon BG et al: Silver-coated endotracheal tubes associated with reduced bacterial burden in the lungs of mechanically ventilated dogs, Chest 121(3):863-870, 2002.
69. Schierholz JM, Rump AF et al: Anti-infective catheters: novel strategies to prevent nosocomial infections in oncology, Anticancer Res 18(5B):3629-3638, 1998.
70. Hartmann M, Guttmann J, Muller B et al: Reduction of the bacterial load by the silver-coated endotracheal tube (SCET), a laboratory investigation, Technol Health Care 7(5):359-370, 1999.
71. Rello J, Kollef M, Diaz E et al: Reduced burden of bacterial airway colonization with a novel silver-coated endotracheal tube in a randomized multiple-center feasibility study, Crit Care Med 34(11):2766-2772, 2006.
72. Valles J, Artigas A, Rello J et al: Continuous aspiration of subglottic secretions in preventing ventilator-associated pneumonia, Ann Intern Med 122:179-186, 1995.
73. Kollef MH, Skubas NJ, Sundt TM: A randomized clinical trial of continuous aspiration of subglottic secretions in cardiac surgery patients, Chest 116:1339-1346, 1999.
74. Bo H, He L, Qu J: Influence of the subglottic secretion drainage on the morbidity of ventilator associated pneumonia in mechanically ventilated patients (in Chinese), Zhonghua Jie He He Hu Xi Za Ahi 23:472-474, 2000.
75. Smulders K, van der Hoeven H, Weers-Pothoff I et al: A randomized clinical trial of intermittent subglottic secretion drainage in patients receiving mechanical ventilation, Chest 121:858-862, 2002.
76. Dezfulian C, Shojania K, Collard HR et al: Subglottic secretion drainage for preventing ventilator-associated pneumonia: a meta-analysis, Am J Med 118:11-18, 2005.
77. Shorr AF, O'Malley PG: Continuous subglottic suctioning for the prevention of ventilator-associated pneumonia: potential economic implications, Chest 119:228-235, 2001.
78. Kollef MH, Skubas NJ, Sundt TM: A randomized clinical trial of continuous aspiration of subglottic secretions in cardiac surgery patients, Chest 116:1339-1346, 1999.
79. Ross A, Crumpler J: The impact of an evidence-based practice education program on the role of oral care in the prevention of ventilator-associated pneumonia, Intensive Crit Care Nurs 2007 Jan 2 [Epub ahead of print].
80. Koeman M, van der Ven AJ, Hak E et al: Oral decontamination with chlorhexidine reduces the incidence of ventilator-associated pneumonia, Am J Respir Crit Care Med 173(12):1348-1355, 2006.
81. Safdar N, Crnich CJ, Maki DG: The pathogenesis of ventilator-associated pneumonia: its relevance to developing effective strategies for prevention, Respir Care 50(6):725-739, 2005.
82. Brennan MT, Bahrani-Mougeot F, Fox PC et al: The role of oral microbial colonization in ventilator-associated pneumonia, Oral Surg Oral Med Oral Pathol Oral Radiol Endod 98(6):665-772, 2004.
83. van Nieuwenhoven CA, Buskens E, Bergmans DC: Oral decontamination is cost-saving in the prevention of ventilator-associated pneumonia in intensive care units, Crit Care Med 32(1):126-130, 2004.
84. Bergmans DC, Bonten MJ, Gaillard CA et al: Prevention of ventilator-associated pneumonia by oral decontamination: a prospective, randomized, double-blind, placebo-controlled study, Am J Respir Crit Care Med 164(3):382-388, 2001.
85. Cooper JD, Grillo HC: The evolution of tracheal injury due to ventilatory assistance through cuffed tubes: a pathologic study, Ann Surg 169:334-348, 1969.
86. Cooper JD, Grillo HC: Experimental production and prevention of injury due to cuffed tracheal tubes, Surg Gynecol Obstet 129:1235-1241, 1969.
87. Grillo HC, Cooper JD, Geffin B et al: A low-pressure cuff for tracheostomy tubes to minimize tracheal injury, J Thorac Cardiovasc Surg 62:898-907, 1971.
88. Knowlson GTG, Bassett HFM: The pressures exerted on the trachea by endotracheal inflatable cuffs, Br J Anaesth 42:834-837, 1970.
89. Dobrin P, Canfield T: Cuffed endotracheal tubes: mucosal and tracheal wall blood flow, Am J Surg 133:562-568, 1977.
90. Pavlin EG, Van Mimwegan D, Hornbein TF: Failure of a high-compliance low-pressure cuff to prevent aspiration, Anesthesiology 42:216-219, 1975.
91. Bernhard WN, Cottrell JE, Sivakumaran C et al: Adjustment of intracuff pressure to prevent aspiration, Anesthesiology 50:363-366, 1979.
92. Hess DR, Branson RD: Airway and suction equipment. In: Branson RD, Hess DR, Chatburn RL, editors: Respiratory care equipment, Philadelphia, Lippincott Williams and Wilkins, 1999, pp 157-186.
93. Crimlisk JT, Horn MH, Wilson DJ et al: Artificial airway: a survey of cuff management practices, Heart Lung 25:225-235, 1996.

94. Off D, Braun SR, Tompkins B et al: Efficacy of the minimal leak technique of cuff inflation in maintaining proper intracuff pressures for patients with cuffed artificial airways, Respir Care 28:1115-1118, 1983.
95. Cox PM, Schatz ME: Pressure measurements in endotracheal cuffs: a common error, Chest 65:84-87, 1974.
96. Ho AM, Contrardi LH: What to do when an endotracheal tube cuff leaks, J Trauma 40:486-487, 1990.
97. Witmer MT, Hess D, Simmons M: An evaluation of the effectiveness of secretion removal with the Ballard closed-circuit suction catheter, Respir Care 36:844-848, 1991.
98. Craig KC, Benson MS, Pierson DJ: Prevention of arterial oxygen desaturation during closed-airway endotracheal suction: effect of ventilator mode, Respir Care 29:1013-1018, 1984.
99. Carlon GC, Fox SJ, Ackerman NJ: Evaluation of a closed-tracheal suction system, Crit Care Med 15:522-525, 1987.
100. Johnson KL, Kearney PA, Johnson SB et al: Closed versus open tracheal suctioning: costs and physiologic consequences, Crit Care Med 22:654-666, 1994.
101. Hrashbarger SA, Hoffman LA, Zullo TG et al: Effects of a closed tracheal suction system on ventilatory and cardiovascular parameters, Am J Respir Crit Care Med 3:57-61, 1992.
102. Deppe SA, Kelly JW, Thoi LL et al: Incidence of colonization, nosocomial pneumonia, and mortality in critically ill patients using a Trach Care closed-suction system versus an open-suction system: prospective, randomized study, Crit Care Med 18:1389-1393, 1990.
103. Cobley M, Atkins M, Jones PL: Environmental contamination during tracheal suction, Anaesthesia 46:957-961, 1991.
104. Ritz R, Scott LR, Coyle MB et al: Contamination of a multiple-use suction catheter in a closed-circuit system compared to contamination of a disposable, single-use suction catheter, Respir Care 31:1086-1091, 1986.
105. Kollef MH, Prentice S, Shapiro SD et al: Mechanical ventilation with or without daily changes of in-line suction catheters, Am J Respir Crit Care Med 156:466-472, 1997.
106. Cereda M, Villa F, Colombo E et al: Closed system endotracheal suctioning maintains lung volume during volume-controlled mechanical ventilation, Intensive Care Med 27(4):648-654, 2001.
107. Maggiore SM, Lellouche F, Pigeot J et al: Prevention of endotracheal suctioning-induced alveolar derecruitment in acute lung injury, Am J Respir Crit Care Med 167(9):1215-1224, 2003.
108. Freytag CC, Thies FL, Konig W et al: Prolonged application of closed in-line suction catheters increases microbial colonization of the lower respiratory tract and bacterial growth on catheter surface, Infection 31(1):31-37, 2003.
109. Combes P, Fauvage B, Oleyer C: Nosocomial pneumonia in mechanically ventilated patients, a prospective randomised evaluation of the Stericath closed suctioning system, Intensive Care Med 26(7):878-882, 2000.
110. Darvas JA, Hawkins LG: The closed tracheal suction catheter: 24 hour or 48 hour change? Aust Crit Care 16(3):86-92, 2003.
111. Stoller JK, Orens DK, Fatica C et al: Weekly versus daily changes of in-line suction catheters: impact on rates of ventilator-associated pneumonia and associated costs, Respir Care 48(5):494-499, 2003.
112. Zeitoun SS, de Barros AL, Diccini S: A prospective, randomized study of ventilator-associated pneumonia in patients using a closed vs. open suction system, J Clin Nurs 12(4):484-489, 2003.
113. Maggiore SM, Iacobone E, Zito G et al: Closed versus open suctioning techniques, Minerva Anestesiol 68(5):360-364, 2002.
114. Anthony JS, Sieniewicz DJ: Suctioning of the left bronchial tree in critically ill patients, Crit Care Med 5:161-162, 1977.
115. Panacek EA, Albertson TE, Rutherford WF et al: Selective left endobronchial suctioning in the intubated patient, Chest 95:885-887, 1989.
116. Haberman PB, Green JP, Archibald C et al: Determinants of successful selective tracheobronchial suctioning, N Engl J Med 313:1060-1063, 1973.
117. Shorten DR, Byrne PJ, Jones RL: Infant responses to saline instillations and endotracheal suctioning, J Obstet Gynecol Neonatal Nurs 20:464-469, 1991.
118. Gray JE, MacIntyre NR, Kronberger WG: The effects of bolus normal-saline instillation in conjunction with endotracheal suctioning, Respir Care 35:785-790, 1990.
119. Hagler DA, Traver GA: Endotracheal saline and suction catheters: sources of lower airway contamination, Am J Crit Care 3:444-447, 1994.
120. Cunha-Goncalves D, Perez-de-Sa V, Ingimarsson J et al: Inflation lung mechanics deteriorates markedly after saline instillation and open endotracheal suctioning in mechanically ventilated healthy piglets, Pediatr Pulmonol 42(1):10-14, 2007.
121. Celik SA, Kanan N: A current conflict: use of isotonic sodium chloride solution on endotracheal suctioning in critically ill patients, Dimens Crit Care Nurs 25(1):11-14, 2006.
122. Ji YR, Kim HS, Park JH: Instillation of normal saline before suctioning in patients with pneumonia, Yonsei Med J 43(5):607-612, 2002.
123. Berman IR, Stahl WM: Prevention of hypoxic complications during endotracheal suctioning, Surgery 63:586-587, 1968.
124. Baker PO, Baker JP, Koen PA: Endotracheal suctioning techniques in hypoxemic patients, Respir Care 28:1563-1568, 1983.
125. Glass C, Grap MJ, Corley MC et al: Nurses' ability to achieve hyperinflation and hyperoxygenation with a manual resuscitation bag during endotracheal suctioning, Heart Lung 22:158-165, 1993.
126. Singer M, Vermaat J, Hall G et al: Hemodynamic effects of manual hyperventilation in critically ill mechanically ventilated patients, Chest 106:1182-1187, 1994.
127. George RB: Duration of suctioning: an important variable, Respir Care 28:457-459, 1983.

128. Baier H, Begin R, Sackner MA: Effect of airway diameter, suction catheters, and the bronchofiberscope on airflow in endotracheal and tracheostomy tubes, Heart Lung 5:235-238, 1976.
129. Amikam B, Landa J, West J et al: Bronchofiberscopic observations of the tracheobronchial tree during intubation, Am Rev Respir Dis 105:747-755, 1972.
130. Landa JF, Chapman GA, Sackner MA: Effects of suctioning on mucociliary transport, Chest 77:202-207, 1980.
131. Sackner MA, Landa JF, Greeneltch N et al: Pathogenesis and prevention of tracheobronchial damage with suction procedures, Chest 64:282-290, 1973.
132. Shim C, Fine N, Fernandez R et al: Cardiac arrhythmias resulting from tracheal suctioning, Ann Intern Med 71:1149-1153, 1969.
133. Winston SJ, Gravelyn TR, Stirin RG: Prevention of bradycardic responses to endotracheal suctioning by prior administration of nebulized atropine, Crit Care Med 15:1009-1011, 1987.
134. Walsh JM, Vanderwarf C, Hoscheit D et al: Unsuspected hemodynamic alterations during endotracheal suctioning, Chest 95:162-165, 1989.
135. Rudy EB, Baun M, Stone K et al: The relationship between endotracheal suctioning and changes in intercranial pressure: a review of the literature, Heart Lung 15:488-494, 1986.
136. Dohi S, Gold I: Pulmonary mechanics during general anesthesia: the influence of mechanical irritation of the airway, Br J Anaesth 51:205-213, 1979.
137. Gugielminotti J, Desmonts J, Dureuil B: Effects of tracheal suctioning on respiratory resistances in mechanically ventilated patients, Chest 113:1335-1338, 1998.
138. AARC Clinical Practice Guideline Group, Patient/Ventilator System Check, 37:882-886, 1992.
139. Akhtar SR, Weaver J, Pierson DJ et al: Practice variation in respiratory therapy documentation during mechanical ventilation, Chest 124(6):2275-2282, 2003.

CHAPTER

4

Humidification and Aerosol Therapy

RICHARD D. BRANSON

OUTLINE

OBJECTIVES

- Explain the physical principles governing humidity.
- Describe the normal structure and function of the respiratory system.
- List the types of devices to add humidity to the respiratory tract during mechanical ventilation.
- Describe the function, application, and limitations of humidification devices.
- Describe the physical principles governing aerosol generation and delivery to the respiratory tract.
- List the types of aerosol delivery devices.
- Discuss the function, application, and limitation of aerosol delivery systems.
- Compare the techniques for monitoring bronchodilator therapy.
- List common pharmacologic agents delivered via aerosol to mechanically ventilated patients.
- Describe the proper technique for metered-dose inhaler use during mechanical ventilation.
- Explain the proper technique for small-volume nebulizer use during mechanical ventilation.

KEY TERMS

absolute humidity
active heat and moisture exchanger
anticholinergics
bronchodilators
β-2 agonists
bubble humidifier
calcium chloride
cascade humidifiers
condensation
dead volume
dry powder inhalers

gravitational sedimentation
heat and moisture exchanger booster
heat and moisture exchanger (HME)
heat and moisture exchanging filter (HMEF)
heated wire circuits
high-flow humidifiers
hygroscopic heat and moisture exchangers (HHMEs)
hygroscopic heat and moisture exchanging filter (HHMEF)
inertial impaction
isothermic saturation boundary (ISB)
lithium chloride
mass median aerodynamic diameter (MMAD)
metered-dose inhaler (MDI)
moisture output
muscarinic receptors
passover humidifiers
rainout
relative humidity
saturated
small-volume nebulizer (SVN)
spacer
vibrating mesh nebulizer
wick humidifiers

PHYSICAL PROPERTIES

Water is found in all three states of matter within a relatively small temperature range. When energy is applied to liquid water, usually in the form of heat, water molecules move independently of one another. As molecules leave the surface of the liquid, they become water vapor. The amount of water vapor present in a gas is commonly referred to as humidity. Water vapor also can be referred to as molecular water.

The amount of water vapor in a gas can be measured and expressed in a number of ways. In medicine, the most common terms are absolute humidity and relative humidity. **Absolute humidity** is the amount of water vapor present in a gas mixture. Absolute humidity is directly proportional to gas temperature, increasing with an increasing gas temperature and decreasing with a decreasing gas temperature (Table 4-1). Absolute humidity typically is expressed in mg/L, g/cm^3, or as a partial pressure (P_{H_2O}). Absolute humidity can be calculated using the equation

$$AH = 16.42 - 0.73T + 0.04T^2$$

where AH is absolute humidity and 100% saturation and T is the gas temperature in °C. Alveolar gas is 37° C and contains 43.9 mg H_2O/L of gas.

A gas mixture holding all the water vapor it is capable of holding is said to be **saturated** or at the maximum capacity of water vapor. The amount of humidity in a gas that is less than saturated can be determined by comparing the absolute humidity (the water vapor present) to the maximum capacity (the maximum possible water vapor) of the gas at a given temperature. This value is known as **relative humidity.** Relative humidity is expressed as a percentage using the following equation:

$$\text{Relative humidity (\%)} = (\text{absolute humidity}) / (\text{maximum capacity}) \times 100$$

These measurements are useful in determining the causes of some common clinical phenomena. For example, if gas leaves a heated humidifier outlet at a temperature of 34°C and 100% relative humidity and is heated by a heated wire circuit to 37° C at the airway, relative humidity decreases because the higher gas temperature has a greater capacity for carrying water. In the previous example, if the gas temperature were 37° C and the absolute humidity measured was 37 mg H_2O/L, then we can determine the relative humidity by comparing this value to the maximum capacity for water vapor at 37° C from Table 4-1.

This explains reports of dried secretions in the endotracheal tubes of patients using heated humidification and heated wire circuits. The greater the difference between temperature at the chamber and temperature at the airway, the lower the relative humidity. This temperature offset is important to keep the circuit free of rainout. Unfortunately, in certain environments (e.g., near windows, fans, heating units, and air conditioning vents) the environmental changes can affect heated wire circuit efficacy. However, clinicians should be careful to ensure that the patient receives adequate relative humidity as a priority over a circuit free from rainout. When a heated humidifier without a heated wire circuit is used, it is often necessary for the temperature of the gas in the humidification chamber to reach temperatures of 50° C for temperature delivered to the airway to approach 37° C. An example of this is shown in Figure 4-1. In this example, the maximum water vapor content of gas at 50° C is 83 mg H_2O/L and the maximum water vapor content of gas at 37° C is 43.9 mg H_2O/L. The difference in water vapor content between the two gases—$83 - 43.9 = 39.1$ mg H_2O/L—represents the amount of condensate or **rainout** that accumulates in the circuit. For a minute ventilation of 10 L/min, this would result in a little more than 0.5 L of rainout in a 24-hour period.

TABLE 4-1 *The Relationship of Gas Temperature, Absolute Humidity, and Water Vapor Pressure*

GAS TEMPERATURE (°C)	ABSOLUTE HUMIDITY (MG H_2O/L)	WATER VAPOR PRESSURE (PH_2O)
0	4.85	4.6
5	6.8	6.5
10	9.4	9.2
15	12.8	12.8
20	17.3	17.5
25	23.0	23.7
30	30.4	31.7
32	33.8	35.5
34	37.6	39.8
36	41.7	44.4
37	43.9	46.9
38	46.2	49.5
40	51.1	55.1
42	56.5	61.3
44	62.5	68.1

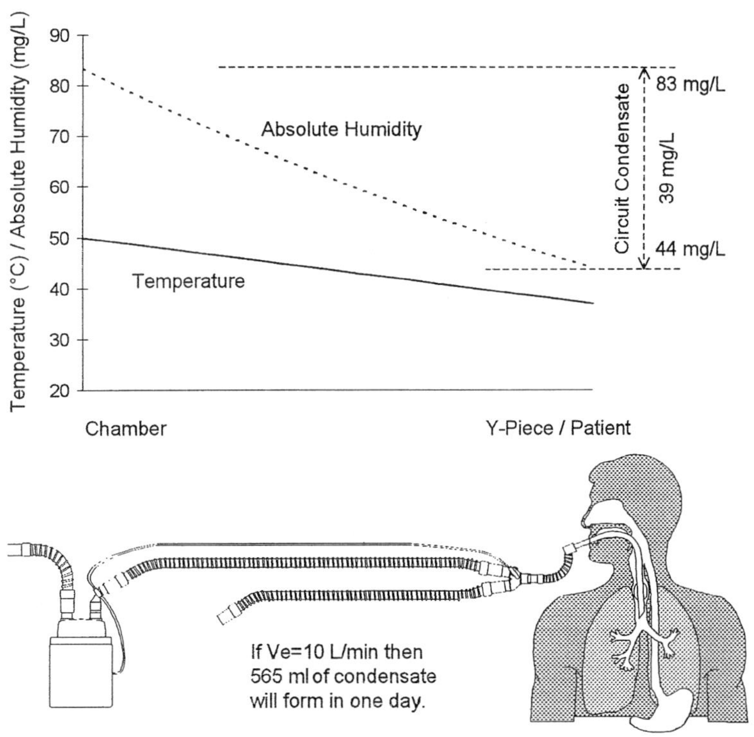

FIGURE 4-1 Gas cooling and condensate formation when a heated humidity generator and unheated delivery system are combined. Gas leaves the humidifier at more than 50° C (83 mg/L) and cools to 37° C (44 mg/L), creating 39 mg/L of condensate. (From Peterson BD: Heated humidifiers: structure and function. Respir Care Clin North Am 4:243-259, 1988.)

If the relative humidity and temperature are known, the water vapor content also can be calculated. For example, if a heat and moisture exchanger (HME) provides 32° C and 95% relative humidity, then the water vapor content can be calculated.

The relative humidity of a gas saturated with water vapor at any temperature is 100%. This point is also commonly known as the dew point.

PHYSIOLOGIC PRINCIPLES

During normal breathing, the upper respiratory tract warms, humidifies, and filters inspired gases. This task is accomplished primarily in the nasopharynx, where gases are exposed to the highly vascular, moist mucus membrane. Upper airway efficiency is enhanced further by the large surface area and turbulent flow afforded by the nasal turbinates. The oropharynx and conducting airways also contribute to this process, but are less efficient because they lack the exquisite architecture of the nasopharynx. During exhalation, the upper airways reclaim a large percentage of the heat and moisture added during inspiration. This function often is overlooked, but the moisture conservation properties of the upper airway rival the humidity properties as part of an extremely efficient countercurrent heat and moisture exchange. Over the course of a normal day, the respiratory tract loses approximately 1470 joules of heat and 250 ml of water.[1] This net loss of heat and moisture is predominantly the result of water vapor escaping in expired gases. Little heat actually is lost through the warming of inspired gas because the specific heat of air is very low.

The efficiency of the normal upper airway is quite remarkable. Even at extremes of inspired temperature and humidity, gas that reaches the alveolar level is 100% saturated at body temperature.[2] Measurements accomplished in patients with an intact upper airway suggest that after passing through the nasopharynx, inspired gases are 29° C to 32° C at nearly 100% relative humidity. As the gases approach the carina, gases are 32° C to 34° C and nearly 100% relative humidity.[3,4] These values become important as a template for deciding which level of heat and humidity to deliver to intubated patients, in whom inspired gases bypass the upper airway and are delivered directly to the lower trachea.

The point at which gases reach alveolar conditions (37° C and 100% relative humidity) is known as the **isothermic saturation boundary (ISB).** Under normal conditions, the ISB resides in the fourth to fifth generation of subsegmental bronchi. The position of the ISB is fairly constant, regardless of environmental temperature and humidity conditions. Position of the ISB also can be shifted by the presence of lung disease and patient fluid status. Above the ISB, the respiratory tract performs the function of a countercurrent **heat and moisture exchanger (HME),** adding heat and moisture on inspiration and conserving heat and moisture during expiration. Below the ISB, temperature and water content remain relatively constant.

After intubation, the ISB is shifted down the respiratory tract as the normal upper airway heat and moisture exchanging structures are bypassed. This places the burden of heat and moisture exchange on the lower respiratory tract, a task for which it is poorly suited. The delivery of cold, anhydrous medical gases further burdens the lower respiratory tract and plunges the ISB down the bronchial tree. The combined effects of intubation and mechanical ventilation with dry gases can result in severe losses of heat and moisture from the respiratory mucosa. In extreme cases, damage to the structure and function of the respiratory epithelium can occur, which has clinical implications.[5-8] Table 4-2 lists the known alterations caused by breathing cool, dry gas via an artificial airway.

The provision of heat and humidity during mechanical ventilation is a standard of care during mechanical ventilation around the world.[9,10] There is

TABLE 4-2 *Structural and Functional Changes in the Respiratory Tract and the Physiologic Effects Caused by Breathing Cool, Dry Gases Via an Artificial Airway*

STRUCTURAL	FUNCTIONAL	PHYSIOLOGIC
Loss of ciliary function	Interruption of the mucociliary escalator	Retained secretions
Destruction of cilia		Mucus plugging of airways
Desiccation of mucus glands	Increased mucus viscosity	Atelectasis
Reduction in cellular cytoplasm	Reduced pulmonary compliance	Increased work of breathing
Ulceration of mucosa	Increased airway resistance	Hypoxemia
Loss of surfactant	Intrapulmonary shunting	Hypothermia

little disagreement about the importance of humidification, but there exists considerable disagreement as to the best method of humidification delivery and the amount of humidification required. The methods for providing humidity include active, microprocessor-controlled, heat and humidifying systems (heated humidifiers) and simple, passive, HMEs (artificial noses).

HIGH-FLOW HUMIDIFIERS

High-flow humidifiers are capable of providing a wide range of temperatures and humidities.[11] High-flow humidifiers generically consist of a heating element, a water reservoir, a temperature control unit (including temperature probe and alarms), and a gas/liquid interface that increases the surface area for evaporation. Most high-flow humidifiers fit into one of the following categories: **passover humidifiers, cascade humidifiers,** or **wick humidifiers.** Because these devices are heated, they also prevent loss of body heat from the patient, which is particularly important in neonatal applications. When heated humidifiers are used, the temperature at the patient's airway should be monitored continuously with a thermometer or thermistor. Although not common, it also may be desirable to monitor the relative humidity at the proximal airway.

With high-flow humidifiers, the water level in the reservoir can be maintained manually by adding water from a bag through a fill-set attached to the humidifier or by a float-feed system that keeps the water level constant. Manual methods tend to increase the risk of reservoir contamination and pose the additional risk of spilling and overfilling. Fill-set and float-feed systems are preferable. The float-feed systems also avoid fluctuations in the temperature of gas delivered, which occurs when a volume of cold water is added to the humidifier.

Most humidifiers are servo-controlled, that is, the operator sets the desired gas temperature at the thermistor, and the system maintains control of patient gas temperature despite changes in gas flow or level of water in the reservoir. These systems also are equipped with audiovisual alarms to alert the user of high temperature conditions. The temperature-monitoring devices used in these systems have a relatively slow response time and only reflect the average temperature of the inspired gas. Actual temperatures fluctuate above and below the average temperature with cyclic gas flow, as may occur in a mechanical ventilator circuit. This creates a situation in which gas in the ventilator circuit cools during inspiration while gas above the humidifier becomes superheated. The resulting gas delivered to the patient begins at a temperature below set temperature, then exceeds set temperature as gas from the humidifier reaches the patient.

Heated wire circuits contain electric wires that impart heat to the gas as it travels down the ventilator circuit. Heated wire circuits prevent a temperature decrease in the tubing, provide a more precise gas temperature delivered to the patient, and prevent **condensation** of water in the tubing. The temperature of the heated wire is controlled by the humidifier in concert with the servo temperature control system. When used with a heated humidifier, the heated wire circuit commonly increases temperature of the gas as it traverses the length of the circuit. This prevents condensate because gas arriving at the patient airway is capable of carrying more moisture then gas exiting the humidifier. This intended positive attribute also causes the relative humidity of delivered gases to decrease. This decrease in relative humidity may result in drying of secretions and endotracheal tube obstruction.[12] Conversely, if the temperature of the tubing is less than the temperature of the gas leaving the humidifier, condensation occurs in the tubing. Because heated wire circuits are commonly a single, nonjointed piece of tubing, placing a water trap in the inspiratory limb is impractical. As such, the presence of condensate in heated wire circuits is discouraged because of difficulties in removing it. However, if set properly, heated wire circuits may develop a small amount of condensate, which requires draining only daily.

The use of servo-controlled heated wire circuits can become complex when the gas is delivered to neonates in an incubator or those under a radiant heater.[13] The problem is related to exposure of the circuit to two temperatures: room temperature and the temperature in the incubator (or under the radiant heater). In these applications, the thermistor should be placed directly outside the incubator (or out from under the radiant heater) rather than at the proximal airway of the patient.

In systems that do not use heated wire circuits, water that collects in the tubing can serve as a potential source of nosocomial infection. Water in the tubing also can result in an accidental lavage of the patient's airway during turning. Condensation in the circuit should be collected in a water trap and disposed of appropriately. The water that condenses in the tubing should be considered contaminated and never should be allowed to drain back into the humidifier.

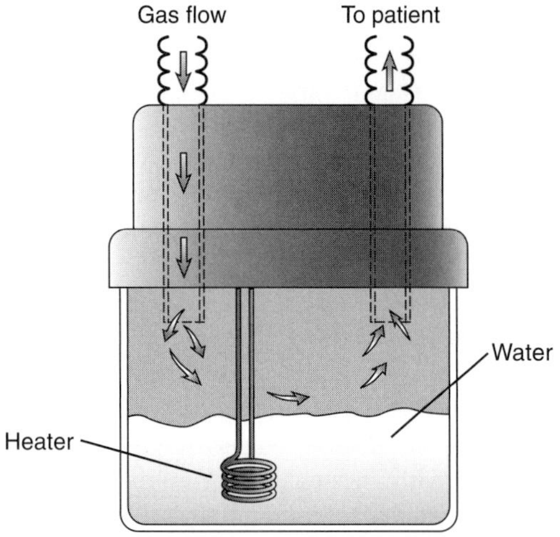

FIGURE 4-2 Passover heated humidifier. (Modified from Hess DR, Branson RD: Humidification. In Branson RD, Hess DR, Chatburn RL: Respiratory Care Equipment, ed 2, Philadelphia, 1999, Lippincott.)

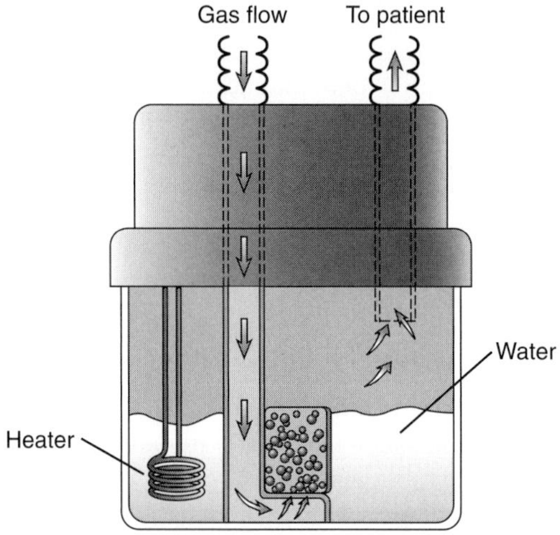

FIGURE 4-3 Bubble heated humidifier. (Modified from Hess DR, Branson RD: Humidification. In Branson RD, Hess DR, Chatburn RL: Respiratory Care Equipment, ed 2, Philadelphia, 1999, Lippincott.)

Types of High-Flow Humidifiers

Passover Humidifier

Gas from the ventilator is introduced into the humidifier chamber, passes over the surface of the water reservoir, and exits to the ventilator circuit. This is the simplest form of heated humidifier (Figure 4-2).

Bubble Humidifier

Gas from the ventilator is directed through a tube that is submerged in the water reservoir. The gas exits under the water through a diffuser or grid and travels into the ventilator circuit (Figure 4-3).

Cascade Humidifier

Gas from the ventilator is directed below the surface of the water reservoir and bubbles upward through a grid. The cascade humidifier is a very efficient **bubble humidifier.** The grid creates a froth of small bubbles that absorb water. Humidifier temperature is maintained by a thermostat. A thermometer or thermistor is used at the patient's airway to monitor the temperature of the gas delivered. Unless the tubing leading to the patient is heated, the temperature of the gas between the humidifier and the patient decreases, resulting in condensation. Although the cascade humidifier delivers water vapor, it also may deliver microaerosols to the patient, which can transmit bacteria to the patient if the reservoir becomes contaminated.[14] However, the temperature in the water reservoir of a system that does not use a heated wire circuit inhibits the growth of pathogens.[15] This is not the case for systems using heated wire circuits. The temperature of the reservoir with heated wire circuit systems approximates body temperature (34° C to 37° C) and can support growth of bacteria[16] (Figure 4-4).

Wick Humidifier

The wick humidifier (Figure 4-5) is a modified passover humidifier that directs gas into a cylinder, lined with a wick of blotter paper. The wick is surrounded by a heating element, and the base of the wick is immersed in water. The wick absorbs water, and as the gas contacts the moist heated wick, the relative humidity of the gas increases. This is a simple method of increasing the temperature and humidification capabilities of the device by increasing the gas or liquid interface without increasing the volume of the reservoir.

PASSIVE HUMIDIFIER

Passive humidifier is a generic term used to describe a group of similar humidification devices that operate without electricity or a supplementary water source. These devices also frequently are called "artificial noses." The name comes from the device's similarity in function to the human nose. By definition, a passive humidifier is a device that collects the patient's expired heat and moisture and returns it during the following inspiration. The term passive humidifier is preferred over artificial nose because it is more specific to function.[11]

There are several types of passive humidifiers. The differences are related to device design. Figure 4-6 depicts the types of passive humidifiers and

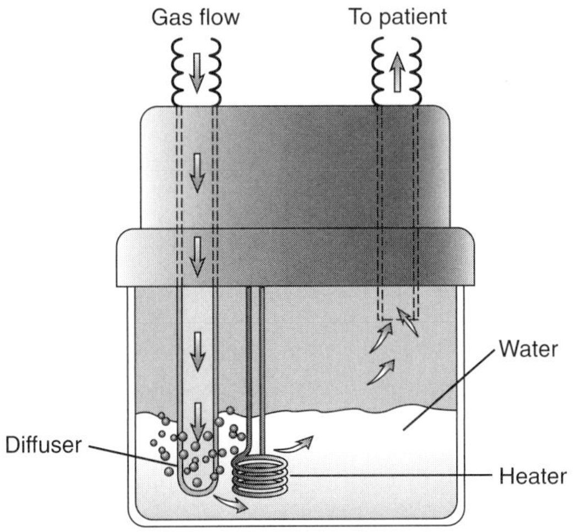

FIGURE 4-4 Cascade heated humidifier. (Modified from Hess DR, Branson RD: Humidification. In Branson RD, Hess DR, Chatburn RL: Respiratory Care Equipment, ed 2, Philadelphia, 1999, Lippincott.)

Figure 4-7 shows an example of these devices. Devices that use only physical principles of heat and moisture exchange are known as HMEs. The addition of a filter to an HME results in a **heat and moisture exchanging filter (HMEF).** Other devices are hygroscopically treated to improve moisture-exchanging properties by adding a chemical means of heat and moisture exchange. These devices are called **hygroscopic heat and moisture exchangers (HHMEs),** and the addition of a filter creates an HHMEF. The term hygroscopic HME is more representative of the actual function of the device and allows differentiation from the HME. These devices frequently have been referred to as hygroscopic condenser humidifiers.

The HME is the simplest of these devices and was the first passive humidifier to be introduced. An HME usually consists of a layered aluminum insert with or without an additional fibrous element. Aluminum exchanges temperature quickly, and during expiration, condensation forms between the aluminum layers. The retained heat and moisture are returned during inspiration. The addition of a fibrous element aids in the retention of moisture and helps reduce pooling of condensate in the dependent portions of the device. HMEs are the least efficient passive humidifiers and often are not used. These devices also tend to be cheaper than other passive humidifiers and may be used in the operating room for short-term humidification. These devices have a

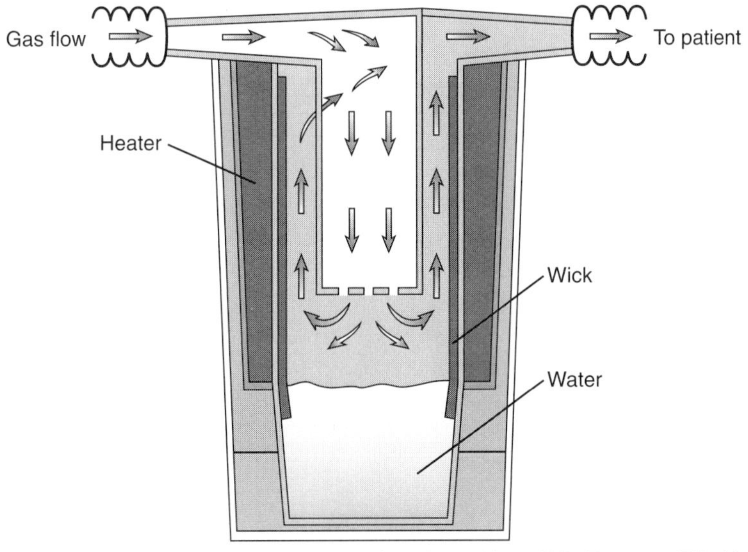

FIGURE 4-5 Heated wick humidifier. (Modified from Hess DR, Branson RD: Humidification. In Branson RD, Hess DR, Chatburn RL: Respiratory Care Equipment, ed 2, Philadelphia, 1999, Lippincott.)

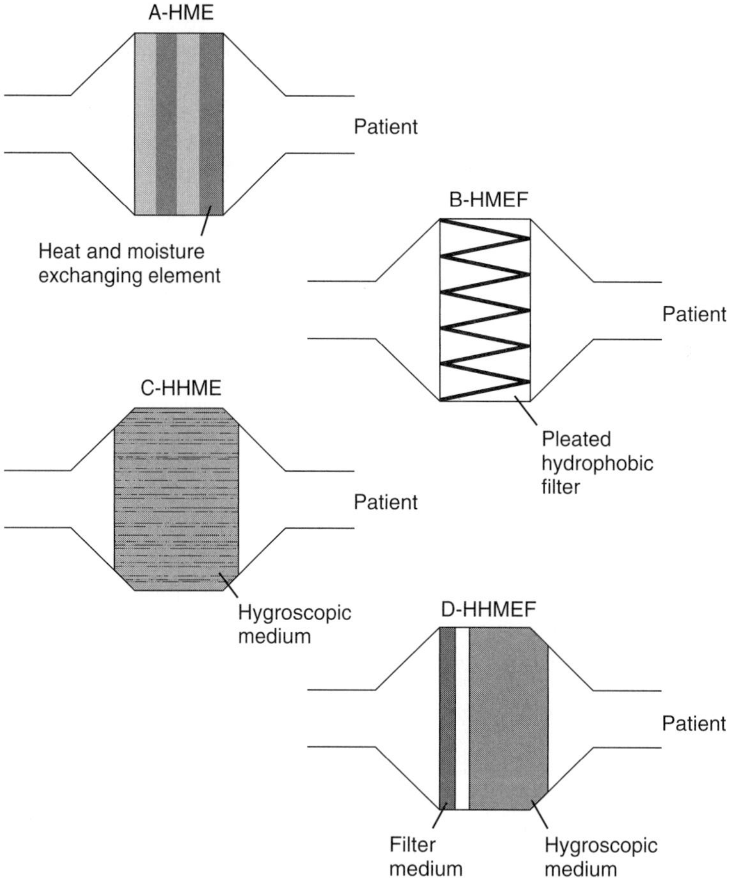

FIGURE 4-6 Types of passive humidifiers. **A,** Heat and moisture exchanger; **B,** heat and moisture exchanging filter; **C,** hygroscopic heat and moisture exchanger; and **D,** hygroscopic heat and moisture exchanging filter.

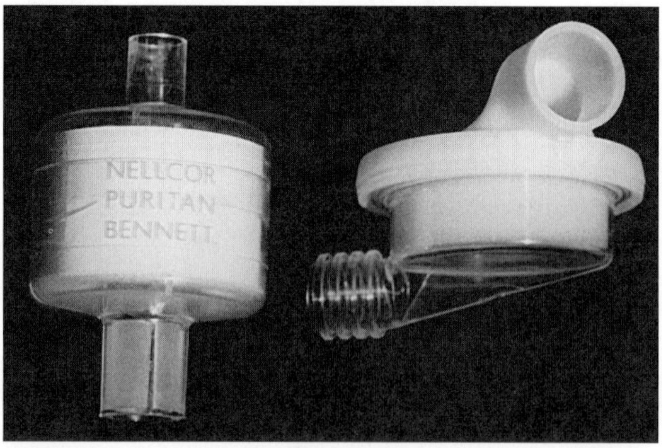

FIGURE 4-7 Typical passive humidifiers used during mechanical ventilation.

nominal moisture output, providing 10 to 14 mg H_2O/L at tidal volumes of 1000 ml to 500 ml.[17,18]

HMEFs have improved performance compared with HMEs secondary to either the presence of a spun filter medium or an increase in the volume (increased surface area) of the medium. Surface area is commonly increased by pleating the medium and increasing its thickness. Laboratory evaluations of these devices demonstrate a moisture output of 18 to 28 mg H_2O/L at a tidal volume of 1000 to 500 ml.[18-28]

The HHME is the most popular style of artificial nose. These devices vary widely in shape, size, and type of medium insert used. Most HHMEs use a paper or polypropylene insert treated with a hygroscopic chemical, usually calcium or lithium chloride, to enhance moisture conservation. Comparative studies have shown that HHMEs can provide a moisture output of 22 to 34 mg H_2O/L at tidal volumes from 500 to 1000 ml. The addition of a filter medium to an HHME creates a **hygroscopic heat and moisture exchanging filter (HHMEF).**[18-28] The filter medium typically is placed between the ventilator connection and the HHMEF's medium insert. This places the hygroscopically treated material between the patient's expired gases and the filter. Typical filtration material is made from spun polypropylene that is electrostatically charged, attracting airborne materials and trapping them. The filter is poorly suited as a heat and moisture exchanging medium, but when combined with the hygroscopic element appears to increase moisture output by 1 to 2 mg H_2O/L. The presence of the filter also increases resistance.

CHARACTERISTICS OF ARTIFICIAL NOSES

Moisture Output

The amount of heat and humidity provided by a passive humidifier typically is referred to as **moisture output.** Moisture output is measured under laboratory conditions and reported in milligrams per H_2O/L. There are currently no standards for the minimum moisture output of a passive humidifier. The standard for heated humidifiers suggests a minimum of 33 mg H_2O/L.[29] Application of this standard to HMEs and HHMEs is not very helpful. The American Association for Respiratory Care (AARC) has recommended that the required moisture output changes with duration of use and application. For example, a patient with normal respiratory function requiring intubation for a 2-hour operation probably only requires 15 to 20 mg H_2O/L. Mechanically ventilated patients with normal secretions appear to require a minimum of 26 mg H_2O/L to prevent drying of secretions and maintain mucociliary function. Patients with an increased secretion production probably require additional heat and moisture, which a passive humidifier cannot supply. In patients with thick, copious amounts of sputum, heated humidification should be used.

The moisture output reported in the package insert is based on a certain tidal volume, inspiratory time, respiratory rate, and temperature.[30] Deviations from these values cause moisture output to change. As tidal volume increases, moisture output decreases. The amount of this decrease depends on the efficiency of the device and the dead space. Larger devices tend to be affected less by an increase in tidal volume due to rebreathing. That is, if an HME with an internal volume of 100 ml is used, 100 ml of each inspiration contains expired gases. An increase in respiratory rate or decrease in inspiratory time also decreases moisture output. Likewise, an increase in expiratory flow due to a decrease in lung compliance causes moisture output to decrease. In each of these instances, the decrease in transit time (gas moves through the medium more quickly) reduces the ability of the device to remove moisture from exhaled gas and add moisture to inspired gas. When using a passive humidifier, there is always a net heat and moisture loss from the respiratory tract.

Resistance

The resistance to gas flow of a passive humidifier increases as medium density increases and as dead space decreases. This increase in resistance may adversely affect the patient's work of breathing.[31-34] However, compared with the added resistance of the endotracheal tube, this increase is small. Most currently manufactured devices have a resistance of less than 3.5 cm H_2O. During use, as the medium absorbs water, resistance increases slightly. After prolonged use, the increase in resistance to expiratory flow may cause air trapping and auto-positive end-expiratory pressure (autoPEEP).

The greatest concern with resistance occurs when the medium becomes occluded with secretions, blood, or water from a secondary source. Several reports have demonstrated an increase in resistance from water and blood accumulating in the medium.[35-39] In one instance, the saline intended to aid in loosening secretions before suctioning accumulated in the HHME medium.[40] Aerosolized drugs also can cause an increase in resistance as the drug or its carrier becomes trapped in the medium or filter. Before delivery of aerosolized medications (delivered by up-draft nebulizer), passive humidifiers should be removed from the airway. During mechanical ventilation, the need for frequent aerosol treatments may necessitate a switch to heated humidification.

Manufacturing defects have resulted in total or partial occlusion of passive humidifiers.[41-44] In each report to date, a remnant from the plastic housing remained in the path of gas flow. Clinicians should visually inspect each device before use.

Dead Space

Placing a passive humidifier on the end of the patient's airway increases dead space. To maintain normal alveolar ventilation, the patient must increase either respiratory rate or tidal volume, or both. If the patient cannot increase alveolar ventilation, arterial CO_2 increases. This effect is most pronounced in spontaneously breathing patients and is related to the relationship between the patient's tidal volume and the dead space.

A 70-kg patient with a spontaneous tidal volume of 350 ml and a respiratory rate of 20 breaths/min has a minute ventilation of 7 L/min.

$$20 \text{ breaths/min} \times 350 \text{ ml} = 7.0 \text{ L/min}$$

If the patient's anatomic dead space is 150 ml, then alveolar ventilation is 20 breaths/min × (350 ml − 150 ml) = 4 L/min.

If an HME with a dead space of 100 ml is added to the airway, while minute ventilation remains the same (7 L/min), alveolar ventilation decreases to 2 L/min.

$$20 \times 350 \text{ ml} - (150 \text{ ml} + 100 \text{ ml}) = 2.0 \text{ L/min}$$

For alveolar ventilation to be restored to 4.0 L/min, minute ventilation must increase via an increase in respiratory rate, tidal volume, or both.

$$20 \times 450 \text{ ml} - 150 \text{ ml} + 100 \text{ ml}) = 4.0 \text{ L/min and minute ventilation} = 9.0 \text{ L/min}$$

Several authors have shown the adverse effects of added dead space on respiratory mechanics.[45-51] In each study, the addition of an HME or an HHME with a dead space of 100 ml resulted in an increase in the work of breathing, an increase in the required minute ventilation, and an increase in autoPEEP. When patients were able to increase respiratory rate and/or tidal volume, arterial CO_2 remained constant. When patients were unable to increase minute ventilation (weak respiratory muscles), arterial CO_2 concentrations increased. Pressure support ventilation can be used to overcome the additional work of breathing, but this can lead to the requirement for higher airway pressures, can increase tidal volumes, and can worsen autoPEEP.

When choosing a passive humidifier, the smallest dead space possible that provides adequate humidification should be selected. Figure 4-8 depicts the added series dead space with use of an HME. This is particularly important in the patient with ARDS requiring low tidal volume ventilation and during spontaneous breathing trials in the patient with marginal respiratory reserves.[48,52,53]

Additives

HHMEs use either **calcium chloride** or **lithium chloride** as hygroscopic additives to increase moisture output. Some manufacturers also add chlorhexidine as a bacteriostatic treatment. Lithium, delivered by mouth or injection, is used in the treatment of psychological disorders, including depression and mania. It has been suggested that lithium from HHME media may be washed into the trachea and absorbed into the bloodstream, where blood levels may increase to a therapeutic level.[54,55] This is a theoretical possibility that has never been conclusively proved. The only report of a patient seen to have elevated serum lithium levels while using an HHME had used lithium by mouth before admission to the hospital. The small amount of lithium in these devices appears to make this concern unwarranted.

Cost

Cost is an important feature of any piece of medical equipment. At the time of this writing, the average cost of an HHME is $3.25. The range of costs is

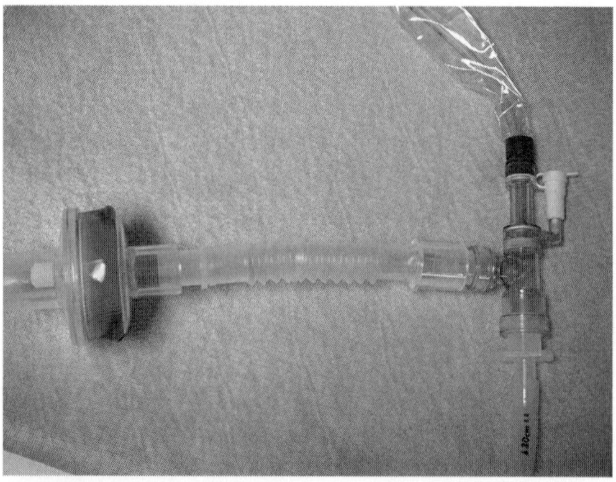

FIGURE 4-8 Series dead space with use of a heat and moisture exchanger.

extensive (\$2.50 to \$6.00), with HHMEFs and HMEFs being the most expensive devices.

Choosing the Right Passive Humidifier

The important features of a passive humidifier were described previously. During mechanical ventilation in the intensive care unit (ICU), important features are moisture output, dead space, resistance, and cost. In this setting, an acceptable passive humidifier should have a minimum moisture output of 30 mg H_2O/L, a dead space of less than 50 ml, a resistance of less than 2.5 cm H_2O/L/sec, and a cost of less than \$2.50 each. Features for devices used in the operating room may be different.

USE OF HUMIDIFICATION DEVICES DURING MECHANICAL VENTILATION

Passive humidifiers function by returning a portion of the heat and moisture exhaled by the patient. As such, there always is a net loss of heat and moisture. The most efficient passive humidifiers return 70% to 80% of the patient's expired humidity. Passive humidifiers are not as efficient as heated humidification devices. We have developed an algorithm for safe and judicious use of passive humidifiers in the ICU[56] (Figure 4-9). This protocol uses contraindications to passive humidifiers use to advise practitioners when to use heated humidification. Contraindications to use of passive humidifiers include thick, copious amounts of sputum; grossly bloody secretions; low tidal volume ventilation; and hypothermia (less than 32° C).

Passive humidifiers are attractive alternatives to heated humidifiers because of their low cost, passive operation, and ease of use. Table 4-3 compares the advantages and disadvantages of heated and passive humidifiers.

Not all patients can use a passive humidifier. Patients with preexisting pulmonary disease characterized by thick, copious secretions should receive heated humidification. The same is true for patients with grossly bloody secretions because blood can occlude the medium or filter and result in excessive resistance, air trapping, hypoventilation, and possibly barotrauma. Patients with hypothermia should receive heated humidification because passive humidifiers can return only a portion of the moisture exhaled. If patient body temperature is only 32° C (absolute humidity of 32 mg H_2O/L), even a very efficient HHME (80%) can only deliver an absolute humidity of 25.6 mg H_2O/L. Patients with bronchopleural fistula or incompetent tracheal tube cuffs also should not use passive humidifiers. Because the device requires the collection of expired heat and moisture, any problem that allows expired gas to escape to the atmosphere without passing through the medium will reduce humidity.

Passive humidifiers should never be used in conjunction with heated humidifiers. Particulate water in the medium increases resistance and prevents adequate delivery of humidity from either device. If water occludes the filter, the patient cannot be ventilated adequately and may be unable to completely exhale during positive pressure ventilation.

In the ICU, passive humidifiers may be used for extended periods of time. Our experience suggests that a 5-day period is safe and effective. This recommendation is based on numerous studies that find that partial or complete obstruction of endotracheal tubes (suggesting inadequate humidity) appears to occur around this time. Patient sputum characteristics should be assessed with every suctioning attempt. If the secretions appear thick on two consecutive suctioning procedures, the patient should be switched to a heated humidifier. Judging the quality of sputum can be done using the following method, described by Suzukawa and colleagues[57]:

- Thin: The suction catheter is clear of secretions after suctioning.
- Moderate: The suction catheter has secretions adhering to the sides after suctioning, which are removed easily by aspirating water through the catheter.
- Thick: The suction catheter has secretions adhering to the sides after suctioning, which are not removed by aspirating water through the catheter.

Recent work has suggested that the presence of condensate in the elbow or flex tube between the HME and the patient implies adequate humidification. This makes sense because the presence of condensate suggests that gases are saturated with water vapor.[58] Using this technique should help clinicians decide on a case-by-case basis when to switch from an artificial nose to a heated humidifier, if ever. Despite this recommendation, many authors report use of artificial noses safely for up to 30 days.

We believe that patients requiring mechanical ventilation for more than 5 days, by definition, are critically ill. At day 5, if lung function has not improved, heated humidification may be considered to prevent secretion retention and maximize mucociliary function. If the patient begins the weaning

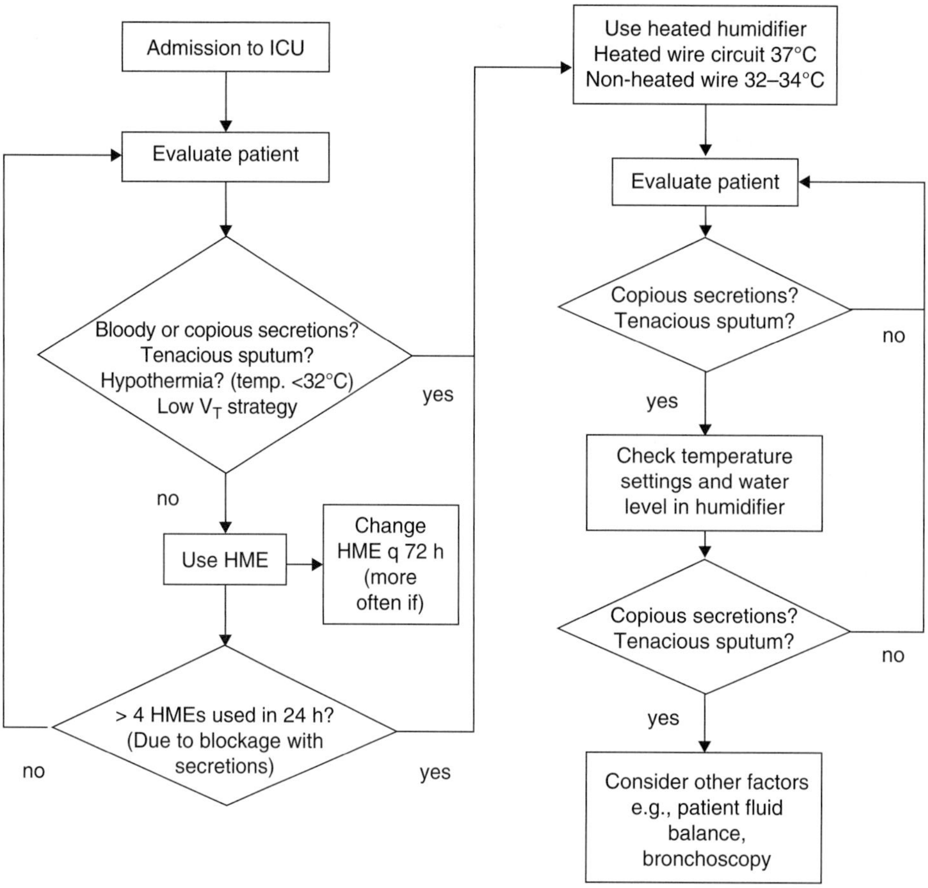

This is the algorithm for choosing humidification devices in the adult intensive care unit.

Check for condensate between the HME and ET tube. If condensate is present, relative humidity is >100%.

HMEs should be avoided when large volumes of secretions may occlude the media – e.g., pulmonary edema or mucopurulent pneumonia. Bloody secretions is intended to cover patients with hemoptysis (secretions appear to be blood). Small streaks of blood are permissible.

Tenacious sputum is related to two consecutive suctioning procedures where sputum is considered 'thick.' Thick is defined as secretions remaining stuck to the walls of the suction catheter after rinsing with saline. This judgement is made without regard to amount (i.e., a small amount of thick sputum also warrants a change to heated humidification). This exclusion concerns inadequate humidification in the face of thickened secretions, not concerns of filter occlusion.

Low tidal volume strategy includes the use of permissive hypercapnia and V_T of 6 ml/kg or less. Removal of the HME in these cases can improve CO_2 elimination and reduce minute ventilation requirement.

FIGURE 4-9 Algorithm to guide clinicians to use the appropriate humidification device.

process at day 5, the added dead space and resistance of the passive humidifier may hinder spontaneous breathing. Although this point may be debated, we believe it to represent the best compromise between cost efficiency, humidification efficiency, and patient safety.[16] Using the clinical evaluation of humidification performance may allow this time period to be extended in some patients.

Most manufacturers suggest changing passive humidifiers every 24 hours. Recent work has shown

TABLE 4-3 *Comparison of the Advantages and Disadvantages of Humidification Devices Used During Mechanical Ventilation*

DEVICE	ADVANTAGES	DISADVANTAGES
Heated humidifiers	Universal application (neonates to adults) Wide range of temperature and humidity Alarms Temperature monitoring Reliability	Cost Water usage Condensation Risk of circuit contamination Overheating Small chance of electric shock/burns
Artificial noses	Cost Passive operation Simple use Elimination of condensate Portable	Not applicable in all patients Increased dead space Increased resistance Potential for occlusion

that if the device remains free of secretions, the change interval can be increased to every 48 or 72 hours, without adverse effect.[59-61] This requires that respiratory care practitioners inspect the device frequently for the presence of secretions and change the device as required. If the device is contaminated frequently by secretions and requires more than three changes daily, the patient should be switched to heated humidification. The frequent soiling of the device suggests that the patient has a secretion problem, and the frequent changes will negate any cost savings.

Early work suggested that the use of passive humidifiers might decrease the incidence of ventilator associated pneumonia (VAP). This concept continues to be debated. In recent years, large studies have failed to demonstrate any advantage of HMEs with regard to reducing VAP.[62-66] In fact, in patients with bacteria already in the sputum, the passive humidifier is readily colonized.

Patients requiring tracheostomy and prolonged mechanical ventilation in subacute care hospitals and long-term care facilities may use artificial noses for much longer periods of time. The maximum duration has yet to be determined. The reason for this prolonged use is multifactorial. Patients requiring tracheostomy have their upper airway permanently bypassed and the morphologic structure of the lower airway may adapt to provide greater heat and moisture exchange capabilities. Additionally, many of these patients have chronic diseases and are not subject to the multitude of homeostasis problems seen in the hospital. The decision to use heated humidification in this setting should, however, be similar to that described previously.

ACTIVE HYGROSCOPIC HEAT AND MOISTURE EXCHANGERS

Passive humidifiers cannot be used in all situations as a consequence of available moisture output and patient disease. As has been discussed, there are patients who require the addition of heat and moisture to the respiratory tract. In an effort to expand the use of HHMEs, Gibeck-Dryden has introduced the active HHME. This device incorporates an HHME that fits inside a heated housing. The housing contains a paper element that acts like a wick to increase the surface area for gas/moisture transfer. A water source continuously drips water onto the wick. Figure 4-10 is a schematic of the **active heat and moisture exchanger (HME).** The wick is warmed by the heated housing, increasing moisture output of the device. This system works much like a wick humidifier, except the source of heat and moisture is added at the airway. This eliminates condensate in the inspiratory limb and the need for water traps. In addition, if the water source runs out, this device continues to operate as an HHME. There is never the possibility of delivering dry gas to the airway, as can occur with a traditional heated humidifier.

In a recent evaluation, it was found that the active HHME provided temperatures of 36° C to 38° C and 90% to 95% relative humidity. Compared with a heated humidifier and a heated humidifier with a heated wire circuit, the active HHME provided equivalent efficiency with lower water usage.[67] These findings have been confirmed in follow-up reports.[68,69] The potential disadvantages of this product are the possibility of skin burns and the increase in dead space compared with a heated humidifier or HHME alone. The external temperature of the housing is

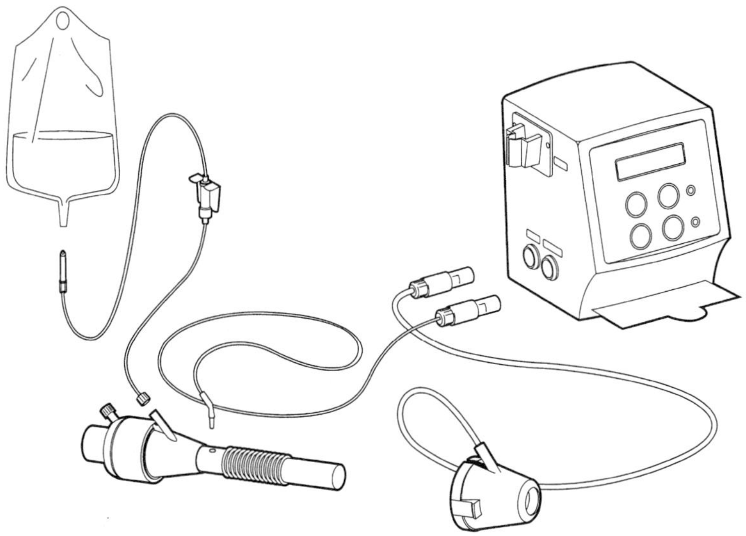

FIGURE 4-10 Schematic of the active heat and moisture exchanger (HME).

near 37° C. Under normal conditions, this temperature is safe. However, patients with peripheral edema or low cardiac output may have reduced blood flow to the skin. In these instances, heat transfer is reduced and modest temperatures can cause local burns.

Heat and Moisture Exchanger Booster

The **heat and moisture exchanger booster** is similar in concept to an active HME, but simpler and less efficient. The booster is a small heating element placed between the passive humidifier and the patient. The heating element is covered with a Gore-Tex membrane. Water flows onto the surface of the heating element and is vaporized (Figure 4-11). The water passes through the membrane and is delivered to the patient during inspiration. During expiration, the additional moisture is trapped in the passive humidifier, serving to "load" the medium with moisture. Some moisture of course escapes through the HME. The water flow is controlled by a small pinhole-sized orifice adjacent to the heating element. This prevents pooling of excess water. Reports of the booster's use are scant. Our laboratory experience suggests that the device can add an additional 2 to 5 mg H_2O/L to inspired gases depending on the tidal volume, inspiratory: expiratory (I: E) ratio, and type of passive humidifier used. Whether this small increase in moisture output is worth the additional equipment and expense remains to be proven.[70-72]

AEROSOL THERAPY DURING MECHANICAL VENTILATION

Physical Properties

Delivery of medications via the respiratory tract has several advantages over systemic therapy in patients with lung disease. Compared with systemic therapy, aerosol therapy provides a more rapid onset of action and similar efficacy at lower doses. Numerous factors affect aerosol delivery to the respiratory tract. These include particle size, inertial impaction, **gravitational sedimentation,** and diffusion.[73-77] A quick review of these subjects is in order before discussing the additional factors present in the mechanically ventilated patient.

Factors Affecting Aerosol Delivery

Aerosols delivered to the respiratory tract can produce the desired clinical effect only if the particle size is appropriate for the application. In ambulatory patients, aerosols with a **mass median aerodynamic diameter (MMAD)** greater than 5 μm are trapped in the naso- and oropharynx. Bronchodilators and drugs meant to act on the airways should have an MMAD of 2 to 5 μm. Drugs intended for peripheral distribution into the lung parenchyma, such as pentamidine, should have an MMAD of 1 to 3 μm. Particles smaller than 1 μm travel into the respiratory tree, but are commonly removed during exhalation without pro-

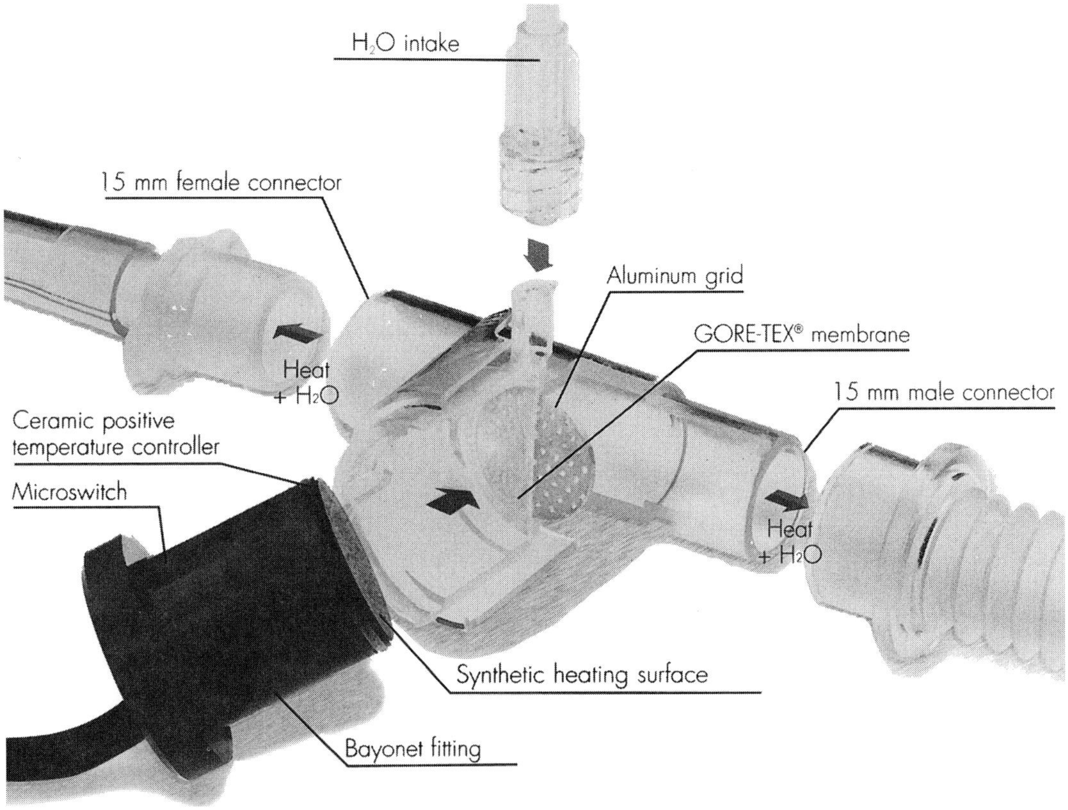

FIGURE 4-11 The heat and moisture exchanger (HME) booster.

ducing any effect. The particles in an aerosol vary greatly in size. The MMAD of an aerosol refers to the point at which half the particles in an aerosol are larger than and half the particles are smaller than the stated value. The aerosol particle size creates a standard bell-shaped curve, which is used to determine MMAD. Bronchodilators are the most common drugs delivered by aerosol therapy in the mechanically ventilated patient. Effective delivery requires an MMAD of 3 to 5 μm.[78-82]

Deposition of aerosol particles primarily results from **inertial impaction.** Inertia is the tendency of an object in motion to remain in motion along a straight trajectory. In the continuously branching tracheobronchial tree, gas carrying an aerosol is constantly changing direction at bifurcations in the airways. The larger the mass of a particle, the greater the particle's inertia. More simply, a large particle approaching a branching airway is less likely to change trajectory with gas flow than a small particle. In essence, the inertia of the particle causes it to collide with the surface of the airway and be deposited. Other factors that affect inertia include inspiratory flow (higher flows increase inertia) and turbulent flow (turbulence increases impaction). These two factors are particularly important during mechanical ventilation.

Particles that enter deep into the respiratory tract tend to lose inertia and are deposited primarily as a result of gravitational sedimentation. During gravitational sedimentation, the larger the particle, the greater the effect of gravity, and the faster it is deposited. Gravitational sedimentation may be an important method of aerosol deposition during breath holding, when airflow has ceased. The role of an inspiratory hold maneuver during aerosol therapy is discussed later in this chapter. Diffusion plays an important role in deposition of small particles (1 to 3 μm) in the periphery of the lung. This can occur by direct deposition onto the mucosa or can result from collision of aerosol particles, causing coalescence and deposition.

Types of Aerosol Generators

Aerosols most commonly are delivered via a **small-volume nebulizer (SVN)** or a **metered-dose**

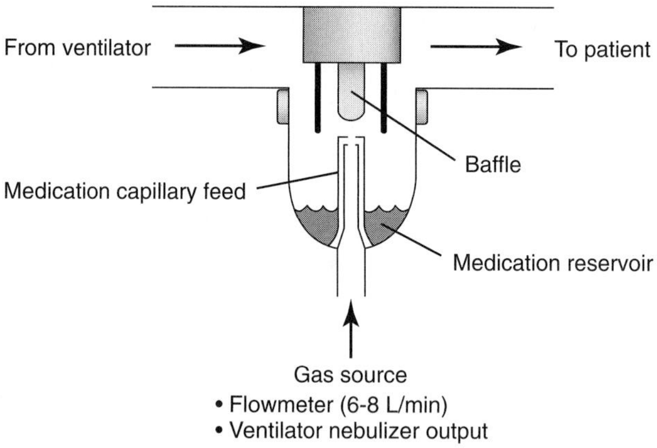

FIGURE 4-12 A typical small-volume nebulizer.

inhaler (MDI) during mechanical ventilation.[11] There are advantages and disadvantages to each device. The SVN has been the traditional device of choice, although evidence suggests that the MDI is as efficient and less expensive.

Small-Volume Nebulizer

The SVN is typically a disposable device consisting of a reservoir, a gas inlet, a baffle, and a Venturi or capillary system that creates the aerosol by combining gas flow and solution at a point of high gas velocity (Figure 4-12). Performance of an SVN can be affected by innumerable factors. These factors include the construction of the nebulizer, the dead volume, the gas flow powering the nebulizer, the drug being nebulized, the volume of solution, the duration of nebulization, and the gas used to power the nebulizer.[78,79]

The **dead volume** refers to the volume of solution that is trapped in the reservoir but that cannot be nebulized. Appropriate construction of the nebulizer can serve to reduce the dead volume. To minimize the effects of the dead volume, a minimum solution of 5 ml is recommended. Increasing flow to the nebulizer results in creation of a smaller particle size, but also speeds the duration of nebulization and results in greater waste (nebulization during the expiratory phase). Because both too low and too high a flow may be problematic, a flow of 8 to 10 L/min is generally used.

Gases with low densities (helium) tend to improve nebulizer function by increasing velocity and creating small particle sizes.[80,81] The low density of helium also may improve aerosol delivery by carrying particles through narrow airways. The ability of helium to carry an aerosol is less than that of gases with higher densities, and nebulization times may be increased. The use of heliox mixtures to power the SVN should be reserved for patients with severe airflow obstruction (e.g., asthma).

Continuous nebulization is sometimes used to deliver large doses of bronchodilators. As nebulization progresses, evaporation of the diluent increases the drug concentration in the remaining solution. When continuous nebulization is used, the reservoir should be emptied of the dead volume between doses.

Metered-Dose Inhalers

An MDI is a simple, single-patient use, drug delivery system that consists of a pressurized, aluminum drug-filled canister and an actuator (Figure 4-13). The device is activated by compressing the canister into the actuator, causing the pressure to release a unit dose (normally called a puff) of medication. The initial particle size of aerosol from an MDI is relatively large (greater than 30 μm), with particle size decreasing as the propellant evaporates. The medication released from the MDI creates a plume of aerosol traveling away from the actuator.[82-84]

The "metered" portion of MDI refers to the metering valve that controls the dose of drug delivered. Each actuation delivers a fixed volume of 25 to 100 μl and results in 15 to 20 ml of aerosol volume. This is accomplished by using a dose-metering chamber that is physically separate from the main reservoir. The metering chamber refills after each actuation and is stored, ready for the next dose.

Factors affecting MDI performance include separation of the drug and propellant, temperature, tail-

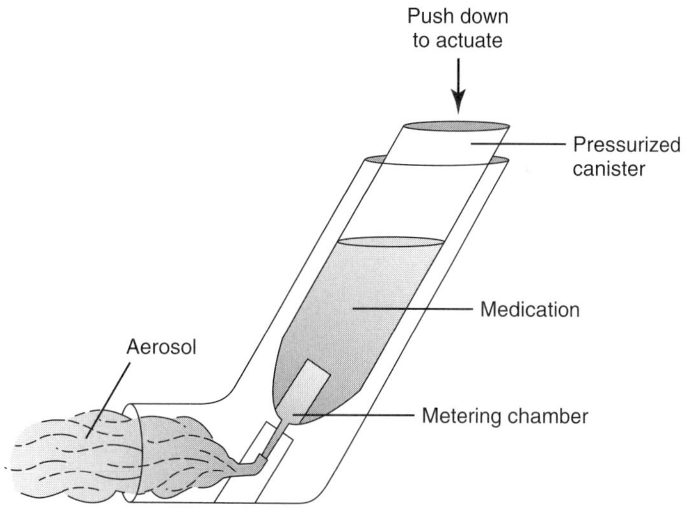

FIGURE 4-13 A metered-dose inhaler.

off, and position. Shaking and warming the canister in the hands help eliminate the first two problems. Tail-off refers to the lower dose delivered near the end of the canister volume.[11] This problem can be remedied by using only the number of doses specified on the canister. The MDI always should be held in an upright position during dosing.

A **spacer** or holding chamber is a device combined with an MDI to improve drug delivery. The spacer serves to reduce the velocity of the dose and reduce MMAD. Factors affecting the efficiency of a spacer include size, shape, and duration of use. Spacers frequently are used in ambulatory patients but have become popular with the use of an MDI during mechanical ventilation. Figure 4-14 depicts spacer devices used during mechanical ventilation.

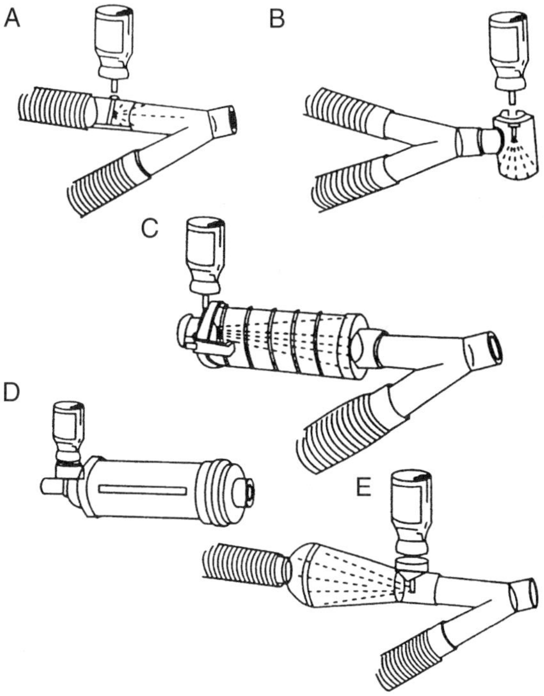

FIGURE 4-14 Different types of commercially available adapters to connect a metered-dose inhaler (MDI) to the ventilator circuit. **A,** In-line adapter; **B,** elbow adapter; **C,** collapsible spacer; **D,** noncollapsible chamber; **E,** chamber where actuation of the MDI delivers aerosol away from the patient. (From Dhand R, Tobin MJ: Bronchodilator delivery with metered dose inhalers in mechanically ventilated patients. Eur J Respir Dis 9:585, 1996.)

Dry Powder Inhalers

Dry powder inhalers (DPIs) are commonly used for drug delivery in ambulatory patients. A DPI creates an aerosol by drawing air through a powder that contains micronized particles.[85] A typical DPI has three components that include the drug formulation, the metering system, and the dispersion mechanism. Current DPIs are passive, that is, the patient provides the energy to aerosolize the particles.

DPI systems are not currently available for delivery during mechanical ventilation, although several authors have reported modifications to allow DPI delivery in the ventilator circuit.[86-89] Three specific problems are associated with DPI use during mechanical ventilation. The first is that most DPIs do not have connections that facilitate connection to the circuit and, as such, modification of the canister is required. Secondly, a method to aerosolize the powder before breath delivery must be devised. Finally, the presence of humidity in the ventilator circuit significantly reduces the drug delivery from a DPI. At present, the use of DPIs during mechanical ventilation is not routine and future use will require addressing these three issues.

Vibrating Mesh Nebulizers

The **vibrating mesh nebulizer** uses a vibrating mesh or plate with multiple apertures to create an aerosol. These devices do not require a gas source for power and eliminate problems associated with the addition of a continuous flow to the ventilator circuit. The vibration frequency and power requirements of the mesh nebulizer allow it to be battery powered and operate at room temperatures without increasing the temperature of the medication. Early trials of the vibrating mesh nebulizers suggest that drug output is up to three times greater than with a traditional SVN.[90]

Aerosol Via an Intratracheal Catheter

In an effort to prevent the baffling effect of the endotracheal tube, one company (Trudell Medical International, London, Ontario, Canada) has introduced an intratracheal catheter (AeroProbe) for aerosol delivery. The coaxial catheter forces the solution to be nebulized to the aerosol tip via a central lumen where gas at 100 psi and 0.1-3 L/min from several lumens surrounding the central lumen impacts the solution and creates an aerosol. This system can use either continuous or intermittent nebulization. This device remains investigational. Initial reports suggest improved drug distribution.[91,92]

Choosing an Aerosol Delivery System

Under routine conditions, the MDI is the preferred method of bronchodilator delivery during mechanical ventilation, if the desired medication is available in an MDI form. The SVN may be preferred when either a high dose or continuous delivery is desired, as the SVN dose is typically up to 10 times the MDI dose. Under these conditions, the SVN offers convenience with similar or improved effectiveness.[93]

Aerosol Delivery During Mechanical Ventilation

Numerous circumstances within the patient/ventilator system affect the efficiency of aerosol delivery using either an SVN or an MDI. These include the artificial airway, the ventilator circuit, humidity, humidification devices, ventilator settings, and position of the aerosol generator in the circuit.[94-117] Each of these is discussed.

The artificial airway typically is considered the major impediment to aerosol delivery to the lower respiratory tract.[96,100] The artificial airway acts as the primary site of aerosol impaction, removing a large portion of the aerosol particles. The ventilator circuit includes the Y-piece, elbow connector, and corrugated tubing, all of which serve as areas of impaction, removing aerosol as a function of circuit length and acuity of angles.[94,96,98,104] The position of the aerosol generator in the circuit also affects efficiency.[98] If the device is too far from the patient, aerosol may be lost because of impaction. If the device is too close to the patient, aerosol may be lost secondary to impaction and through the expiratory side of the breathing circuit. When the aerosol generator is placed approximately 25 to 30 cm from the Y-piece, the circuit serves as a spacer, improving aerosol delivery. The addition of a spacer only marginally improves aerosol delivery with an SVN.

When an MDI is used, the actuator adapter may be paced in-line in the inspiratory limb of the circuit, at the elbow, or directly onto the airway. The use of a spacer in the inspiratory limb significantly improves aerosol delivery with an MDI.[97,100,101] The MDI can be actuated during expiration such that the plume is carried to the patient on the subsequent breath or, in some cases, synchronized with breath delivery. Some authors have suggested that synchronization with inspiration improves aerosol delivery by one third.[94] Numerous methods for improving aerosol delivery during use of an MDI have been suggested.

Humidity in the ventilator circuit tends to result in an increase in particle size and diminished aerosol delivery.[96] The amount of alteration in particle size is a function of relative humidity. During heated humidification, the dose may be diminished by half. Heated humidification with a nonheated wire circuit has the highest relative humidity and greatest adverse effect on aerosol delivery. In these cases, it may be wise to bypass the heated humidifier during use of an SVN. Heated humidification with a heated wire circuit generally has a relative humidity of less than 100% and has less effect. The ventilator circuit has no humidity when a passive humidifier is used. However, the presence of a passive humidifier acts as a filter, removing aerosol particles. In the case of the SVN, nebulization of solutions into a passive humidifier may result in occlusion. When a passive humidifier is used, it must be removed during use of the SVN. If an MDI is used, it should be removed unless the actuator adapter is between the patient and the passive humidifier. Patients requiring continuous nebulization of bronchodilators never should use a passive humidifier.[11]

Ventilator settings, mode, the presence of continuous flow, and the source of gas flow all may affect aerosol delivery.[95,98,99] Spontaneous breaths tend to improve aerosol delivery over mandatory breaths when tidal volume is sufficient. Sufficient tidal volume means a volume greater than the volume of the ventilator circuit and artificial airway. In adults, a tidal volume of greater than 500 ml generally improves aerosol delivery. A longer inspiratory duty cycle (longer inspiratory time) also improves aerosol delivery because a greater volume from the aerosol generator is delivered with each breath. Prolonged inspiratory times also may improve aerosol delivery by enhancing deposition in the airways.

When flow-triggering systems are used, a continuous flow of gas from 2 to 20 L/min may travel through the ventilator circuit. This continuous flow of gas increases aerosol being washed through the ventilator circuit and out to the atmosphere. When using an SVN, the continuous flow should be disabled, if possible. When using an MDI, the actuation should be synchronized with inspiration.[94]

When using an SVN treatment, time can affect total aerosol deposition. Generally the longer the treatment time, the greater the dose of drug that is deposited. This concept is the pretext for using continuous nebulization of bronchodilators with an SVN in patients with severe airway obstruction.

Use of the mechanical ventilator nebulizer option also may influence SVN efficiency. McPeck and associates found that the flow-through delivered via the ventilator's nebulizer port varied considerably.[99] Lower flow can result in large particle size and prolonged nebulization times. The activation of ventilator nebulizers is also different from manufacturer to manufacturer. In some instances, only mandatory breaths result in initiation of the nebulizer. In others, every breath triggers the nebulizer flow. The duration of nebulizer flow also changes with inspiratory flow waveform (Box 4-1). Nebulization systems were designed to prevent augmentation of tidal volume during aerosol delivery using an SVN and a continuous flow of gas. Sophisticated ventilator algorithms also maintain inspired O_2 concentration (F_{IO_2}) and tidal volume constant during nebulizer function.

Interestingly, the continuous flow of an SVN powered by an external flowmeter can complicate ventilator triggering and volume monitoring. During flow triggering, the additional external flow prevents triggering by forcing the patient to increase effort to overcome both the ventilator continuous flow and the external continuous flow.[107] This additional flow also passes through the expiratory flow transducer, causing the ventilator to overestimate actual tidal

BOX 4-1 *Factors Influencing the Deposition of Aerosol Delivery in Intubated, Mechanically Ventilated Patients*

Ventilator-related factors
- Mode of mechanical ventilation
- Tidal volume
- Respiratory frequency
- Inspiratory time (duty cycle)
- Inspiratory flow waveform
- Presence of continuous flow (flow triggering)

Device-related factors
- Position of nebulizer in circuit—SVN
- Position of adapter and/or spacer in the circuit—MDI
- Timing of actuation—MDI
- Type of nebulizer (SVN) or adapter (MDI)
- Duration of operation and continuous vs. intermittent nebulization (SVN)

Ventilator circuit-related factors
- Endotracheal tube size
- Presence of angles in the circuit (90-degree elbow, flex tubes)
- Relative humidity of inspired gases
- Density of inspired gases (heliox)
- Presence of a passive humidifier

Drug-related factors
- Dose
- Aerosol particle
- Duration of action

Patient-related factors
- Severity of airway obstruction
- Mechanism of airway obstruction (mucus, bronchospasm, mechanical)
- Presence of dynamic hyperinflation
- Patient-ventilator synchrony

Modified from Dhand R, Tobin MJ: Bronchodilator delivery with metered dose inhalers in mechanically ventilated patients, Eur J Respir Dis 9:585, 1996.
MDI, Metered-dose inhaler; *SVN,* small-volume nebulizer.

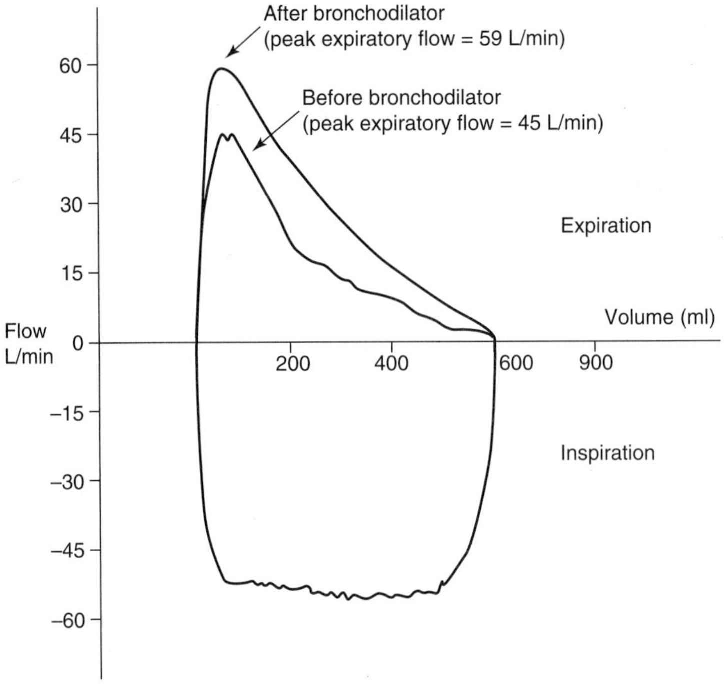

FIGURE 4-15 Flow-volume loops before and after bronchodilator therapy in a mechanically ventilated patient with chronic obstructive pulmonary disease.

volume. In these instances, aerosol delivery affects the efficacy of mechanical ventilation, the opposite effect of our previous discussions. Additionally, the presence of aerosolized medications in the expiratory limb of the ventilator may affect the accuracy of some flow sensors. This usually is seen only when continuous nebulization using an SVN is used. Filters often are placed in the expiratory limb of the ventilator circuit to protect these devices. When this is done, it is imperative to change the filters regularly, otherwise they become partially occluded, prevent triggering, retard exhalation, and cause air trapping.

Monitoring Bronchodilator Efficacy

Determining the effect of aerosolized bronchodilators commonly is done simply by listening to breath sounds and observing patient comfort. The actual response to bronchodilator therapy depends on a multitude of factors, including the severity of airflow obstruction, the reversibility of bronchospasm, the volume of secretions, the degree of inflammation, and the use of concomitant parenteral bronchodilators.[108-117]

Monitoring the shape of the expiratory flow-volume curve may be useful in detecting a reduction in expiratory airway resistance (Figure 4-15). Subtle improvements may not be detected in this manner, but most ventilators provide this measurement, making it readily available. When observing the expiratory flow-volume curve, both the peak expiratory flow and the shape of the curve may show signs of reduced airway resistance. When bronchodilation is successful, the peak expiratory flow commonly increases and the duration of expiratory flow may be diminished. These observations are frequently all that is necessary in routine clinical decision making.

More accurate measurements of bronchodilator response are available, although routine application may not be warranted. The equipment and expertise to measure these variables are not routinely available. Measurements of inspiratory parameters (peak inspiratory pressure, inspiratory resistance) are rarely helpful because positive pressure and lung inflation alter resistance by mechanical means. Measurements of expiratory parameters are more sensitive and are described subsequently.

Expiratory airway resistance is measured by delivering a constant flow, passive inflation coupled with an inspiratory plateau.[112,113] If the flow is not constant or if the patient contributes inspiratory or expiratory effort, the measurement is invalid. The duration of

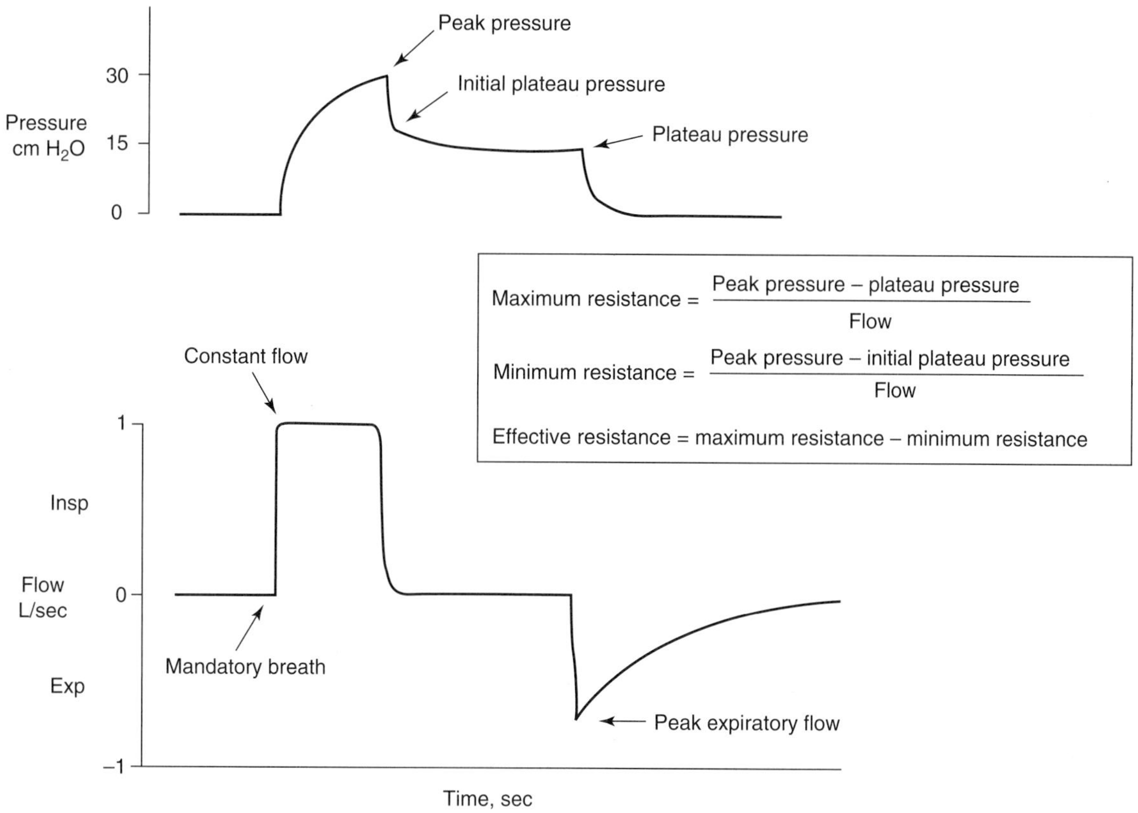

FIGURE 4-16 Measurement of minimum and maximum expiratory resistance using flow and pressure waveforms.

the required inspiratory pressure plateau depends on the degree of airway obstruction. Typically, 2 to 3 seconds are sufficient. However, in some cases, up to 5 seconds are necessary to reach a plateau. Dhand and colleagues have proposed the measurement of both minimal and maximal resistance.[113] These measurements are shown in Figure 4-16. During passive inflation, the peak inspiratory pressure is measured as is the initial pressure at the beginning of the plateau pressure. This initial pressure change (peak pressure – initial plateau pressure/flow) represents ohmic resistance. By use of the difference between peak pressure and final plateau pressure divided by flow, the maximum or total expiratory resistance can be determined. The difference between the minimum and maximum airway resistance measurements can provide some insight into the degree of airway obstruction. Alveolar units with inhomogeneous time constants require different times before reaching the steady state plateau pressure. The greater the difference between minimum and maximum resistance, the greater the inhomogeneties.

Changes in autoPEEP also can provide evidence of reduced expiratory resistance as a response to bronchodilator therapy (Figure 4-17). As expiratory resistance diminishes, the lung empties more rapidly, resulting in a decrease in autoPEEP. AutoPEEP is measured more simply than expiratory resistance, but is not as sensitive as the expiratory resistance measurement.

The required dose of bronchodilator to achieve the desired effect depends on the patient factors previously discussed. Routine administration of 2.5 mg of albuterol by SVN or 4 puffs of albuterol by MDI provides the maximum effect with minimum side effects (tachycardia, dysrhythmias). In patients with refractory bronchospasm, continuous nebulization by SVN may be necessary. Monitoring of bronchodilator therapy for dose response using these measurements in routine cases is probably more trouble than it is worth. MDI therapy is cheap, and monitoring in routine cases can be accomplished with simple patient assessment. In severe cases, particularly when continuous nebulization is used, more intensive monitoring is justified.

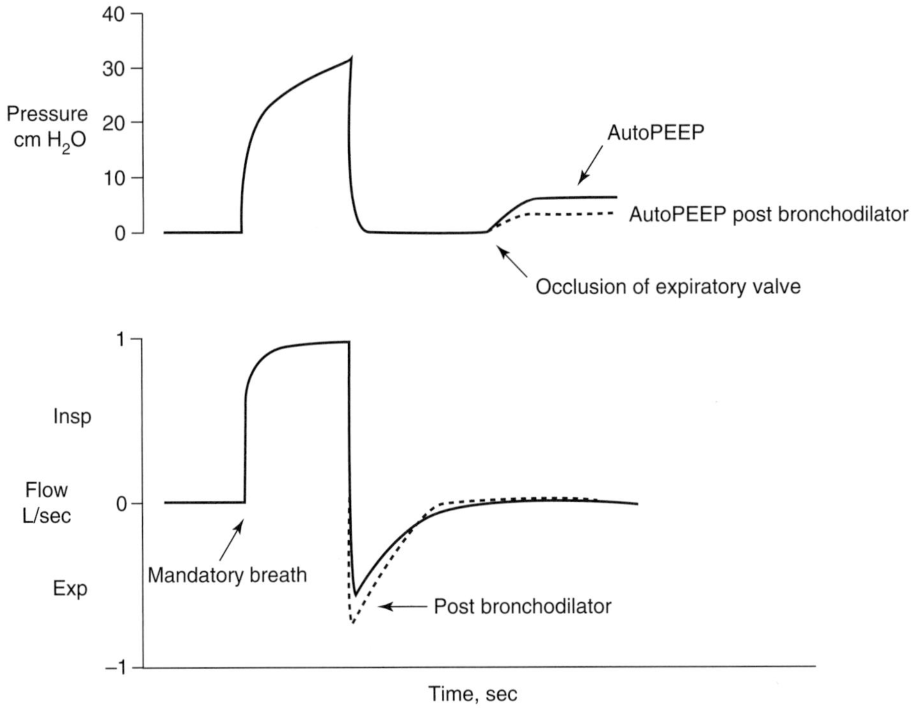

FIGURE 4-17 Measurement of auto-positive end-expiratory pressure (autoPEEP) before and after delivery of a bronchodilator.

Recommendations for Aerosol Therapy in Mechanically Ventilated Patients

Based on the aforementioned data, MDI should be used to deliver aerosol therapy during mechanical ventilation. There is no evidence to support the widely held belief that an SVN improves drug delivery or provides faster relief than an MDI. In fact, the MDI is cheaper and requires less time to administer. Use of the SVN is complicated by variation in device performance, dead volume, driving gas flow, and the potential for contamination. SVNs should be used to deliver drugs not available in an MDI system or when continuous nebulization is required for severe airway obstruction.

Recommendations for SVN and MDI use are shown in Table 4-4.

AEROSOLIZED PHARMACOLOGIC AGENTS

Bronchodilators are the most frequently delivered aerosolized medication during mechanical ventilation. However, antibiotics, antivirals, and a host of other drugs are becoming more popular. Inhaled drug delivery is preferred when the drug can be delivered directly to the site of action, maximizing effect while minimizing the required dose. The inhaled route also reduces systemic side effects compared with intravenous administration. The nature of the airway is such that inhaled pharmacologic agents also have a rapid onset of action.

Bronchodilators

The most common aerosolized bronchodilators used during mechanical ventilation are β-adrenergic agonists and **anticholinergics.** The mechanism of action of **β_2-agonists** is understood to involve interaction of the drug with a receptor that leads to exchange of guanosine triphosphate (GTP) for guanosine diphosphate (GDP). The GTP-activated G protein then activates adenylate cyclase, leading to the formation of cyclic adenosine monophosphate (cAMP). Among the initial events that result in a cellular response is the activation of protein kinase A, which phosphorylates various cellular proteins and regulates their activities.

Tissue responses after beta receptor stimulation include relaxation of bronchial smooth muscle, prevention of release of mediators from mast cells,

TABLE 4-4 *Recommendations for Small-Volume Nebulizer (SVN) and Metered-Dose Inhaler (MDI) Use*

PROPER TECHNIQUE FOR USING SVN	PROPER TECHNIQUE FOR USING MDI
Fill nebulizer with medication and diluent to appropriate fill volume (4-6 ml)	Choose appropriate MDI adapter/spacer and place in the inspiratory limb of the ventilator circuit
Place nebulizer in the inspiratory limb of the ventilator circuit 25-35 cm from the patient (circuit acts as a spacer)	Adjust ventilation parameters for optimum drug delivery (increase tidal volume, decrease respiratory frequency, lengthen inspiratory time—reset alarms if necessary)
Establish appropriate flow for nebulizer operation (6-8 L/min)—intermittent flow from the ventilator's nebulization system is preferred	Warm MDI with hands and shake vigorously
Adjust ventilation parameters for optimum drug delivery (increase tidal volume, decrease respiratory frequency, lengthen inspiratory time—reset alarms if necessary)	Remove passive humidifier or bypass heated humidifier
If a pediatric continuous flow ventilator is used, reduce ventilator flow to maintain constant tidal volume	Actuate MDI with mandatory breath delivery (adapter)
Turn off continuous flow, if possible	Actuate MDI near end-exhalation (spacer)
Remove passive humidifier or bypass heated humidifier	Wait 30-60 sec between actuations
Observe nebulization, tap sides to reduce dead volume, and continue until all solution is delivered	Remove MDI from circuit adapter and maintain the MDI clean
Remove SVN from circuit and maintain the SVN clean	Monitor patient for signs of improvement or complications
Monitor patient for signs of improvement or complications	

increased mucus secretion from submucosal glands, and increased mucociliary transport. The acute bronchodilator properties of β-agonists are regarded as the most useful to the practitioner.[118,119]

The goal of acute bronchodilation is best achieved through the inhalation of β_2-agonists. Bronchodilator effects typically outweigh the known and suspected adverse effects of both short- and long-acting agents.[120,121] Potential adverse effects from beta receptor stimulation include tachycardia, skeletal muscle tremors, and hypokalemia (Figure 4-18). Patients with preexisting cardiovascular disease—particularly the elderly—may be more prone to such reactions. Because these patients often represent a substantial portion of ventilated patients, one must monitor therapy, particularly with any dose titration regimens.

The provision of optimal pharmacotherapy is paramount in the goals of modern-day asthma therapy, and a stepwise approach currently is outlined in clinical practice guidelines.[122] Short-acting clinical agents are indicated for relief of acute symptoms, whereas long-acting β-agonists added to anti-inflammatory agents are indicated for long-term symptom prevention (especially nocturnal symptoms). In chronic obstructive pulmonary disease (COPD), current pharmacologic care standards[123,124] recognize the role of β-agonists for the relief of symptoms. Again, the potential for arrhythmias should be considered in using these agents in patients with cardiac disease, although serious complications with conventional dosages in the stable patient are regarded as rare.[125] The most commonly used bronchodilators are listed in Table 4-5 along with trade names, duration of action, and dose.

Significant bronchodilation can be achieved with β-agonists when they are employed optimally in patients requiring mechanical ventilation. Consensus statements presently support the use of either the nebulizer or the MDI as an acceptable method of delivery in mechanically ventilated patients.[126] Many, but not all, trials have demonstrated an improvement in airway pressure responses (e.g., airway resistance) after MDI administration of albuterol[127-131] or

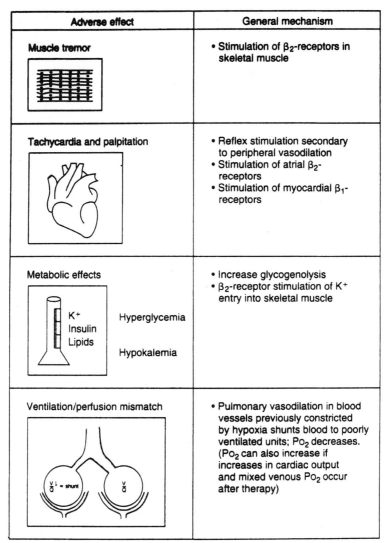

Adverse effect	General mechanism
Muscle tremor 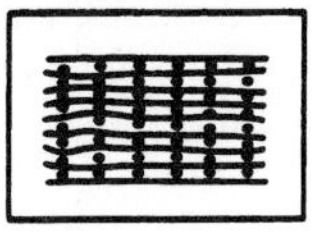	• Stimulation of β_2-receptors in skeletal muscle
Tachycardia and palpitation 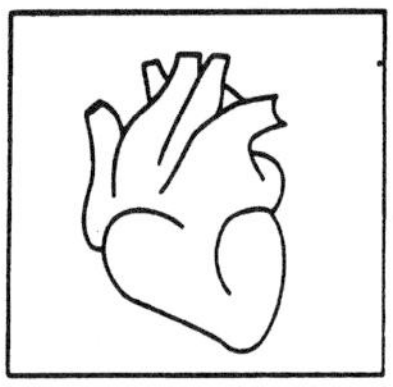	• Reflex stimulation secondary to peripheral vasodilation • Stimulation of atrial β_2-receptors • Stimulation of myocardial β_1-receptors
Metabolic effects 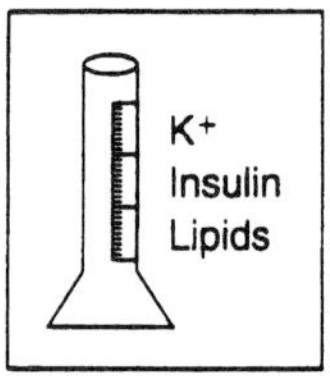 Hyperglycemia Hypokalemia	• Increase glycogenolysis • β_2-receptor stimulation of K^+ entry into skeletal muscle
Ventilation/perfusion mismatch 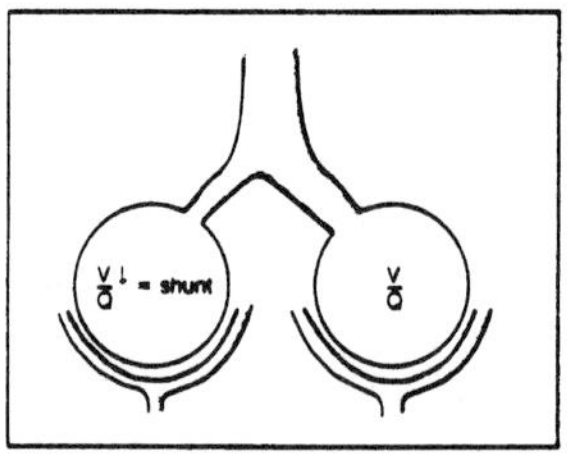 	• Pulmonary vasodilation in blood vessels previously constricted by hypoxia shunts blood to poorly ventilated units; Po_2 decreases. (Po_2 can also increase if increases in cardiac output and mixed venous Po_2 occur after therapy)

FIGURE 4-18 Adverse effects and their general mechanisms associated with β-2 agonists.

TABLE 4-5 *Commonly Used Bronchodilators, Trade Names, Dose, and Action*

			ACTION		
AGENT	**TRADE NAMES**	**DOSE**	**ONSET**	**PEAK**	**DURATION**
Albuterol	Proventil Proventil HFA Ventolin	SVN: 0.5% solution, 2.5 mg MDI: 90 μg/puff 2 puffs Both given tid or qid	5-15 min	30-60 min	5-8 hr
Levalbuterol	Xopenex	SVN: 0.63 mg q 6-8 h	15 min	30-60 min	5-8 hr
Terbutaline	Brethine	MDI: 200 μg/puff 2 puffs q 4 h	5-30 min	30-60 min	3-6 hr
Ipratropium	Atrovent	SVN: 0.02% solution, 2.5 mg MDI: 18 μg/puff, 2 puffs BID	15 min	90-120 min	6-8 hr

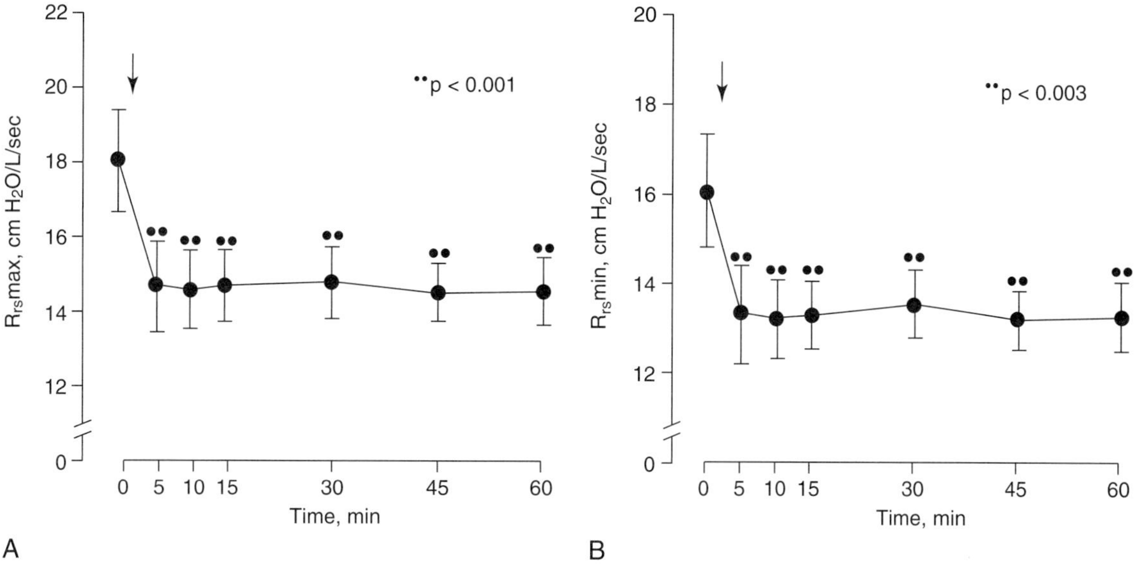

FIGURE 4-19 Effect of administration of four puffs on R_{rs}max **(A)** and R_{rs}min **(B)** in seven patients. A significant decrease in R_{rs}max and R_{rs}min occurred within 5 minutes of albuterol administration ($p < 0.003$ for both). The effect of albuterol persisted for 60 minutes ($p < 0.003$ for both R_{rs}max and R_{rs}min). R_{rs}, respiratory system resistance. (From Dhand R, Duarte AG, Jubran A et al: Dose response to bronchodilator delivered by metered-dose inhaler in ventilator-supported patients. Am J Respir Crit Care Med 154:388-393, 1996. © American Lung Association.)

metaproterenol[132] in mechanically ventilated patients. In these trials, cohorts were generally small (N = 7-20) and included patients with COPD,[128,129-131] acute respiratory distress syndrome (ARDS),[133] or mixed conditions.[128-132] The doses of β-agonists used in these studies varied (0.2-3 mg), as did the administrative and assessment techniques.

Dose response to MDI albuterol has been evaluated in patients who require mechanical ventilation. Manthous and associates[130] administered albuterol with cumulative exposure as high as 100 puffs (90 μg/puff) from an MDI and did not observe significant bronchodilator or toxic effects. In a subsequent trial with the use of a spacer,[133] they observed significantly reduced pressure responses after cumulative doses of 15 puffs (90 μg/puff) that were not improved further with 15 more puffs (total = 30 puffs). Dhand and coworkers[131] observed significant differences in airway resistance in 12 patients with COPD after 4 puffs of albuterol (90 μg/puff) (Figure 4-19) that were comparable to those seen after cumulative doses of both 12 and 28 puffs. Because heart rate was increased significantly after the cumulative dose of 28 puffs (mean of 89 beats/min after 28 puffs, 84 beats/min after 12 puffs, and 81 beats/min after 4 puffs; no increases greater than 110 beats/min) (Figure 4-20), the investigators concluded that 4 puffs was the best dosage.

Taken together, the observations with albuterol administered to mechanically ventilated patients via MDI highlight several important aspects of therapeutics. First, the technique of delivery, the assessment of response, and the disease characteristics of the study population need to be considered in evaluating existing data. Second, the clinician must carefully assess the individual therapeutic outcome by monitoring both the desired effect (e.g., decreased airway resistance, lower auto-PEEP) and the unwanted pharmacodynamic responses (e.g., tachycardia).

Anticholinergics

Anticholinergic agents achieve bronchodilation by competitively inhibiting the action of acetylcholine on **muscarinic receptors.** This effect not only relaxes bronchial smooth muscle, but may produce a bronchoprotective effect against new bronchoconstriction.[134,135] Like β-agonists, bronchodilatory properties of this class of drugs have been known for centuries. The prototype agent atropine, although occasionally administered via aerosol in the modern

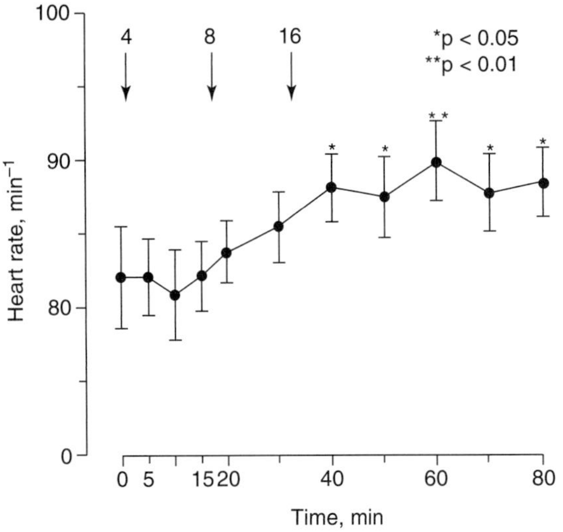

FIGURE 4-20 **Effect of doubling doses of albuterol (4, 8, and 16 puffs) on heart rate. Heart rate did not change after administration of 4 puffs or a cumulative dose of 12 puffs ($p > 0.05$). After a cumulative dose of 28 puffs, heart rate increased significantly ($p < 0.01$) and was significantly higher at 80 minutes ($p < 0.05$) when compared with baseline values. Bars represent standard error* p less than 0.05;[†] p less than 0.01.** (From Dhand R, Duarte AG, Jubran A et al: Dose response to bronchodilator delivered by metered-dose inhaler in ventilator-supported patients. Am J Respir Crit Care Med 154:388-393, 1996. © American Lung Association.)

era, was hampered by its side effects. Antimuscarinic bronchodilators were introduced into current practice with the development of ipratropium bromide. By contrast, the inability of ipratropium bromide to be absorbed across biologic membranes widens its therapeutic window; this has resulted in its widespread use for relief of the obstructed airway.[135]

Antimuscarinic pharmacology has been advanced over the past decade. Five muscarinic receptors have been cloned, four of which have been defined pharmacologically, and three of which have known functions.[136,137] Mediation of cholinergic bronchoconstriction and glandular secretion occurs via the respiratory M_3 receptor. M_3 stimulation, via a G protein, activates phospholipase C (PLC) to release inositol 1,4,5-triphosphate (IP_3) and diacylglycerol (DAG). IP_3 results in release of intracellular calcium, whereas DAG activates protein kinase C (PKC), which leads to smooth muscle contraction. The bronchodilatory role of antimuscarinic drugs such as ipratropium bromide is based on inhibition of these postreceptor events.

Ipratropium bromide has been used most extensively as a bronchodilator in the treatment of COPD,[138] for which treatment guidelines highlight its role in maintenance treatment. Ipratropium bromide is not indicated for rapid relief of bronchospasm because its onset is somewhat slower than that of short-acting β-agonists (see Table 4-5). Because many patients with COPD are prescribed ipratropium bromide concurrently with a β-agonist, a single MDI with both agents has been developed and introduced.[139]

Ipratropium bromide is used extensively in maintenance care of stable patients with COPD. There is one report[127] that describes significant improvements in pressure responses both 30 and 60 minutes after MDI administration of 0.04 mg of ipratropium bromide in COPD patients, most of whom had acute exacerbations of their underlying lung disease. Cardiovascular monitoring did not identify any significant changes, with the exception of a slight increase in systolic blood pressure that the authors speculated was related to sedation differences.

Tiotropium is a long acting muscarinic bronchodilator delivered once daily, which is currently only available as a DPI.[140] The onset of action is approximately 30 minutes with a duration of action lasting 24 hours. Tiotropium has not been studied in mechanically ventilated patients.

Anti-inflammatory Agents

Oral and intravenous corticosteroid therapies remain effective and often life-saving forms of treatment for patients with a variety of acute and chronic pulmonary disorders. The long-term use of these agents, however, is limited by undesirable systemic effects. These include a large array of reactions, some potentially serious, such as adrenal insufficiency, fluid and electrolyte imbalances, glucose intolerance, gastric ulceration, osteoporosis, and growth impairment in children. The severe systemic side effects of chronic oral corticosteroid use prompted the development of inhaled preparations, with the goal of achieving a therapeutic effect in the lungs without the untoward systemic effects. Given the safety profile of inhaled therapy, increasingly widespread use of these agents has occurred over the past 2 decades.

Current guidelines for the treatment of obstructive lung disease indicate a primary role for inhaled corticosteroid therapy in asthma[121-123] but a limited role in COPD. The use of inhaled corticosteroids in the treatment of asthma is dictated by disease severity and is directed toward suppression of airway inflammation. The efficacy of these agents in the management of asthma is probably the result of their wide range of cellular anti-inflammatory effects. Details of proposed cellular and molecular pathophysiologic mechanisms of airway inflammation and the therapeutic activity of corticosteroids can be found in several reviews.[141-143]

Aerosolized corticosteroids, although effective as a maintenance therapy, have no role in the acute management of asthma exacerbations. As recommended in the Asthma Management Guidelines and observed in clinical practice, intravenous steroids are essential for the successful management of asthma patients with acute respiratory failure who require mechanical ventilation. After resolution of the acute episode, strategies for the transition to oral steroids and ultimately inhaled agents are based on the patient's clinical response to therapy.

For the most part, the use of inhaled corticosteroids in mechanically ventilated patients is not indicated. An exception to this practice would be in patients who require maintenance inhaled corticosteroid therapy and who are on mechanical ventilation for reasons other than acute respiratory failure. In these situations, inhaled corticosteroids could be administered via the endotracheal tube. However, to date, no clinical studies have been conducted that support the therapeutic value of inhaled corticosteroids in patients requiring ventilatory assistance.

Aerosolized Antibiotics

The conceptual basis for delivering antibiotics to the lower respiratory tract via aerosolization is compelling. Namely, aerosol administration of antibiotics to the lungs may enable very high concentrations of antibiotics to be delivered directly to the site of lung infection with minimal systemic absorption and therefore minimal systemic side effects. However, the hoped-for improvements in therapeutic efficacy generally have not been achieved with this form of therapy, mostly because of factors that affect the aerosol characteristics of antibiotics (e.g., surface tension, viscosity, and osmolality).[144]

Clinical trials with aerosolized antibiotics have yielded inconsistent results. As noted previously, these inconsistencies are due in part to physical and chemical factors that affect antibiotic aerosol delivery and that may limit the amount of antibiotic that reaches the lower respiratory tract.[145-147] Optimally, an antibiotic that is to be aerosolized should not be readily susceptible to oxidation and must not have an excessively high (will not form droplets) or low (causes foaming and diminishes aerosol production) surface tension. Likewise, as the concentration of antibiotic increases in the nebulized solution, there is a greater likelihood that osmolality and viscosity will also increase, leading to cough and a lower nebulization rate, respectively.[148] Finally, the distribution and extent of lung consolidation may affect antibiotic distribution because the antibiotic will not be optimally delivered to lung units that are consolidated and/or poorly ventilated.[147]

Given these diverse factors affecting antibiotic aerosol delivery, it perhaps is not surprising that results of clinical trials have been inconsistent. Nonetheless, aerosolization of antibiotics has been shown to be clinically useful in the prevention of lung infection in stable patients with cystic fibrosis and may be useful as an adjunct to intravenous antibiotic therapy in cystic fibrosis patients with acute infection.[146] In this regard, Touw and colleagues[147] recently reviewed all studies published between 1965 and 1995 in which inhaled antibiotics were used to treat cystic fibrosis. Among the 12 studies in which inhaled antibiotics were used as maintenance therapy in stable outpatients, an improvement in lung function and/or a reduction in the number of hospital admissions was reported in four uncontrolled studies and in six of eight placebo-controlled studies. By contrast, antibiotic aerosol therapy did not add to the clinical efficacy of intravenous antibiotics in cystic fibrosis patients hospitalized with acute infection. Thus, despite the conceptual appeal of aerosol antibiotic therapy, its role in cystic fibrosis appears limited to preventive and maintenance therapy.

Experimentally, conditions can be defined in which at least certain antibiotics achieve lung concentrations after aerosol delivery that exceed those that occur after intravenous infusion. Specifically, Hashimoto and associates[148] showed that aerosolized imipenem-cilastatin produced greater bronchoalveolar lavage (BAL) antibiotic concentrations in rats than did the intravenous infusions. More importantly, these investigators showed that aerosolizing antibiotics resulted in better bacterial killing and less lung injury than intravenous antibiotics in rats with *Pseudomonas aeruginosa* lung injury.[149] By contrast, aerosolized antibiotics used in mechanically ventilated ICU patients have not been effective and may, at times, be associated with deleterious consequences. Namely, although aerosolized antibiotics can reduce gram-negative colonization rates in intubated patients, their routine use in this patient population also can lead to the emergence of resistant bacteria and an increase in ICU mortality.[150,151]

Currently, aerosolized antibiotics do not have an established role in the prevention or treatment of lower respiratory tract infections in mechanically ventilated patients. However, recent studies have shown that in cases of tracheobronchitis, a pulmonary infection difficult to distinguish from VAP, the use of aerosolized antibiotics can reduce secretion volume.[151-154] The mechanism of action here is thought to be impregnation of secretions and reduction in bacterial colony counts. Repetitive short term aerosolized antibiotics might reduce the bacterial burden in tracheobronchial secretions and prevent VAP. This regimen has been successful in small numbers of patients without the emergence of antibiotic resistance. Additional findings include high levels of drug concentration in the sputum, decreased sputum volume, reduced bacterial growth, and lower cytokine concentrations, suggesting reduced airway inflammation.[152,153] Establishing appropriate clinical end points remains a significant challenge in studies designed to prevent or treat VAP.

KEY POINTS

- Heat and humidification of inspired gases during mechanical ventilation is a standard of care.
- Absolute humidity describes the amount of water vapor present in a gas mixture.
- Relative humidity describes the amount of water vapor present in a gas compared with the maximum amount of water vapor that gas can carry.
- As gas temperature increases, the amount of water vapor a gas can carry increases.
- The HME has an increased risk for occlusion compared with the heated humidifier.
- HMEs may not be indicated for all patients.
- The dead space of an HME can adversely affect the patient's respiratory status.
- The type of humidifier appears to have no effect on the incidence of ventilator associated pneumonia.
- An MDI and an SVN are equally effective for bronchodilator delivery during mechanical ventilation.
- Use of a chamber with the MDI placed in the inspiratory limb enhances aerosol delivery.
- Monitoring bronchodilator response is best accomplished using expiratory measurements.
- Aerosol delivery during mechanical ventilation is affected by device-related, ventilator-related, drug-related, and patient-related factors.
- β_2-agonists are the most frequently used aerosolized bronchodilators during mechanical ventilation.
- Before aerosol delivery, if an HME is being used it must be removed from the circuit.
- Dry powder inhalers (DPIs) are currently not designed for delivery to mechanically ventilated patients.

ASSESSMENT QUESTIONS

1. The point at which gases reach alveolar conditions (37° C and 100% relative humidity) is known as:

A. the humidity deficit.
B. absolute humidity.
C. rainout.
D. the isothermic saturation boundary.

2. The formula for relative humidity is:

A. (absolute humidity)/(maximum capacity) × 37.
B. (absolute humidity)/(maximum capacity) × 100.
C. (absolute humidity)/(minimum capacity) × 100.
D. (absolute humidity)/(maximum capacity) + 37.

ASSESSMENT QUESTIONS—cont'd

3. Over the course of a normal day, the respiratory tract loses approximately:
A. 1470 joules of heat and 250 ml of water.
B. 1470 joules of heat and 0.5 L of water.
C. 1470 joules of heat and 25 ml of water.
D. 1470 joules of heat and 250 g of water.

4. During use of a heated humidifier and heated wire circuit, if the chamber temperature is 34° C and the proximal airway temperature is 39° C, which of the following are true?
I. Absolute humidity increases
II. Relative humidity decreases
III. The risk of drying secretions in the large airways increases
IV. Rainout increases
V. Absolute humidity decreases
A. I, II, and IV
B. II, III, and V
C. II and III only
D. I and II only
E. II and V only

5. Contraindications to heated humidifier use include:
I. Bloody secretions
II. Small tidal volumes
III. Thick secretions
IV. Leaks around the tracheal tube cuff
A. All of the above
B. None of the above
C. I, III, and IV
D. I and III only

6. Contraindications to HME use include:
I. Bloody secretions
II. Small tidal volumes
III. Thick secretions
IV. Leaks around the tracheal tube cuff
A. All of the above
B. None of the above
C. I, III, and IV
D. I and III only

7. True or False. HMEs are ideal for use during face mask ventilation.

8. True or False. The risk of endotracheal tube occlusion is increased with HMEs compared with heated humidifiers.

9. The active HME combines what components:
I. An HME
II. A heated humidifier
III. A filter
IV. An MDI adapter
A. All of the above
B. I and II only
C. I and III only
D. I and IV only

10. The additional dead space of an HME can result in:
I. Elevated $Paco_2$
II. Increased work of breathing
III. Decreased Pao_2
IV. Weaning failure
A. I only
B. II only
C. I, II, and III
D. I, II, and IV

11. Which of the following affect aerosol delivery with an MDI during mechanical ventilation?
I. Type of spacer or adapter used with an MDI
II. Position of the spacer in the circuit
III. Timing of actuation
IV. Type of MDI
A. I, II, and III
B. I, III, and IV
C. II, III, and IV
D. All of the above

12. Which of the following affect aerosol delivery with an SVN during mechanical ventilation?
I. Fill volume
II. Position in the circuit
III. Continuous vs. intermittent nebulization
IV. Type of nebulizer
A. I, II, and III
B. I, III, and IV
C. II, III, and IV
D. All of the above

13. True or False. Evaluation of expiratory parameters are more sensitive than inspiratory parameters when evaluating bronchodilator response.

14. True or False. A vibrating mesh nebulizer works at ultrasonic frequencies.

Continued

ASSESSMENT QUESTIONS—cont'd

15. Agents delivered by the inhaled route have what potential advantages?
- **I.** Rapid onset
- **II.** High drug concentrations at the site of action
- **III.** Reduced systemic side effects
- **IV.** Less frequent dosing
  - **A.** I and III
  - **B.** I, III, and IV
  - **C.** I, II, and III
  - **D.** I, II, and IV

16. True or False. Anti-inflammatory agents such as corticosteroids should be routinely aerosolized in the mechanically ventilated patient.

17. True or False. An MDI is more effective than an SVN for delivery of a bronchodilator during mechanical ventilation.

18. Use of an SVN may be superior to an MDI under what conditions?
- **I.** Faster duration of action
- **II.** Continuous delivery
- **III.** Longer duration of action
- **IV.** Desire to deliver high drug concentrations
  - **A.** I and II
  - **B.** II and III
  - **C.** I, II, and III
  - **D.** II and IV

19. True or False. Aerosolized antibiotics are not routinely used for the treatment of VAP.

20. Potential side effects of β_2-agonists include:
- **I.** Tachycardia
- **II.** Skeletal muscle tremors
- **III.** Hypokalemia
- **IV.** Hypernatremia
  - **A.** I, II, and III
  - **B.** I, II, and IV
  - **C.** I and IV
  - **D.** I and III

21. True or False. Dry powder inhalers are commonly used during mechanical ventilation.

22. Anticholinergic agents achieve bronchodilation by:
- **A.** competitively inhibiting the action of acetylcholine on muscarinic receptors.
- **B.** increasing cyclic GMP.
- **C.** increasing nitric oxide concentrations.
- **D.** stimulating β-2 receptors.

REFERENCES

1. Walker AKY, Bethune DW: A comparative study of condenser humidifiers, Anaesthesia 31:1086-1093, 1976.
2. Drery R: The evolution of heat and moisture in the respiratory tract during anaesthesia with a non-rebreathing system, Can Anaesth Soc J 20:269-277, 1967.
3. Ingelstedt S: Studies on conditioning of respired air in the respiratory tract, Acta Otolarygol 131(suppl):7-21, 1956.
4. Drery R, Pelletier J, Jacques A et al: Humidity in anesthesiology III: heat and moisture exchange in the respiratory tract during anesthesia with the semi-closed system, Can Anaesth Soc J 14:287-295, 1967.
5. Burton JDK: Effects of dry anaesthetic gases on the respiratory mucous membrane, Lancet 1:235-238, 1962.
6. Chalon J, Loew DAY, Malenbranche J: Effects of dry anesthetic gases on tracheobronchial epithelium, Anesthesiology 37:338-343, 1972.
7. Fonkalsrud EW, Sanchez M, Higgashijima I et al: A comparative study of the effects of dry vs humidified ventilation on canine lungs, Surgery 78:373-380, 1975.
8. Forbes AR: Humidification and mucus flow in the intubated trachea, Br J Anaesth 45:874-878, 1973.
9. American Association for Respiratory Care Clinical Practice Guidelines: Humidification during mechanical ventilation, Respir Care 37:887-890, 1992.
10. American Association for Respiratory Care: Consensus statement on the essentials of mechanical ventilators-1992, Respir Care 37:1000-1008, 1992.
11. Hess DR, Branson RD: Humidification: humidifiers and nebulizers. In: Branson RD, Hess DR, Chatburn RL, editors: Respiratory care equipment, Philadelphia, JB Lippincott, 1995.
12. Miyao H, Hirokawa T, Miyasaka K et al: Relative humidity, not absolute humidity, is of great importance when using a humidifier with a heating wire, Crit Care Med 20:674-679, 1992.
13. Chatburn R: Physiologic and methodologic issues regarding humidity therapy (editorial), J Pediatr 114:416-420, 1989.
14. Rhame FS, Streifel A, McComb C et al: Bubbling humidifiers produce microaerosols which can carry bacteria, Infect Control 7:403-407, 1986.
15. Goularte TA, Manning MT, Craven DE: Bacterial colonization in humidifying cascade reservoirs after 24 and 48 hours of continuous mechanical ventilation, Infect Control 8:200-203, 1987.
16. Branson RD, Davis K Jr, Brown R et al: Comparison of three humidification techniques during mechanical ventilation: patient selection, cost, and infection considerations, Respir Care 41:809-816, 1996.

17. Shanks CA: Clinical anesthesia and the multiple gauze condenser humidifier, Br J Anaesth 46:773-777, 1974.
18. Mapelson WW, Morgan JG, Hillard ER: Assessment of condenser humidifiers with special reference to the multiple gauze model, Br Med J 1:300-305, 1963.
19. Branson RD, Davis K Jr: Evaluation of 21 passive humidifiers according to the ISO 9360 standard: moisture output, deadspace, and flow resistance, Respir Care 41:736-743, 1996.
20. Medical Devices Directorate Evaluation. Department of Health, Scottish Home and Health Department, Welsh Office and Department of Health and Social Services Northern Ireland, London, 1994.
21. Cigada M, Elena A, Solca M et al: The efficiency of twelve heat and moisture exchangers: an in vitro evaluation, Intensive Care World 7:98-101, 1990.
22. Shelly M, Bethune DW, Latimer RD: A comparison of five heat and moisture exchangers, Anaesthesia 41:527-532, 1986.
23. Weeks DB, Ramsey FM: A laboratory investigation of six artificial noses for use during endotracheal anesthesia, Anesth Analg 62:758-763, 1981.
24. Mebius CA: A comparative evaluation of disposable humidifiers, Acta Anaesthesiol Scand 27:403-409, 1983.
25. Hayes B: Evaluation report: heat and moisture exchangers, J Med Eng Technol 11:117-128, 1987.
26. Ogino M, Kopotic R, Mannino FL: Moisture-conserving efficiency of condenser humidifiers, Anaesthesia 40:990-995, 1985.
27. Heat and moisture exchangers, Health Devices 12:155-166, 1983.
28. Unal N, Pompe JC, Holland WPJ et al: An experimental set-up to test heat-moisture exchangers, Intensive Care Med 21:142-148, 1995.
29. Annual Book of ASTM Standards: F1690-96 Standard Specification for Humidifiers for Medical Use-Part 1: General Requirements for Active Humidification Systems. Section 13: Medical Devices and Services, Volume 13.01: Medical Devices: Emergency Medical Services, West Conshohocken, Pa, American Society for Testing and Materials, 1996, pp 1078-1092.
30. International Organization for Standardization 1992: ISO 9360. Anaesthetic and Respiratory Equipment-Heat and Moisture Exchangers for Use in Humidifying Respired Gases in Humans, Geneva, Switzerland, International Organization for Standardization, 1992.
31. Ploysongsang Y, Branson RD, Rashkin MC et al: Effect of flowrate and duration of use on the pressure drop across six artificial noses, Respir Care 34:902-907, 1989.
32. Nishimura M, Nishijima MK, Okada T et al: Comparison of flow-resistive work load due to humidifying devices, Chest 97:600-604, 1990.
33. Manthous CA, Schmidt GA: Resistive pressure of a condenser humidifier in mechanically ventilated patients, Crit Care Med 22:1792-1795, 1994.
34. Chiaranda M, Verona L, Pinamonti O et al: Use of heat and moisture exchanging (HME) filters in mechanically ventilated ICU patients: influence on airway flow-resistance, Intensive Care Med 19:462-466, 1993.
35. McEwan AI, Dowell L, Karis JH: Bilateral tension pneumothorax caused by a blocked bacterial filter in an anesthesia breathing circuit, Anesth Analg 76:440-442, 1993.
36. Loeser EA: Water induced resistance in disposable respiratory-circuit bacterial filters, Anesth Analg 57:269-271, 1978.
37. Buckley PM: Increase in resistance of in-line breathing filters in humidified air, Br J Anaesth 56:637-643, 1984.
38. Tenaillon A, Cholley G, Boiteau R et al: Heat and moisture exchanging bacterial filters versus heated humidifier in long term mechanical ventilation, Care Critically Ill 7:56-66, 1991.
39. Prasad KK, Chen L: Complications related to the use of a heat and moisture exchanger, Anesthesiology 72:958, 1990.
40. Martinez FJ, Pietchel S, Wise C et al: Increased resistance of hygroscopic condenser humidifiers when using a closed circuit suction system, Crit Care Med 22:1668-1673, 1994.
41. Stacey MRW, Asai T, Wilkes A et al: Obstruction of a breathing system filter, Can J Anaesth 43:1276, 1996.
42. Smith CE, Otworth JR, Kaluszyk P: Bilateral tension pneumothorax due to a defective anesthesia breathing circuit filter, J Clin Anesth 3:229-234, 1991.
43. Yoga Y, Iwatsuki N, Takahashi M et al: A hazardous defect in a humidifier, Anesth Analg 71:712, 1990.
44. Prados W: A dangerous defect in a heat and moisture exchanger, Anesthesiology 71:804, 1989.
45. Iotti GA, Olivei MC, Palo A et al: Unfavorable mechanical effects of heat and moisture exchangers in ventilated patients, Intensive Care Med 23:399-405, 1997.
46. Pelosi P, Solca M, Ravagnan I et al: Effects of heat and moisture exchangers on minute ventilation, ventilatory drive, and work of breathing during pressure-support ventilation in acute respiratory failure, Crit Care Med 24:1184-1188, 1996.
47. Conti G, De Blasi RA, Rocco M et al: Effects of heat-moisture exchangers on dynamic hyper-inflation of mechanically ventilated COPD patients, Intensive Care Med 16:441-443, 1990.
48. Le Bourdelles G, Mier L, Fiquet B et al: Comparison of the effects of heat and moisture exchangers and heated humidifiers on ventilation and gas exchange during weaning trials from mechanical ventilation, Chest 110:1294-1298, 1996.
49. Campbell RS, Davis K Jr, Johannigman JA et al: The effects of passive humidifier dead space on respiratory variables in paralyzed and spontaneously breathing patients, Respir Care 45(3):306-312, 2000.
50. Prin S, Chergui K, Augarde R et al: Ability and safety of a heated humidifier to control hypercapnic acidosis in severe ARDS, Intensive Care Med 28(10):1756-1760, 2002.
51. Prat G, Renault A, Tonnelier JM et al: Influence of the humidification device during acute respiratory distress syndrome, Intensive Care Med 29(12):2211-2215, 2003.

52. Natalini G, Bardini P, Latronico N et al: Impact of heat and moisture exchangers on ventilatory pattern and respiratory mechanics in spontaneously breathing patients, Monaldi Arch Chest Dis 49(6):561-564, 1994.
53. Girault C, Breton L, Richard JC et al: Mechanical effects of airway humidification devices in difficult to wean patients, Crit Care Med 31(5):1306-1311, 2003.
54. Rathberger J, Zielman S, Kietzman D et al: Is the use of lithium chloride coated "Heat and Moisture Exchangers" (artificial noses) dangerous for patients? Der Anaesthesist 41:204-207, 1992.
55. Rosi R, Buscalferri A, Monfregola MR et al: Systemic lithium reabsorption from lithium chloride coated heat and moisture exchangers, Intensive Care Med 18:97-100, 1992.
56. Branson RD, Davis K, Campbell RS et al: Humidification in the intensive care unit: prospective study of a new protocol utilizing heated humidification and a hygroscopic condenser humidifier, Chest 104:1800-1805, 1993.
57. Suzukawa M, Usuda Y, Numata K: The effects of sputum characteristics of combining an unheated humidifier with a heat-moisture exchanging filter, Respir Care 34:976-984, 1989.
58. Beydon L, Tong D, Jackson N et al: Correlation between simple clinical parameters and the in vitro humidification characteristics of filter heat and moisture exchangers, Chest 112:739-744, 1997.
59. Djedaini K, Billiard M, Mier L et al: Changing heat and moisture exchangers every 48 hours rather than 24 hours does not affect their efficacy and the incidence of nosocomial pneumonia, Am J Respir Crit Care Med 152:1562-1569, 1995.
60. Kollef MH, Shapiro SD, Boyd V et al: A randomized clinical trial comparing an extended use hygroscopic condenser humidifier with heated water humidification in mechanically ventilated patients, Chest 113:759-767, 1998.
61. Davis K Jr, Evans SL, Campbell RS et al: Prolonged use of heat and moisture exchangers does not effect efficiency or incidence of nosocomial pneumonia, Crit Care Med 28:1412-1418, 2000.
62. Memish ZA, Oni GA, Djazmati W et al: A randomized clinical trial to compare the effects of a heat and moisture exchanger with a heated humidifying system on the occurrence rate of ventilator-associated pneumonia, Am J Infect Control 29(5):301-305, 2001.
63. Misset B, Escudier B, Rivara D et al: Heat and moisture exchanger vs heated humidifier during long-term mechanical ventilation: a prospective randomized study, Chest 100(1):160-163, 1991.
64. Kranabetter R, Leier M, Kammermeier D et al: The effects of active and passive humidification on ventilation-associated nosocomial pneumonia, Anaesthesia 53(1):29-35, 2004 (Article in German).
65. Kola A, Eckmanns T, Gastmeier P: Efficacy of heat and moisture exchangers in preventing ventilator-associated pneumonia: meta-analysis of randomized controlled trials, Intensive Care Med 31(1):5-11, 2005.
66. Lacherade JC, Auburtin M, Cerf C et al: Impact of humidification systems on ventilator-associated pneumonia: a randomized multicenter trial, Am J Respir Crit Care Med 172(10):1276-1282, 2005.
67. Branson RD, Campbell RS, Davis K Jr et al: Comparison of a new active heat and moisture exchanger to conventional heated humidification, Respir Care 44:912-917, 1999.
68. Larsson A, Gustafsson A, Svanborg L: A new device for 100 per cent humidification of inspired air, Crit Care 4(1):54-60, 2000.
69. Chiumello D, Pelosi P, Park G et al: In vitro and in vivo evaluation of a new active heat moisture exchanger, Crit Care 8:281-288, 2004.
70. Branson RD, Campbell RS, Johannigman JA et al: Laboratory evaluation of two novel methods of humidification (abstract), Crit Care Med 27(suppl): A71, 1999.
71. Thomachot L, Vialet R, Viguier JM et al: Efficacy of heat and moisture exchangers after changing every 48 hours rather than 24 hours, Crit Care Med 26(3):477-481, 1998.
72. Thomachot L, Viviand X, Boyadjiev I et al: The combination of a heat and moisture exchanger and a booster: a clinical and bacteriological evaluation over 96 h, Intensive Care Med 28(2):147-153, 2002.
73. Newhouse MT, Dolovich MB: Control of asthma by aerosols, N Engl J Med 315:870-874, 1986.
74. Dhand R, Tobin MJ: Bronchodilator delivery with metered-dose inhalers in mechanically ventilated patients, Eur J Respir Dis 9:585-595, 1996.
75. Brain JD, Valberg PA: Deposition of aerosol in the respiratory tract, Am Rev Respir Dis 120:1325-1373, 1979.
76. Dhand R: Bronchodilator therapy. In: Tobin MJ, editor: Principles and practice of mechanical ventilation, New York, McGraw-Hill, 2006, pp 1277-1310.
77. Dolovich M: Physical principles underlying aerosol therapy, J Aerosol Med 2:171-186, 1989.
78. Hess D, Horney D, Snyder T: Medication delivery performance of eight small volume, hand-held nebulizers: effects of diluent volume, nebulizer flow, and nebulizer model, Respir Care 34:717-723, 1989.
79. Hess D, Fisher D, Williams P et al: Medication nebulizer performance: effects of diluent volume, nebulizer flow, and nebulizer brand, Chest 110:498-505, 1996.
80. Svartengren M, Anderson M, Philipson K et al: Human lung deposition of particles suspended in air or in helium/oxygen mixture, Exp Lung Res 15:575-585, 1989.
81. Anderson M, Svartengren M, Bylin G et al: Deposition in asthmatics of particles inhaled in air or in helium/oxygen, Am J Respir Crit Care Med 47:524-528, 1993.
82. Dhand R, Malik SK, Balakrishnan M et al: High speed photographic analysis of aerosols produced by metered dose inhalers, J Pharm Pharmacol 40:429-430, 1988.
83. Dolovich M, Ruffin RE, Roberts R et al: Optimal delivery of aerosols from metered dose inhalers, Chest 80:911-915, 1981.

84. Fuller HD, Dolovich MB, Posmituck G et al: Pressurized aerosol versus jet aerosol delivery to mechanically ventilated patients: comparison of dose to the lungs, Am Rev Respir Dis 141:440-444, 1990.
85. Dhand R, Fink J: Dry powder inhalers, Respir Care 44(8):940-951, 1999.
86. Mitchell JP, Nagel MW, Wiersema KJ et al: The delivery of chlorofluorocarbon-propelled versus hydrofluoroalkane-propelled beclomethasone dipropionate aerosol to the mechanically ventilated patient: a laboratory study, Respir Care 48(11):1025-1032, 2003.
87. Jashnani RN, Byron PR, Dalby RN: Testing of dry powder aerosol formulations in different environmental conditions, Int J Pharm 113:123-130, 1995.
88. Lindsay DA, Russell NL, Thompson JE et al: A multicenter comparison of the efficacy of terbutaline Turbuhaler and salbutamol pressurized metered dose inhaler in hot, humid regions, Eur Respir J 7(2):342-345, 1994.
89. Dhand R: Inhalation therapy with metered-dose inhalers and dry powder inhalers in mechanically ventilated patients, Respir Care 50(10):1331-1334, 2005.
90. Rink JB, Barraza P, Bisgaard J: Aerosol delivery during mechanical ventilation with high frequency oscillation: an in vitro evaluation (abstract) Chest 120: S277, 2001.
91. Tronde A, Baran G, Eirefelt S et al: Miniaturized nebulization catheters: a new approach for delivery of defined aerosol doses to the rat lung, J Aerosol Med 15:283-296, 2002.
92. Dhand R: New frontiers in aerosol delivery during mechanical ventilation, Respir Care 49:666-677, 2004.
93. Dhand R: Inhalation therapy with metered dose inhalers and dry powder inhalers in mechanically ventilated patients, Respir Care 50(10):1331-1344, 2005.
94. Fink JB, Dhand R, Grychowski J et al: Reconciling in vitro and in vivo measurements of aerosol delivery from a metered dose inhaler during mechanical ventilation and defining efficiency enhancing factors, Am J Respir Crit Care Med 159:63-68, 1999.
95. Fuller HD, Dolovich MB, Chambers C et al: Aerosol delivery during mechanical ventilation: a predictive in vitro lung model, J Aerosol Med 5:251-259, 1992.
96. O'Riordan TG, Greco MJ, Perry RJ et al: Nebulizer function during mechanical ventilation, Am Rev Respir Dis 145:1117-1122, 1992.
97. Rau JL, Harwood RJ, Groff JL: Evaluation of a reservoir device for metered dose bronchodilator delivery to intubated adults: an in vitro study, Chest 102:924-930, 1993.
98. Hughes JM, Saez J: Effects of nebulizer mode and position in a mechanical ventilator circuit on dose efficiency, Respir Care 32:1131-1135, 1987.
99. McPeck M, O'Riordan TG, Smaldone GC: Choice of mechanical ventilator influence on nebulizer performance, Respir Care 38:887-895, 1993.
100. Bishop MJ, Larson RP, Buschman DL: Metered dose inhaler aerosol characteristics are affected by the endotracheal tube actuator/adapter used, Anesthesiology 73:1263-1265, 1990.
101. Fuller HD, Dolovich MB, Turpie FH et al: Efficiency of bronchodilator aerosol delivery to the lungs from the metered dose inhaler in mechanically ventilated patients: a study comparing four different actuator devices, Chest 105:214-218, 1994.
102. Manthous CA, Hall JB, Schmidt GA et al: Metered dose inhaler versus nebulized albuterol in mechanically ventilated patients, Am Rev Respir Dis 148:1567-1570, 1993.
103. Ahrens RC, Ries RA, Popendorf W et al: The delivery of therapeutic aerosols through endotracheal tubes, Pediatr Pulmonol 2:19-26, 1986.
104. O'Riordan TG, Palmer LB, Smaldone GC: Aerosol deposition in mechanically ventilated patients: optimizing nebulizer delivery, Am J Respir Crit Care Med 149:214-219, 1994.
105. Thomas SHL, O'Doherty MJ, Fidler HM et al: Pulmonary deposition of a nebulized aerosol during mechanical ventilation, Thorax 48:154-159, 1993.
106. MacIntyre NR, Silver RM, Miller CW et al: Aerosol delivery in intubated, mechanically ventilated patients, Crit Care Med 13:81-84, 1985.
107. Beaty CD, Ritz RH, Benson MS: Continuous in-line nebulizers complicate pressure support ventilation, Chest 96:1360-1363, 1989.
108. Duarte AG, Dhand R, Reid R et al: Serum albuterol levels in mechanically ventilated patients and healthy subjects after metered dose inhaler administration, Am J Respir Crit Care Med 54:1658-1663, 1996.
109. Fernandes A, Lazaro A, Garcia A et al: Bronchodilators in patients with chronic obstructive pulmonary disease on mechanical ventilation: utilization of metered dose inhalers, Am Rev Respir Dis 141:164-168, 1990.
110. Manthous CA, Chatila W, Schmidt GA et al: Treatment of bronchospasm by metered dose inhaler albuterol in mechanically ventilated patients, Chest 107:210-213, 1995.
111. Dhand R, Jubran A, Tobin MJ: Bronchodilator delivery by metered dose inhaler in ventilator supported patients, Am J Respir Crit Care Med 151:1827-1833, 1995.
112. Dhand R, Duarte AG, Jubran A et al: Dose response to bronchodilator delivered by metered dose inhaler in ventilator supported patients, Am J Respir Crit Care Med 154:388-393, 1996.
113. Gay PC, Rodarte JR, Tayyab M et al: Evaluation of bronchodilator responsiveness in mechanically ventilated patients, Am Rev Respir Dis 136:880-885, 1987.
114. Gay PC, Patel HG, Nelson SB et al: Metered dose inhalers for bronchodilator delivery in intubated, mechanically ventilated patients, Am Rev Respir Dis 99:66-71, 1991.
115. Pepe PE, Marini JJ: Occult positive end expiratory pressure in mechanically ventilated patients with airflow obstruction: the auto PEEP effect, Am Rev Respir Dis 26:166-170, 1982.

116. Turner JR, Corkery KJ, Eckman D et al: Equivalence of continuous flow nebulizer and metered dose inhaler with reservoir bag treatment of acute airflow obstruction, Chest 93:476-481, 1988.
117. Bowton DL, Goldsmith WM, Haponik EF: Substitution of metered dose inhalers for hand held nebulizers: success and cost savings in a large, acute care hospital, Chest 101:305-308, 1992.
118. Graham RM: Adrenergic receptors: structures and function, Cleve Clin J Med 57:481-491, 1990.
119. Rasmussen H, Kelley G, Douglas JS: Interaction between Ca^{2+} and cAMP messenger system in regulation of airway smooth muscle contraction, Am J Physiol Lung Cell Mol Physiol 258:L279-L288, 1990.
120. Price AH, Clissold SP: Salbutamol in the 1980s: a re-appraisal of its clinical efficacy, Drugs 38:77-122, 1989.
121. AAAI Committee on Drugs: Position statement: safety and appropriate use of salmeterol in the treatment of asthma, J Allergy Clin Immunol 98:475-480, 1996.
122. National Heart, Lung and Blood Institute and World Health Organization: Global Initiative for Asthma, Bethesda, Md: National Institutes of Health, 1995, NIH Publication #95-3659.
123. American Thoracic Society: Standards for the diagnosis and care of patients with chronic obstructive pulmonary disease, Am J Respir Crit Care Med 152: S77-S120, 1995.
124. Siafakas NM, Vermeire P, Pride NB et al: Optimal assessment and management of chronic obstructive pulmonary disease (COPD), Eur Respir J 8:1398-1420, 1995.
125. Dhand R, Tobin MJ: Bronchodilator delivery with metered dose inhalers in mechanically ventilated patients, Eur Respir J 9:585-595, 1996.
126. American Association for Respiratory Care: Aerosol consensus statement-1991, Respir Care 36:916-921, 1991.
127. Fernandez A, Lazaro A, Garcia A et al: Bronchodilators in patients with chronic obstructive pulmonary disease on mechanical ventilation: utilization of metered-dose inhalers, Am Rev Respir Dis 141:164-168, 1990.
128. Mancebo J, Amaro P, Lorino H et al: Effects of albuterol inhalation on the work of breathing during weaning from mechanical ventilation, Am Rev Respir Dis 144:95-100, 1991.
129. Dhand R, Jubran A, Tobin MJ: Bronchodilator delivery by metered-dose inhaler in ventilator-supported patients, Am J Respir Crit Care Med 151:1827-1833, 1995.
130. Manthous CA, Chatila W, Schmidt GA et al: Treatment of bronchospasm by metered-dose inhaler albuterol in mechanically-ventilated patients, Chest 107:210-213, 1995.
131. Dhand R, Duarte AG, Jubran A et al: Dose response to bronchodilator delivered by metered-dose inhaler in ventilator-supported patients, Am J Respir Crit Care Med 154:388-393, 1996.
132. Wright PE, Carmichael LC, Bernard GR: Effect of bronchodilators on lung mechanics in the acute respiratory distress syndrome (ARDS), Chest 106:1517-1523, 1994.
133. Manthous CA, Hall JB, Schmidt GA et al: Metered-dose inhaler versus nebulized albuterol in mechanically-ventilated patients, Am Rev Respir Dis 148:1567-1570, 1993.
134. Fryer AD: The cholinergic control of the airways. In: Barnes PJ, editor. Autonomic control of the respiratory system, Amsterdam: Harwood Academic Publishers, 1997:59-86.
135. Coulson FR, Fryer AD: Muscarinic acetylcholine receptors in airway disease, Pharmacol Ther 98:59-69, 2003.
136. Baraniuk JN: Muscarinic receptors. In: Leff AR, editor: Pulmonary and critical care pharmacology, New York, McGraw-Hill, 1996, pp 97-104.
137. Barnes PJ: New developments in anticholinergic drugs, Eur Respir Rev 6:290-294, 1996.
138. Ferguson GT, Cherniack RM: Management of chronic obstructive pulmonary disease, N Engl J Med 328:1017-1022, 1993.
139. Wilson JD, Serby CW, Menjoge SS et al: The efficacy and safety of combination bronchodilator therapy, Eur Respir Rev 6:286-289, 1996.
140. Casburi R, Briggs DD Jr., Donohue JF et al: The spirometric efficacy of once-daily dosing with tiotropium in stable COPD: a 13 week multicenter trial. The US Tiotropium study Group, Chest 118:1294-1302, 2000.
141. Barnes PJ, Pederson S, Busse WW: Efficacy and safety of inhaled corticosteroids in asthma: new developments, Am J Respir Crit Care Med 157:S1-S53, 1998.
142. National Asthma Education and Prevention Program: Expert panel report II: guidelines for the diagnosis and management of asthma, February 1997.
143. Robinson DS, Geddes DM: Inhaled corticosteroids: benefits and risks, J Asthma 33:5-16, 1996.
144. Smith AL, Ramsey B: Aerosol administration of antibiotics, Respiration 62:19-24, 1995.
145. Weber A, Morlin G, Cohen M et al: Effect of nebulizer type and antibiotic concentration on device performance, Pediatr Pulmonol 23:249-260, 1997.
146. Coates AL, MacNeish CF, Meisner D et al: The choice of jet nebulizer, nebulizing flow and the addition of albuterol affects the output of tobramycin aerosols, Chest 111:1206-1212, 1997.
147. Touw DJ, Brimicombe RW, Hodson ME et al: Inhalation of antibiotics in cystic fibrosis, Eur Respir J 8:1594-1604, 1995.
148. Hashimoto S, Wolfe E, Guglielmo B et al: Aerosolization of imipenem/cilastatin prevents *Pseudomonas*-induced acute lung injury, J Antimicrob Chemother 38:809-818, 1996.
149. Greenfield S, Teres D, Bushnell LS et al: Prevention of gram-negative bacillary pneumonia using aerosol polymyxin as prophylaxis: effect on colonization pattern of the upper respiratory tract of seriously ill patients, J Clin Invest 52:2935-2940, 1973.
150. Feeley TW, DuMoulin GC, Hedley-Whyte J et al: Aerosol polymyxin and pneumonia in seriously ill patients, N Engl J Med 293:471-475, 1975.

151. Smaldone GC: Aerosolized antibiotics in mechanically ventilated patients, Respir Care 49(6):635-639, 2004.
152. Palmer LB, Smaldone GC, Simon SR et al: Aerosolized antibiotics in mechanically ventilated patients: delivery and response, Crit Care Med 26(1):31-39, 1998.
153. Smaldone GC, Palmer LB: Aerosolized antibiotics: current and future, Respir Care 45(6):667-675, 2000.
154. Singh N, Rogers P, Atwood CW et al: Shortcourse empiric antibiotic therapy for patients with pulmonary infiltrates in the intensive care unit: a proposed solution for indiscriminate antibiotic prescription, Am J Respir Crit Care Med 162(2 Pt 1):505-511, 2000.

CHAPTER 5

Ventilator Monitors and Displays

Neil R. MacIntyre

OUTLINE

- PRESSURE AND FLOW SENSORS
  - Pressure Sensors
  - Flow and Volume Sensors
  - Output from Pressure/Flow/Volume Sensors
  - Monitoring Maneuvers
- GAS ANALYZERS AND GAS EXCHANGE MONITORS
- DISPLAY SCREENS
- FUTURE SENSORS AND MONITORS
- VENTILATOR ALARM SYSTEMS
  - Levels of Events and Alarm Requirements
  - Alarm Cost Effectiveness

OBJECTIVES

- Discuss the principles of monitoring.
- Describe pressure flow and volume measuring devices.
- Explain the principles of alarm functioning.
- Describe modern graphical interfaces.

KEY TERMS

airway pressure
alarm
esophageal pressure
events
flow
inspired O_2 concentrations (FIO_2)
manometers
monitors
pulse oximeter
transducers
volume

Monitoring is the process of continued or repetitive measurement of a parameter.[1] With mechanical ventilators, the purpose of monitoring is generally to detect patient or machine events or trends that require management changes. In addition, the sensors used for monitoring can also be used for various feedback functions on the ventilator. Monitoring patients on mechanical ventilators is usually done in one of three locations: the ventilator itself, the patient-ventilator interface (usually in the ventilator circuitry), or on the patient.

Typical **monitors** inside the ventilator include continuous assessments of electrical, software, and pneumatic functions. Typical interface monitors include measurements of airway/circuit/tracheal pressures, circuit gas flow, delivered/returned volume, and circuit gas concentrations. Typical direct patient monitors include measurements of arterial oxygenation, pulmonary vascular pressures, invasive and noninvasive assessments of cardiac output, hemoglobin content, and tissue perfusion.

Although all the aforementioned monitoring capabilities can be important, the remainder of this chapter focuses only on clinical monitoring capabilities integral to the ventilator system. Specifically, the following sections describe the various sensors in the patient-ventilator interface, their displays of both real-time and trend data, and how these monitors can affect patient-ventilator management. A consensus conference described the importance of these ventilator integral monitors for patients receiving various levels of mechanical ventilatory support (Table 5-1).[1]

TABLE 5-1 *Ventilator Consensus Statement-1992 Essential, Recommended, and Optional Variables* to Be Monitored on Mechanical Ventilators*†

	PRINCIPAL VENTILATOR APPLICATION		
VARIABLE	**CRITICAL CARE**	**TRANSPORT**	**HOME CARE**
Pressure			
P_{PEAK}	Essential	Essential	Essential
P_{MEAN}	Essential	Optional	Optional
P_{PLAT}	Essential	Optional	Optional‡
Intrinsic PEEP (auto-PEEP)	Recommended	Optional	Optional
Volume			
V_T expired machine	Essential	Recommended	Optional
$\dot{V}_E$ machine	Essential	Optional	Optional
V_T expired spontaneous	Essential	Recommended	Optional
$\dot{V}_E$ spontaneous	Essential	Optional	Optional
V_T inspired spontaneous	Recommended	Optional	Optional
Timing			
Flow mechanical	Recommended	Optional	Optional
Flow spontaneous	Optional	Optional	Optional
I:E ratio	Essential	Recommended	Optional
Rate mechanical	Essential	Recommended	Optional
Rate spontaneous	Essential	Recommended	Optional
Gas concentration			
FIO_2	Essential	Optional‡	Optional‡
Lung mechanics			
Effective compliance	Optional	Optional	Optional
Inspiratory airways resistance	Optional	Optional	Optional
Expiratory airways resistance	Optional	Optional	Optional
Maximal inspiratory pressure	Optional	Optional	Optional
Circuit characteristics			
Tubing compliance	Recommended	Optional	Optional

From American Association for Respiratory Care Consensus Group: Essentials of mechanical ventilation, Respir Care 37:1001-1009, 1992.

PEEP, Positive end-expiratory pressure; *V_T,* tidal volume; *V_E,* minute volume; *I:E,* inspiratory : expiratory time; FIO_2, O_2 concentration delivered by device.

*Essential, considered necessary for safe and effective operation in most patients in the specified setting; recommended, considered necessary for optimal management of virtually all patients in the specified setting; optional, considered possibly useful in limited situations, but not necessary for most patients in the specified setting.

†Monitors need not be integral part of ventilator.

‡Essential if feature is used on a patient at risk for hypoxemia.

PRESSURE AND FLOW SENSORS

Pressure Sensors

Pressure generally is measured by either aneroid **manometers** or electromechanical **transducers.**[2] Aneroid manometers use an expandable chamber that responds to pressure changes by changing its volume and moving a gear that rotates a needle around a calibrated dial. Electromechanical transducers convert pressure into an electrical current. Standard specifications for ventilator pressure monitors are of ±10% accuracy.[3]

Pressure can be monitored in the ventilator, the ventilator circuitry (often the patient wye connector), the distal endotracheal tube, and the esophagus. The actual pressure transducers are often within the ventilator and connected to the sensing site by low-compliance, air-filled tubing. By convention, pressures measured in the ventilator or ventilator circuitry are often considered as **airway pressure** or airway opening pressures (P_{AW} or P_{AO}, respectively). Pressures in the distal endotracheal tube often are considered tracheal pressures (P_{TR}), and pressures from a balloon in the midesophagus (P_{ES}) generally are considered reflective of pleural pressures if it has been positioned properly (Figure 5-1).[4]

Airway or ventilator circuit pressures reflect the pressures to overcome airway resistance and

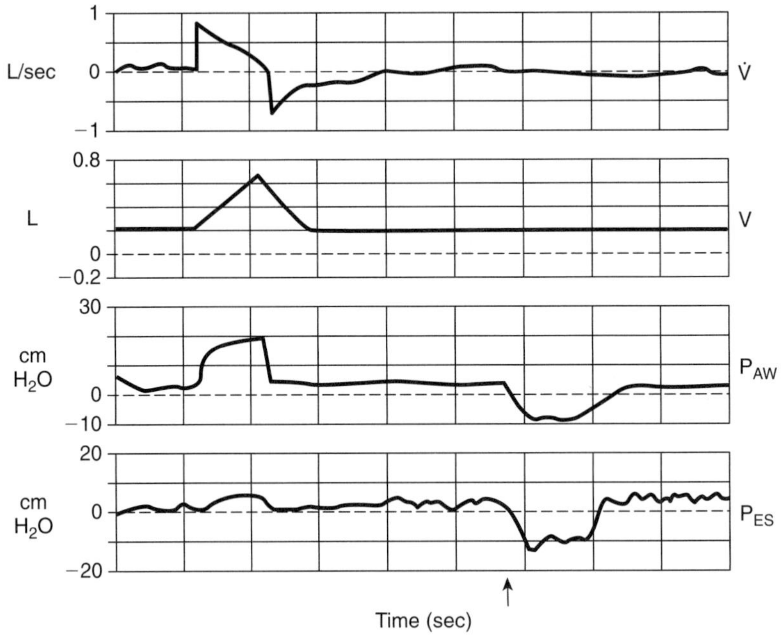

FIGURE 5-1 The "sniff" test to ensure proper placement of an esophageal balloon. Flow *(upper panel)*, tidal volume *(2nd panel)*, airway pressure *(3rd panel)*, and esophageal pressure *(bottom panel)* are plotted over time. The tracings demonstrate a positive pressure breath followed by a sniff test (a maneuver performed by an inspiratory effort against an occluded airway [i.e., no flow or volume change, *arrow*]). If the balloon is positioned properly, similar pressure swings are observed in the airway and in the esophagus.

respiratory system compliance (see Chapter 6). Tracheal pressure monitoring can provide similar information to airway pressure monitoring although the pressure due to flow through the endotracheal tube is eliminated. **Esophageal pressure** changes during a control breath will reflect the compliance of the chest wall; esophageal pressure changes during a spontaneous breath will reflect inspiratory muscle effort (see Chapter 6).

Flow and Volume Sensors

Older ventilators usually would monitor only exhaled volume by either volume-displacing spirometers or turbines. Most modern systems, however, monitor **flow** with various types of pneumotachometers and integrate flow to obtain **volume.** The most common pneumotachometers work on one of the three following principles: differential pressure flowmeters, hot wire flowmeters, or ultrasonic flowmeters.[2,5]

Differential Pressure Flowmeters

Differential pressure flowmeters determine flow from the pressure drop across a known resistance. The most widely used types incorporate either a screen or a series of capillary tubes (Fleisch) as the resistance element. Advantages of these flowmeters include a nearly linear bidirectional pressure-flow relationship and a high-frequency response. An important disadvantage of these types of flowmeters in the intensive care setting is that they are highly sensitive to moisture and mucus accumulation if placed in the patient's airway. Additional disadvantages are that a large housing is often necessary to produce the required laminar flow, and gas viscosity affects calibration (e.g., an error of 12% occurs if 100% O_2 is used on a flowmeter calibrated with 21% O_2). Because of these limitations, screen and Fleisch flowmeters usually are not maintained for prolonged periods near the patient's airway but rather are placed elsewhere in the ventilator circuitry.

Another type of differential pressure flowmeter more applicable to patient airway application uses either a fixed or variable orifice resistor. A fixed resistor results in turbulent flow and thus is inherently nonlinear. These types of flowmeters are affected less by mucus and moisture than are Fleisch or screen devices. Another alternative is the variable orifice resistor, which mechanically linearizes flow through an elastic "flap." These devices have low resistance and dead space characteristics, and they provide reasonable clinical accuracy.

Hot Wire Flowmeters

Hot wire flowmeters operate on the principle that cooling of a heated wire or film is proportional to gas flow past it. The rate of cooling also depends on gas viscosity and thermal conductivity. Advantages to these devices are that dead space and resistance are very small, a very high frequency response is possible, and mucus-moisture effects are lessened because the sensor is heated. Disadvantages are that only unidirectional flow can be sensed by a single sensor and that different gas mixtures can have different thermal conductivities.

Ultrasonic Flowmeters

Ultrasonic flowmeters use an ultrasonic transmitter-receiver and function on the principle that ultrasonic transit times are proportional to gas flow. A variation of this approach is to produce small air-flow obstructions, which create vortices. The intensity of an ultrasonic signal across these vortices is proportional to flow. Advantages are low resistance to flow, little impact by viscosity or mucus-moisture, and a high-frequency response to the ultrasonic transmitter-receiver system. A disadvantage is that ultrasonic signal transmission is affected by both gas composition and temperature.

One final point to make about flow sensors is that they usually are calibrated to deal only with O_2/nitrogen mixtures. This is important when using heliox, a much lower density gas. Under these conditions care must be taken to adjust the monitoring outputs to account for potential inaccuracies. Alternatively, an additional volume displacement monitor (not affected by gas density) could be incorporated in the ventilator exhalation assembly.

Output from Pressure/Flow/ Volume Sensors

Pressure, flow, and volume are usually monitored continuously during the delivery of mechanical ventilation and the signals can be displayed either graphically or digitally (Figure 5-2). Specific airway pressure measurements that are usually made and displayed over the ventilatory cycle include: peak pressure (the highest pressure during inspiration [P_{PEAK}]), inspiratory plateau pressure (end-inspiratory pressure under no-flow conditions [P_{PLAT}]), mean inspiratory pressure (average pressure during inspiration [inspP_{MEAN}]), positive end-expiratory pressure (circuit pressure just before delivery of the next breath [PEEP]), and mean airway pressure (average pressure throughout the ventilatory cycle [P_{MEAN}]). In addition, during a no-flow pause or hold at end expiration, a measurement of total end-expiratory alveolar pressure (intrinsic plus applied PEEP) can be made.

When flow is measured over the ventilatory cycle (see Figure 5-2), specific measurements that can be digitally displayed include peak inspiratory flow, mean inspiratory flow, the inspiratory flow pattern, peak expiratory flow, and mean expiratory flow. Specific volume measurements over time include the delivered (inspired) and the expired tidal volume (V_T). Importantly, differences in inspired and expired tidal volume can signal a circuit leak or bronchopleural fistula (inspired volume greater than expired volume) or can reflect additional inspired gas flow from a nebulizer or other source (expired volume greater than inspired volume if the flow sensor is proximal to the added gas source). Integrating pressure over time (pressure-time product) or volume (work) can quantify and display loads on either the patient's muscles (using esophageal pressure) or on the ventilator (using airway pressure). These are discussed in more detail in Chapter 6.

Pressure, flow, and volume signals are also used by the ventilator for alarm functions (see below) and to drive various feedback mechanisms (e.g., pressure-regulated volume control, volume support, automatic tube or airway compensation, synchronized intermittent mandatory ventilation, proportional assist ventilation, and minimum minute ventilation).[6]

Monitoring Maneuvers

In addition to continuous monitoring, the pressure, flow, and volume sensors can be used to display information during both automated and manual maneuvers. The two simplest maneuvers are the control "test" breath and the inspiratory or expiratory hold maneuver. Pressure volume plotting, automated spontaneous breathing trials, and automated airway occlusion maneuvers are more complex monitoring maneuvers. All of these are discussed in more detail below.

Although control breaths are an inherent component of assist-control ventilation modes, additional control breaths can be delivered by either the clinician or automatically as part of a specific monitoring process. These control breaths are used to calculate respiratory system mechanics as described in Chapter 6 and can be used for straightforward monitoring or be incorporated into various feedback algorithms (e.g., pressure-regulated volume control or propor-

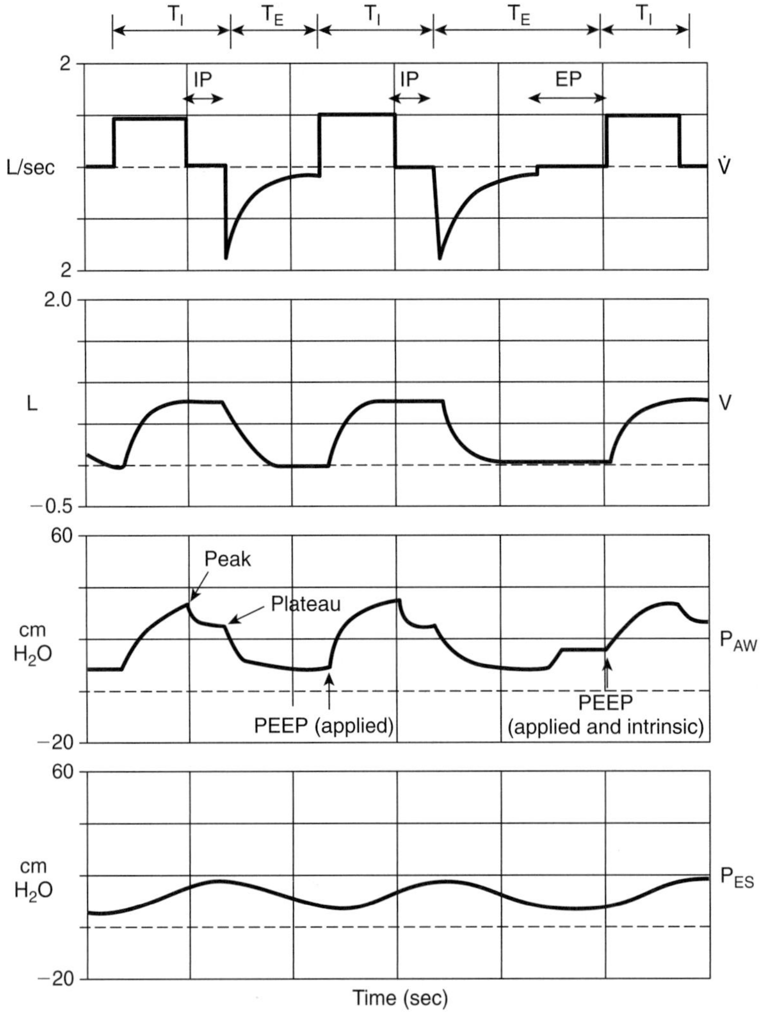

FIGURE 5-2 Ventilator circuit flow ($\dot{V}$), volume (V), and airway pressure (P_{AW}) over time illustrating various measurements during controlled ventilation. In this example, the inspiratory phase (T_I) has both a flow delivery phase and an inspiratory pause (IP). In addition, during expiration (T_E) of the second breath, an expiratory pause also is illustrated (EP). During inspiration, the highest pressure is the peak airway pressure, the P_{AW} during the inspiratory pause is the plateau pressure, and the mean P_{AW} during the entire inspiratory phase is the mean inspiratory pressure. During expiration, the end-expiratory P_{AW} is positive end-expiratory pressure (PEEP). If the expiratory circuit is occluded before the next breath delivery (expiratory pause), this PEEP reflects both applied and intrinsic PEEP. Without such an occlusion, the measured PEEP is only the applied one. The average P_{AW} over the entire steady state inspiratory and expiratory phases is the mean airway pressure.

tional assist ventilation). When used as part of a feedback control system, the size of the control tidal volume may vary ("test breaths") to provide additional information to the feedback algorithm. Control breaths can also be used in comparison with assisted breaths to assess patient muscle loading (see Chapter 6).

Hold maneuvers prevent flow from occurring in the ventilator circuit and are only useful during controlled mechanical breaths. As described above, hold maneuvers at end inspiration and end expiration allow for measurements of P_{PLAT} and total PEEP (applied plus intrinsic), respectively.

On some ventilators, an automated static pressure volume plot can be constructed using either frequent automated holds or else multiple tidal breaths of different sizes. A simpler variation of this is to plot the single-breath dynamic pressure volume relationship during a "slow flow" maneuver. When this is done, a very slow, constant inspiratory flow (e.g., 3 to 10 L/min) is delivered for up to 10 seconds. Because this flow is so slow, the pressures related to flow are minimal and the curve thus approximates the static pressure volume relationships, reflecting only respiratory system compliance[7] (see Chapter 6, Figure 6-3).

Modern ventilators can also be set to perform spontaneous breathing trials (SBTs) and monitor them automatically. Clinicians can select the ventilator settings during the trial (e.g., pressure support or continuous positive airway pressure [CPAP]), the duration of the trial, and the parameters to be monitored (e.g., minute ventilation, frequency, tidal volume, the frequency/tidal volume ratio). During a spontaneous effort, inspiratory pressure against a closed demand valve after 100 milliseconds of effort ($P_{0.1}$) and with maximal effort (MIF) also can also be determined with automated airway occlusion techniques.

GAS ANALYZERS AND GAS EXCHANGE MONITORS

Gas concentrations in the ventilator circuitry can be assessed through either mainstream (in-line) or sidestream analyzers. Probably the most important measurement is the **inspired O_2 concentration (F_{IO_2})** to ensure that the O_2 supply system is performing properly. O_2 concentration in the inspired gas is most commonly measured using fuel cell technology.

Another common gas concentration measurement is the exhaled CO_2 concentration using infrared absorption technology. The CO_2 at end expiration (end-tidal CO_2) correlates with arterial P_{CO_2} and can be used to trend ventilation effectiveness when tidal volume and expiratory time are held nearly constant.[8,9] The mixed expired CO_2 can be used in the Bohr equation to calculate functional dead space (V_D/V_T = [arterial or end tidal CO_2 − mixed expired CO_2]/arterial or end tidal CO_2). Trends in exhaled CO_2 can also be plotted over time.

The most commonly used oxygenation monitor is the **pulse oximeter.** Pulse oximeters use infrared light absorption technology through the skin to assess O_2-hemoglobin saturation. The use of pulse oximeters is increasingly being incorporated into the ventilator both for monitoring and for driving feedback systems such as F_{IO_2} control in neonates.[10] These devices are reasonably accurate but problems can occur in the setting of poor perfusion and sensor misplacement. Accuracy is also reduced at low levels of hemoglobin saturation. It must also be remembered that the pulse oximeter measures a saturation, not a partial pressure, and thus significant decreases in P_{O_2} can occur before the saturation notably drops.

DISPLAY SCREENS

Display screens on mechanical ventilators have developed rapidly since the first cathode ray tube systems were introduced in the 1980s. Modern screens can display both digital and analog data in real time, in comparison with previous times (including trend plots), and in plots versus other selected parameters (Figure 5-3). The screen can also be used to display an array of information that can include the user manual, imbedded protocols, decision support technology, hospital information system, and the Internet.

Modern display screens not only display measured data but also provide touch screen technology to operate the ventilator. Indeed, the most common design on current ventilators is a comprehensive touch screen (often layered with more advanced features displayed only on screens available to selected clinicians) and a single knob or dial to adjust the selected parameter on the screen.

FUTURE SENSORS AND MONITORS

There are a number of exciting developments on the horizon for monitoring patients receiving mechanical ventilation. More sophisticated analysis of exhaled CO_2 and O_2 can provide several types of information. First, exhaled CO_2, when analyzed over a brief rebreathing period, can be used to calculate cardiac output.[11] Second, by comparing both O_2 and CO_2 concentrations in inspired and expired gas, O_2 consumption and CO_2 production can be calculated (indirect calorimetry). Many argue that these values can guide nutritional support strategies although strong consensus is lacking.[12]

Ventilators in the future also may have integral monitors for other gases that could measure lung volumes (e.g., methane or helium), pulmonary capillary blood flow (e.g., acetylene), and inflammatory biomarkers (e.g., nitric oxide).[13] An interesting (but currently cumbersome) technique uses blood and gas measurements of six inert gases of different solubilities to describe ventilation-perfusion relationships.[14] In the future, this may become more "user friendly" and provide important information that may guide ventilator settings.

There are a number of other potential ventilator monitors on the horizon. One is the use of

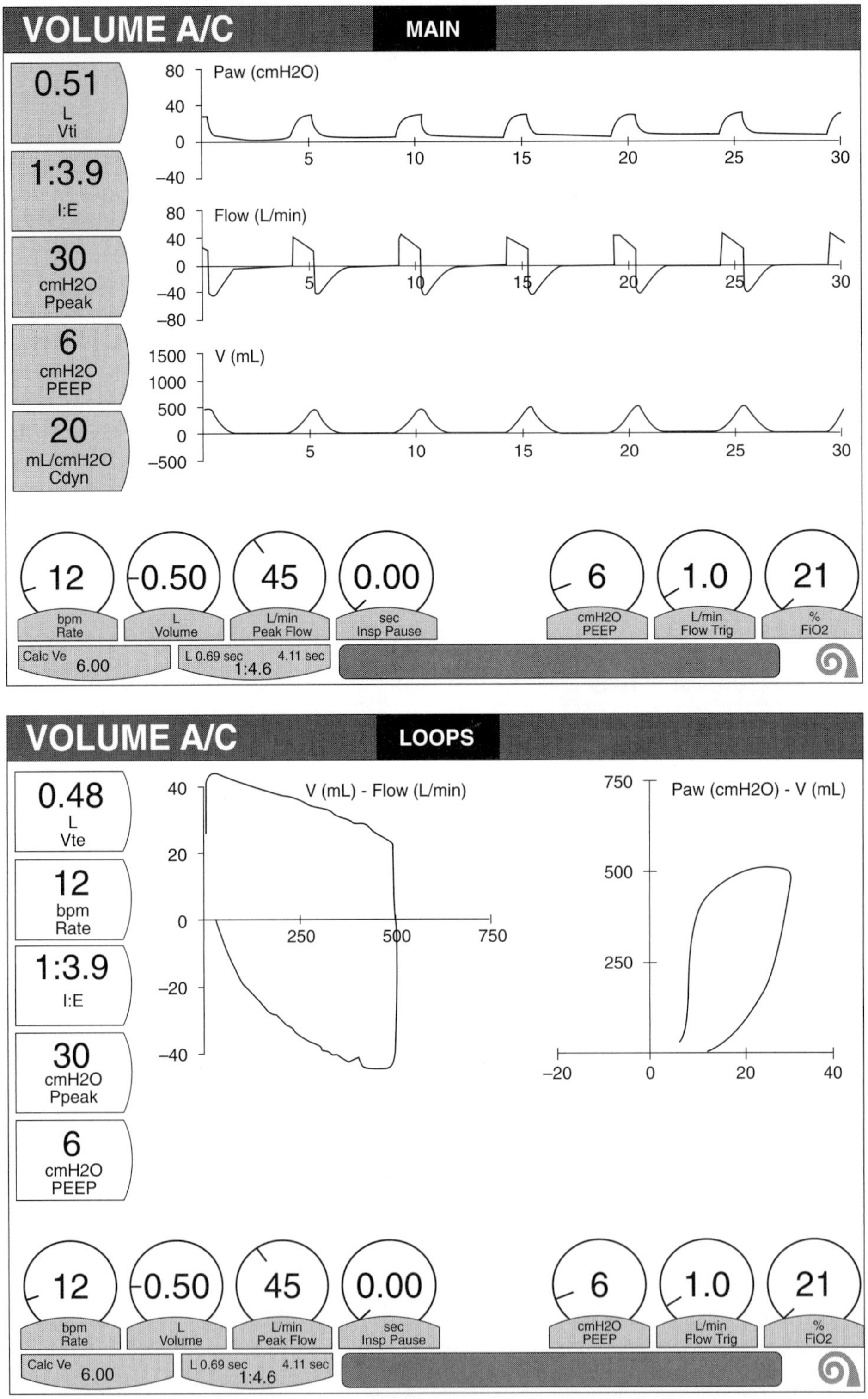

FIGURE 5-3 Examples of modern ventilator displays. **A,** Pressure, flow, and volume are plotted over time. **B,** Flow is plotted against volume on the left and pressure is plotted against volume on the right. Digital displays can represent monitored values (vertical, upper left on each screen) or set values (horizontal, bottom of each screen).

electromyograms of the respiratory muscles to better synchronize flow delivery with patient effort.[15] A particularly interesting anatomic assessment technique in development is electrical impedance tomography (EIT). EIT measures electrical impedance across 17-34 electrodes placed on the chest to construct two-dimensional cross-sectional images that resemble a single slice of the standard radiographic computerized chest tomogram (CT scan).[16] Another potential class of monitors might involve analyses of lung lavage fluids or breath condensates to assess a wide array of inflammatory and infectious biomarkers. Finally, transcutaneous sensors for not only O_2 and CO_2 but also a variety of other metabolic markers are under development for possible incorporation into mechanical ventilators.[13]

VENTILATOR ALARM SYSTEMS

The goal of a mechanical ventilator **alarm** is to warn clinicians of **events.** An event is any condition or occurrence that requires clinician awareness or action. Events can be divided conceptually into two broad categories—mechanical/technical events and patient-generated events.

Mechanical/technical events involve the ventilator system itself. Because these systems replace or support the patient's life-sustaining ventilatory efforts, an alarm is required for every potential mechanical event that could impact on this function.[1,17,18] Moreover, the alarm must occur in time for prompt correction.

In contrast, a patient event involves a change in the patient's clinical status. This may be a consequence of a mechanical/technical malfunction but more often reflects changes in the patient's underlying disease process. Monitors and alarms are reasonable for such patient events but should not be a required integral component of a mechanical ventilator system. Rather, these alarms should be individualized for each patient as a supplement to clinical decision making.

Levels of Events and Alarm Requirements

Alarm goals and strategies should be categorized by the events that they are designed to warn of rather than by any technical features they may have. The discussion of ventilator system alarm strategies that follows, therefore, considers four levels, or priorities, of alarmed mechanical and patient events (Table 5-2).

Level 1

A Level 1 event describes immediate life-threatening consequences to a ventilator malfunction. The expectation for a Level 1 alarm is that it will warn of every event in time for prompt corrections (Table 5-3). Because of the essential nature of this type of warning, alarms with redundant or overlapping function should be present. For instance, a failure to deliver gas should cause a low-volume alarm, a low-pressure alarm, and, if practical, even a gas exchange alarm (e.g., capnography). This type of event should not be considered

TABLE 5-2 *Alarm Features for Different Event Priorities*

	EVENT PRIORITIES				
ALARM FEATURES	INTEGRAL PART OF VENTILATOR	MUST BE REDUNDANT	ALARM SITES	AUTOMATIC RESPONSE NEEDED	CLINICAL FOCUS
Level 1—ventilator malfunction, life-threatening	Yes	Yes	1, 2, 3*	Yes	Machine
Level 2—ventilator malfunction, not immediately life-threatening	Yes	No	1, 2*	No	Machine
Level 3—patient event affecting ventilator-patient interface	Yes	No	2, 3*	No	Machine and patient
Level 4—patient event not affecting ventilator-patient interface	No	No	3*	No	Patient

From Day S, MacIntyre NR: Ventilator alarm system. Prob Respir Care 4:118-126, 1991.
*Site 1, Ventilator system; site 2, patient-ventilator interface; site 3, patient.

TABLE 5-3 *Level 1 Events and Alarms: Ventilator Events, Life-Threatening (Mandatory, Redundant, Noncanceling)*

EVENT	ALARM SENSOR
No gas delivery to patient	Pressure/flow transducer, CO_2 monitor, timing device
Excessive gas delivery to patient	Pressure/flow transducer, timing device
Exhalation valve failure	Pressure/flow transducer, mandatory rate
Loss of electric power	Battery-powered alarm

From Day S, MacIntyre NR: Ventilator alarm systems, Prob Respir Care 4:118-126, 1991.

to have a "mild" form; it is a serious failure every time it occurs. The alarms in this category are thus mandatory, redundant, and noncanceling. The goal is to provide virtually 100% reliability of the life-support functions of the ventilator. Although machine failure is unavoidable, appropriate alarms should alert users to technical breakdowns.

With a Level 1 event, machines should not simply alarm and shut down; rather, they should default to a condition in which the patient is at the very least not "locked out" and is able to breathe from a fresh gas source. A more sophisticated default condition could be a backup minimum ventilation mode. Both responses are designed to alert users to immediately replace the ventilator with as little harm as possible done to the patient during mechanical failure. Ventilators also should have battery-backed alarms for Level 1 events in case of power source failure.

Level 2

The events in the Level 2 category can range from mild irregularities in the mechanical function of the ventilator to dangerous situations that, under the proper circumstances, could threaten the patient's safety or life if left uncorrected for a period of time (Table 5-4). An example of a Level 2 event would be a circuit leak. A small leak (less than 10 ml/breath) would not harm most adult patients, whereas a large leak (several hundred ml/breath) may cause serious hypoventilation. These alarms are important and are included in some form on all modern ventilators. There may not be redundant counterparts for each, however, and alarm-canceling capabilities often exist.

TABLE 5-4 *Level 2 Events and Alarms: Ventilator Event Not Immediately Life-Threatening*

EVENT	ALARM SENSOR
Blender failure	FIO_2 sensor
Loss of PEEP or excessive PEEP	Pressure transducer
Autocycling	Timer/flow transducer, CO_2 sensor
Circuit leak	Flow transducer, pressure transducer
Circuit partially occluded	Pressure, flow transducer
Inappropriate I:E ratio	Timer, flow transducer
Inappropriate heater/humidifier function	Temperature probe

From Day S, MacIntyre NR: Ventilator alarm systems, Prob Respir Care 4:118-126, 1991.
FIO_2, Inspired O_2 concentration; *PEEP,* positive end-expiratory pressure; *I:E,* inspiratory : expiratory time.

TABLE 5-5 *Level 3 Events and Alarms: Patient Events Affecting Ventilator-Patient Interface*

EVENT	ALARM SENSOR
Change in ventilatory drive (CNS, peripheral nerves, or muscle function)	Timer, flow transducer, pressure transducer, CO_2 analyzer
Change in compliance/resistance (air trapping, barotrauma)	Pressure transducer, flow transducer
AutoPEEP	Pressure transducer, flow transducer

From Day S, MacIntyre NR: Ventilator alarm systems, Prob Respir Care 4:118-126, 1991.
CNS, Central nervous system; *PEEP,* positive end-expiratory pressure.

Level 3

Level 3 events can have significant impact on the level of support given and on the pressure and volume consequences of that support (Table 5-5). Examples include changes in patient compliance or resistance. Sensors for these events are generally in the ventilator circuitry (e.g., pressure/flow/volume sensors), although direct patient monitors also are used. Modern ventilators usually include alarms for Level 3 events, although redundancy is not considered essential.

Level 3 events often trigger the same alarms as those in Levels 1 and 2, and the clinician must be

TABLE 5-6 *Level 4 Events and Alarms: Patient Events Not Affecting Ventilator-Patient Interface*

EVENT	ALARM SENSOR
Change in gas exchange	
$\dot{V}/\dot{Q}$	Capnograph
V_D/V_T	Oximeter, metabolic calculations
$\dot{V}O_2$ demands	Arterial blood gases
Change in respiratory system impedances	Mechanics measurements
Change in muscle function	Respiratory pressures, ventilatory capabilities
Change in cardiovascular function	Hemodynamic measurements

From Day S, MacIntyre NR: Ventilator alarm systems, Prob Respir Care 4:118-126, 1991.
V_D/V_T, Dead space volume/tidal volume; $\dot{V}/\dot{Q}$, ventilation perfusion; $\dot{V}O_2$, O_2 consumption.

capable of quickly determining the nature of the alarmed event. Because patient status can change either abruptly or more insidiously, the alarms for these events must be adjusted carefully for each patient and changed often to correlate with patient conditions to remain accurate enough to warn of significant problems.

Level 4

Level 4 events are not a function of ventilator system malfunction, nor do they impact ventilator behavior. Alarm sites are thus only on the patient. Because of this, many modern ventilators may not contain any such alarm system as an integral part of the device. These events, however, can have significant clinical impact, but they often must be detected by other types of critical care monitors, such as free-standing oximeters, cardiac monitors, or blood gas analyzers (Table 5-6).

Alarm Cost-Effectiveness

Ventilator setup involves selecting alarm parameters that should maximize sensitivity (i.e., percentage of events alarmed) and specificity (i.e., percentage of non-events not alarmed). A high sensitivity, however, often leads to a loss of specificity and a high rate of false-positive alarms. This false-positive rate may be quite acceptable for a single alarm (e.g., 5%), but if a number of alarms are used together with similar specificity, the chances of a false-positive alarm can rise dramatically.[19] False-positive alarms produce two important problems. First, a high rate of false-positive alarms can lead to clinicians ignoring alarms. Indeed, in one study of mechanical ventilation hazards, 9% of ventilator alarms had been disabled by clinicians, ostensibly to reduce noise "pollution."[20] A second problem is the costs and patient risks of inappropriate therapy or unnecessary diagnostic tests in response to the false-positive alarm condition.

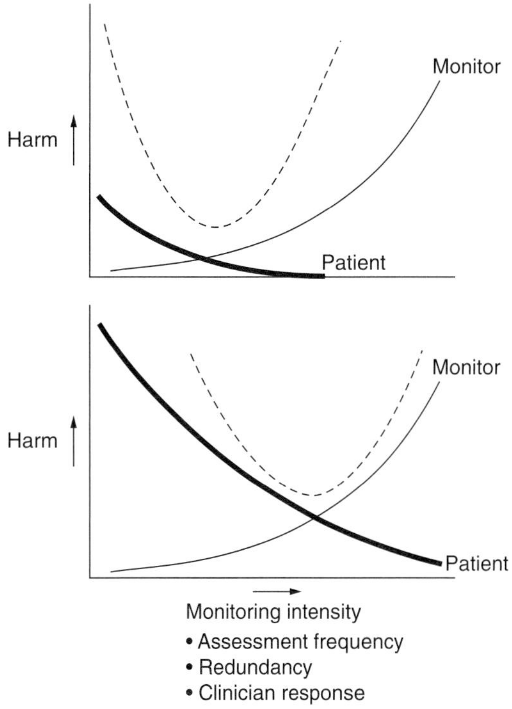

FIGURE 5-4 The cost-effectiveness of monitoring intensity is determined by patient risk and monitoring system properties. Harm can come from both patient disease events ("patient" line) and monitoring system events ("monitor" line). As monitoring intensity increases, patient harm should decrease. Increasing monitoring intensity, however, increases costs, the risk of monitor-induced injury, and the false-positive rate—all forms of potential patient harm. The dotted curve represents net harm when these different factors are considered. The upper panel depicts a situation in which risk of harm due to patient disease is low, such that a lower level of monitoring intensity produces lowest net harm. The bottom panel depicts a situation in which patient harm due to patient disease is high, such that a higher level of monitoring intensity is cost-effective. (From MacIntyre NR: Levels of intensity of intensive care unit monitoring. In: Tobin M, editor: Principles and practices of intensive care monitoring, New York, 1997, McGraw-Hill.)

Balancing sensitivity and specificity is the goal of setting appropriate alarm parameters (Figure 5-4).[18]

TABLE 5-7 *Examples of Alarm Auto-Set Parameters*

ALARM	AUTO-SETTING
Low exhaled mandatory tidal volume	–25% to a minimum of 30 ml
Low exhaled spontaneous tidal volume	–25% to a minimum of 30 ml
Low exhaled minute volume	–25% to a minimum of 0.3 L
High exhaled minute volume	+25% or 1000 ml, whichever is greater
Low breath rate	–5 bpm to a minimum of 3 bpm
High breath rate	+5 bpm
Low peak normal pressure	–5 cm H_2O or preset PEEP/CPAP, whichever is greater, to a minimum of 3 cm H_2O
Low mean airway pressure	–5 cm H_2O
Low PEEP/CPAP pressure	–5 cm H_2O or 20%, whichever is less, to a minimum margin of 2 cm H_2O

From Day S, MacIntyre NR: Ventilator alarm systems, Prob Respir Care 4:118-126, 1991.
PEEP/CPAP, Positive end-expiratory pressure/continuous positive airway pressure.

One approach would be to arbitrarily set alarm parameters as a "standard" percentage of the targeted values (Table 5-7).[21] Although this approach is reasonable, the clinician still may want to individualize certain alarm ranges. In doing this, the clinician must consider the likelihood of an otherwise undetected event, the potential harm from such an event, and the precision with which the alarm setting can distinguish a real event from simple physiologic variability or artifact. In general, the higher the likelihood of an undetected event causing serious harm, the more sensitive (at the expense of specificity) an alarm setting should be.

Interpreting and Responding to Alarm Conditions

Even if an alarm is set properly, clinical skills are vital in determining the cause of the alarm and in responding appropriately. It is of no use to have alarms if a clinical response is not readily available. As noted earlier, automated responses such as backup modes are available on some ventilators. These, however, should not be considered a substitute for prompt clinical assessment.

Other Alarm Issues

Two other issues are related to alarm cost-effectiveness: costs and reliability. Alarms have direct costs associated with the actual hardware and software involved. Costs also are involved in equipment maintenance and staff training. These costs must be balanced against the potential patient harm (with its attendant costs) of unrecognized events.

Alarm systems are generally quite reliable. However, like any other component of the ventilatory support system, an alarm can malfunction. This has been reported to occur in as many as 3.7% of patients[22] and is one of the reasons for redundancy in Level 1 event strategies (see section on Level 1 events).

KEY POINTS

- Integral to all modern ventilators are sophisticated sensors, monitors, displays, and data analysis packages.
- The sensors, monitors, displays, and data analysis packages can produce a sometimes bewildering array of data for the clinician that must be properly prioritized and understood for safe and effective operation of the ventilator.
- More sophisticated data analysis can be reserved for advanced practitioners to more carefully evaluate patient status and device function.
- Alarms are critical for safe operation.
- Alarms must be prioritized so as to maximally protect the patient from ventilator malfunctions but not be so sensitive that clinicians are overwhelmed by nuisance alarms that could drown out more serious alarms.

ASSESSMENT QUESTIONS

1. True or False. Pressure sensors in the esophagus are taken to represent pleural pressures.
2. True or False. Ventilator circuit pressure is often taken to represent airway pressure.
3. True or False. Circuit compliance is so low that it is usually ignored in assessing delivered volume.
4. True or False. Ultrasonic flowmeters use a pressure drop across an orifice to calculate flow.
5. True or False. Helium O_2 mixtures have no impact on any modern flow sensors.
6. True or False. Inspiratory and expiratory hold maneuvers (no-flow periods) allow ventilator circuit pressure to equilibrate with alveolar pressures.
7. True or False. Pulse oximeters use absorption of ultraviolet light to detect hemoglobin saturation.
8. True or False. Modern graphical display screens often allow for touch screen technology to operate the ventilator.
9. True or False. Alarms designed to detect and warn of immediate life-threatening consequences from ventilator malfunction should be redundant.
10. True or False. Overly sensitive alarms can lead to noise "pollution" and can result in clinicians either not paying attention to the alarm or disabling the alarm.

REFERENCES

1. American Association for Respiratory Care Consensus Group: Essentials of mechanical ventilation, Respir Care 37:1001-1009, 1992.
2. Tobin MJ: Monitoring of pressure, flow, and volume during mechanical ventilation, Respir Care 37:1081-1096, 1992.
3. American Society for Testing and Materials: F29: standard specification for ventilators intended for use in critical care F1100. In: Annual Book for ASTM Standards, Philadelphia: American Society for Testing and Materials, 1993.
4. Baydur A, Behrakis K, Zin A et al: A simple method for assessing the validity of esophageal balloon technique, Am Rev Respir Dis 126:788-791, 1982.
5. Sullivan WJ, Peters GM, Enright PL: Pneumotachographs: theory and clinical application. Respir Care 29:736-749, 1984.
6. Iotti GA, Braschi A: Closed-loop support of ventilatory workload: the P0.1 controller. Respir Care Clin N Am 7:441-464, 2001.
7. Ranieri VM, Giuliani R, Fiore T et al: Volume-pressure curve of the respiratory system predicts effects of PEEP in ARDS: "occlusion" versus "constant flow" technique, Am J Respir Crit Care Med 149:19-27, 1994.
8. Rebuck AS, Chapman KR: Measurement and monitoring of exhaled carbon dioxide. In: Nochomovitz ML, Cherniack NS, editors: Non-invasive respiratory monitoring, New York, 1986, Churchill Livingstone, pp 189-201.
9. McLellan PA, Goldstein RS, Ramcharan V et al: Transcutaneous carbon dioxide monitoring, Am Rev Respir Dis 124:199-201, 1981.
10. Claure N, Gerhardt T, Everett R et al: Closed-loop controlled inspired oxygen concentration for mechanically ventilated very low birth weight infants with frequent episodes of hypoxemia, Pediatrics 107:1120-1124, 2001.
11. Odenstedt H, Stenqvist O, Lundin S: Clinical evaluation of a partial CO_2 rebreathing technique for cardiac output monitoring in critically ill patients, Acta Anaesth Scand 46:152-159, 2002.
12. Reid CL: Nutritional requirements of surgical and critically-ill patients: do we really know what they need? Proc Nutr Soc 63:467-472, 2004.
13. Tobin M, editor: Principles and practice of intensive care monitoring, New York, 1997, McGraw-Hill.
14. Wagner PD, Saltzman HA, West JB: Measurement of continuous distributions of ventilation-perfusion ratios: theory, J Appl Phys 36:588-599, 1974.
15. Spahija J, Beck J, de Marchie M et al: Closed-loop control of respiratory drive using pressure-support ventilation: target drive ventilation, Am J Respir Crit Care Med 171:1009-1014, 2005.
16. Riedel T, Richards T, Schibler A: The value of electrical impedance tomography in assessing the effect of body position and positive airway pressures on regional lung ventilation in spontaneously breathing subjects, Intensive Care Med 31:1522-1528, 2005.
17. Day S, MacIntyre NR: Ventilator alarm systems, Prob Respir Care 4:118-126, 1991.

18. MacIntyre NR: Levels of intensity of intensive care unit monitoring. In: Tobin M, editor: Principles and practice of intensive care monitoring, New York, 1997, McGraw-Hill.
19. Hess D: Noninvasive monitoring in respiratory care—present, past, and future: an overview, Respir Care 35:482-499, 1990.
20. Zwillich CW, Pierson DJ, Creagh CE et al: Complications of assisted ventilation: a prospective study of 354 consecutive episodes, Am J Med 57:161-170, 1974.
21. The Bear® Ventilator Instruction Manual, Riverside, Calif: Bear Intermed, 1990.
22. Watson H, MacIntyre NR: Mechanical ventilator failure, Prob Respir Care 4:127-135, 1991.

SECTION II PHYSIOLOGY

CHAPTER 6

Respiratory System Mechanics

Neil R. MacIntyre

OUTLINE

OBJECTIVES

- Explain the equation of motion as it applies to mechanical ventilation.
- Discuss the measurement of compliance, resistance, pressure time products, and work.
- Describe the principles of a pressure volume graph.
- Recognize the interactions of respiratory system mechanics and ventilatory settings.

KEY TERMS

compliance
elastance
hysteresis
intrinsic positive end-expiratory pressure (PEEPi)
minute ventilation ($\dot{V}_E$)
positive end-expiratory pressure (PEEP)
pressure-time product (PTP)
resistance
tidal volumes
ventilation distribution
work (W)

During normal spontaneous ventilation, fresh gas is exchanged with alveolar gas by a convective to-and-fro pumping action. This "bulk flow" gas transport is driven by pressure gradients created by the ventilatory muscles and respiratory system elastic recoil.[1] Most current modes of mechanical ventilation tend to mimic this pattern. Specifically, a positive pressure ventilator produces a periodic pressure gradient across the lungs to drive discrete volumes **(tidal volumes)** of gas into the lung, whereas respiratory system elastic recoil pressure and expiratory muscle activity drive these volumes back out of the lungs. Understanding these processes is critical in understanding mechanical ventilatory support. This chapter is divided into two broad areas of discussion: (1) a basic review of respiratory system mechanics and (2) a discussion of the interaction of ventilator settings and/or patient effort with these mechanical properties.

MEASUREMENTS

The key parameters that are commonly measured during mechanical ventilation are ventilator and respiratory system pressures, gas flow in and out of the lung, and the consequent tidal volume delivered and returned.[2-4] Ventilator pressures are usually measured in the ventilator circuitry and often are expressed

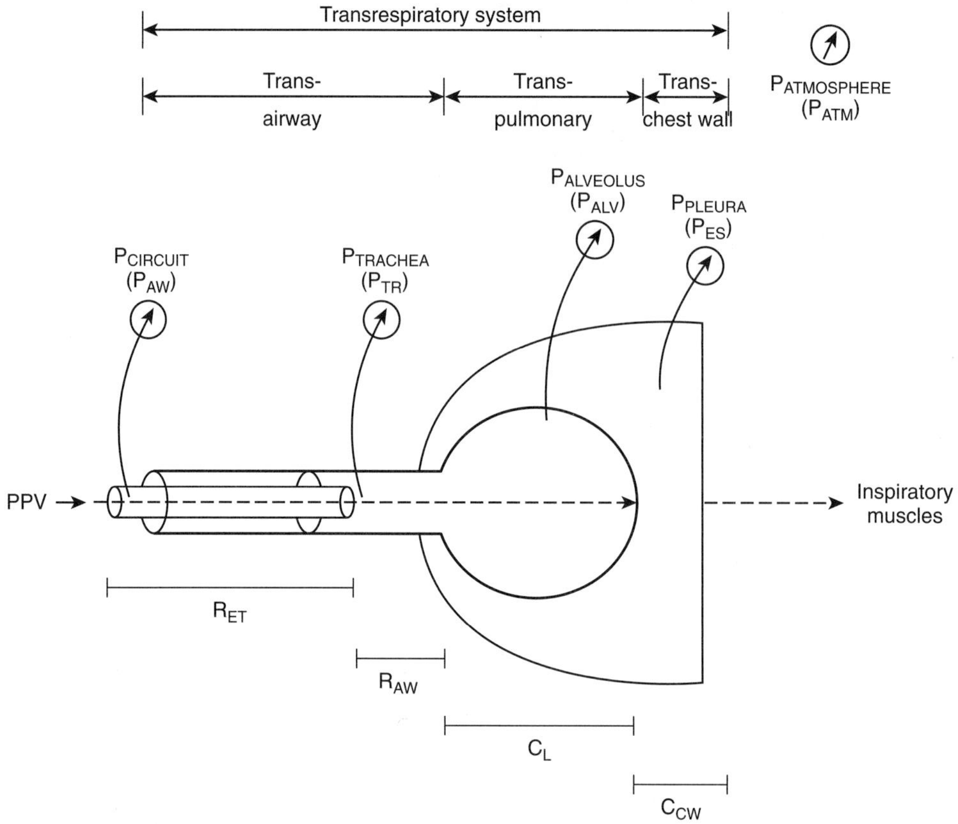

FIGURE 6-1 Sites of pressure measurements in intubated patients during either positive pressure ventilation (PPV; "pushing" gas into the respiratory system) or spontaneous ventilation (inspiratory muscles "pulling" gas into the respiratory system). Commonly measured pressures are: ventilator circuit pressure ($P_{CIRCUIT}$, often taken to represent airway pressure or P_{AW}), tracheal pressure (P_{TR}), alveolar pressure (P_{ALV}), and pleural pressure (usually approximated by esophageal pressure or P_{ES}). These pressures can be referenced to each other or to atmospheric pressure (P_{ATM}, usually considered to be zero) to determine transairway pressure, transrespiratory system pressure, transpulmonary pressure, and transchest wall pressure *(horizontal arrows)*. Mechanical properties (i.e., resistance of the endotracheal tube (R_{ET}), resistance of the natural airways (R_{AW}), compliance of the lung (C_L), and compliance of the chest wall (C_{CW}) can be determined by analyzing these pressure gradients in conjunction with flow and volume measurements (see text for details).

as airway pressures (P_{AW}). Pressure also can be measured in the trachea at the distal end of the artificial airway (tracheal pressure or P_{TR}), and the esophagus (P_{ES})—a reasonable approximation of pleural pressure (Figure 6-1). From these measurements, various pressure gradients (ΔP) can be calculated: ΔP between P_{AW} and alveolar pressure (P_{ALV}) is transairway pressure (subdivided into artificial and natural airways using P_{TR}); ΔP between P_{AW} and atmospheric pressure (P_{ATM}—generally considered to be zero in this context) is transrespiratory system pressure; ΔP between P_{ES} and atmospheric pressure (again considered to be zero) is transchest wall pressure, and ΔP between P_{ALV} and P_{ES} is transpulmonary pressure or the stretching pressure across the lung.[5]

These pressure gradients generated during a positive pressure breath without spontaneous activity reflect different mechanical properties during different phases of the respiratory cycle. These are depicted in Figure 6-2, left panel, by pressures "f" through "j." During inspiratory flow, the difference between P_{AW} and P_{ALV} (transairway ΔP or pressure "f" minus "g") reflects pressure required for flow. Conversely, under no-flow conditions (i.e., during an inspiratory or expiratory "hold" or "pause") there are no flow-related pressure gradients and this transairway ΔP

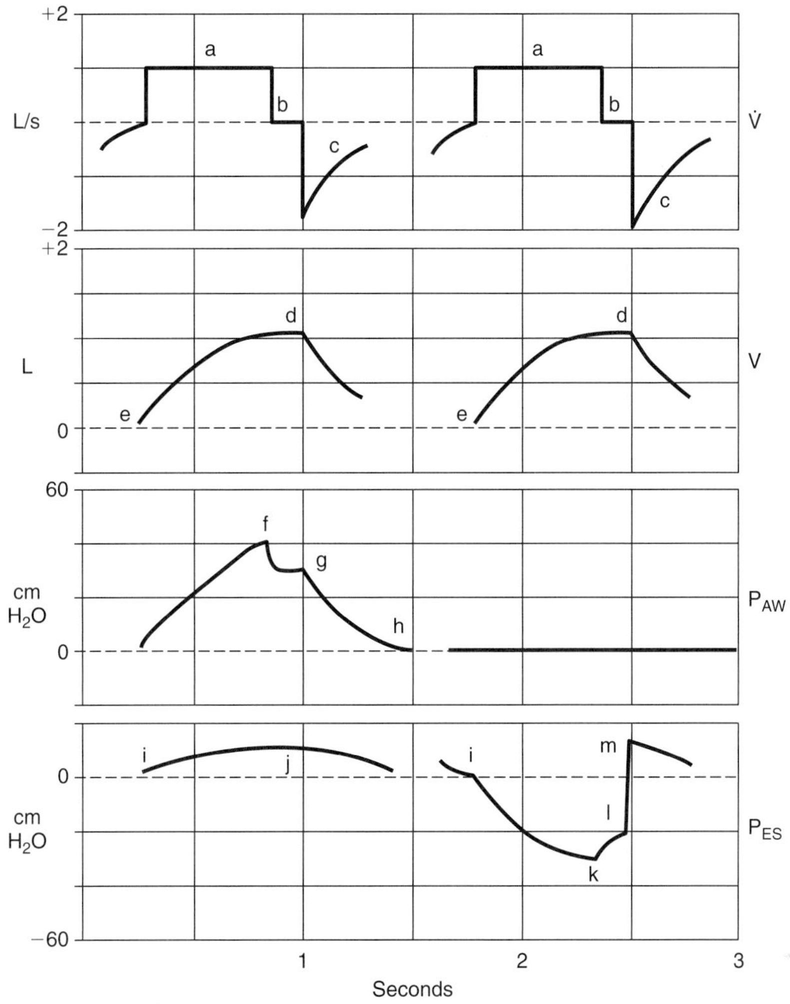

FIGURE 6-2 Flow ($\dot{V}$—*upper panel*), volume (V—*second panel*), airway pressure (P_{AW}—*third panel*) and esophageal pressure (P_{ES}) during either a machine delivered positive pressure breath (left panels) or an unassisted spontaneous breath (right panels). In the flow tracings, "a" represents inspiratory flow, "b" represents an end inspiratory hold (which, during the spontaneous breath, has both an active breath-hold component from inspiratory muscle contraction followed by a passive breath-hold component against a closed airway shutter), and "c" represents expiratory flow. In the volume tracings, "d" represents end inspiratory volume and "e" represents end expiratory volume. In the P_{AW} tracings, "f" represents peak P_{AW}, "g" represents plateau P_{AW}, and "h" represents expiratory P_{AW}. Note that during spontaneous breaths, the P_{AW} tracing remains constant as no ventilator pressure is applied. In the P_{ES} tracings, "i" represents end expiratory P_{ES} and "j" represents end inspiratory P_{ES} during a mechanical breath. During a spontaneous breath, "i" again represents end expiratory P_{ES}, "k" represents peak P_{ES}, "l" represents a plateau P_{ES} during the active breath-hold, and "m" represents a plateau P_{ES} during the passive breath-hold. Note that "m" and "j" are identical since both are reflecting the passive chest wall recoil pressure after delivery of a similar tidal volume.

becomes zero. Under these circumstances, P_{AW} becomes equal to P_{TR} and to P_{ALV}. The absolute value for P_{AW} then reflects the end inspiratory stretching pressure on the respiratory system (pressure "g") while end inspiratory P_{AW} pressure minus end expiratory P_{AW} (pressure "g" minus "h") reflects the tidal stretching pressure. Note that this transrespiratory system stretching ΔP can be separated into the lung and chest wall components by measuring the ΔP between airway (alveolus) and the pleura during the inspiratory hold (P_{AW} minus P_{ES} or pressure "g" minus "j") to reflect the transpulmonary pressure; and P_{ES} at end inspiration minus P_{ES} at end expiration (pressure "j" minus "i") to reflect trans chest wall stretching pressure.

During a passive expiration, P_{AW} at end expiration can be atmospheric or can be elevated by the application of **positive end-expiratory pressure (PEEP)** to the ventilator circuit. Like the inspiratory hold, flow can be stopped at any point during expiration producing an expiratory hold and the P_{AW} then reflects the pressure (P_{ALV}) remaining in the respiratory system. If lung emptying is complete at the time the expiratory hold is applied, the P_{ALV} will equal P_{AW} and there will be no change in measured pressure during the hold; if lung emptying is not complete, the P_{AW} during the hold will rise to equal the higher remaining P_{ALV}. This higher P_{ALV} under these conditions is often termed **intrinsic PEEP** or PEEPi.

Note that the above discussion uses pressures generated by a positive pressure ventilator without any patient respiratory muscle activity (i.e., the chest wall acts as a passive structure). These same principles, however, can also be used during a spontaneous patient effort where the respiratory muscles supply the pressure for gas movement and the ventilator circuit pressure (P_{AW}) remains constant (i.e., equal during inspiration and expiration). These are depicted in Figure 6-2, right panel, with pressures "i" through "m." Under these active conditions, P_{ES} during inspiration represents the driving transpulmonary pressures created by inspiratory muscle contraction. During expiration, however, inspiratory muscles are not active and P_{ES} now reflects only chest wall stretching or recoil pressure. If a muscle-generated hold is created at end inspiration (active breath-hold) that is then followed by relaxation against an occluded airway (relaxed breath-hold) (pressures "l" and "m," respectively), all the pressure gradients described above for the passive breath can be measured (and, given the same flow and tidal volume, these gradients should be the same). ΔP_{ES} during inspiratory flow referenced to the active breath-hold period is transairway pressure (pressure "k" minus "l"). ΔP_{ES} between the active breath-hold period and end expiration is transpulmonary pressure (pressure "l" minus "i"). ΔP_{ES} between the passive breath-hold period and end expiration is the transchest wall stretching or passive recoil pressure (pressure "m" minus "i"). ΔP_{ES} between the active and the passive breath-hold period is the transrespiratory system stretching pressure (pressure "l" minus "m").

LUNG INFLATION AND RESPIRATORY SYSTEM MECHANICS: EQUATION OF MOTION

Lung inflation occurs when pressure and flow are applied at the airway opening during mechanical ventilation. These applied forces interact with respiratory system compliance (both lung and chest wall components), airway resistance, respiratory system inertness, and lung tissue resistance. For simplicity, because inertness and tissue resistance are relatively small, they generally are ignored and the interactions of pressure flow and volume with respiratory system mechanics can be expressed by the simplified equation of motion:

$$\text{Driving pressure} = (\text{flow} \times \text{resistance}) + (\text{volume/system compliance})$$

In the passive mechanically ventilated patient, this relationship is expressed as:

$$\Delta P_{RS} = \Delta P_{AW} = (\dot{V} \times R) + (V_T/C_{RS})$$

where ΔP_{RS} is the transrespiratory system pressure change during inspiration; $\dot{V}$ is the flow into the patient's lungs; R_{AW} is the resistance of the ventilator circuit, artificial airway, and natural airways; V_T is the tidal volume; and C_{RS} is the respiratory system compliance. These mechanical components are discussed subsequently in more detail.

Compliance (Elastance)

Static **compliance** (and its inverse, **elastance**) describes the "willingness" of the structural components of the respiratory system to expand in response to delivery of pressure and volume.[1,3] Static compliance of the respiratory system is expressed as the ratio of volume added to pressure applied in the alveoli ($C_{RS} = \Delta V/\Delta P_{ALV}$), and elastance is the inverse of compliance and is expressed as the ratio of pressure applied to volume added ($E_{RS} = \Delta P_{ALV}/\Delta V$). A so-called "dynamic compliance" can be calculated using $\Delta V/\Delta P_{AW}$ while flow is occurring. Because the P_{AW}

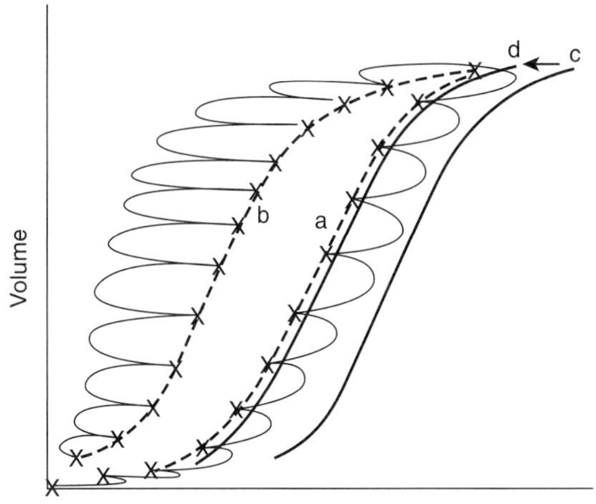

FIGURE 6-3 Pressure volume (PV) plots of the respiratory system. Pressure is measured in the airway (horizontal axis—P_{AW}), and volume (vertical axis—V) represents the volume change in the respiratory system. Dashed lines "a" and "b" represent a static PV plot during inflation and deflation, respectively. These lines are constructed by connecting the measured pressures during multiple inspiratory and expiratory pauses or holds as the lung is inflated and deflated (solid thin lines). During each pause or hold, airflow is not occurring and thus $P_{AW} = P_{ALV}$ (alveolar pressure). Solid thick line "c" represents a PV plot during a single constant inflation from a positive pressure breath with a physiologic inspiratory time. It is shifted rightward from the static PV plot because of the additional pressure required for flow delivery. Note, however, that if the inspiratory flow during this continuous inflation is significantly reduced (e.g., less than 10 L/min), the flow resistive pressures are minimal and the "slow flow" PV plot (solid thick line "d") approximates the static inspiratory PV plot.

under these conditions reflects both compliance and airway resistance properties of the respiratory system, this measurement should not be used as a substitute for static compliance.

To fully understand respiratory system compliance properties, a plot of $\Delta V/\Delta P_{ALV}$ from residual volume to total lung capacity can be very helpful[6-9] (Figure 6-3). As noted above, however, the measured P_{AW} must be a reflection of P_{ALV} and thus have no flow-related pressures present. This is called a "static" pressure volume plot and is constructed using a range of small discrete lung volume changes and measurements of corresponding values for P_{AW} under no-flow conditions during both inflation and deflation (see Figure 6-3, curves "a" and "b").[10] Because this procedure is time consuming and often requires patient paralysis, alternative strategies have been proposed. One approach during the inflation phase is to minimize flow-related pressures during a single slow (e.g., <10 L/min) positive pressure inspiration. Under these conditions, P_{TR} or P_{AW} can be used as a close approximation of P_{ALV} to construct a reasonable facsimile of the inflation limb of the static pressure volume plot (see Figure 6-3, curve "d").[11] This technique can be made even more accurate by correcting for known airway resistance.

In practice, C_{RS} is often reported as a single value that usually is determined during a passive inflation over the operational range of tidal ventilation ($C_{RS} = V_T/(P_{PLAT} - \text{PEEP})$ or volume "d" minus "e" divided by pressure "g" minus "h" in Figure 6-2). Similar calculations, however, can be done during a spontaneous breath where $V_T/\Delta P_{ES}$ between the active breath-hold and the passive breath-hold represents C_{RS} (volume "d" minus "e" divided by pressure "l" minus "m" in Figure 6-2). A normal value for C_{RS} is 100 ml/cm H_2O while severe lung injury is often associated with values for C_{RS} less than 20 ml/cm H_2O. Several features of C_{RS}, however, must be considered in its interpretation. Specifically, C_{RS} reflects two compliances in *series* (i.e., lung and chest wall), C_{RS} has *volume dependency*, C_{RS} has *hysteresis*, and the lung component of $C_{RS}/(C_L)$ is actually a reflection of multiple *regional* compliances.

Respiratory System Compliance Reflects Two Compliances in Series

The lung sits within the thoracic cage and both structures have their own compliance: lung compliance (C_L) and chest wall compliance (C_{CW}) (see Figure 6-1).[1,12] Lung compliance is the volume change/pressure change across the alveolar structure. Chest wall compliance is the volume change/pressure change across the thoracic cage and diaphragm structures. Measurements of ΔP across the lung and across the chest wall as described above can be used to calculate these different compliances.

Because lung and chest wall structures represent compliances in series, their reciprocals are additive:

Normal values for C_L and C_{CW} are 200 ml/cm H_2O each with C_{RS} thus equal to 100 ml/cm H_2O as noted above.

Compliance Is Volume Dependent

In the human respiratory system, compliance is nonlinear and volume dependent.[3,4,5,7,10] At low lung volumes and applied pressure, alveolar units may be collapsed and $\Delta V/\Delta P_{ALV}$ may be quite low ("flat"). With further application of pressure, these alveolar units open and the already open alveolar units distend. $\Delta V/\Delta P_{ALV}$ thus becomes higher ("steeper"). Finally, at high volumes and pressures, the structural properties of the respiratory system become unable to expand further and thus $\Delta V/\Delta P_{ALV}$ begins to fall again ("flattens" again). Thus, the plot of $\Delta V/\Delta P_{ALV}$ over the full range of lung volumes is usually sigmoid in shape (see Figure 6-3) with lower and upper inflection points. For this reason, the volume at which C_{RS} is measured must be considered when assessing or comparing C_{RS} values.

Compliance Has Hysteresis

Hysteresis refers to the difference in compliance during inflation versus deflation. In the respiratory system, compliance is higher during a deflation from near total lung capacity compared with inflation from near residual volume (note the difference in inflation and deflation shown in Figure 6-3).[8] This is because the inflation maneuver may require a level of pressure to initially recruit collapsed alveoli and stabilize the surfactant layer. This "extra" pressure is not needed to prevent de-recruitment in alveoli during deflation. As a consequence of these effects, ventilation on the deflation limb is the most mechanically advantageous (i.e., requires the least pressure application).[7,8] This is the rationale behind incorporating sigh breaths or "recruitment maneuvers" in the approach to setting PEEP.[3,7]

Compliance Is Determined by Many Different Regional Compliances

The measured $\Delta V/\Delta P_{ALV}$ value treats the respiratory system as a single compliance structure. The respiratory system, however, consists of millions of units, often with quite different mechanical properties. Even in the normal upright human lungs, gravitational effects on lung water, lung stretch, and blood flow create lower compliance units in the base and higher compliance units in the apices.[1,13] These differences account for the sequential filling and emptying of basilar and apical units.[11,14] In lungs with parenchymal injury, there are often heavily injured regions with very poor compliance interspersed with healthier regions with more normal compliance.[15]

Regional volume expansion from a positive pressure breath is heavily affected by these regional compliances. Specifically, severely injured lungs may have little ventilation delivered to stiffer regions and potential overdistention of healthier regions.[15,16] This has given rise to the concept that parenchymal injury effectively creates "baby lungs," a description that emphasizes the fact that only small portions of the lung may be available for ventilation. Regional compliance differences, by producing regional differences in resting volume (functional residual capacity), also may create the potential for shearing injury if one unit is filling proportionately faster or with markedly different volumes. The overall measured $\Delta V/\Delta P_{ALV}$ relationship should thus be considered a weighted mean value for the behavior of millions of alveolar units in the respiratory system rather than the behavior of a single structure. Because of this, predicting optimal ventilator settings from $\Delta V/\Delta P_{ALV}$ relationships may not be as simple as sometimes claimed.

Resistance

Resistance to airflow (R_{AW}) is caused by both the natural and the artificial airways (see Figure 6-1).[1,3,7] The determinants of resistance depend on whether flow is turbulent or laminar. Gas flow in the major airways is often turbulent, but in the majority of the airways flow is laminar. As a consequence, during positive pressure ventilation, gas flow is usually treated as laminar and thus flow related $P_{AW} \propto R_{AW} \times \dot{V}$.[3,7] Note that under these conditions, airway diameter is the major determinant of resistance in that R_{AW} varies inversely with the fourth power of the airway radius.

Clinically, airflow resistance can be measured during either inspiration or expiration. Inspiratory resistance generally is determined by using a constant flow breath and then calculating the driving pressure as the difference between the P_{AW} during flow and without flow (e.g., so called "peak to plateau" pressure gradient or pressures "f" minus "g" or "k" minus "l" in Figure 6-2).[4] Expressing this result with respect to volume (i.e., "specific resistance") takes into account the effects of lung volume described below.[1,4] Normal values are 4 to 6 cm H_2O/L/sec. Expiratory resistance is calculated in several ways.[2,3] A common approach is to use P_{PLAT} − PEEP at end inspiration (pressures "g" minus "h" or pressures "l" minus "m" in Figure 6-2) and divide peak expiratory flow by this value. Flow interrupters could be used to make similar calculations at different lung volumes during expiration. A more complex approach is to analyze the exponential decay characteristics of expiratory flow to calculate a time constant (resistance times compliance or $R_{AW} \times C_{RS}$) for a one-compartment model (or two time constants for a two-compartment model). One then can use a known compliance value to solve for resistance.

Like compliance, R_{AW} varies with lung *volume*, R_{AW} differs during *inspiration* and *expiration*, R_{AW} is a reflection of two resistances in *series* (i.e., artificial and natural airways), and R_{AW} can have significant *regional* variation.[17]

Resistance Varies With Lung Volume

The effects of lung volume on total airway resistance largely depend upon the behavior of the smaller membranous airways, as the larger central airways have cartilaginous structures that keep airway caliber relatively constant. In general, at larger lung volumes, smaller airways are either "pulled open" by the negative pleural pressures of a spontaneous effort or "pushed open" by the positive airway pressures of a mechanical breath.[1,3,10] The magnitude of these effects, however, differs during inspiration and expiration as described below.

Resistance Differs During Inspiratory and Expiratory Flow

At any given lung volume, inspiratory flow resistance tends to be lower than expiratory flow resistance. This is because during expiration, collapsing smaller membranous airways behave like Starling resistors, creating flow-limited segments.[18] In these segments, elastic recoil pressure is the only effective driving force for gas flow because increases in pleural pressure greater than this pressure only serve to further compress these airways and increase resistance. It is thus easier to fill the lung than empty the lung and this explains why air trapping and PEEPi can develop under certain circumstances.[19,20]

Total Resistance Reflects Two Resistances (Artificial and Natural Airways) in Series

In mechanically ventilated lungs, measured airflow resistance is influenced heavily by the properties of the artificial airways.[21] Indeed, long narrow endotracheal tubes (ET) can produce air flow resistance several times higher than normal airway resistance.[21] This ET resistance (R_{ET}) can have a number of important effects. First, R_{ET} creates an inspiratory muscle load. Indeed, the loading imposed by R_{ET} may be of sufficient magnitude to fatigue a spontaneously breathing patient who otherwise might be able to tolerate extubation. This is the rationale for using small amounts of pressure support in intubated patients during spontaneous breathing trials.[22] Second, R_{ET} creates a delay in achieving airway pressurization compared with circuit pressurization during ventilator gas delivery. In an actively breathing patient, this may cause discomfort.[23] To address this problem, a novel approach to triggering is to move the ventilator-sensing site (and thus, pressure-targeting site) to the distal end of the ET.[24] This can also be done mathematically as automatic tube compensation.[25] Finally, R_{ET} also produces both an expiratory muscle load and an increased risk for air trapping.[20]

Resistance Has Regional Differences

In normal lungs, gravitational effects on lung water and required stretch make airway resistance slightly higher at the bases than at the apices.[13,14] In disease states, airway resistance may have marked regional inhomogeneities and like compliance inhomogeneities may contribute to regional overdistention, shearing in adjacent units, and lung injury.

MECHANICAL LOADS

Mechanical loads describe the mechanical aspects of ventilation with a single number—an expression either of **work (W)** or of a **pressure-time product (PTP)** (Figures 6-4 and 6-5).[26] Work expresses load as the integral of pressure over volume (W = PdV). Thus, compliance, resistance, and the size of the breath all contribute to the magnitude of the work per breath. During a machine-controlled breath, integrating P_{AW} over V_T describes the work performed on the respiratory system by the ventilator; integrating P_{ES} over V_T describes the work performed on the chest wall by the ventilator.[3,10] During spontaneous breaths, integrating P_{ES} over V_T (referenced to the passive recoil pressure of the chest wall) describes the work performed on the respiratory system by the inspiratory muscles; integrating P_{ES} over V_T (referenced to end expiratory pressure) describes the work performed on the lungs by the inspiratory muscles. For a given $\dot{V}$, V_T, and set of respiratory system mechanics, measured total work should be identical regardless of whether measured during a spontaneous breath (patient work), a controlled breath (ventilator work), or an interactive breath (shared work).[27]

Normal values for work are 4 to 6 joules/min. Normal respiratory muscles generally do not fatigue with work less than 20 to 25 joules/min; abnormal respiratory muscles, however, may fatigue with even normal workloads.[26,28,29] Note that a common expression in the literature is work per liter of ventilation. This expression, however, is a misnomer in that since work is PdV, dividing this value by volume (V) per minute converts this work per liter expression to a simple mean pressure over time.

The PTP expresses load as the integral of pressure over inspiratory time (PTP = Pdt [see Figure 6-5]).

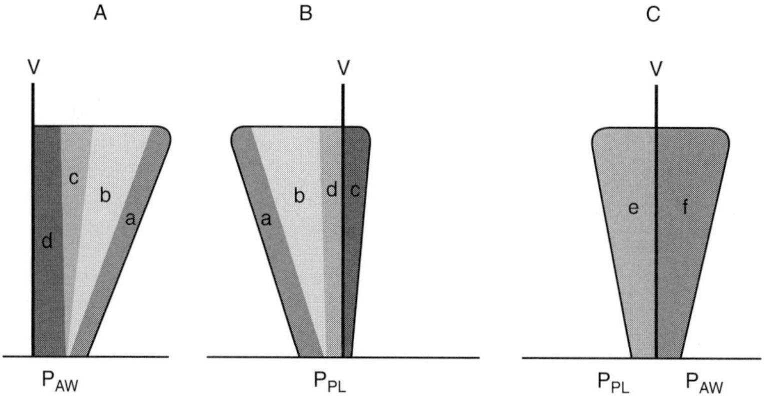

FIGURE 6-4 Loads expressed as work (W) during machine-controlled breaths *(panel A)*, spontaneous breaths *(panel B)*, and interactive or shared breaths *(panel C)*. P_{AW} is airway pressure, and P_{PL} is pleural pressure (often approximated as esophageal pressure). Both are plotted against V, the volume in and out of the lungs, and the integral of the pressure over volume (all the shaded areas) is the W. Depicted are the components of W due to airway resistance (R_{AW}, area "a"), lung compliance (C_L, area "b"), chest wall compliance (C_{CW}, area "c"), and intrinsic PEEP (PEEPi, area "d"). In the interactive breath, areas "e" and "f" represent patient (area e) and ventilator (area f) contributions to the W.

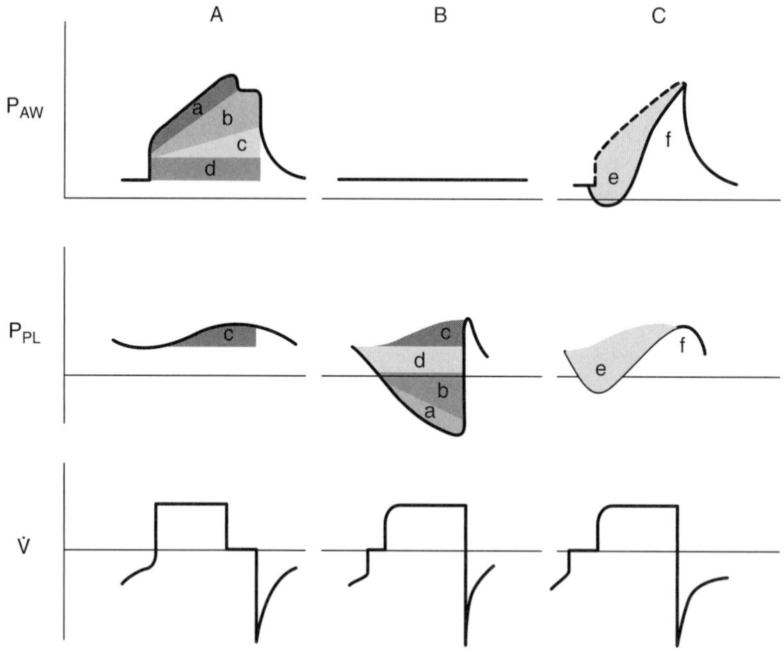

FIGURE 6-5 Loads expressed as pressure time products (PTP) during machine controlled breaths *(panel A)*, spontaneous breaths *(panel B)*, and interactive or shared breaths *(panel C)*. P_{AW} is airway pressure, P_{PL} is pleural pressure (often approximated as esophageal pressure), and $\dot{V}$ is flow in and out of the lungs. All are plotted versus time. The integral of the pressure over time (all of the shaded areas) is the PTP. Depicted are the components of PTP due to airway resistance (R_{aw}, area "a"), lung compliance (C_L, area "b"), chest wall compliance (C_{CW}, area "c"), and intrinsic PEEP (PEEPi, area "d"). In the interactive breath, areas "e" and "f" represent patient (area e) and ventilator (area f) contributions to the PTP.

Depending on whether the measured breath is spontaneous or machine controlled and whether pressure is P_{AW} or P_{ES}, the PTP (as in the aforementioned work discussion) can reflect properties of the lung, the chest wall, or the entire respiratory system and whether the load is borne by the patient, by the ventilator, or is shared. Normal values for the respiratory system are 4 to 6 cm $H_2O \times$ seconds per breath.[29]

A simple way of calculating work or PTP for a given tidal volume uses a machine-controlled breath with a constant flow. Mean inflation pressure can be calculated from simple geometric relationships or read directly from the ventilator monitor, and this pressure can be multiplied by either V_T (to calculate work per breath) or inspiratory time (to calculate PTP per breath).[30] If the tidal volume and inspiratory time selected for these measurements match the patient's spontaneous pattern, one can infer that these machine load calculations are equal to the loads borne by the patient during spontaneous breaths.

The concept of load is particularly useful in considering the inspiratory muscle energy requirement during spontaneous or interactive partial ventilatory support as mechanical loads correlate well with inspiratory muscle O_2 demands.[26] Importantly, duration of pressure (i.e., the PTP) correlates better with muscle energetics and fatigue potential than does the volume moved with pressure (i.e., work).[28,29,31] Moreover, the PTP, when referenced to muscle strength and/or endurance properties, may be a useful guide to set levels of partial ventilatory support or predict the spontaneous breathing capabilities. One particularly well studied index references the PTP and the inspiratory/total time fraction (T_I/Ttot) with respect to maximal diaphragmatic pressure (PDImax) to calculate a pressure time index (PTI = (PTP $\times$ T_I/Ttot)/PDImax). PTI values above 0.15 suggest a high likelihood of muscle overload and fatigue.[28]

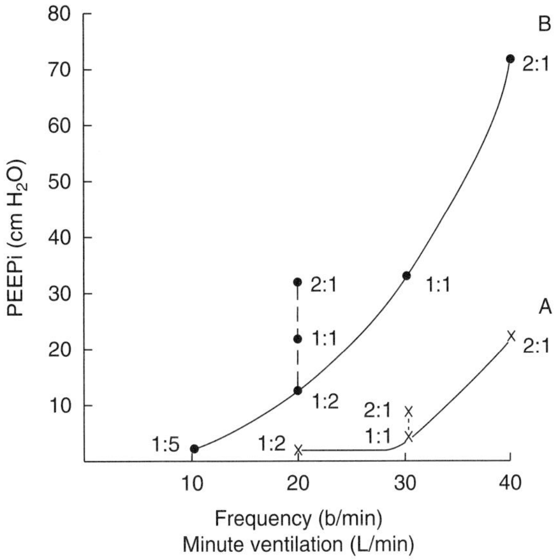

FIGURE 6-6 Examples of how intrinsic positive end-expiratory pressure (PEEPi) is a function of lung mechanics, minute ventilation, and I:E ratio. On the vertical axis is PEEPi predicted from a lung model and on the horizontal axis is frequency (f). In this model, tidal volume is set at 1 L and inspiratory time is 1 second such that minute ventilation ($\dot{V}_E$) is determined by frequency. I:E increases as f and $\dot{V}_E$ increase (representative I:E ratios are listed). Curve A illustrates the behavior of moderately restricted lung with only a slightly elevated resistance (C_L = 30 ml/cm H_2O, inspiratory R_{AW} = 10 cm H_2O/L/s, and expiratory R_{AW} = 10 cm H_2O/L/s). Note that significant PEEPi does not develop until f and $\dot{V}_E$ exceed 30. Curve B illustrates the behavior of a severely obstructed lung (C_L = 70 ml/cm H_2O, inspiratory R_{AW} = 20 cm H_2O/L/s, and expiratory R_{AW} = 40 cm H_2O/L/s). Note now that significant PEEPi develops at f and $\dot{V}_E$ values of 20 (Model B). Dotted lines depict the development of PEEPi as inspiratory flow is reduced and inspiratory time is lengthened with a constant minute ventilation. (From Marini JJ, Crooke PS: A general mathematical model for respiratory dynamics relevant to the clinical setting, Am Rev Respir Dis 147:14-24, 1993.)

INTERACTION OF RESPIRATORY SYSTEM MECHANICS WITH VENTILATOR SETTINGS

Mechanical Determinants of Delivered Ventilation

For a given frequency and tidal volume setting, the main limitations on gas delivery are the machine's pressure and volume capabilities (generally not an issue on modern machines), the high pressure alarm limits (especially in the setting of severe compliance and resistance abnormalities), and the development of intrinsic PEEP (PEEPi).

The mechanical effects of PEEPi are particularly important to understand, as the effects may not always be obvious. The three determinants of PEEPi are the total **minute ventilation ($\dot{V}_E$)**, the inspiratory/expiratory (I:E) ratio, and the mechanical factors involved in lung emptying (i.e., expiratory R_{AW} and the elastic recoil driving pressure C_{RS}) (Figure 6-6).[32] The lung-emptying mechanical factors are often expressed as a time constant (recall that the time constant is the

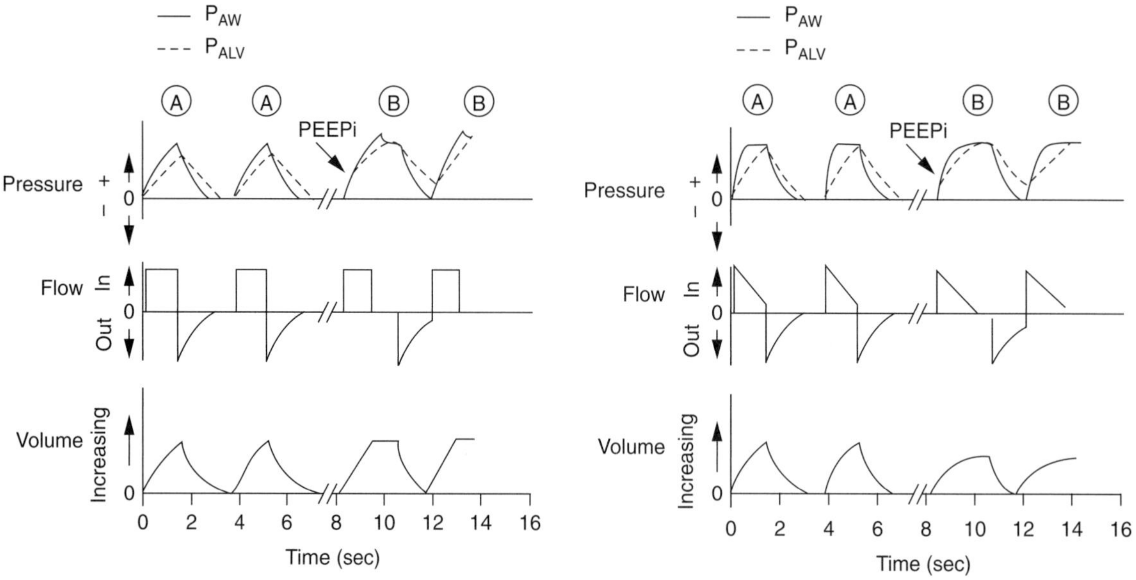

FIGURE 6-7 Effects of intrinsic PEEP (PEEPi) on flow-targeted/volume-cycled *(left panel)* and pressure-targeted *(right panel)* ventilation. P_{ALV} = alveolar pressure, P_{AW} = airway pressure. In both panels, the first two breaths have adequate expiratory times and, thus, no trapping. In contrast, the second two breaths in both panels have inadequate expiratory times, and airway trapping (PEEPi) develops. With volume-targeted breaths, this increases airway pressures. With pressure-targeted breaths, this reduces tidal volume. (From Fulkerson WJ, MacIntyre NR: Problems in respiratory care complications of mechanical ventilation, Philadelphia, 1991, Lippincott Williams & Wilkins.)

product of $C_{RS} \times R_{AW}$). Short time constants favor rapid emptying and occur when C_{RS} and R_{AW} are low (e.g., fibrosis). In contrast, long-time constants favor slow emptying and occur when C_{RS} and R_{AW} are high (e.g., emphysema).[32]

PEEPi may be either intentional (see discussion of airway pressure release ventilation in Chapter 22) or may be inadvertent (especially in patients with obstructive airway physiology). PEEPi has different effects on pressure-targeted and flow-targeted/volume-cycled ventilation; Figure 6-7). In pressure-targeted ventilation, intrinsic PEEP results in tidal volume loss, whereas in flow-targeted/volume-cycled ventilation, it results in airway pressure elevations. Other signs of PEEPi developing are the expiratory flow signal not returning to baseline before the next breath is triggered and the expiratory hold maneuver in the passive patient in whom a rise in airway pressure indicates the residual pressure (PEEPi) remaining in the lungs at that point in expiration.

Pressure vs. Flow Targeting and Respiratory System Mechanics

With pressure targeting, the clinician sets an inspiratory pressure target (with either time or flow as the cycling criterion) such that flow and volume are dependent variables (i.e., varying with lung mechanics and patient effort to maintain the pressure target). With flow targeting/volume cycling, the clinician sets an inspiratory flow and volume such that airway pressure is the dependent variable. Changes in compliance, resistance, PEEPi, or effort cause a change of tidal volume (but not P_{AW}) with the pressure-targeted breath. In contrast, similar changes in compliance, resistance, PEEPi, or effort change P_{AW} (but not flow or volume) with a flow-targeted/volume-cycled breath.

Respiratory System Mechanics and Ventilation Distribution

A positive pressure tidal breath must distribute itself among the millions of alveolar units in the lung. Factors affecting this distribution include regional resistances, compliances, functional residual capacities, PEEPi, and the delivered flow pattern (including inspiratory pause). As noted above, distribution inhomogeneities are a major factor in creating regional overdistention in "healthier" units during a positive pressure breath, which can lead to regional lung injury.

In general, slower flows tend to distribute more evenly in obstructive inhomogeneities (although consequent shorter expiratory times may worsen air trapping) whereas faster flows (especially decelerating flows) tend to distribute more evenly in compliance inhomogeneities.[33] Inspiratory pauses also allow pendelluft action to fill slow-filling alveoli. It should be noted, however, that more uniform ventilation distribution does *not* necessarily mean better ventilation-perfusion matching (i.e., more even ventilation distribution actually may worsen ventilation-perfusion matching in a lung with perfusion inhomogeneities). Because of all these considerations, predicting which flow pattern and I:E ratio will optimize ventilation-perfusion matching is difficult and often an empirical trial-and-error exercise.

KEY POINTS

- Respiratory system mechanics involve the interactions of resistance, compliance, patient effort, and positive pressure breath delivery strategy.
- Regional mechanical behavior influences the distribution of ventilation and consequent ventilation-perfusion matching.
- The integration of mechanical factors allows for calculation of loads on the ventilatory muscles.
- Understanding these relationships is important in optimizing ventilatory support.[34]

ASSESSMENT QUESTIONS

1. True or False. The key mechanical parameters that are measured during mechanical ventilation are ventilator respiratory system pressures and gas flow.
2. True or False. The stretching pressure across lung tissue is the difference between alveolar pressure and pleural pressure.
3. True or False. Airway pressure during expiratory flow reflects the driving alveolar pressure for gas out of a lung.
4. True or False. The equation of motion only applies to a mechanical breath delivered by the ventilator.
5. True or False. Respiratory system compliance reflects lung compliance and chest wall compliance in that series.
6. True or False. Airway resistance does not change with lung volume.
7. True or False. Ventilator work is the integral of pressure over time.
8. True or False. Ventilator work on the chest wall can be measured using the esophageal pressure catheter.
9. True or False. Intrinsic PEEP during controlled ventilation can be estimated from an expiratory hold maneuver.
10. True or False. Intrinsic PEEP development during flow- and volume-targeted ventilation will increase the plateau pressure.

CASE STUDIES

For additional practice, refer to Case Study 9 in the appendix at the back of this book.

REFERENCES

1. Murry JF: The normal lung, ed 2, Philadelphia, 1986, WB Saunders.
2. Truwit JD, Marini JJ: Evaluation of thoracic mechanics in the ventilated patient: part I, primary measurements, J Crit Care 3:133-150, 1988.
3. Truwit JD, Marini JJ: Evaluation of thoracic mechanics in the ventilated patient: part II, applied mechanics, J Crit Care 3:192-213, 1988.
4. American Association of Respiratory Care Consensus Group. Essentials of mechanical ventilation, Respir Care 37:999-1130, 1992.
5. Brander L, Ranieri VM, Slutsky AS: Esophageal and transpulmonary pressure help optimize mechanical ventilation in patients with acute lung injury, Crit Care Med 34:1556-1558, 2006.
6. Beydon L, Lemaire F, Jonson B: Lung mechanics in ARDS: compliance and pressure-volume curves. In: Zapol WM, Lemaire F, editors: Adult respiratory

distress syndrome, New York, 1991, Marcel Dekker, pp 139-161.
7. Servillo G, Svantesson C, Beydon L et al: Pressure volume curves in acute respiratory failure, Am J Respir Crit Care Med 155:1629-1636, 1997.
8. Salmon RB, Primiano FP, Saidel GM et al: Human pressure-volume relationships: alveolar collapse and airway closure, J Appl Physiol 51:353-362, 1981.
9. Sharp JT, Johnson FN, Goldberg NB et al: Hysteresis and stress adaption in the human respiratory system, J Appl Physiol 23:487-497, 1967.
10. Harris RS: Pressure-volume curves of the respiratory system, Respir Care 50:78-98, 2005.
11. Ranieri VM, Giuliani R, Fiore T et al: Volume-pressure curve of the respiratory system predicts effects of PEEP in ARDS: "occlusion" versus "constant flow" technique, Am J Respir Crit Care Med 149:19-27, 1994.
12. Ranieri VM, Brienza N, Santostasi S et al: Impairment of lung and chest wall mechanics in patients with acute respiratory distress syndrome: role of abdominal distension, Am J Respir Crit Care Med 156:1082-1091, 1997.
13. Milic-Emili J, Henderson JAN, Dolovich MB et al: Regional distribution of inhaled gas in the lung, J Appl Physiol 21:749-759, 1966.
14. Anthonisen NR, Robertson PC, Ross WRD: Gravity dependent sequential emptying of lung regions, J Appl Physiol 28:589-595, 1970.
15. Gattinoni L, Pesenti A, Torresin A et al: Adult respiratory distress syndrome profiles by computed tomography, J Thorac Imaging 3:25-30, 1988.
16. Gattinoni L, Caironi P, Pelosi P et al: What has computed tomography taught us about the acute respiratory distress syndrome? Am J Respir Crit Care Med 164:1701-1711, 2001.
17. Briscoe WA, Dubois AB: The relationship between airway resistance, airway conductance and lung volume in subjects of different age and body size, J Clin Invest 37:1279-1285, 1958.
18. Pride NB, Permutt S, Riley RL et al: Determinants of maximal expiratory flow from the lungs, J Appl Physiol 23:646-662, 1967.
19. Pepe PE, Marini JJ: Occult positive end-expiratory pressure in mechanically ventilated patients with airflow obstruction, Am Rev Respir Dis 126:166-170, 1982.
20. Tobin MJ, Ladato RF: PEEP, auto-PEEP, and waterfalls (editorial), Chest 96:449-451, 1989.
21. Wright PW, Marini JJ, Bernard GF: In vitro versus in vivo comparison of endotracheal tube airflow resistance, Am Rev Respir Dis 140:10-16, 1989.
22. Fiastro JF, Habib MP, Quan SF: Pressure support compensation for inspiratory work due to endotracheal tubes and demand continuous positive airway pressure, Chest 93:499-505, 1988.
23. Sasoon CSH: Mechanical ventilator design and function: the trigger variable, Respir Care 37:1056-1069, 1992.
24. Banner MJ, Blanch PB, Kirby RR: Imposed work of breathing and methods of triggering a demand flow CPAP system, Crit Care Med 21:183-191, 1993.
25. Guttmann J, Haberthur C, Mols G: Automatic tube compensation, Respir Care Clin N Amer 7:475-501, 2001.
26. MacIntyre NR, Leatherman NE: Mechanical loads on the ventilatory muscles, Am Rev Respir Dis 144:139-143, 1989.
27. Banner MJ, Kirby RR, MacIntyre NR: Patient and ventilator work of breathing and ventilatory muscle loads at different levels of pressure support ventilation, Chest 100:531-533, 1991.
28. Bellemare F, Grassino A: Effect of pressure and timing or contraction on human diaphragm fatigue, J Appl Physiol 57:44-51, 1984.
29. Field S, Sanci S, Grassino A: Respiratory muscle oxygen consumption estimated by the diaphragm pressure-time index, J Appl Physiol 57:44-51, 1984.
30. Marini JJ, Rodriguez M, Lamb V: Bedside estimation of the inspiratory dynamics relevant to mechanical ventilation, Chest 89:56-62, 1986.
31. Collett PW, Perry C, Engel LA: Pressure time product, flow, and oxygen cost during resistive breathing in humans, J Appl Physiol 58:1263-1272, 1985.
32. Marini JJ, Crooke PS: A general mathematical model for respiratory dynamics relevant to the clinical setting, Am Rev Respir Dis 147:14-24, 1993.
33. Macklem PT: Relationship between lung mechanics and ventilation distribution, Physiology 16:580-588, 1973.

CHAPTER 7

Alveolar-Capillary Gas Transport

NEIL R. MACINTYRE

OUTLINE

OBJECTIVES

- Describe alveolar capillary gas transport.
- Explain ventilation-perfusion relationships.
- Discuss the effects of increasing F_{IO_2}.
- Identify effects of positive end-expiratory airway pressure and gas distribution.

KEY TERMS

airway pressure release ventilation (APRV)
inspiratory : expiratory ratios (I:E)
inverse ratio ventilation (IRV)
O_2 delivery (D_{O_2})
positive end-expiratory pressure (PEEP)
pressure gradient
ventilation-perfusion relationship ($\dot{V}/\dot{Q}$)

Alveolar capillary gas transport is one of several steps that take place in the overall process of delivering O_2 to and removing CO_2 from the tissue (Figure 7-1). Metabolic demands are quantified by tissue O_2 consumption (V_{O_2}) and tissue CO_2 production (V_{CO_2}).[1] In oxidative metabolism, depending on the caloric substrate, V_{CO_2} is generally 0.7 to 0.9 of V_{O_2} (the "R" value). The demands on the alveolar-capillary transport system thus are to provide for an influx of O_2 to equal metabolic V_{O_2} and to provide an efflux of CO_2 to equal metabolic V_{CO_2}. Calculated values for V_{O_2} and V_{CO_2} generally are referenced to body surface area. Representative normal values for V_{O_2} are 100 to 150 ml/min/m^2 and for V_{CO_2} are 80 to 120 ml/min/m^2.

STEADY-STATE ALVEOLAR-CAPILLARY PRESSURE GRADIENTS

The steady-state **pressure gradient** for capillary-alveolar CO_2 transport is the incoming mixed venous P_{CO_2} (P_{VCO_2}) with respect to the mean alveolar P_{CO_2} (P_{ACO_2}). Under normal conditions, P_{VCO_2} is 45 mm Hg and P_{ACO_2} is 40 mm Hg. The determinant of P_{ACO_2} is V_{CO_2} with respect to the ventilation delivered to perfused alveoli (functional or alveolar ventilation [VA]). This relationship often is expressed in terms of alveolar P_{CO_2}:[1]

$$P_{ACO_2} \propto \frac{V_{CO_2}}{VA} \quad (1)$$

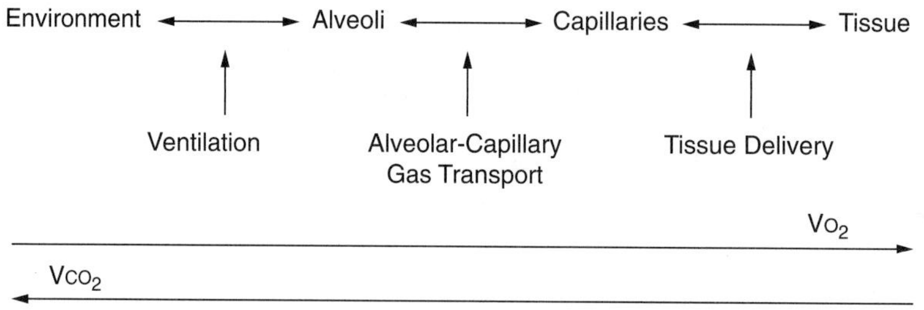

FIGURE 7-1 The respiratory chain. VCO_2, tissue CO_2 production; VO_2, tissue O_2 consumption.

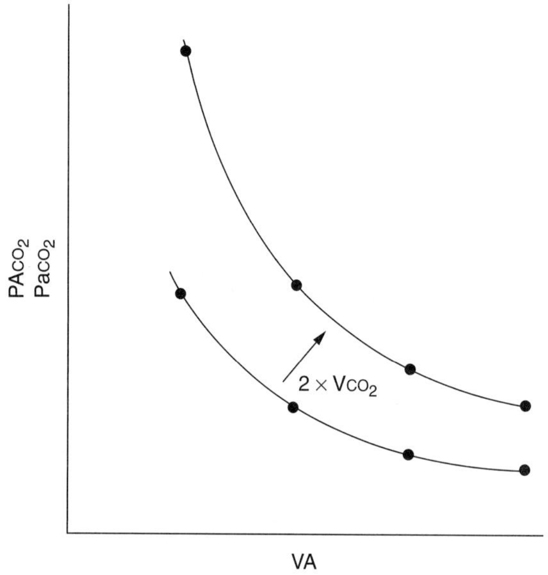

FIGURE 7-2 The relationship of alveolar (and arterial) partial pressure of CO_2 to VCO_2 and alveolar ventilation (VA).

This relationship is plotted in Figure 7-2 and, as can be seen, $PACO_2$ is related linearly to VCO_2 and related inversely to VA. Thus, for example, doubling VCO_2 ($2 \times VCO_2$ in Figure 7-2) doubles the $PACO_2$, whereas doubling the VA halves the $PACO_2$.

Because of the high diffusibility of CO_2 and the near linear relationship of PCO_2 and CO_2 content in blood, CO_2 alveolar-capillary gas transport is affected only minimally by the **ventilation-perfusion relationship ($\dot{V}/\dot{Q}$)**[1-3] (see later discussion). Thus in both normal and abnormal lungs, arterial PCO_2 ($PaCO_2$) is virtually identical to $PACO_2$. Because of this, $PaCO_2$ can be used in place of $PACO_2$ in Equation 1 and in Figure 7-2.

The steady-state pressure gradient for alveolar-capillary O_2 transport is mean alveolar PO_2 (PAO_2) and the incoming mixed venous PO_2 ($P\bar{v}O_2$). Under normal conditions, $P\bar{v}O_2$ is 40 mm Hg and PAO_2 is 100 mm Hg. Like $P\bar{v}CO_2$, $P\bar{v}O_2$ is affected by tissue O_2 consumption (VO_2), and PAO_2 is affected by ventilation delivered to perfused alveoli (VA). PAO_2 also is affected by the inspired PO_2 (PIO_2). The interaction of these factors is expressed as:

$$PAO_2 \propto PIO_2 \frac{VO_2}{VA} \qquad (2)$$

This relationship is plotted in Figure 7-3. Note that in contrast to CO_2, decreases in VO_2 and/or increases in VA increase PAO_2, but PAO_2 will asymptote on PIO_2 (partial pressure of inspired O_2). This is why increasing alveolar ventilation has progressively less effect on PAO_2 and O_2 transport. Equation 2 also can be rearranged using R as the ratio of VCO_2/VO_2 and VA as a function of $PaCO_2$ (Equation 1), to give the simplified alveolar gas equation for PAO_2:

$$PAO_2 = PIO_2 - \frac{PACO_2}{R} \qquad (3)$$

$\dot{V}/\dot{Q}$ matching has much more effect on alveolar-capillary O_2 transport than on CO_2 transport. As discussed subsequently in more detail, this is because the relationship between PaO_2 and O_2 content is not linear (O_2 content depends heavily on hemoglobin, which is fully saturated at $PO_2 \sim 100$ mm Hg) and the fact that O_2 is less diffusible than CO_2. Substantial differences in alveolar and arterial O_2 pressure thus can develop in the presence of $\dot{V}/\dot{Q}$ mismatch. Arterial PO_2 therefore cannot be substituted into Equation 2 or 3 for PAO_2. Instead, an "alveolar-arterial O_2 difference" ($A\text{-}aDO_2$) can be calculated to reflect this phenomenon:

$$A - aDO_2 = \left(PIO_2 - \frac{PACO_2}{R}\right) - PAO_2 \qquad (4)$$

A small $A\text{-}aDO_2$ gradient exists even in normal lungs (up to 25 mm Hg with room air breathing), but it can increase many times in disease states.[3,4] Thus

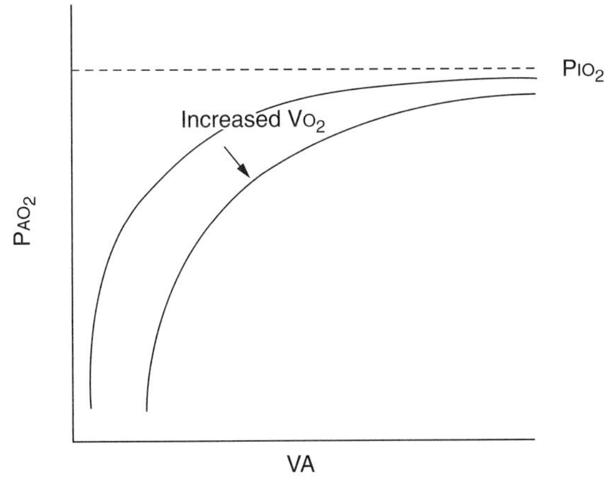

FIGURE 7-3 The relationship of alveolar partial pressure of O_2 (P_{AO_2}) to V_{O_2}, inspired O_2 (P_{IO_2}), and VA.

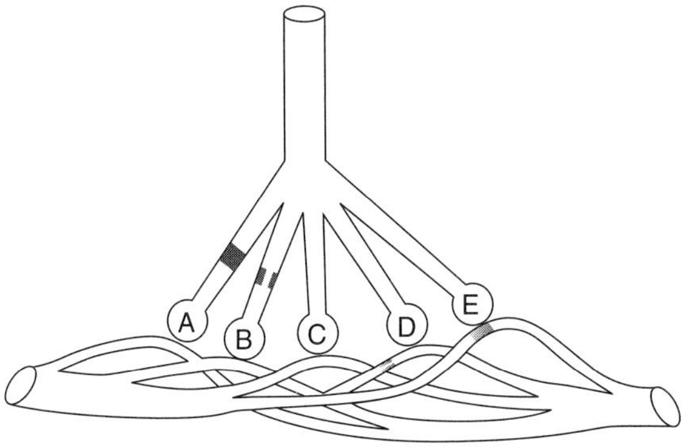

FIGURE 7-4 Conceptual depiction of ventilation-perfusion ($\dot{V}/\dot{Q}$) matching using a 5-unit lung model. Unit A is a $\dot{V}/\dot{Q}$ of 0 (a shunt), unit B is a low $\dot{V}/\dot{Q}$ unit (less than 1), unit C is a normal $\dot{V}/\dot{Q}$ unit of 1, unit D is a high $\dot{V}/\dot{Q}$ unit (greater than 1), and unit E is a $\dot{V}/\dot{Q}$ of ∞ (dead space).

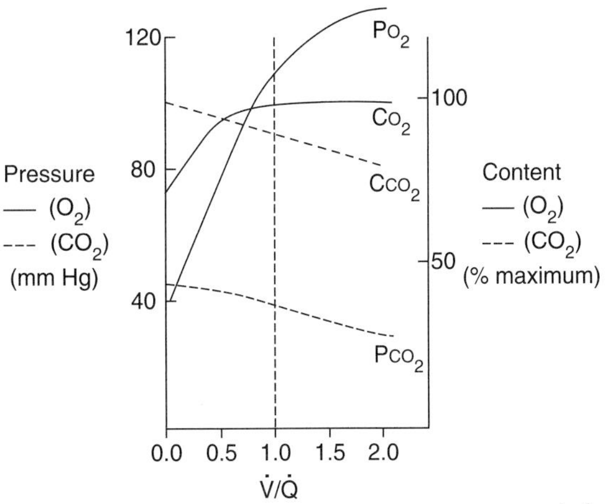

FIGURE 7-5 Effect of ventilation-perfusion ($\dot{V}/\dot{Q}$) ratios on arterial P_{O_2}, P_{CO_2}, O_2 content, and CO_2 content. Note that CO_2 pressure and content vary linearly with $\dot{V}/\dot{Q}$. High $\dot{V}/\dot{Q}$ units thus can "compensate" for low $\dot{V}/\dot{Q}$ units in overall CO_2 transport. In contrast, because hemoglobin is fully saturated with O_2 at $\dot{V}/\dot{Q}$ near 1, high $\dot{V}/\dot{Q}$ cannot "compensate" for low $\dot{V}/\dot{Q}$ in overall O_2 transport. *C_{CO_2}*, CO_2 content.

the A-aD_{O_2} gradient can be used to quantify the degree of lung injury.

VENTILATION-PERFUSION MATCHING

The concept of $\dot{V}/\dot{Q}$ matching is depicted in Figure 7-4.[2,5-7] Ideal $\dot{V}/\dot{Q}$ is near 1 (i.e., ventilation and perfusion are equal to each other). At the extremes are shunts ($\dot{V}/\dot{Q} = 0$) and dead space ($\dot{V}/\dot{Q} = \infty$). In normal upright human lungs, gravitational effects on lung water, perfusion, and ventilation create a vertical distribution of $\dot{V}/\dot{Q}$ relationships ranging from near 5 at the apex to near 0.5 at the bases.[2,5-7] In diseased lungs, this distribution can be many times larger.[2,5-7] A useful way to express this distribution is to use six gases of different solubilities and measure their lung and blood concentrations to construct a lung model with 50 $\dot{V}/\dot{Q}$ units.[5] The logarithmic standard deviation (sigma or σ) of this distribution then is used to quantify the degree of $\dot{V}/\dot{Q}$ inhomogeneities in the lung. Normal values for σ are less than 0.5, whereas values for σ of 2 or greater can be seen in severe disease.[2,5-7]

The effects of $\dot{V}/\dot{Q}$ mismatching on P_{CO_2} and P_{O_2} are different. In general, as noted previously, CO_2 is more diffusible than O_2, and its partial pressure in blood is roughly linearly related to its content. High $\dot{V}/\dot{Q}$ units thus can "compensate" for low $\dot{V}/\dot{Q}$ units such that even moderately abnormal $\dot{V}/\dot{Q}$ distributions have only small effects on Pa_{CO_2} (Figure 7-5). Because of this behavior, CO_2 is the gas used to quantify functional or alveolar ventilation (VA). Specifically, as long as there is measurable ventilation and perfusion to a lung unit, CO_2 transport occurs, and that alveolar-capillary unit can be considered functional. Extending this concept, physiologic dead space is defined as alveolar-capillary units in which no measurable CO_2 transport occurs. This is the basis for the Bohr equation that separates alveolar (functional) ventilation from wasted or dead-space ventilation (i.e., ventilation going to units with $\dot{V}/\dot{Q} = \infty$):[1]

$$\frac{V_D}{V_T} = \frac{Pa_{CO_2} - P_{ECO_2}}{Pa_{CO_2}} \quad (5)$$

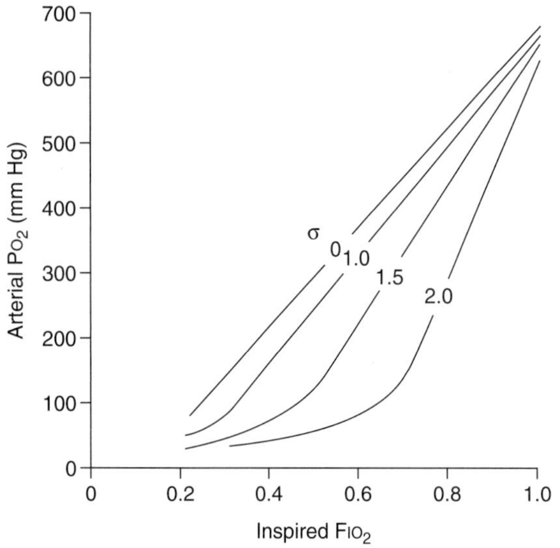

FIGURE 7-6 Graph showing the effects of changing inspired O_2 concentration (FIO_2) on arterial PO_2 in the presence of varying amounts of ventilation-perfusion inequality. When ventilation and perfusion are evenly matched (δ near 0), the relationship between inspired FIO_2, from 0.21 to 1.0, is linear. As ventilation-perfusion inequalities worsen (δ = 1 – 2), the effect of breathing a given FIO_2 is progressively less. Note that when the ventilation-perfusion abnormality is severe (δ = 2), breathing gas with an FIO_2 as high as 0.7 has little effect on arterial PO_2. (From West JB, Wagner PD: Pulmonary gas exchange. In: West JB, Wagner PD, editors: Bioengineering aspects of the lung, New York, 1977, Marcel Dekker, pp 361-457.)

where V_D/V_T is the dead space/tidal volume ratio and $PECO_2$ is mixed expired PCO_2. When the tidal volume and respiratory frequency (f) are known, alveolar ventilation can be expressed as the proportion of total delivered ventilation (VE) that is not "wasted" in dead-space ventilation:

$$VA = VE - (f \times V_D) \qquad (6)$$

In contrast to CO_2 behavior, O_2 is more sensitive to $\dot{V}/\dot{Q}$ abnormalities. The most important reason for this is the fact that hemoglobin, the major transport vehicle for O_2, is nearly fully saturated at $\dot{V}/\dot{Q}$ values near 1. PO_2 and O_2 content thus are not related linearly. This means that, unlike CO_2, high $\dot{V}/\dot{Q}$ units cannot compensate for low $\dot{V}/\dot{Q}$ units (see Figure 7-5) and a widened $A\text{-}aDO_2$ develops in disease states.[4,6,7] For this same reason, increasing the inspired O_2 concentration (FIO_2) has progressively less effect on PaO_2 as $\dot{V}/\dot{Q}$ worsens (Figure 7-6).[3]

As already noted, O_2 transport abnormalities can be quantified by the $A\text{-}aDO_2$ gradient. A simpler (although less precise) reflection of this same phenomenon is the PaO_2/FIO_2 ratio (P/F ratio). This ratio has been used by a number of consensus groups to define and quantify lung injury.[8] Specifically, acute lung injury can be defined by a P/F ratio of less than 300, whereas acute respiratory distress syndrome (ARDS) requires a P/F less than 200. Although easy to use and conceptually appealing, the P/F ratio is problematic as a severity indicator in that it can be affected by FIO_2, levels of end-expiratory pressure, and $PaCO_2$.

Another technique to quantify alveolar-capillary O_2 transport abnormalities is to calculate an effective shunt. A relatively simple way to do this requires breathing 100% O_2. As long as arterial blood has near 100% hemoglobin saturation, the resultant PaO_2 can be used in the simplified shunt equation[1]:

$$\frac{Q_s}{Q_T} = \frac{(A - aDO_2\ \text{gradient})(0.0031)}{(A - aDO_2\ \text{gradient}) + (0.0031)} \qquad (7)$$

where Q_S/Q_T is the fraction of total pulmonary blood flow that is "shunted" through $\dot{V}/\dot{Q}$ units near zero.

POSITIVE PRESSURE VENTILATION EFFECTS ON VENTILATION-PERFUSION MATCHING

Positive pressure ventilation can affect $\dot{V}/\dot{Q}$ relationships in a number of ways. Following are discussions on inspiratory and expiratory positive pressure, the inspiratory-expiratory flow relationships, and the perfusion effects of intrathoracic pressure.

Inspiratory and Expiratory Positive Pressure

At end exhalation, perfused alveolar units can be gas-less (i.e., flooded or collapsed), can be partially collapsed or fluid filled, can be open and normal sized, or can be overinflated. In the collapsed units (Figure 7-7), applying positive pressure below the required alveolar opening pressure delivers no gas to the units, the pressure-volume (PV) relationship is flat, and $\dot{V}/\dot{Q}$ is zero. Once the applied pressure exceeds the required alveolar opening pressure, gas is delivered, the PV relationship steepens and $\dot{V}/\dot{Q}$ rises. In overdistended units produced by either excessive applied positive pressure or because of air trapping, additional application of positive pressure will further overdistend the

A

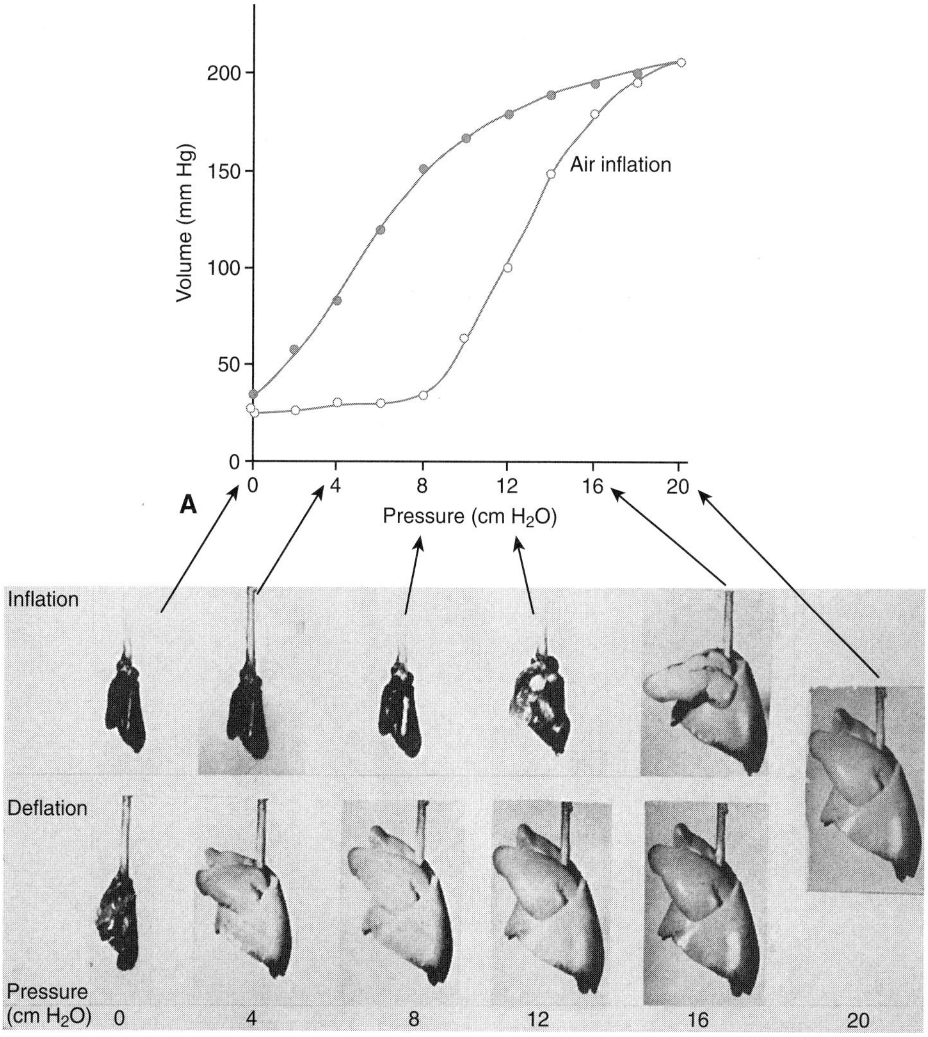

B

FIGURE 7-7 A, **A pressure-volume plot (PV) plot with pressure on the horizontal axis and volume on the vertical axis) of an initially collapsed animal lung during inflation and deflation with a positive pressure breath. B, Depicts the state of lung inflation. Note that pressures to open the lungs during inflation are much higher than the pressures required to keep them open during deflation.** (Modified from Mead J, Milic-Emili J: Theory and methodology in respiratory mechanics. In: Fenn WO, Rahn H, editors: Handbook of physiology. Section 3, Respiration. Vol. 1, Washington DC, 1964, American Physiological Society, p. 363.)

units, the PV relationship becomes flattened, and, because both ventilation and perfusion will fall in overdistended regions, $\dot{V}/\dot{Q}$ is variable. The overall inspiratory PV relationship and $\dot{V}/\dot{Q}$ behavior of the lung is an amalgam of these regional properties.

During expiration, PV relationships are shifted leftward (lower pressures are required to maintain a volume [see deflation limb in Figure 7-7]) because the surfactant monolayer produced when collapsed units are opened stabilizes the alveoli during deflation. Alveolar volumes and good $\dot{V}/\dot{Q}$ matching are thus maintained at lower applied pressure during expiration.

Positive end-expiratory pressure (PEEP) is defined as an elevation of transpulmonary pressures at the end of expiration. PEEP is generally produced in one of two ways: applied or intrinsic.[9] Applied PEEP is produced in the ventilator circuitry generally

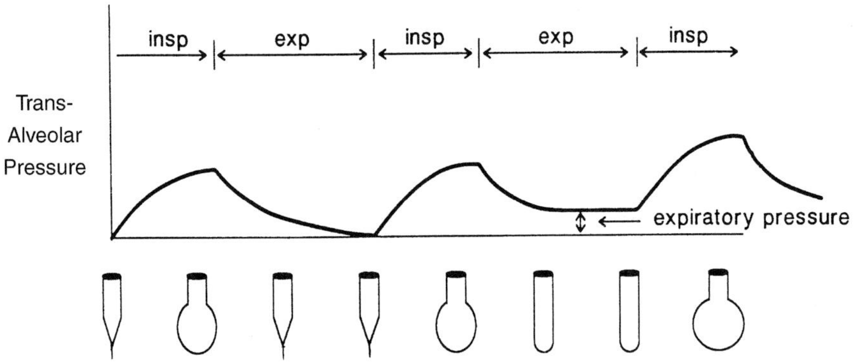

FIGURE 7-8 **Conceptual action of positive end-expiratory pressure (PEEP) to prevent de-recruitment and maintain alveolar patency throughout the ventilatory cycle.** (From MacIntyre NR: Oxygenation support. In: Dantzker D, MacIntyre NR, Bakow E, editors: Comprehensive respiratory care, Philadelphia, 1995, Saunders.)

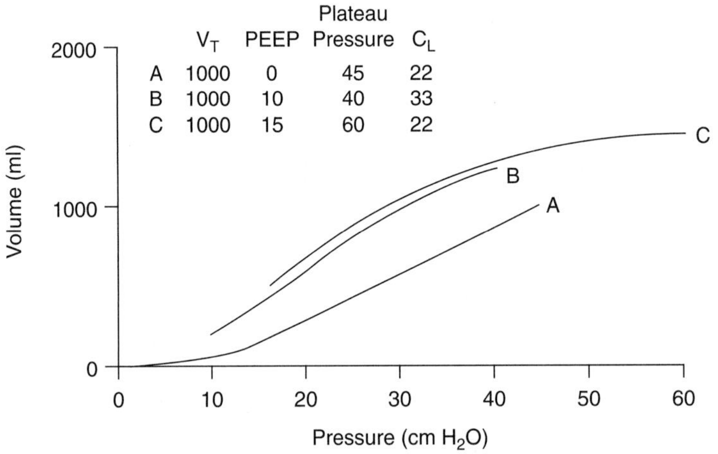

FIGURE 7-9 **Mechanical changes in collapsed alveoli when ventilated with increasing levels of positive end-expiratory pressure (PEEP). Curve A represents alveoli that remain collapsed until 5 to 10 cm H_2O pressure is applied (opening pressure). Subsequent delivery of a 1000 ml tidal volume (V_T) produces a plateau pressure of 45 cm H_2O, and a calculated compliance (C_L) of 22 ml/cm H_2O PEEP improves C_L (curve B). Levels of PEEP above this opening pressure, however, serve only to overdistend the alveoli, thereby worsening C_L (curve C).** (From MacIntyre NR: Oxygenation support. In: Dantzker D, MacIntyre NR, Bakow E, editors: Comprehensive respiratory care, Philadelphia, 1995, Saunders.)

through expiratory valves. Intrinsic PEEP is produced either when expiratory time is inadequate to return the lung to its physiologic functional residual capacity (FRC) or when airway obstruction prevents alveoli from fully emptying.[9,10] Expiratory muscle contraction can also raise intrathoracic pressures at end expiration, but this should not be considered PEEP because it is not a transpulmonary pressure (i.e., alveolar-pleural pressure).

PEEP is often employed in infiltrative lung diseases where alveolar inflammation and edema coupled with dysfunctional surfactant produce poorly ventilated regions and in regions that actually collapse during all or part (i.e., end-expiratory phase) of the ventilatory cycle. Functionally, these units behave as low $\dot{V}/\dot{Q}$ units or shunts.[9,11,12] The rationale behind applying PEEP is that if such units can be opened with a tidal breath or recruitment maneuver, the PEEP will prevent subsequent recollapse. PEEP thus doesn't recruit alveoli but rather prevents de-recruitment (Figure 7-8).

Maintaining alveolar recruitment provides several benefits (Figure 7-9, curve B versus A).[9] First, recruited alveoli improve $\dot{V}/\dot{Q}$ matching and gas exchange.[11,12] Second, as discussed in more detail in Chapter 10, patent alveoli throughout the ventilatory cycle appear to have less risk of injury from the shear stress of repeated opening and closing.[13] Third, alveoli recruited throughout the ventilatory cycle do not have to repeatedly construct the surfactant monolayer and this improves overall lung compliance.[14]

PEEP can also be detrimental (see Figure 7-9, curve C versus B). Because the tidal breath is delivered on top of the baseline PEEP, end-inspiratory pressures are raised by PEEP application. This must be considered if the lung is at risk for overstretch injury (Chapter 10). Moreover, because alveolar injury is often quite heterogeneous, appropriate PEEP in one region may be suboptimal in another and excessive in yet another[15] (see Figure 7-9). Thus optimizing PEEP is a balance between recruiting the recruitable alveoli in diseased regions without overdistending already recruited alveoli in healthier regions.[16] Another potential detrimental effect of PEEP is that it also raises mean intrathoracic pressure. This can compromise cardiac filling in susceptible patients (see Chapter 9).[17]

Inspiratory Flow Pattern and Inspiratory-Expiratory Time Relationship

Inspiration from a positive pressure breath consists of a flow magnitude, a flow profile, and, if desired, a pause (inspiratory hold). Each of these can affect $\dot{V}/\dot{Q}$ matching to a certain extent. In general, rapid initial flows (a consequence of set decelerating flow profiles

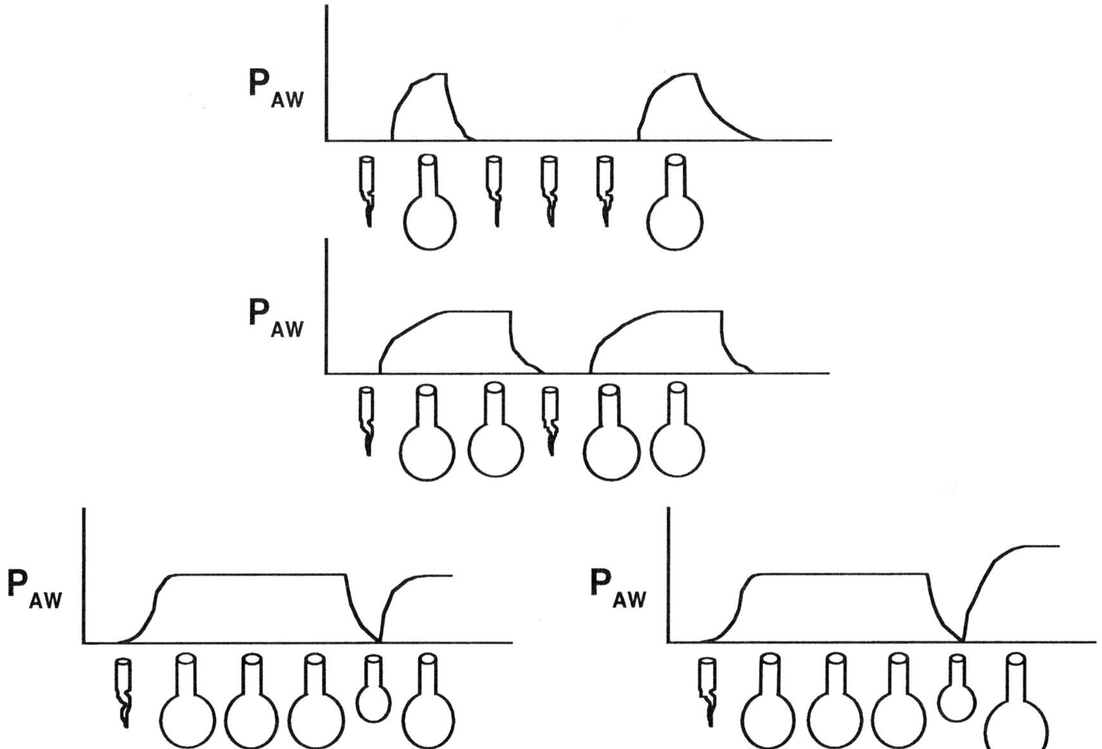

FIGURE 7-10 Airway pressure effects of longer inspiratory times. Plotted are airway pressure (P_{AW}) tracings over time with corresponding depictions of alveolar volume. In the top panel, the inspiratory and expiratory ratios are such that alveoli are at baseline volume for three fourths of the time. In the middle panel, inspiratory time has been extended so that alveoli are at inspiratory volume for a longer fraction of time, yet expiratory time is adequate for return to baseline volume. Under these circumstances, mean alveolar pressure is increased, but peak and baseline alveolar pressures are not affected. In the bottom panels, inspiratory time has been extended to the point that expiratory time is inadequate for a return to baseline volume. Under these circumstances, mean alveolar pressure has increased further. However, baseline alveolar pressure also has increased (i.e., "intrinsic" positive end-expiratory pressure [PEEP]), which either reduces tidal volume (pressure-targeted breath in left panel) or increases end inspiratory alveolar pressures (volume-targeted breath in right panel).

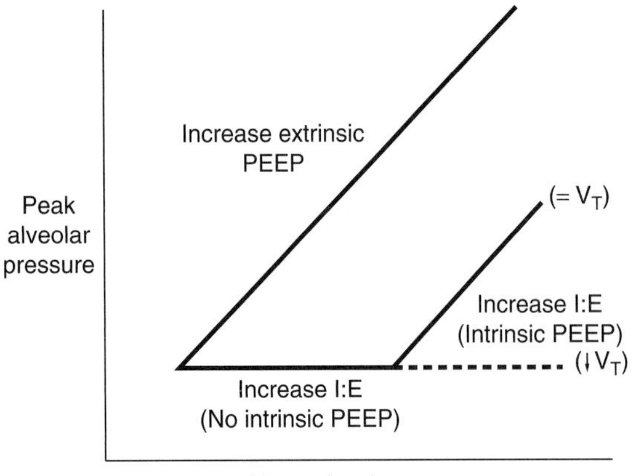

FIGURE 7-11 Relationship of peak alveolar pressure to mean alveolar pressure using various strategies to increase mean alveolar pressure. With increases in extrinsic or applied positive end-expiratory pressure (PEEP), the relationship is linear. With increases in inspiratory time that do not produce air trapping (intrinsic PEEP), mean airway pressure is increased without increases in peak alveolar pressure. However, when air trapping and intrinsic PEEP develop, either a higher peak alveolar pressure is needed for a constant V_T *(solid line)* or V_T diminishes for a constant peak alveolar pressure *(dotted line)*. (From MacIntyre NR: Oxygenation support. In: Dantzker D, MacIntyre NR, Bakow E, editors: Comprehensive respiratory care, Philadelphia, 1995, Saunders.)

or pressure-targeted breaths) pressurize the lung most rapidly and thus produce the highest *mean* inspiratory alveolar pressure for a given end-inflation pressure. Although theoretically this may affect $\dot{V}/\dot{Q}$, studies showing improved gas exchange with this rapid filling strategy are few.[18]

Prolonging inspiratory time, generally by adding a pause and often used in conjunction with a rapid decelerating flow (i.e., pressure targeted breath), also increases mean inflation pressure and lengthens gas-mixing time in the lung. Moreover, if the resultant expiratory time is inadequate for the lung to return to its relaxed volume (i.e., FRC), intrinsic PEEP (air trapping) develops. These effects are depicted in Figures 7-10 and 7-11.

There are several physiologic effects of prolonging inspiratory time. First, the aforementioned increased gas-mixing time may improve $\dot{V}/\dot{Q}$ matching in infiltrative lung disease.[18,19] Second, intrinsic PEEP has similar effects to applied PEEP and, indeed, much of the improvement in gas exchange associated with long inspiratory time strategies may be merely a PEEP phenomenon.[20] Third, because these long inspiratory times significantly increase total intrathoracic pressures, cardiac filling and cardiac output also may be reduced.

Importantly, **inspiratory : expiratory ratios (I:E)** that exceed 1 : 1 (so-called **inverse ratio ventilation [IRV]**) with conventional assist-control modes are uncomfortable, and patient sedation/paralysis often is required.[20] On many newer ventilators, however, a pressure relief (or release) feature has been added that allows spontaneous breathing during a pressure-targeted inflation period. This has led to the strategy of **airway pressure release ventilation (APRV),** which uses very long I:E ratios, lower tidal pressure swings, and encourages patients to breathe spontaneously (Figure 7-12).[21,22] In addition to the recruitment effects of the long I:E ratios, the required spontaneous breathing has been shown to better distribute ventilation to dependent lung regions and thus further improve $\dot{V}/\dot{Q}$ relationships.[21,22] Whether this approach should replace more conventional techniques remains controversial, as good clinical outcome data are lacking. APRV is discussed further in Chapter 22.

Intrathoracic Pressures and Perfusion

In addition to affecting ventilation and ventilation distribution, intrathoracic pressure applications from positive pressure ventilation can also affect both total perfusion and perfusion distribution. In general, as mean intrathoracic pressure is increased, cardiac filling is decreased and cardiac output/pulmonary perfusion decreases.[17,23] Reduced perfusion, however, can sometimes make $\dot{V}/\dot{Q}$ matching better even though total O_2 delivery may fall (i.e., reduced blood flow may reduce shunt flow).[23,24]

Intrathoracic pressures also can influence distribution of perfusion.[25] In the spontaneously breathing supine human lung, most capillaries are perfused. However, as intrathoracic pressures are raised with positive pressure ventilation, perfusion to nondependent lung regions may decrease, creating high $\dot{V}/\dot{Q}$ units and dead space.

ALVEOLAR-CAPILLARY GAS TRANSPORT IN THE CONTEXT OF OVERALL OXYGEN DELIVERY

Thus far, the discussion has focused on the alveolar-capillary gas transport—the "middle link" in the respiration chain shown in Figure 7-1. This discussion

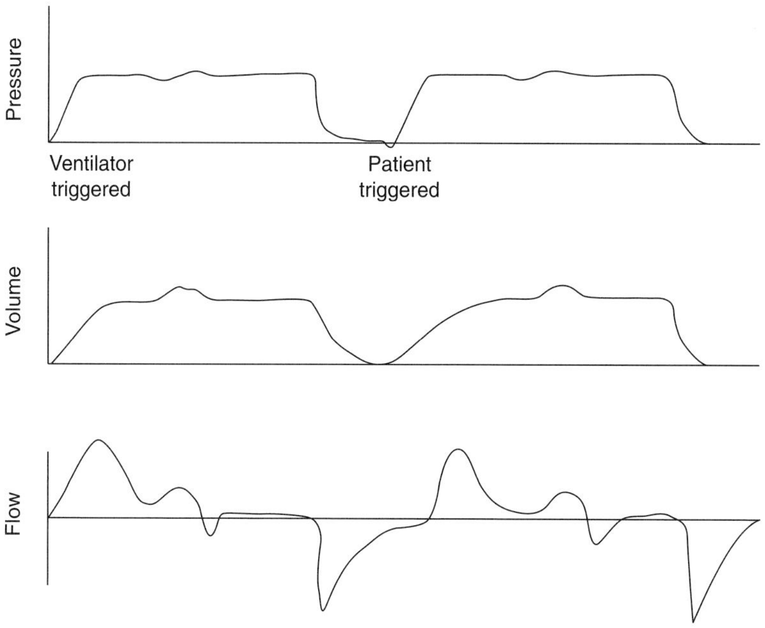

FIGURE 7-12 Pressure (upper panel), flow (middle panel), and volume (bottom panel) over time during airway pressure release ventilation (APRV). These breaths can be either machine (left breath) or patient (right breath) triggered, and are then pressure targeted and time cycled. The pressure release mechanism during inflation allows spontaneous breathing during both the inflation and deflation phases. This allows long inflation : deflation time ratios with spontaneous breathing during the inflation period as depicted here. See text for details.

would be incomplete, however, without a brief discussion of O_2 transport from the alveolar capillaries to the ultimate use site for O_2—the tissues.

Tissue delivery is the product of content times blood flow. **O_2 delivery (Do_2)** is thus the product of arterial hemoglobin saturation (Sao_2) times hemoglobin concentration (Hb) times Hb-O_2 affinity (1.34 ml O_2/dl Hb) times cardiac output (CO). Thus:

$$Do_2 = Sao_2 \times Hb \times 1.34 \times CO \quad (8)$$

Normal values generally are referenced to body surface area and are 300 to 400 ml/min/m^2. Do_2 can be increased several fold through increases in cardiac output or O_2 content. However, cardiac output manipulations or hemoglobin increases have the greatest effect on O_2 delivery. Indeed, this is the reason that aggressively pushing the Pao_2 above 60 mm Hg (a level that avoids pulmonary vasoconstriction and tissue hypoxia) usually offers little clinical Do_2 benefit.

O_2 delivery often is assessed in reference to O_2 consumption. Generally, O_2 consumption is 25% of O_2 delivery. This is the so-called extraction ratio that also can be expressed as the arterial-venous O_2 difference (a-vo_2). The normal a-vo_2 is 5 ml/dl of blood. Normal tissues can increase the extraction ratio to 50% or more when O_2 demands are high or O_2 delivery is low. In conditions such as the systemic inflammatory response syndrome (SIRS), however, this capability to increase extraction is lost.[26] Thus tissue hypoxia may exist even in the setting of high O_2 delivery. This is the reason that the a-vo_2 difference, although useful in managing patients with primary cardiovascular compromise, becomes potentially misleading in SIRS. For example, a narrow a-vo_2 difference (i.e., less than 5 ml O_2/dl) in a patient with cardiogenic shock suggests good function, whereas this same a-vo_2 difference in a septic patient may reflect poor extraction capabilities from the systemic disease.

Cardiorespiratory support strategies using Do_2 can be useful. This may depend, however, on the patient population being treated. Specifically, strategies aimed at "supranormal" Do_2 have shown benefit in young surgical or trauma patients.[27,28] In contrast, medical patients may have untoward complications from excessive cardiac stimulation and thus may be managed better using a more normal Do_2 target.[29] A recently reported "goal directed" approach to managing septic shock targets hemoglobin (greater than 10 mg/dl) and mixed venous O_2 saturation (greater than 70%) as therapy guides and has shown improved survival.[30]

Finally, in disease states with severe reduction in Do_2, a concomitant reduction in Vo_2 has been reported ("supply dependency").[31] Whether this represents a tissue metabolic response or a measurement artifact (mathematical "coupling" because Do_2 and Vo_2 share several common measurements) is not clear. Thus managing patients using Do_2/Vo_2 relationships probably is not justified at the present time.

KEY POINTS

- Alveolar capillary gas transport refers to the process of O_2 and CO_2 movement from alveolar gas to capillary blood.
- Arterial CO_2 is directly related to CO_2 production, inversely related to alveolar ventilation, and only minimally affected by $\dot{V}/\dot{Q}$ relationships.
- Arterial O_2 is directly related to inspired O_2, directly (but not linearly) related to alveolar ventilation, inversely related to O_2 production, and heavily influenced by $\dot{V}/\dot{Q}$ relationships.
- Intrathoracic pressures can have profound effects on $\dot{V}/\dot{Q}$ relationships and thus on O_2 transport.

ASSESSMENT QUESTIONS

1. True or False. Alveolar Po_2 rises in a linear fashion with increasing ventilation.
2. True or False. The determinants of the arterial CO_2 are CO_2 production and alveolar ventilation.
3. True or False. Because hemoglobin is virtually 100% saturated at a Po_2 of 100, high $\dot{V}/\dot{Q}$ units cannot compensate for low $\dot{V}/\dot{Q}$ units.
4. True or False. The multiple inert gas elimination technique can be used to describe $\dot{V}/\dot{Q}$ distributions.
5. True or False. Increasing Fio_2 has the same effect on Po_2 in normal lungs as it does in lungs with abnormal $\dot{V}/\dot{Q}$ distributions.
6. True or False. Expiratory pressure in itself does not recruit the lung; it only maintains recruitment that has already been achieved.
7. True or False. Applied PEEP and intrinsic PEEP distribute in a similar fashion.
8. True or False. The deflation limb and inflation limb of a pressure volume measurement in a patient with parenchymal lung disease are identical.
9. True or False. The dynamic pressure volume plot (i.e., with flow occurring) can mimic the static pressure volume plot if the applied flows are very slow (e.g., less than 10 L/min).
10. True or False. Conceptually, increasing PEEP should be preceded by a recruitment maneuver.

CASE STUDIES

For additional practice, refer to Case Studies 7 and 8 in the appendix at the back of this book.

REFERENCES

1. Roughton FJW: Transport of oxygen and carbon dioxide. In: Fenn WO, Rahn H, editors: Handbook of physiology, Section 3. Respiration. Vol I. Washington, DC: American Physiological Society, 1964, pp 767-825.
2. West JB: Ventilation-perfusion relationships, Am Rev Respir Dis 116:919-943, 1977.
3. West JB, Wagner PD: Pulmonary gas exchange. In: West JB, Wagner PD, editors: Bioengineering aspects of the lung, New York, 1977, Marcel Dekker, pp 361-457.
4. Mellemgaard K: The alveolar-arterial oxygen difference: its size and components in normal man, Acta Physiol Scand 67:10-20, 1966.
5. Wagner PD, Laravuso RB, Uhl RR et al: Continuous distributions of ventilation-perfusion ratios in normal subjects breathing air and 100% O_2, J Clin Invest 54:54-68, 1974.

6. West JB: Ventilation-perfusion inequality and overall gas exchange in computer models of the lung, Respir Physiol 7:88-110, 1969.
7. Wagner PD: Ventilation-perfusion relationships, Annu Rev Physiol 42:235-247, 1980.
8. Steinberg KP, Hudson LD: Acute lung injury and acute respiratory distress syndrome: the clinical syndrome, Clin Chest Med 21:401-417, 2000.
9. Kacmarek RM, Pierson DJ, editors: AARC conference on positive end expiratory pressure, Respir Care 33:419-527, 1988.
10. Pepe PE, Marini JJ: Occult positive end expiratory pressure in mechanically ventilated patients with airflow obstruction, the auto-PEEP effect, Am Rev Respir Dis 126:166-170, 1982.
11. Gattinoni L, Pelosi P, Crotti S et al: Effects of positive end expiratory pressure on regional distribution of tidal volume and recruitment in adult respiratory distress syndrome, Am J Respir Crit Care Med 151:1807-1814, 1995.
12. Suter PM, Fairley HB, Isenberg MD: Optimum end-expiratory pressure in patients with acute pulmonary failure, N Engl J Med 292:284-289, 1975.
13. Webb HH, Tierney DF: Experimental pulmonary edema due to intermittent positive pressure ventilation with high inflation pressures: protection by positive end-expiratory pressure, Am Rev Respir Dis 110:556-565, 1974.
14. Wyszogodski I, Kyei-Aboagye K, Taeusch HW Jr et al: Surfactant inactivation by hyperventilation: conservation by end-expiratory pressure, J Appl Physiol 38:461-466, 1975.
15. Gattinoni L, Pesenti A: The concept of "baby lung," Intensive Care Med 31:776-784, 2005.
16. Gattinoni L, Caironi P, Pelosi P et al: What has computed tomography taught us about the acute respiratory distress syndrome? Am J Respir Crit Care Med 164:1701-1711, 2001.
17. Pinsky MR, Guimond JG: The effects of positive end-expiratory pressure on heart-lung interactions, J Crit Care 6:1-15, 1991.
18. Abraham E, Yoshihara G: Cardiorespiratory effects of pressure controlled ventilation in severe respiratory failure, Chest 98:1445-1449, 1990.
19. Armstrong BW, MacIntyre NR: Pressure controlled inverse ratio ventilation that avoids air trapping in ARDS, Crit Care Med 23:279-285, 1995.
20. Cole AGH, Weller SF, Sykes MD: Inverse ratio ventilation compared with PEEP in adult respiratory failure, Intensive Care Med 10:227-232, 1984.
21. Putensen C, Wrigge H: Clinical review: biphasic positive airway pressure and airway pressure release ventilation, Crit Care (London) 8:492-497, 2004.
22. Habashi NM: Other approaches to open-lung ventilation: airway pressure release ventilation, Crit Care Med 33(3 Suppl):S228-240, 2005.
23. Lynch JP, Mhyre JG, Dantzker DR: Influence of cardiac output on intrapulmonary shunt, J Appl Physiol 46:315-321, 1979.
24. Pinsky MR: The hemodynamic consequences of mechanical ventilation: an evolving story, Intensive Care Med 23:493-503, 1997.
25. Hughes JM, West J, Wagner P et al: Effect of lung volume on the distribution of pulmonary blood flow in man, Respir Physiol 4:58-72, 1968.
26. Vincent JL: The relationship between oxygen demand, oxygen uptake and oxygen supply, Intensive Care Med 16:s145-s148, 1990.
27. Astiz ME, Rackow EC, Falk JL et al: Oxygen delivery and consumption in patients with hyperdynamic septic shock, Crit Care Med 15:26-28, 1987.
28. Shoemaker WC, Appel PL, Kram HB et al: Prospective trial of supranormal values of survivors as therapeutic goals in high risk surgical patients, Chest 94:1176-1186, 1988.
29. Hayes MA, Timmins AC, Yau EHS et al: Elevation of systemic oxygen delivery in the treatment of critically ill patients, N Engl J Med 330:1717-1722, 1994.
30. Rivers E, Nguyen B, Havstad S et al: Early Goal-Directed Therapy Collaborative Group. Early goal-directed therapy in the treatment of severe sepsis and septic shock, N Engl J Med 345:1368-1377, 2001.
31. Danek SJ, Lynch JP, Weg JG et al: The dependence of oxygen uptake on oxygen delivery in the adult respiratory distress syndrome, Am Rev Respir Dis 122:387-395, 1980.

CHAPTER

8 Patient-Ventilator Interactions

Lawrence R. Tom; Catherine S. H. Sassoon

OUTLINE

OBJECTIVES

- Describe the determinants of spontaneous ventilation and how they relate to mechanical ventilation.
- Explain the factors involved in patient-ventilator interactions.
- Identify the underlying mechanisms of patient-ventilator dyssynchrony.
- Discuss available interventions to potentially synchronize the patient and ventilator.
- Describe novel ventilator modes that may improve patient-ventilator interactions.

KEY TERMS

auto-triggering
dead space
dynamic hyperinflation (DH)
dyssynchrony
flow triggering
flow-waveform triggering
functional residual capacity (FRC)
ineffective triggering
pressure support ventilation (PSV)
pressure triggering
proportional assist ventilation (PAV)
spontaneous ventilation
synchronous intermittent mandatory ventilation (SIMV)
time cycling
trigger variable
volume cycling
volume triggering

One third of patients admitted to the intensive care unit (ICU) require supportive therapy in the form of mechanical ventilation.[1,2] In the proper setting, the ventilator can contribute to the successful treatment of respiratory failure by improving gas exchange and unloading respiratory muscle work. Ventilators can provide complete or partial support. With complete ventilator support, the ventilator totally assumes the patient's respiratory muscle work. Because the patient's respiratory system is completely passive, no interaction exists between the patient and ventilator. With partial ventilator support, the patient and the ventilator interact in unloading respiratory muscle work. Ideally the ventilator should be sensitive and responsive to continual changes in a patient's effort and breath (inspiratory and expiratory) timing to synchronize the interactions between itself and the patient. **Dyssynchrony** occurs when the patient's breath and ventilator timing are out of phase, or when ventilator gas delivery is inadequate to match the patient's ventilatory demand. Patient-ventilator interactions extend into the weaning period until the patient resumes autonomous breathing without ventilator assistance.

Synchronizing patient-ventilator interactions is important to prevent unnecessary "imposed" muscle loading, which may manifest as the patient's "fighting" the ventilator. The latter potentially dictates the administration of sedation with its adverse outcomes: a longer duration of mechanical ventilation, weaning time, and intensive care unit (ICU) stay.[3,4] Furthermore, patient-ventilator synchrony has the potential to decrease the sensation of dyspnea, to prevent hypocapnia, and increase the likelihood of periodic breathing during sleep.[5]

The goals of this chapter are to describe (1) the determinants of spontaneous ventilation and how it relates to mechanical ventilation, (2) the response of patient effort to ventilator-delivered breaths, (3) the response of the mechanical ventilator to patient effort, and (4) novel methods of artificial ventilation to improve patient-ventilator interaction.

DETERMINANTS OF SPONTANEOUS VENTILATION

Respiratory Control System

The patient's biologic respiratory control system is responsible for control of **spontaneous ventilation** and is composed of four components[6]: (1) a central controller, (2) connecting nerves, (3) the ventilatory pump and upper airway muscles, and (4) sensors (chemoreceptors and mechanoreceptors) (Figure 8-1). The central controller is located in the brainstem, and after integrating information relayed from the sensors and the cerebral cortex (which conveys voluntary influences, such as talking, singing, and

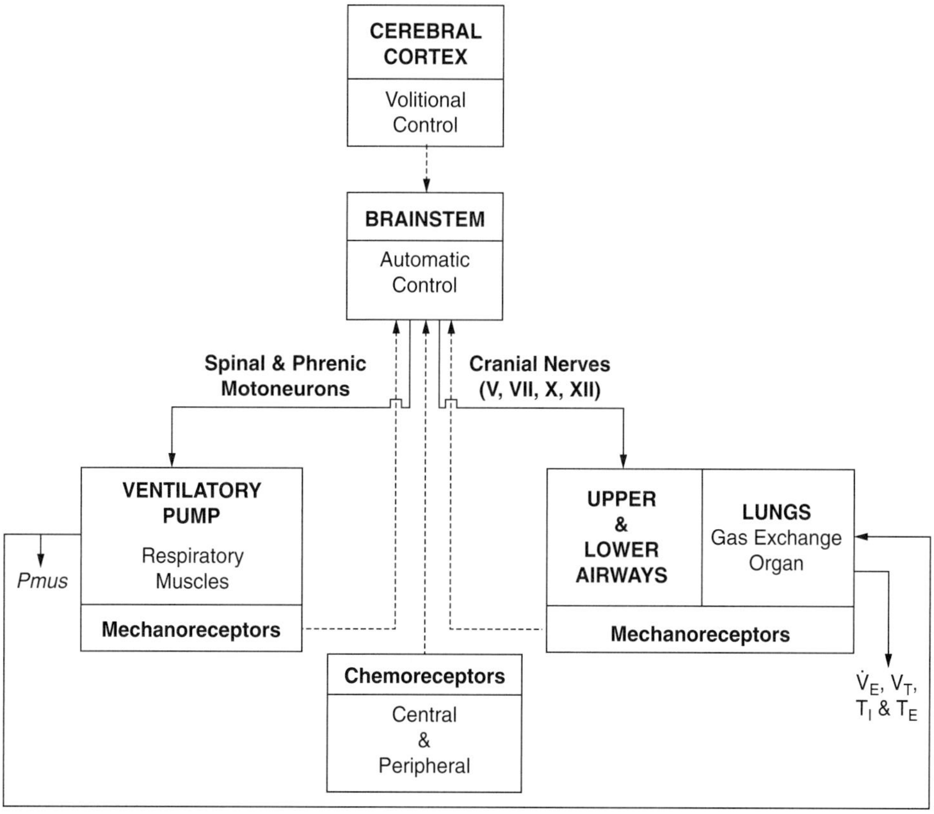

FIGURE 8-1 Schematic diagram of the respiratory control system. Solid lines indicate output signal from the central controller in the brainstem, transmitted to the ventilatory pump and upper airways via the connecting nerves. Output from the ventilator pump, *Pmus,* drives the gas exchange organ (lungs), and is translated into tidal volume (V_T). The product of V_T and frequency is total ventilation ($\dot{V}_E$), while frequency is 60 divided by the sum of inspiratory (T_I) and expiratory (T_E) time. Dashed lines indicate input signals from the cerebral cortex and sensors; chemoreceptors and mechanoreceptors to the central controller.

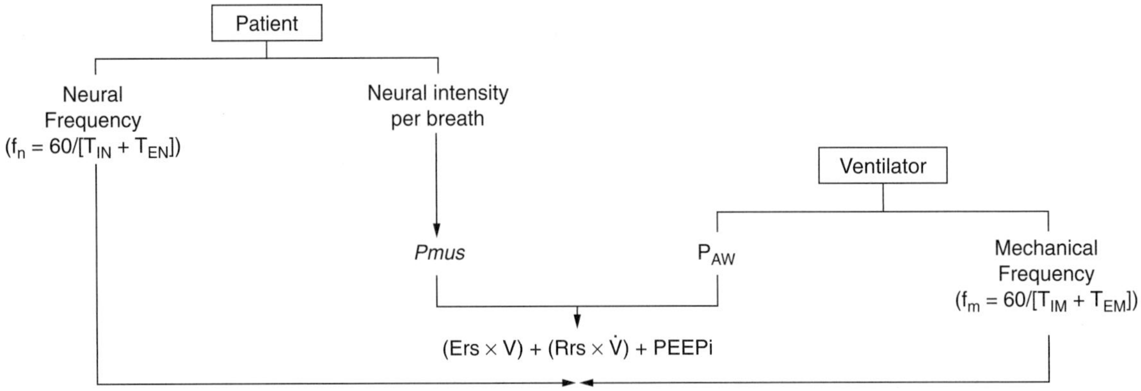

FIGURE 8-2 Schematic diagram of the interaction between patient's neural intensity per breath *(Pmus)* and neural frequency (f_n), and ventilator's driving pressure (P_{AW}) and mechanical frequency (f_m). Both *Pmus* and P_{AW} are the pressures to overcome the respiratory system's elastance (Ers), resistance (Rrs), and intrinsic positive end-expiratory pressure (PEEPi). V is volume above the passive functional residual capacity; $\dot{V}$ is inspiratory flow. The patient's breath or neural timing components are neural inspiratory (T_{IN}) and expiratory (T_{EN}) time; and those of the ventilator are mechanical inspiratory (T_{IM}) and expiratory (T_{EM}) time. Both f_n and f_m can be derived from the respective timing components as shown.

laughing), transmits the information to the ventilatory pump, causing the respiratory muscle to contract and generate pressure *(Pmus)*. *Pmus* reflects the output neural intensity of the central controller and is dissipated to overcome the respiratory system's elastic recoil (Pel), and resistive pressure (Pres) (see below). In addition to *Pmus*, the central controller regulates neural frequency (f_n) and its components, neural inspiratory (T_{IN}) and expiratory (T_{EN}) timing. *Pmus* is translated into tidal volume (V_T) per breath, and when multiplied by frequency, determines total ventilation ($\dot{V}_E$). The central controller's output to the respiratory muscles is coordinated with its output to the upper airways. The sensors transmit to the central controller via a variety of sources, including chemoreceptors located in the carotid body and the brainstem, and mechanoreceptors located in the lungs, chest wall, and upper airway. The chemoreceptors are influenced by changes in pH, $Paco_2$, and Pao_2. Specific mechanoreceptors are influenced by changes in lung inflation, pressure, flow rate, fluid congestion within the lungs, irritants in the airway, changes in muscle length, and muscle loading.

Equation of Motion

During spontaneous ventilation, *Pmus* is required to overcome Pel, Pres, and the respiratory system's inertia.[7,8] Because the last is negligible, the equation of motion can be rendered simply as *Pmus* = Pel + Pres. Since Pel is the product of respiratory system elastance (Ers) and volume (V) above the passive **functional residual capacity (FRC)** and Pres is the product of respiratory system resistance (Rrs) and inspiratory flow ($\dot{V}$), we can substitute these components for Pel and Pres. Therefore in the event of detectable intrinsic positive end-expiratory pressure (PEEPi), the equation of motion can be rendered as *Pmus* = (Ers × V) + (Rrs × $\dot{V}$) + PEEPi.

How does *Pmus* generated during spontaneous ventilation relate to pressure provided by the ventilator? During mechanical ventilation, the pressure supplied by the ventilator (P_{AW}) is added to *Pmus*, and therefore the sum of *Pmus* and P_{AW} becomes the driving pressure for inspiratory flow. Thus, the driving pressure required for inspiratory flow can be described as: P_{AW} + *Pmus* = (Ers × V) + (Rrs × $\dot{V}$) + PEEPi. Rearranging the equation, we obtain: P_{AW} = (Ers × V) + (Rrs × $\dot{V}$) + PEEPi − *Pmus*. Hence, during partial ventilator support, the ventilator pushes (P_{AW}) and the patient pulls fresh gas (−*Pmus*), and the combined ventilator- and patient-generated pressures are essential to overcome Ers, Rrs, and PEEPi. Thus the interactions between the patient and ventilator encompass (1) the patient's effort to pull ventilator-delivered breath (patient-related factors), and (2) the ventilator's response to the patient's effort (ventilator-related factors). In the context of patient-ventilator interactions, in addition to *Pmus* and neural frequency (f_n), mechanical frequency (f_m) and its components, ventilatory inspiratory time and ventilatory expiratory time (T_{IM} and T_{EM}) are important factors (Figure 8-2).

PATIENT-VENTILATOR INTERACTIONS

Patient-Related Factors

Pmus generation rate, intensity, and duration during mechanical ventilation are affected by chemoreceptor-mediated (chemical), mechanoreceptor-mediated (mechanical), and cortical-mediated (behavioral) feedback.

Chemical Feedback

Chemical feedback is the respiratory controller's response to levels of PaO_2, $PaCO_2$, and pH in the patient's blood. The feedback allows maintenance of blood gas tensions that would otherwise disrupt homeostasis due to changes in metabolic rate or gas exchange. In spontaneously breathing or mechanically ventilated patients, chemical feedback is an important determinant of *Pmus* during both wakefulness and sleep.[9] However, in mechanically ventilated patients, the ability of chemical feedback to compensate for changes in blood gas tensions depends on the mechanical ventilation mode, irrespective of wakefulness or sleep.

In mechanically ventilated awake healthy subjects randomized to three modes of support—**proportional assist ventilation (PAV),** assist-control volume-cycled ventilation (ACV), and **pressure support ventilation (PSV)**—Mitrouska and coworkers[10] studied the chemical feedback response to increasing levels of fractional inspired CO_2. PAV is a mechanical ventilation mode in which *Pmus* is proportional to ventilator P_{AW}; as patient effort increases or decreases, P_{AW} proportionately increases or decreases, respectively.

With all modes, the ventilator was set at the highest comfortable level of assist, providing significant muscle unloading, although the unloading was higher with ACV and PSV than with PAV. With PAV, patients were noted to have eucapnia (i.e., the same $P_{ET}CO_2$ as that during spontaneous ventilation), whereas hypocapnia was observed with either ACV or PSV. V_T was greater with ACV and PSV compared with PAV, whereas respiratory frequency was similar with all modes. Despite hypocapnia, which in some cases was severe, the subjects continued to trigger the ventilator. Hence, at high-assist levels with ACV or PSV, the central controller is insensitive to chemical feedback of hypocapnia. With PAV, the prevention of a further drop in $P_{ET}CO_2$ was due to the preserved neuroventilatory coupling (i.e., the output of neural intensity or patient's effort is proportionately translated into $\dot{V}_E$).[10]

As with healthy subjects, the chemical feedback response of critically ill patients who are ready to wean depends on the ventilation modes.[11,12] When challenged with added **dead space**[11] or mechanical load[12] to increase $PaCO_2$, the response with PSV differs from that with PAV. With PSV, added dead space caused little change in V_T, but an increase in respiratory rate and breathing discomfort. In contrast, with PAV, V_T increased, but respiratory frequency was unchanged.[11] With PSV, added mechanical load resulted in decreased V_T and an increased respiratory rate, whereas with PAV the decrease in V_T was smaller (10% versus 29%), as was the increase in respiratory rate (14% versus 58%).[12] With both modes of ventilation, $\dot{V}_E$ was preserved. This observation suggests that when the ability to increase V_T is limited to defending changes in blood gas tensions, the remaining option is to increase respiratory frequency, with consequently greater breathing discomfort.

When patients are asleep or under sedation, chemical feedback is the most important factor in determining the patient's breathing pattern.[13,14] Under this condition, a drop in $PaCO_2$ by a few mm Hg induces apnea. Assisted ventilation with high V_T with ACV or PSV results in hypocapnia and increases the likelihood of apneas and periodic breathing,[15] the latter of which may result in hypoxemia. Whereas periodic breathing is observed with both PSV and ACV, it is less frequent with PAV,[9] where V_T is maintained relatively constant at different assist levels due to appropriate adjustments in *Pmus*.[9]

Mechanical Feedback

Mechanical feedback is the response of the patient's respiratory controller to changes in delivered volume, pressure, or (flow). This nonchemical feedback manifests as inhibitory or excitatory alterations in respiratory rate and *Pmus*, and is qualitatively similar during wakefulness and sleep.[16] In awake healthy subjects on ACV, when the increase in V_T (100% change from initial V_T) was balanced by an increase in ventilator $\dot{V}$ to maintain ventilator inspiratory time constant (T_{IM}), respiratory rate decreased very little (~12%).[17,18] As a result, severe hypocapnia may ensue as the patient continues to trigger the ventilator. Georgopoulos et al[19] demonstrated that when V_T increased with the application of PAV and CO_2 challenge, the decrease in *Pmus* was small (14%). Hence, during mechanical ventilation, the effect of neuromechanical inhibition with increasing V_T on respiratory rate and *Pmus* is small. However, a high ventilator V_T or pressure may result in significant mismatching between T_{IN} and T_{IM}, causing asynchrony in the breath's cycling off. When ventilator inflation extends into neural expiration, the time available for expiratory flow, before the next inspiratory effort, is reduced. If passive FRC is not reached during the abbreviated expiratory phase, **dynamic hyperinflation (DH)** results or is aggravated. DH is the presence of end-expiratory lung volume above the passive FRC; in this case alveolar pressure can remain positive throughout expiration because of the respiratory system's persistent inward elastic recoil pressure (PEEPi). Healthy subjects evoke compensatory responses by recruiting the expiratory muscles and prolonging neural expiratory time (T_{EN}) to enhance expiratory flow and lungs emptying. Younes et al[22] demonstrated that in patients with acute respiratory failure these compensatory responses are weak despite their ability to prolong T_{EN} with increasing V_T or pressure,[21] and therefore extending ventilator inflation into T_{EN} tends to exacerbate DH.

Increasing ventilator $\dot{V}$ elicits excitatory effects in both healthy subjects[23,23] and patients with acute respiratory failure[21,24] in the form of increased respiratory rate and an association with decreased *Pmus*.[20] However, during mechanical ventilation the imposed T_{IM} (for example, by increasing pause time) can determine respiratory rate independent of delivered $\dot{V}$ and V_T.[22] The increased respiratory rate with increasing $\dot{V}$ is accomplished by shortening of T_{IN}.[25] In healthy subjects, the shortening of T_{IN} is associated with shortening of T_{EN}. However, in patients with chronic obstructive pulmonary disease (COPD), these responses differ.[18] Increased ventilator $\dot{V}$ caused shortening of T_{IM}, increased respiratory rate, and tachypnea, yet the time available for exhalation was slightly prolonged, with small decreases in PEEPi. The neural pathway mediating this excitatory effect is unclear, but probably is vagally mediated.

Behavioral Feedback

Behavioral feedback is the respiratory controller response to patient anxiety, fear, or pain as a result of environmental stressors or ventilator settings, and manifests as breathing discomfort, air hunger, or dyspnea. In mechanically ventilated patients, a 30-minute session of listening to classical music (or music of the patient's preference) significantly decreased anxiety, heart rate, blood pressure, and respiratory rate, promoting patient comfort.[26]

Ventilator settings can either induce or alleviate the sensation of discomfort. In healthy subjects breathing on ACV, dyspnea develops when the ventilator $\dot{V}$ is set either lower or higher than that of spontaneous breathing.[27] Manning et al[28] demonstrated an inverse relation between V_T and the sensation of air hunger for a constant $P_{ET}CO_2$ in patients with a high spinal cord injury. Similarly, in patients with COPD, a high PSV level may cause ventilator inflation to encroach into T_{EN}, exacerbating DH and inducing dyspnea.[29] During sleep or sedation, behavioral factors are absent; hence, ventilator settings that appear satisfactory under those conditions may be inadequate during wakefulness or when sedation is discontinued.

Ventilator-Related Factors

Ventilator-related factors include three variables: (1) the **trigger variable** to initiate gas delivery; (2) the variable to control gas delivery throughout inspiration; and (3) the cycle-off variable to terminate gas delivery and allow exhalation.

Trigger Variable

The ventilator can be triggered by a change in pressure, flow, volume, or flow waveform.[7] **Pressure triggering** requires patient effort, with the demand valve closed, to decrease pressure in the ventilator circuit to a preset value; whereas **flow or volume triggering** requires patient effort, with the demand valve partially opened, to produce a preset flow or volume for the ventilator to deliver fresh gas flow. It is generally believed that the work of breathing is less with flow than with pressure triggering; however, differences in patient total effort are small and of questionable clinical significance.

The **flow-waveform triggering** combines the volume and shape-signal methods. The flow-waveform method requires patient effort to generate flow until 6 ml of volume accumulates above the baseline flow (volume method), or when patient effort distorts the expiratory flow waveform to a certain extent, whichever occurs first (shape-signal method).[30] The latter is based on the generation of a new flow signal by offsetting the signal from the actual flow by 0.25 L/sec and delaying it for 300 msec. The intentional delay causes the flow shape-signal to be slightly behind the patient's flow rate. As the patient generates an inspiratory effort, the sudden decrease in expiratory flow crosses the flow shape-signal, creating a signal to trigger the ventilator. Likewise, the flow shape-signal can be used to cycle off the ventilator. Compared with flow triggering, flow-waveform triggering is more sensitive to patient effort, resulting in fewer ineffective efforts but more auto-triggerings.[30] Using a lung model with controlled DH and inspiratory effort, the simulated patient effort to trigger the ventilator is ~50% less with the flow-waveform method than with flow triggering.[30] Hence, compared with flow triggering, flow-waveform triggering improves trigger synchrony and requires less effort for triggering, but because of the improved sensitivity, is susceptible to auto-triggering.

With ventilator triggering, patient-ventilator dyssynchrony can manifest as auto-triggering or ineffective triggering.[31] **Auto-triggering** is automatic delivery of mechanical breaths without inspiratory efforts. A highly sensitive triggering system increases the risk of auto-triggering, for example, with the shape-signal method (see previous discussion). Other factors causing auto-triggering include random noise or water in the circuit, leaks, and cardiogenic oscillations. Respiratory center depression with low breathing frequency is susceptible to auto-triggering. It allows zero flow for an extended duration, making the system vulnerable to triggering from changes in airway pressure within the ventilator circuit that are not caused by patient effort (Figure 8-3).

The converse of auto-triggering is **ineffective triggering**, in which the ventilator is insensitive to patient effort. Ineffective triggering occurs in patients

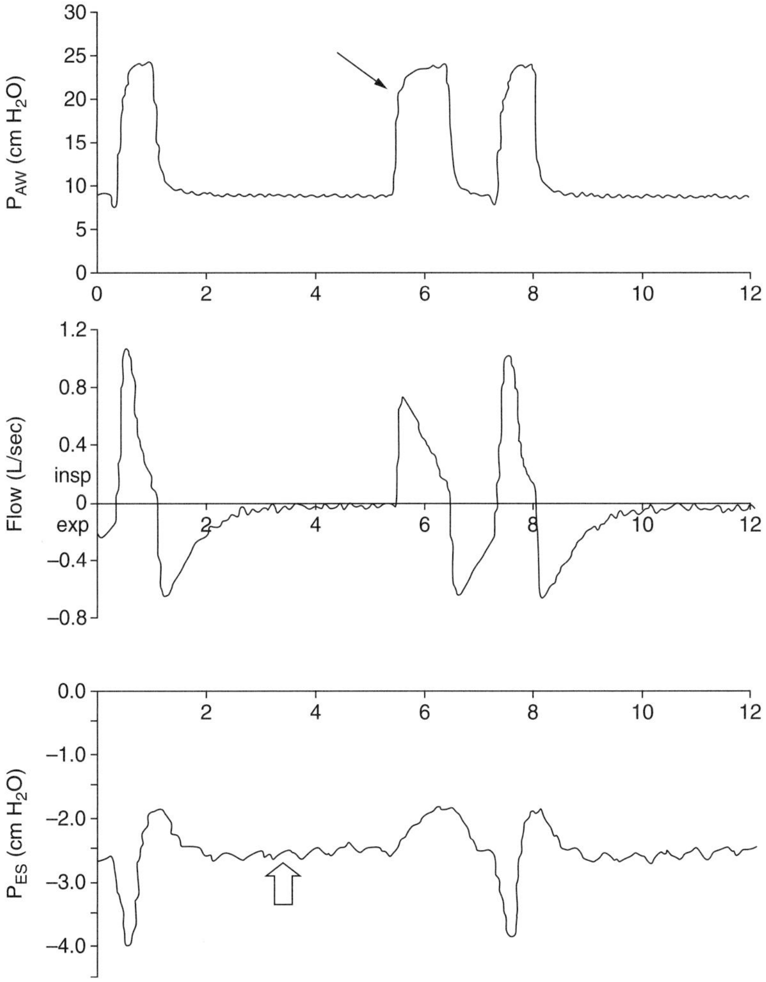

FIGURE 8-3 Auto-triggering. Airway pressure (P_{AW}), flow, and esophageal pressure (P_{ES}) in a patient on pressure support ventilation. The second breath is auto-triggered *(solid arrow);* note the absence of an abrupt decrease in P_{AW} and P_{ES}. Note the flow distortion due to cardiogenic oscillations and/or secretions clearly detected on the P_{ES} waveform *(open arrow)*, and that before the auto-triggered breath the flow remains zero for some time. Insp and exp denote inspiration and expiration, respectively. (Modified from Georgopoulos D, Prinianakis G, Kondili E: Bedside waveform interpretation as a tool to identify patient-ventilator asynchronies, Intensive Care Med 32:34, 2006.)

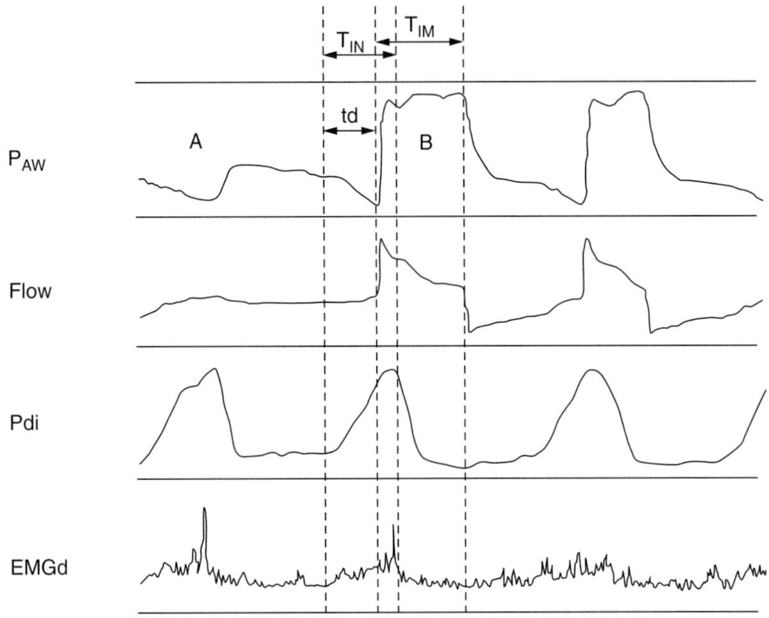

FIGURE 8-4 Trigger delay (td). Airway pressure (P_{AW}), flow, transdiaphragmatic pressure (Pdi), and diaphragmatic electrical activity in a patient with COPD and intrinsic positive end-expiratory pressure (PEEPi). Note that patient effort as reflected by Pdi is dissipated to overcome PEEPi before onset of flow delivery. The time needed to trigger the ventilator occupies the majority of neural inspiratory time (T_{IN}). Ineffective or wasted effort **(A)** precedes triggered breath **(B)**. T_{IM} is ventilator inspiratory timing. (Modified from Tassaux D, Gainnier M, Battisti A et al: Impact of expiratory trigger setting on delayed cycling and inspiratory muscle workload, Am J Respir Crit Care Med 172:1283, 2005.)

with DH and PEEPi (elastic threshold load), or low *Pmus*.[32] With DH and PEEPi, the patient must first generate a *Pmus* equivalent to PEEPi to be able to decrease alveolar pressure below the applied PEEP (PEEPe) to trigger the ventilator. The time for *Pmus* to overcome PEEPi results in triggering delay (Figure 8-4). Triggering can be completely ineffective when the PEEPi is too high or *Pmus* is too low because of respiratory muscle weakness, or the neural drive is decreased as a result of high ventilatory assistance (Figure 8-5).[8,32] Changes in ventilator settings may improve the frequency of ineffective triggering. With PSV, the frequency of ineffective trigger efforts decreases when PEEPe is set at 75% of the PEEPi (measured under static conditions).[33] With ACV at a constant V_T, by increasing ventilator inspiratory flow, the time for exhalation increases as T_{IM} decreases, resulting in decreased DH and PEEPi, and improved effective triggering (Figure 8-6).[8]

Variable Controlling Gas Delivery

The variable controlling gas delivery during inspiration consists of volume, flow, or pressure. With ACV, the variable controlling gas delivery is flow, and when the preset volume is reached, the ventilator cycles off **(volume-cycling).** The inflation time depends on the preset flow and volume. At a constant volume, increasing flow increases the ventilatory assistance, and therefore decreases *Pmus* and is associated with decreased T_{IM} (see previous discussion). As patient effort increases, the increased *Pmus* results in a decrease in airway pressure (P_{AW}) over time and is shown as distorted P_{AW} waveform (Figure 8-7). Thus there is an inverse relationship between P_{AW} and *Pmus*. With pressure assist-control ventilation (PACV) or PSV, the variable controlling gas delivery is pressure. In some ventilators, the clinician can adjust the initial pressure increase rate to meet patient flow demand.[34] Because pressure is set constant, changes in *Pmus* do not result in changes in P_{AW} (see Figure 8-7); hence, there is no relationship between P_{AW} and *Pmus*. Inflation time depends on a preset inspiratory time for PACV and on flow inputs from both patient and ventilator for PSV (flow-cycled). With PAV as with PSV, the variable controlling gas delivery is pressure; however, the pressure delivered is

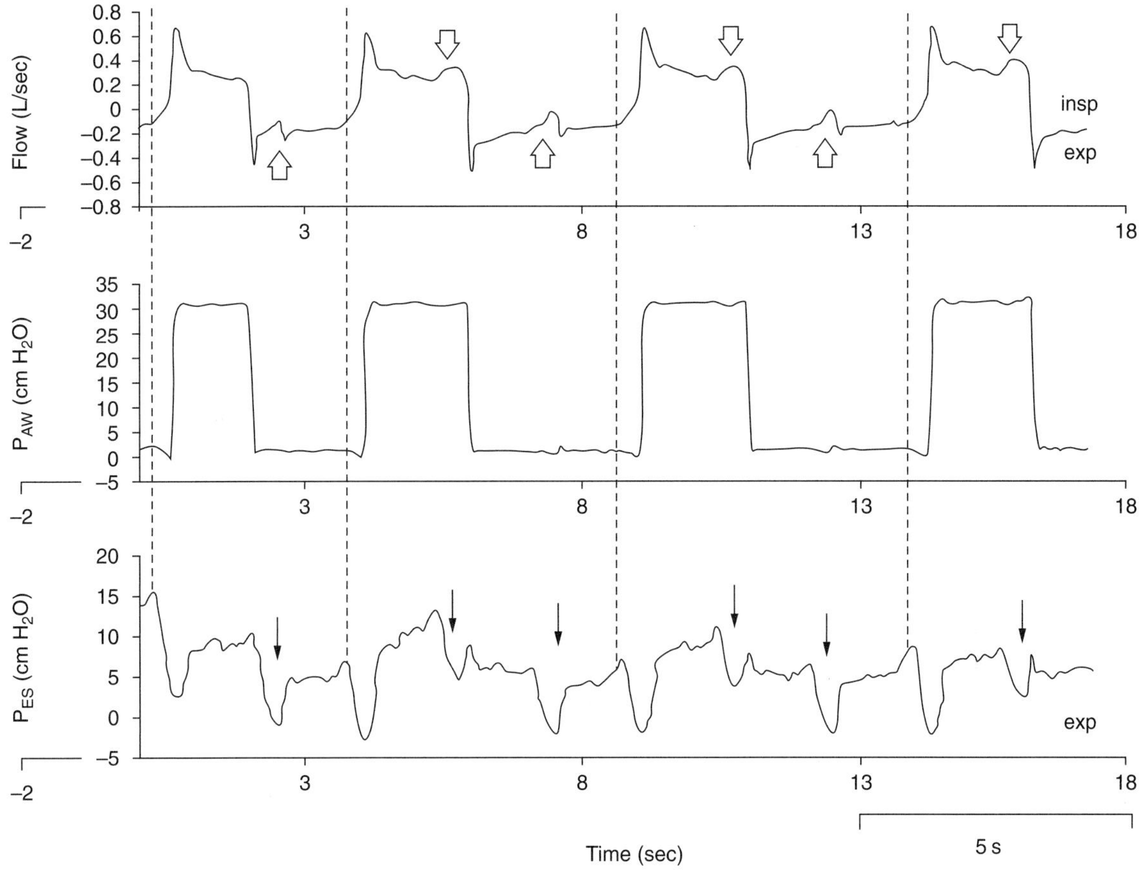

FIGURE 8-5 Ineffective or wasted efforts. Flow, airway pressure (P_{AW}), and esophageal pressure (P_{ES}) waveforms of a patient with severe COPD on pressure support ventilation. Dotted vertical lines indicate the beginning of inspiratory efforts that triggered the ventilator. Closed arrows indicate ineffective efforts. These ineffective efforts may be identified easily on the flow tracing *(open arrows)*. Note that ineffective efforts occurred during both mechanical inspiration and expiration. Ineffective efforts during mechanical inspiration result in an abrupt increase in inspiratory flow, whereas during mechanical expiration they result in an abrupt decrease in expiratory flow *(open arrows)*. The ventilator frequency is 12 breaths/min, and that of the patient is 33 inspiratory efforts/min. Insp and exp denote inspiration and expiration, respectively. (Modified from Kondili E, Prinianakis G, Georgopoulos D: Patient-ventilator interaction, Br J Anaesth 91:106, 2003.)

proportional to patient-derived flow (flow-assist) and volume (volume-assist). As patient effort or *Pmus* increases, P_{AW} increases proportionately (see Figure 8-7). With PAV, the patient has control of ventilator inflation time. Modern ventilators have the capability to combine the variables controlling gas delivery, called hybrid or dual control modes.[35] MacIntyre et al[36] demonstrated that ACV coupled with the pressure-limited breath feature (pressure augmentation) to some extent improves the patient-ventilator dyssynchrony observed with ACV alone (Figure 8-8). This is because the initial high flow delivery of the pressure-limited breath meets the patient's early ventilatory demand while maintaining a constant V_T, a feature of ACV.

As with ACV, the variable controlling gas delivery with **synchronous intermittent mandatory ventilation (SIMV)** can be either flow (volume-cycled) or pressure **(time-cycling).** With SIMV, ventilator breaths are interspersed among spontaneous breaths. Down-regulation of inspiratory muscle activity during the ventilator breath does not occur at low-to-medium assistance level.[37] For ventilatory support of patients in acute respiratory failure, SIMV is

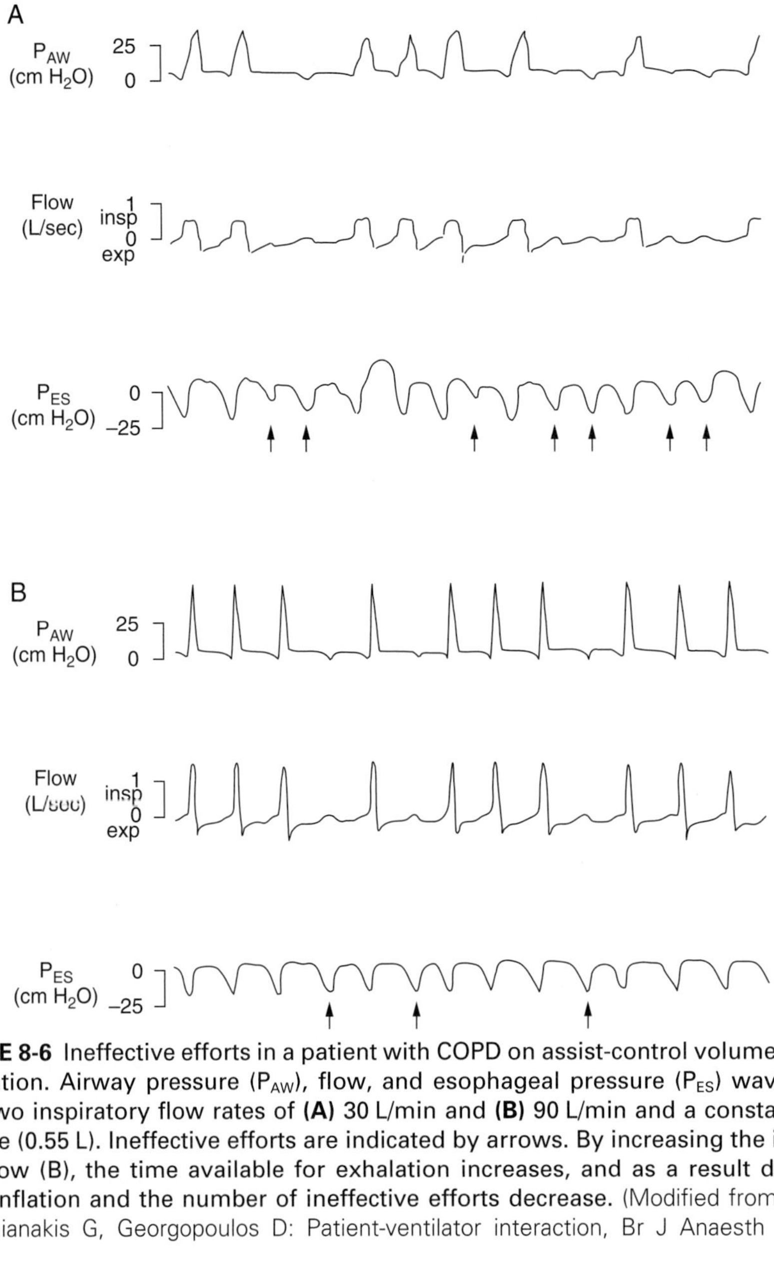

FIGURE 8-6 Ineffective efforts in a patient with COPD on assist-control volume-cycled ventilation. Airway pressure (P_{AW}), flow, and esophageal pressure (P_{ES}) waveforms with two inspiratory flow rates of **(A)** 30 L/min and **(B)** 90 L/min and a constant tidal volume (0.55 L). Ineffective efforts are indicated by arrows. By increasing the inspiratory flow (B), the time available for exhalation increases, and as a result dynamic hyperinflation and the number of ineffective efforts decrease. (Modified from Kondili E, Prinianakis G, Georgopoulos D: Patient-ventilator interaction, Br J Anaesth 91:106, 2003.)

commonly combined with PSV.[1] When used alone, a decrease in the number of ventilator breaths produced a decrease in the average V_T of the intervening spontaneous breaths, with an inevitable increase in the dead space–to–tidal volume ratio.[32] To avoid a decrease in alveolar ventilation, patient neural drive, inspiratory effort, and frequency increased. Adding pressure support (PS) of 10 cm H_2O decreased effort at any given SIMV rate. The decrease in effort during the ventilator breaths was related to the decrease in neural drive during the intervening spontaneous breaths. Thus the reduction in drive during the intervening breaths achieved by adding PS was carried over to the ventilator breaths, facilitating greater unloading with PSV.[32] As a weaning modality, SIMV is less advantageous than PSV, but whether the reason is related to differences in muscle unloading remains to be determined. From 0 to 60% of maximum assistance, the decrease in pressure-time product per minute (PTP/min) was greater with PSV than with SIMV. PTP/min reflects patient's effort and an indirect estimate of the respiratory muscles' metabolic

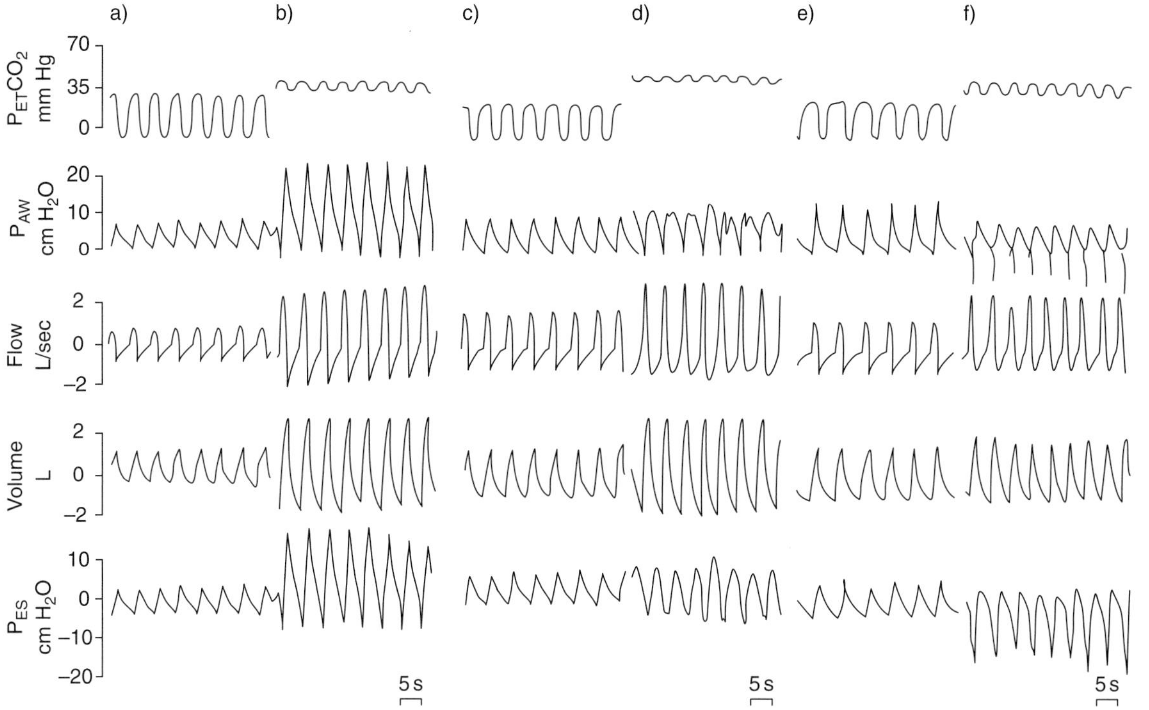

FIGURE 8-7 The different response of airway pressure (P_{AW}) without and with CO_2 stimulation among the three ventilation modes in a healthy subject breathing on proportional assist ventilation (**A** and **B**, respectively), pressure support ventilation (**C** and **D**), and assist-control volume-cycled ventilation (**E** and **F**). End tidal PCO_2 ($P_{ET}CO_2$); airway pressure (P_{AW}); and flow, volume, and esophageal pressure (P_{ES}) waveforms are shown. (Modified from Mitrouska J, Xirouchaki N, Patakas D et al: Effects of chemical feedback on respiratory motor and ventilatory output during different modes of assisted mechanical ventilation, Eur Respir J 13:873, 1999.)

rate. At higher assistance level, the converse was observed (Figure 8-9). Frequency decreased linearly with an increase in PSV. With SIMV, frequency changed little until a high assistance level was provided (see Figure 8-9). Thus, when a high assistance level is needed, both SIMV and PSV provide comparable assistance. At low to medium assistance levels, PSV provides a greater decrease in patient effort, making it more clinically useful than SIMV.

Cycling-off Variable

The ideal cycling off or flow termination of the ventilator, also known as the expiratory trigger (ETr), should coincide with the end of patient T_{IN}.[38] More commonly, however, ventilator flow ceases before or after the end of T_{IN}, termed expiratory dyssynchrony. With ACV, flow and V_T are preset, and therefore T_{IM} is constant with every breath. Similarly, with assist-control pressure-limited (ACP) ventilation, T_{IM} is preset, and the patient has no influence on ventilator flow termination. With PSV, ventilator flow termination is determined by both patient and ventilator. For the same ventilator ETr sensitivity, a patient with a high time constant (high compliance and resistance, COPD) requires a longer time for the ventilator flow to cease than a patient with a normal time constant. The ventilator cycling off algorithm uses a preset criterion, either as a percentage (5%, 25%, or 30%) of peak inspiratory flow or an absolute value (i.e., when inspiratory flow decreases to 5 L/min, at which time the ventilator cycles off). Some ventilators employ a clinician-adjustable expiratory trigger as a percentage of peak inspiratory flow. Flow-waveform triggering for inspiratory trigger (see previous discussion) is also used for expiratory triggering.[20] With this method, relaxation of the inspiratory muscles and/or contraction of the expiratory muscles result in a sudden decrease in inspiratory flow that crosses the correspondingly created inspiratory flow shape-signal, causing ventilator flow termination. With PAV, the

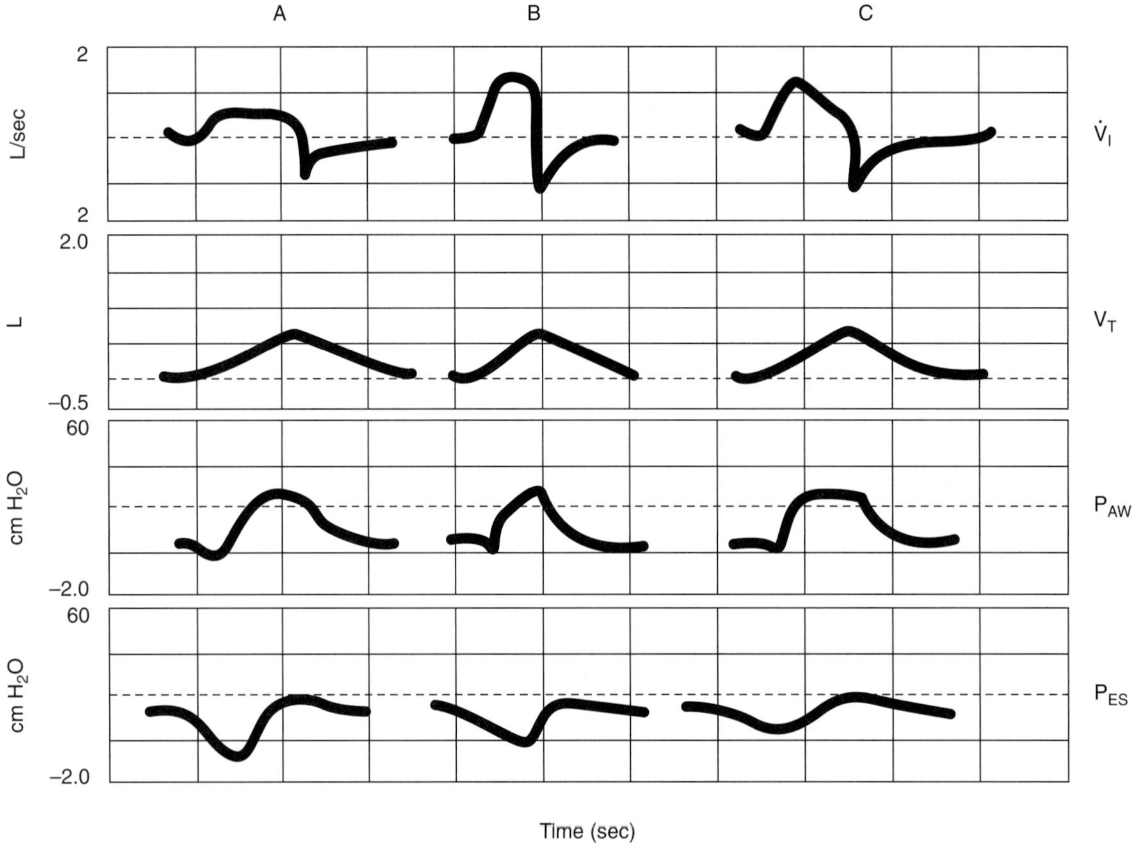

FIGURE 8-8 Ventilator flow ($\dot{V}$), tidal volume (V_T), airway pressure (P_{AW}), and esophageal pressure (P_{ES}) waveforms in a ventilated patient. The patient is receiving ventilator flow set at 30 L/min to induce flow dyssynchrony *(left panels)*. This dyssynchrony is demonstrated by a markedly negative P_{ES} tracing during inspiration. The airway pressure tracing also appears "pulled" down. When the set ventilator flow has been increased to 75 L/min, the P_{ES} tracing can be seen to improve *(middle panels)*. A pressure-targeted breath of 22 cm H_2O has been given *(right panels)*. With this approach, the dyssynchronous esophageal pressure can be seen to improve even further. (From MacIntyre NR, McConnell R, Cheng KG et al: Patient-ventilator flow dys-synchrony: Flow limited versus pressure limited breaths, Crit Care Med 25:1671, 1997.)

patient has control over ETr, and theoretically ETr should coincide with the end of T_{IN}. However, all ventilator modes are not exempt from expiratory dyssynchrony.[7,38] The cause of expiratory dyssynchrony in PAV is attributed to a delay between ventilator control system input and output, and an overestimation of patient respiratory system mechanics.[38,39] Expiratory dyssynchrony increases both the inspiratory and expiratory work of breathing, and a delay in ventilator triggering.

Expiratory dyssynchrony may occur as premature or delayed termination of ventilator flow relative to the end of T_{IN}. When ventilator flow ceases prematurely, the inspiratory muscles continue to contract into the ventilator exhalation phase (T_{EM}). The *Pmus* generated may be dissipated to overcome the elastic recoil, which causes airway pressure to decrease below PEEP and triggers the ventilator, causing double triggering[31] (Figure 8-10) and increased inspiratory muscle work. When ventilator flow termination is delayed relative to the end of T_{IN}, ventilator inflation continues into T_{EN}, and expiratory muscle recruitment occurs in an attempt to terminate inspiration, increases expiratory muscle work, and manifests as the patient "fighting" the ventilator, which may dictate the use of sedation. In patients with COPD, the continued ventilator inflation into T_{EN} exacerbates DH because of the limited exhalation time and, consequently,

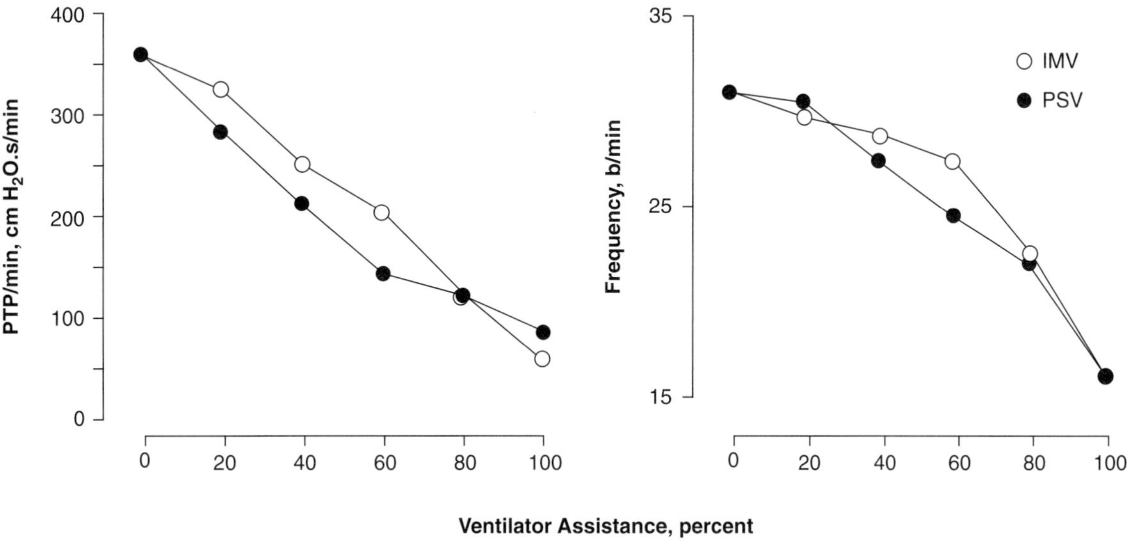

FIGURE 8-9 Changes in pressure-time product per minute (PTP/min) *(left panel)* and frequency *(right panel)* as intermittent mandatory ventilation (IMV) and pressure-support ventilation (PSV) were progressively increased. A PSV of 100% represents the level necessary to achieve a V_T equivalent to that during assist-control volume-cycled ventilation (10 ml/kg); 100% IMV, the same ventilator rate and V_T as during assist-control volume-cycled ventilation. (Modified from Leung P, Jubran A, Tobin MJ: Comparison of assisted ventilator modes on triggering, patients' effort, and dyspnea, Am J Respir Crit Care Med 155:1940, 1997 and Tobin MJ, Jubran A, Laghi F: Patient-ventilator interaction, Am J Respir Crit Care Med 163:1059, 2001.)

increases ineffective trigger efforts. In these patients, when expiratory trigger was set equal or greater than 50% of peak flow, expiratory dyssynchrony improved; PEEPi, frequency of ineffective triggering, and patient effort to trigger the ventilator decreased compared with the low percentage of peak flow.[40] Recently, automated expiratory trigger sensitivity has been described.[41] It is based on a closed-loop control system in which the controller automatically adjusts ETr based on the measured respiratory time constant and supra-plateau pressure of the previous breaths. Supra-plateau pressure is the pressure above the set target pressure level at the end of inspiration. The higher the time constant or the supra-plateau pressure, the higher the ETr sensitivity the ventilator controller selects for the upcoming breath. Automated ETr has yet to be compared with preset ETr in patients with various underlying diseases.

THE FUTURE

Conventional modes of mechanical ventilation are constrained by the need to adapt to instantaneous changes in patient ventilatory demand and respiratory timing. Improvements in inspiratory triggering,[20] flow delivery,[35] and expiratory triggering[38,41] have been developed in modern ventilators based on a closed-loop feedback system using respiratory mechanics as the feedback signal (Table 8-1). Some of these systems or ventilator modes are available for clinical application, and some have not undergone rigorous clinical trials in comparison with conventional systems or ventilator modes; hence, their efficacy remains to be determined. The closer the system is to the patient's biologic respiratory controller, the less the system delays in responding to the patient's ventilatory demand, and the better the synchrony that is expected between the patient and ventilator. A small step toward the patient's respiratory controller is the transdiaphragmatic pressure (Pdi)-driven servoventilator, which uses a preset rise in Pdi or flow, whichever occurs first, to trigger the ventilator while pressurization is provided proportional to the change in Pdi from the baseline.[42] The ventilator cycles off according to a preset flow threshold. Moving closer to the biologic respiratory controller is the neurally adjusted ventilatory assist (NAVA), in which diaphragmatic electrical activity (EMGd) is

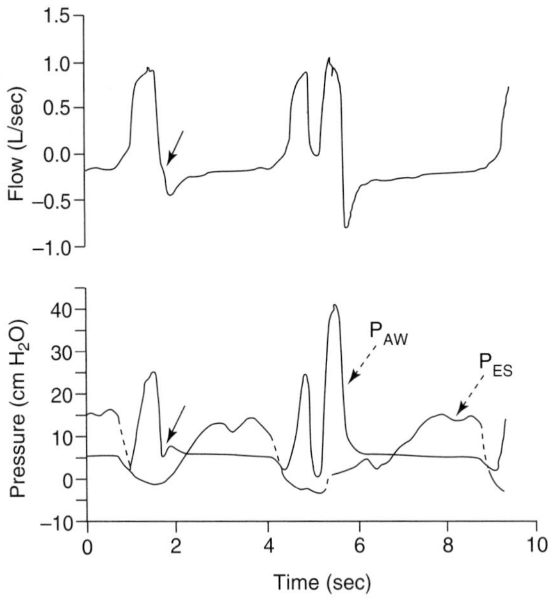

FIGURE 8-10 Double triggering. Flow, airway pressure (P_{AW}), and esophageal (P_{ES}) pressure waveforms in a patient on assist-control volume-cycled ventilation. In the first breath, the retardation of early expiratory flow and the distortion of P_{AW} after opening the exhalation valve *(solid arrows)* are signs that mechanical ventilation has been terminated prematurely. This is clearly shown in the second breath, in which tidal volume (volume was not shown) is decreased at the same inspiratory flow. As a result, mechanical inflation time is further reduced, exaggerating the premature termination of mechanical inspiration. Because the inspiratory muscles continue to contract with the open exhalation valve, the pressure developed is adequate to overcome the elastic recoil at the end of inspiration. As a result, P_{AW} decreases below the triggering threshold, and the ventilator delivers a new mechanical breath. The ventilator is triggered three times by the two inspiratory efforts. Notice the high P_{AW} of the third mechanical breath due to high lung volume (the volume of the third breath was added to that of the second). Note also that the total breath duration of the patient's second inspiratory effort is considerably longer than that of the first because the high volume activates the Hering-Breuer reflex. (Modified from Georgopoulos D, Prinianakis G, Kondili E: Bedside waveforms interpretation as a tool to identify patient-ventilator asynchronies, Intensive Care Med 32:34, 2006.)

used to trigger the ventilator. Flow delivery is provided by means of continuous ventilatory assist in proportion to the neural drive, both within and between breaths.[43] Because the ventilator is triggered directly by the diaphragm's electrical activity, the synchrony between T_{IN} and T_{IM} is guaranteed at both the onset and end of inspiration. With both the Pdi-driven ventilator and NAVA, ventilator triggering is independent of respiratory mechanics, PEEPi, and leaks; however, because the gain factor for intrabreath assist is fixed, to receive more support within a given breath, the patient must increase Pdi or EMGd. Unlike NAVA, targeted-neural drive pressure support is based on closed-loop ventilation, in which a target EMGd is the feedback signal for adjusting the pressure support level.[44] EMGd activity or flow triggering is used to trigger the ventilator, whichever occurs first. The ventilator cycling off takes place when the EMGd activity drops to 80% of the peak activity for a given breath. The above described modes probably improve patient-ventilator interactions; however, clinical application may be hampered by the relatively invasive procedure of catheter insertions to measure Pdi and EMGd and the signals' possible long-term instability. Currently, all of the above ventilation modes remain investigational tools.

TABLE 8-1 *Triggering Methods and Ventilator Modes to Improve Patient-Ventilator Synchrony Based on Closed-Loop System With Respiratory Mechanics As Feedback Signal*

TRIGGERING METHODS AND VENTILATOR MODES	FEEDBACK SIGNAL
INSPIRATORY TRIGGERING	
Flow-waveform triggering (shape-signal method)	Flow
FLOW DELIVERY	
Proportional assist ventilation (PAV)	Patient's effort
Adaptive support ventilation (ASV)	Volume and respiratory frequency
Automatic tube compensation (ATC)	Resistance of endotracheal tube
Dual control breath-to-breath: pressure-regulated volume control or autoflow	Delivered volume
Dual control within breath: volume assured pressure support (VAPS) or pressure augmentation (PA)	Delivered volume
Volume support (VS) and variable pressure support (VPS)	Delivered volume
Pressure support controlled by airway occlusion pressure	Occlusion pressure measured in 0.1 sec and alveolar ventilation
Automode (volume support/pressure regulated volume control or variable pressure support/ variable pressure control)	Patient's effort
EXPIRATORY TRIGGERING	
Automated expiratory trigger	Respiratory system time constant and supra-plateau pressure

KEY POINTS

- At a high-assist level with ACV or PSV, the respiratory controller is insensitive to low $PaCO_2$; hence despite hypocapnia the subject continues to trigger the ventilator.
- Extending the ventilator inflation into the patient's or neural expiratory time, by increasing tidal volume or pressure, tends to exacerbate dynamic hyperinflation.
- Increasing ventilator flow rate exhibits excitatory effects in the form of increased respiratory rate.
- Flow-waveform triggering improves trigger sensitivity and synchrony, but is susceptible to auto-triggering.
- Frequency of ineffective trigger efforts improves when PEEP equal to 75% of PEEPi, measured under static conditions, is applied, or when inspiratory flow rate is increased.
- With ACV, P_{AW} is inversely related to *Pmus*; with PSV, P_{AW} is unrelated to *Pmus*; with PAV, P_{AW} is proportionate to *Pmus*.
- In patients with COPD and dynamic hyperinflation, high expiratory trigger sensitivity improves expiratory dyssynchrony.
- To improve patient-ventilator interactions, novel modes of ventilation employ closed-loop systems using Pdi or EMGd as a feedback signal.

ASSESSMENT QUESTIONS

1. What are the ramifications of sedating a patient who appears to be "fighting" the mechanical ventilator?
2. What are the three feedback signals to the patient's biologic respiratory controller that can affect the respiratory muscles' pressure (*Pmus*) generation during mechanical ventilation?
3. What is the meaning of the respiratory central controller's insensitivity to hypocapnia during ACV or PSV?
4. What effect does increasing ventilator flow rate have on a patient's respiratory rate?
5. Which method of triggering has been demonstrated to be more sensitive than flow-triggering?

Continued

ASSESSMENT QUESTIONS—cont'd

6. What is the difference between auto-triggering and ineffective triggering? What applicable methods may decrease the frequency of ineffective triggering?
7. What is the relationship between airway pressure (P_{AW}) and respiratory muscle pressure *(Pmus)* in ACV, PSV, and PAV?
8. What is meant by expiratory dyssynchrony, and what are the consequences?
9. In patients with COPD, what level of expiratory trigger sensitivity can potentially decrease PEEPi and frequency of ineffective triggering?
10. What are the feedback signals employed in NAVA, transdiaphragmatic pressure-driven servo-ventilator, and targeted-neural drive pressure support?

CASE STUDIES

For additional practice, refer to Case Studies 5, 6, 9, and 13 in the appendix at the back of this book.

REFERENCES

1. Esteban A, Anzueto A, Alia I et al: How is mechanical ventilation employed in the intensive care unit? An international utilization review, Am J Respir Crit Care Med 161:1450-1458, 2000.
2. Tobin MJ: Advances in mechanical ventilation, N Engl J Med 344:1986-1996, 2001.
3. Arroliga A, Frutos-Vivar F, Hall J et al: International Mechanical Ventilation Study Group. Use of sedatives and neuromuscular blockers in a cohort of patients receiving mechanical ventilation, Chest 128:496-506, 2005.
4. Kress JP, Pohlman AS, O'Connor MF et al: Daily interruption of sedative infusions in critically ill patients undergoing mechanical ventilation, N Engl J Med 342:1471-1477, 2000.
5. Ramar K, Sassoon CSH: Potential advantages of patient-ventilator synchrony, Respir Care Clin N Am 11:307-317, 2005.
6. Corne S, Bshouty Z: Basic principles of control of breathing, Respir Care Clin N Am 11:147-172, 2005.
7. Prinianakis G, Kondili E, Georgopoulos D: Patient-ventilator interaction: An overview, Respir Care Clin N Am 11:201-224, 2005.
8. Kondili E, Prinianakis G, Georgopoulos D: Patient-ventilator interaction, Br J Anaesth 91:106-119, 2003.
9. Meza S, Giannouli E, Younes M: Control of breathing during sleep assessed by proportional assist ventilation, J Appl Physiol 84:3-12, 1998.
10. Mitrouska J, Xirouchaki N, Patakas D et al: Effects of chemical feedback on respiratory motor and ventilatory output during different modes of assisted mechanical ventilation, Eur Respir J 13:873-882, 1999.
11. Ranieri VM, Giuliani R, Mascia L et al: Patient-ventilator interaction during acute hypercapnia: pressure-support vs. proportional-assist ventilation, J Appl Physiol 81:426-436, 1996.
12. Grasso S, Puntillo F, Mascia L et al: Compensation for increase in respiratory workload during mechanical ventilation. Pressure-support versus proportional-assist ventilation, Am J Respir Crit Care Med 161:819-826, 2000.
13. Skatrud JB, Dempsey JA: Interaction of sleep state and chemical stimuli in sustaining rhythmic ventilation, J Appl Physiol 55:813-822, 1983.
14. Dempsey JA, Skatrud JB: A sleep-induced apneic threshold and its consequences, Am Rev Respir Dis 133:1163-1170, 1986.
15. Meza S, Mendez M, Ostrowski M et al: Susceptibility to periodic breathing with assisted ventilation during sleep in normal subjects, J Appl Physiol 85:1929-1940, 1998.
16. Georgopoulos D, Mitrouska I, Bshouty Z et al: Effects of non-REM sleep on the response of respiratory output to varying inspiratory flow, Am J Respir Crit Care Med 153:1624-1630, 1996.
17. Puddy A, Patrick W, Webster K et al: Respiratory control during volume-cycled ventilation in normal humans, J Appl Physiol 80:1749-1758, 1996.
18. Laghi F, Segal J, Choe WK et al: Effect of imposed inflation time on respiratory frequency and hyperinflation in patients with chronic obstructive pulmonary disease, Am J Respir Crit Care Med 163:1365-1370, 2001.
19. Georgopoulos D, Mitrouska I, Webster K et al: Effects of inspiratory muscle unloading on the response of respiratory motor output to CO_2, Am J Respir Crit Care Med 155:2000-2009, 1997.
20. Younes M, Kun J, Webster K et al: Response of ventilator-dependent patients to delayed opening of exhalation valve, Am J Respir Crit Care Med 166:21-30, 2002.
21. Kondili E, Prinianakis G, Anastasaki M et al: Acute effects of ventilator settings on respiratory motor output in patients with acute lung injury, Intensive Care Med 27:1147-1157, 2001.
22. Laghi F, Karamchandani K, Tobin MJ: Influence of ventilator settings in determining respiratory frequency

during mechanical ventilation, Am J Respir Crit Care Med 160:1766-1770, 1999.
23. Puddy A, Younes M: Effect of inspiratory flow rate on respiratory output in normal subjects, Am Rev Respir Dis 146:787-789, 1992.
24. Corne S, Gillespie D, Roberts D et al: Effect of inspiratory flow rate on respiratory rate in intubated ventilated patients, Am J Respir Crit Care Med 156:304-308, 1997.
25. Fernandez R, Mendez M, Younes M: Effect of ventilator flow rate on respiratory timing in normal humans, Am J Respir Crit Care Med 159:710-719, 1999.
26. Lee OK, Chung YF, Chan MF et al: Music and its effect on the physiological responses and anxiety levels of patients receiving mechanical ventilation: A pilot study, J Clin Nurs 14:609-620, 2005.
27. Manning HL, Molinary EJ, Leiter JC: Effect of inspiratory flow rate on respiratory sensation and pattern of breathing, Am J Respir Crit Care Med 151:751-757, 1995.
28. Manning HL, Shea SA, Schwartzstein RM et al: Reduced tidal volume increases "air hunger" at fixed PCO_2 in ventilated quadriplegics, Respir Physiol 90:19-30, 1992.
29. Jubran A, Van de Graaff WB, Tobin MJ: Variability of patient-ventilator interaction with pressure support ventilation in patients with chronic obstructive pulmonary disease, Am J Respir Crit Care Med 152:129-136, 1995.
30. Prinianakis G, Kondili E, Georgopoulos D: Effects of the flow waveform method of triggering and cycling on patient-ventilator interaction during pressure support, Intensive Care Med 29:1950-1959, 2003.
31. Georgopoulos D, Prinianakis G, Kondili E: Bedside waveform interpretation as a tool to identify patient-ventilator asynchronies, Intensive Care Med 32:34-47, 2006.
32. Leung P, Jubran A, Tobin MJ: Comparison of assisted ventilator modes on triggering, patients' effort, and dyspnea, Am J Respir Crit Care Med 155:1940-1948, 1997.
33. Nava S, Bruschi C, Rubini F, Palo A et al: Respiratory response and inspiratory effort during pressure support ventilation in COPD patients, Intensive Care Med 21:871-879, 1995.
34. Chiumello D, Pelosi P, Taccone P et al: Effect of different inspiratory rise time and cycling off criteria during pressure support ventilation in patients recovering from acute lung injury, Crit Care Med 31:2604-2610, 2003.
35. Branson RD, Johannigman JA, Campbell RS et al: Closed-loop mechanical ventilation, Respir Care 47:427-451, 2002.
36. MacIntyre NR, McConnell R, Cheng KG et al: Patient-ventilator flow dyssynchrony: Flow limited versus pressure limited breaths, Crit Care Med 25:1671-1677, 1997.
37. Imsand C, Feihl F, Perret C et al: Regulation of inspiratory neuromuscular output during synchronized intermittent mechanical ventilation, Anesthesiology 80:13-22, 1994.
38. Du HL, Yamada Y: Expiratory asynchrony, Respir Care Clin N Am 11:265-280, 2005.
39. Du HL, Ohtsuji M, Shigeta M et al: Expiratory asynchrony in proportional assist ventilation, Am J Respir Crit Care Med 165:972-977, 2002.
40. Tassaux D, Gainnier M, Battisti A et al: Impact of expiratory trigger setting on delayed cycling and inspiratory muscle workload, Am J Respir Crit Care Med 172:1283-1289, 2005.
41. Yamada Y, Du HL: Analysis of the mechanisms of expiratory asynchrony in pressure support ventilation: A mathematical approach, J Appl Physiol 88:2143-2150, 2000.
42. Sharshar T, Desmarais G, Louis B et al: Transdiaphragmatic pressure control of airway pressure support in healthy subjects, Am J Respir Crit Care Med 168:760-769, 2003.
43. Sinderby C, Navalesi P, Beck J et al: Neural control of mechanical ventilation in respiratory failure, Nat Med 5:1433-1436, 1999.
44. Spahija J, Beck J, de Marchie M et al: Closed-loop control of respiratory drive using pressure-support ventilation: Target drive ventilation, Am J Respir Crit Care Med 171:1009-1014, 2005.

CHAPTER

9 Cardiopulmonary Interactions

David N. Hager; Henry E. Fessler

OUTLINE

MECHANICAL FORCES DURING VENTILATION
- Venous Return
- Ventricular Interdependence
- Pulmonary Vascular Resistance
- Pulmonary Vascular Capacitance
- Ventricular Afterload
- Stress on Abdominal Vessels

CLINICAL APPLICATIONS: TRANSIENT EFFECTS
- Valsalva Maneuver
- Respiratory Changes in Pulse Pressure

CLINICAL APPLICATIONS: STEADY-STATE EFFECTS
- PEEP
- Weaning

OBJECTIVES

- Describe the fundamental mechanical forces acting on circulation during mechanical ventilation.
- Explain how these forces affect determinants of preload and afterload of the right and left ventricle.
- Infer cardiovascular function or volume status in patients by observation of the circulatory response.
- State the cardiovascular consequences of PEEP and weaning.

KEY TERMS

afterload
pleural pressure
positive pressure ventilation (PPV)
preload
pulmonary artery wedge pressure (PAWP)
pulmonary vascular resistance (PVR)
pulse pressure
pulsus paradoxus
stroke volume
Valsalva maneuver
venous return

Because the heart is surrounded by pleural pressure and pumps its entire output through the lungs, the mechanics of ventilation and circulation are intimately related. When either system is diseased, the normally subtle effects of this relationship can be exaggerated. Informed observation of the effects of ventilation on the circulation can provide insight into the status of both systems and into underlying diagnoses. This chapter will discuss (1) the basic mechanical forces during ventilation, (2) how these forces interact with the circulation during spontaneous and **positive pressure ventilation** (spontaneous ventilation [SV] and **PPV**), (3) examples of what the transient circulatory response to ventilation reveals about cardiovascular function, and (4) examples of the mechanisms behind the steady-state responses to positive end-expiratory pressure (PEEP) or weaning.

For simplicity, we will consider PPV only as represented by controlled ventilation in a relaxed patient. Modes in which inspiratory effort triggers a positive pressure breath or that alternate machine and spontaneous breaths add complexity, but do not alter the underlying mechanisms we describe.

MECHANICAL FORCES DURING VENTILATION

Ventilation changes only two fundamental mechanical factors: pressure and lung volume. For effects on the heart, the most important pressure is pleural pressure. In the transition from SV to PPV, pleural pressure goes from being negative to positive during inspiration. The tidal volume and the pleural pressure at end-expiration might be, but need not be, identical during SV and PPV. Other interventions, such as use of PEEP or continuous positive airway pressure (CPAP), will increase mean lung volume and mean pleural pressure.

Pleural pressure and lung volume vary continuously during the respiratory cycle, and these changes engender cyclic, transient responses in the circulatory system. In addition, steady-state changes in mean pleural pressure and lung volume, as occur when transitioning from SV to PPV or with the addition of PEEP, cause steady-state circulatory responses. We will consider in greater detail how these fundamental mechanical factors impact the circulatory system. Although our focus will be on mechanical forces, it should be remembered that these forces are modified in complex ways by vascular reflexes and humoral responses, which remain incompletely characterized.

Venous Return

Because the heart cannot pump out more blood than it receives, **venous return** is a primary determinant of cardiac output. Venous return is driven by a pressure gradient, the downstream end of which is right atrial pressure (Pra). The functional upstream pressure for venous return has been called the mean circulatory filling pressure or mean systemic pressure (Pms). This conceptual pressure is the weighted average of all pressures throughout all parts of the systemic circulation. In experimental models, it equals the vascular pressure measured during transient asystole or ventricular fibrillation.[1,2] The elastic properties of blood vessels and the volume of blood they contain determine the magnitude of Pms. In normal humans and many animal species, Pms is relatively low (about 7 mm Hg).[1-4] Therefore, the entire cardiac output is returned to the heart by a very small pressure gradient, indicating a very low resistance in the venous system. An increase in Pms, or decrease in Pra, will increase venous return. Conversely, a reduction in Pms or increase in Pra decreases venous return[5,6] (Figure 9-1). As will be seen, ventilation can change both Pms and Pra. Because the total pressure gradient driving flow is so small, even relatively small changes in Pms and Pra can have substantial effects on venous return.

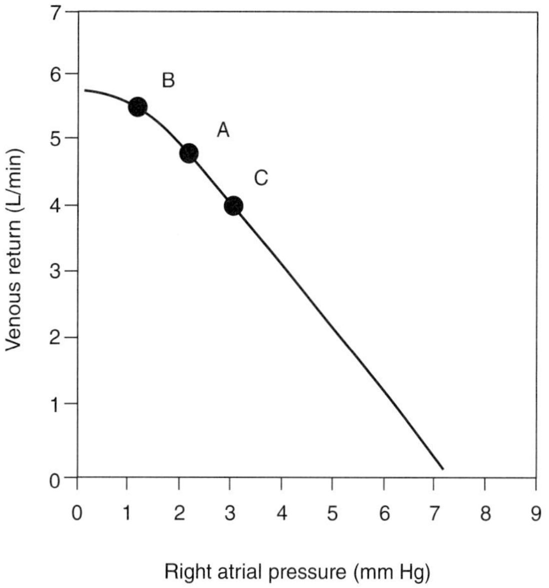

FIGURE 9-1 The relationship between right atrial pressure and venous return. Right atrial pressure is the downstream pressure against which venous return flows back to the heart. Under relaxed normal conditions, right atrial pressure is about 2 mm Hg and venous return about 5 L/min *(Point A)*. Spontaneous inspiration lowers right atrial pressure and transiently increases venous return *(Point B)*. Positive pressure inspiration raises atrial pressure and thereby decreases venous return *(Point C)*. Note also that the zero-flow intercept is about 7 mm Hg. At that right atrial pressure, there is no venous return (for a moment until vascular reflexes are activated). Since there is no flow, there must be no gradient for flow, indicating that Pms is 7 mm Hg. Finally, note that the slope of this relationship is quite steep. Small changes in driving pressure cause large changes in flow (i.e., resistance to venous return is quite low). See references 5 and 6 for details.

Ventricular Interdependence

Because the right and left ventricles share the space of the pericardium, an increase in the size of one chamber requires a decrease in the size, shape, and function of the other. For example, an increased volume of the right ventricle during spontaneous inspiration pushes the interventricular septum to the left. This decreases left ventricular volume and makes it less compliant.[7] Left ventricular filling is impeded, and **stroke volume** may be reduced.

Pulmonary Vascular Resistance

Pulmonary vascular resistance (PVR) is a composite of the resistances of all pulmonary vessels, which are arranged both in parallel and in series. Functionally, this myriad of vessels can be divided into two categories based on the pressure that acts on their surface. *Alveolar vessels* are those vessels exposed to the pressure in the alveoli and correspond anatomically to the capillaries in the alveolar walls. *Extra-alveolar vessels* behave as if surrounded by pleural pressure. These are represented by larger vessels, which feed or drain capillaries, and vessels in the corners of alveolar junctions. These two classes of vessels respond differently to changing lung volume. As lung volume increases and alveoli expand, alveolar vessels are compressed. In contrast, the extra-alveolar vessels are pulled open. Because the alveolar vessels greatly outnumber the extra-alveolar vessels, effects on alveolar vessels usually predominate. Therefore, an increase in lung volume above functional residual capacity leads to an increase in PVR.[8]

Pulmonary Vascular Capacitance

Lung inflation also affects pulmonary blood volume, and this effect depends upon the absolute pulmonary vascular blood content and its relative distribution between alveolar and extra-alveolar vessels.[9] Recall that as the lung inflates, the alveolar vessels are compressed (decreased capacitance) and extra-alveolar vessels are pulled open (increased capacitance). If the alveolar capillaries are engorged, as occurs during hypervolemic states or congestive heart failure, inspiration causes a discharge of alveolar blood volume into the left atrium. However, if alveolar capillaries are less full, as in the case of hemorrhagic shock or dehydration, lung inflation will result in a transient decrease in pulmonary venous outflow as blood pools in the enlarged extra-alveolar vessels.

Ventricular Afterload

Right and left ventricular ejection are also affected by changes in pleural pressure or lung volume during ventilation. For the right ventricle, increased lung volume increases **afterload.** This is due to the increase in PVR as described above. It is also due to the fact that the right ventricle is surrounded by pleural pressure, while it must pump through alveolar vessels surrounded by alveolar pressure. With inspiration (either SV or PPV), alveolar pressure rises *relative to pleural pressure*, increasing the pressure gradient against which the right ventricle works.

For the left ventricle, the situation is somewhat different. The left ventricle, like the right, is surrounded by pleural pressure, but it ejects into the systemic circulation, which is unaffected by pleural pressure or lung volume. Therefore, when pleural pressure decreases, the left ventricle must generate more muscular force to eject blood from the thorax.[10] When pleural pressure rises, the converse is true. From the perspective of the ventricular muscle, increased pleural pressure (at constant arterial pressure) decreases afterload in a fashion exactly analogous to decreased arterial pressure (at constant pleural pressure).

For either ventricle, the impact of changes in afterload on ejection depends on the state of myocardial contractility. Hearts with normal function are relatively insensitive to afterload changes, whereas failing hearts can be quite sensitive.

Stress on Abdominal Vessels

A final mechanical result of ventilation that can affect the circulatory system (and is frequently overlooked) is the increase in abdominal pressure that accompanies descent of the diaphragm.[11,12] For a given tidal volume, this increase is greater during SV due to active contraction of the diaphragm, compared to PPV when the diaphragm is passively displaced. As with the pulmonary vessels, the effects of diaphragmatic descent on the capacitance vessels of the abdominal cavity depend on how full these vessels are. In a hypervolemic state, a transient bolus of blood is returned to the heart, whereas no such bolus is seen in hypovolemic states.[12]

CLINICAL APPLICATIONS: TRANSIENT EFFECTS

Valsalva Maneuver

Transient cardiopulmonary interactions due to increased pleural pressure at constant lung volume have been used to gain information about volume status and myocardial function. In a cooperative patient, pleural pressure can be increased volitionally by contracting expiratory muscles against a closed glottis or an occluded endotracheal tube **(Valsalva maneuver).** The associated increase in Pra decreases venous return. Initially, the left ventricle continues to fill from the pulmonary capacitance vessels. The increased pleural pressure also immediately decreases left ventricular afterload. These effects cause typical changes in arterial pressure in the early seconds of a Valsalva maneuver. If cardiac function is normal and left atrial pressure low, stroke volume and arterial pressure briefly rise in response to decreased afterload. However, stroke volume then quickly falls once the decreased venous return transits through the lungs and decreases left ventricular filling. In contrast, if the left ventricle is failing and left atrial pressure is elevated, the ventricle is more responsive to afterload reduction, and the ongoing discharge from the engorged pulmonary vessels can sustain ventricular filling for many seconds. Stroke volume and arterial pressure rise during the onset of the Valsalva maneuver and then remains elevated as the maneuver is maintained. This so-called plateau response has been shown to correlate with pulmonary artery occlusion pressure.[13,14]

Respiratory Changes in Pulse Pressure

Transient effects during a respiratory cycle are more complex because both pleural pressure and lung volume are changing. During relaxed SV in normal humans and animals, the dominant mechanical factor is the change in pleural pressure and its effects on venous return. Venous return rises during inspiration and falls during expiration. Because of the time lag as blood transits through the lungs, these changes in venous return are out of phase with respiration by the time they affect arterial pressure. Thus, arterial pressure falls slightly during inspiration and rises during expiration. An exaggeration of this normal respiratory variation in systolic blood pressure (a change of greater than 10 mm Hg) is termed **pulsus paradoxus.** This has been associated with diverse conditions, including severe asthma, upper airway obstruction, hypovolemia, and pericardial tamponade. In these conditions, other factors such as ventricular interdependence, afterload, etc., contribute to the variability in stroke volume. The relative importance of each contributory mechanical factor varies with each condition and is beyond the scope of this chapter.

A common question during management of a critically ill patient is whether cardiac output will respond to further fluid loading. Careful analysis of the transient changes in arterial pressure during a PPV respiratory cycle can help answer this question. For a relaxed patient receiving a PPV breath, nearly all of the individual mechanical effects are invoked with each inspiration. Pleural pressure increases, which would tend to decrease venous return and left ventricular afterload. Lung volume increases, which raises right ventricular afterload and PVR, and could either increase or decrease blood flow into the left atrium, depending upon volume status. Left ventricular inflow will also vary with filling of the right ventricle through ventricular interdependence. Lastly, abdominal pressure increases, and in a hypervolemic patient, this could attenuate the effects of elevated Pra on venous return. With expiration, all of these effects are reversed.

The summated action of these individual stresses changes left ventricular stroke volume. Stroke volume is best reflected in the arterial waveform by the **pulse pressure,** the difference between systolic and diastolic arterial pressure. In patients who are fully volume replete or hypervolemic, positive and negative effects of ventilation on stroke volume tend to balance each other, so that the pulse pressure remains relatively constant. In patients who are relatively hypovolemic, the positive and negative effects on left ventricular stroke volume predominate during separate phases of the respiratory cycle. This exaggerates the changes in pulse pressure. When studied quantitatively, the change in pulse pressure across the respiratory cycle has been shown to predict the improvements in cardiac output following a fluid bolus.[15] Similarly, a decrease in cardiac output following the application of PEEP can be predicted[16] (Figure 9-2). It should be noted that the positive and negative predictive values of changes in pulse pressure during a PPV breath exceed other traditional indices of volume status, including the Pra and **pulmonary artery wedge pressure (PAWP).**[17]

This index can be easily measured in any patient with an arterial cannula, with two important caveats. First, the patient must be in a regular cardiac rhythm. Second, the patient must be fully relaxed or paralyzed, neither triggering assisted breaths nor tensing expiratory muscles. This index has not been validated during patient-triggered ventilatory modes and may also be less reliable in patients receiving small tidal volumes.[18]

CLINICAL APPLICATIONS: STEADY-STATE EFFECTS

PEEP

The circulatory effects of PEEP have been studied for more than 50 years, beginning when positive pressure breathing was used to prevent syncope from hypoxia in high altitude flight before cabin pressurization. However, positive pressure breathing with PEEP was soon found to itself lead to syncope due to inhibition of venous return and the associated reduction in blood pressure. This is a known limiting

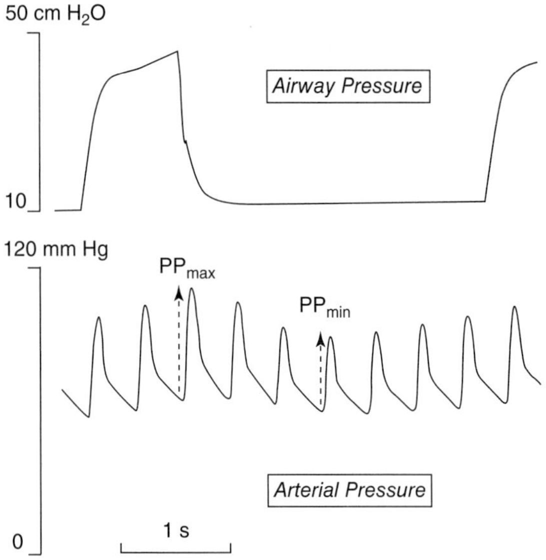

FIGURE 9-2 Example of the change in arterial pulse pressure (PP) during a respiratory cycle of a passive patient receiving PPV. The relatively large changes between PPmax and PPmin indicate a patient likely to increase cardiac output with a fluid bolus or decrease cardiac output with application of PEEP. (From Michard F, Chemla D, Richard C et al: Clinical use of respiratory changes in arterial pulse pressure to monitor the hemodynamic effects of PEEP, Am J Respir Crit Care Med 159:935-939, 1999.)

factor in the use of PEEP in the critical care setting.

PEEP (and CPAP during SV) elevates airway pressure above atmospheric pressure at end-expiration. By so doing, PEEP increases both lung volume and pleural pressure, and affects the circulation in much the same way as the transient elevations in airway pressure associated with PPV during inspiration. However, because PEEP is applied continuously, it can also activate neurohumoral reflex compensations for the purely mechanical effects described above. Despite these reflexes, PEEP often causes sustained, and therefore clinically important, decreases in cardiac output.

PEEP increases Pra, and this is commonly believed to decrease venous return (and cardiac output) by decreasing the gradient between Pms and Pra. However, studies in animals[1,2] and humans[3] have shown that PEEP also increases Pms. The increases in Pms and Pra are of similar magnitude, such that the pressure gradient driving venous return is unaltered. The increase in Pms is attributable in part to a shift of blood from the pulmonary capacitance vessels to the systemic circulation,[19] and in part to the activation of neurovascular reflexes.[1] Because the pressure gradient is unaltered, decreased venous return, when it occurs, must be due to an increase in the resistance to venous return. In canine studies, direct compression of the inferior vena cava by hyperinflated lungs was observed, and provides a possible explanation for increased venous resistance.[20] Though it is not known whether this occurs in humans on PEEP, a similar phenomenon has been observed in patients hyperinflated from severe emphysema.[21]

Another important effect of PEEP is the associated decrease in left ventricle (LV) afterload. Consistent with this mechanism, CPAP has been used effectively to treat acute cardiogenic pulmonary edema.[22] One study has even shown small increases in ejection fraction after chronic home use of CPAP in patients with congestive heart failure and sleep apnea.[23] CPAP and PEEP decrease both **preload** (through their effects on venous return) and left ventricular afterload, which mechanically mimics diuresis and vasodilation. In patients with obstructive sleep apnea, the associated reductions in blood pressure and loss of the afterload stress of obstructed inspiratory efforts likely also contributed to the observed improvements in ejection fraction.

PEEP is typically applied to patients with acute lung injury (ALI) or acute respiratory distress syndrome (ARDS). In such patients whose lung compliance is reduced, the increase in lung volume and pleural pressure induced by PEEP is attenuated. In contrast, intrinsic PEEP commonly occurs in patients with obstructive lung disease who have normal or increased lung compliance. For a given increase in alveolar pressure at end-expiration, their hyperinflation is greater. Furthermore, such patients may arrive at the hospital hypovolemic from several days of fever, poor oral intake, and increased minute ventilation. This would make them more sensitive to hemodynamic effects of PEEP. However, their vigorous inspiratory efforts while breathing spontaneously can obscure many of the hemodynamic effects of the intrinsic PEEP. These effects can be revealed, with disastrous results, when they are sedated and placed on PPV.[24] Inappropriate attempts to normalize CO_2 by increasing ventilation will lead to further hyperinflation and hypotension.[25,26]

Somewhat paradoxically, patients with intrinsic PEEP may be protected from the negative hemodynamic effects of applied PEEP. Patients whose obstructive lung disease is sufficiently severe to necessitate intubation are often flow limited during their passive expiration. A characteristic of flow-limited systems is that pressures downstream of the site of flow limitation do not affect flow. Application of low levels of PEEP has been shown to neither retard expiratory flow, cause further hyperinflation, nor decrease cardiac output in ventilated patients with intrinsic PEEP from obstructive lung disease. It is only higher levels of PEEP, sufficient to exceed the characteristic closing pressures of the flow-limited airways, that cause further hyperinflation and hypotension.[27]

Weaning

The major change in respiratory mechanics when switching from PPV to SV is a fall in mean pleural pressure. Since the pleural pressure is transmitted to Pra, venous return will increase. This may shift the interventricular septum to the left. The decrease in pleural pressure will also increase left ventricular afterload. Respiratory muscle effort increases and requires a higher nutritive blood flow than during PPV. Cardiac output is therefore redistributed to the diaphragm. A final effect of diaphragmatic contraction is an increase in abdominal pressure, particularly the surface pressure over the liver.[12] As has been described, this can also contribute to an increase in venous return.

In patients with normal cardiac function, these changes are well tolerated and cardiac output typically increases during spontaneous breathing trials. If patients fail their spontaneous breathing trial, it is usually attributed to poor lung function and respiratory muscle weakness. However, some patients fail breathing trials despite respiratory mechanics that appear to predict success. In one group of such patients with both lung disease and cardiac dysfunction, central venous pressure was observed to rise when the patients were switched from PPV to SV. An increase in central venous pressure cannot be attributed to decreased pleural pressure. However, a likely explanation for the rise in central venous pressure is compression of engorged abdominal vessels by the contracting diaphragm.[28] In this study, these patients with poor cardiac reserve were intolerant of the increased preload and increased afterload, and spontaneous breathing initiated a spiral of vascular congestion and ultimately weaning failure. However, after 1 week of empiric diuresis with a mean weight loss of 5 kg, half the patients were successfully weaned.[29] In patients with known cardiac dysfunction who fail weaning for enigmatic reasons, a trial of empiric diuresis may be considered.

KEY POINTS

- All of the circulatory effects of mechanical ventilation can be traced to two mechanical factors: changes in pleural pressure and changes in lung volume.
- These fundamental factors have numerous downstream circulatory effects upon:
  - Upstream and downstream pressures driving venous return
  - Resistance to venous return
  - Pulmonary vascular resistance and capacitance
  - Right and left ventricular filling
  - Ventricular interdependence
  - Right and left ventricular afterload
  - Stress on the surface of the abdominal vessels
  - Compensatory neurovascular reflexes
- The integrated response to these numerous effects varies with cardiac function and intravascular volume.
- Cardiopulmonary interactions during mechanical ventilation can be used to assist diagnosis and therapy. Patients with poor cardiac function and hypervolemia tend to be more tolerant of PPV, and hypovolemic patients with normal cardiac function tend to be less tolerant of PPV.

ASSESSMENT QUESTIONS

1. Define mean systemic pressure and its significance.
2. What effect does increased venous return have on right ventricular size and left ventricular filling?
3. How does lung inflation alter right ventricular afterload?
4. How does positive pressure inspiration alter left ventricular afterload? What about spontaneous inspiration?

Continued

ASSESSMENT QUESTIONS—cont'd

5. What is a normal variation in systolic arterial pressure? Why does it occur? What is it called when it exceeds the normal range?

6. Why might a patient with an exacerbation of obstructive lung disease become hypotensive shortly after being placed on PPV?

7. What are the two physiologic categories of pulmonary blood vessels? How does the capacitance of each change with lung inflation?

8. Does PVR increase or decrease during expiration? Is this change in resistance different for patients breathing spontaneously compared with those on PPV?

9. What mechanisms contribute to the decrease in cardiac output commonly seen when patients are placed on PEEP?

10. A hypotensive patient on controlled ventilation has a pulse pressure that changes substantially (by 20%) with each respiratory cycle. Would this patient be (likely/unlikely) to respond to a fluid bolus?

11. Would a patient with decompensated congestive heart failure be (likely/unlikely) to experience syncope while straining on the toilet?

REFERENCES

1. Fessler HE, Brower RG, Wise RA et al: Effects of positive end-expiratory pressure on the gradient for venous return, Am Rev Respir Dis 143:19-24, 1991.
2. Nanas S, Magder S: Adaptations of the peripheral circulation to PEEP, Am Rev Respir Dis 146:688-693, 1992.
3. Jellinek H, Krenn H, Oczenski W et al: Influence of positive airway pressure on the pressure gradient for venous return in humans, J Appl Physiol 88:926-993, 2000.
4. Samar RE, Coleman TG: Measurement of mean circulatory filling pressure and vascular capacitance in the rat, Am J Physiol 234:H94-H100, 1978.
5. Guyton AC, Lindsey AW, Kaufmann BN et al: Effect of blood transfusion and hemorrhage on cardiac output and on the venous return curve, Am J Physiol 194:263-267, 1958.
6. Guyton AC, Lindsey AW, Abernathy B et al: Venous return at various right atrial pressures and the normal venous return curve, Am J Physiol 189:609-615, 1957.
7. Amoore JN, Santamore WP: Model studies of the contribution of ventricular interdependence to the transient changes in ventricular function with respiratory efforts, Cardiovasc Res 23:683-694, 1989.
8. Burton AC, Patel DJ: Effect on pulmonary vascular resistance of inflation of the rabbit lungs, J Appl Physiol 12:239-246, 1958.
9. Permutt S, Howell JBL, Proctor DF et al: Effect of lung inflation on static pressure-volume characteristics of pulmonary vessels, J Appl Physiol 16:64-70, 1961.
10. Buda AJ, Pinsky MR, Ingels NB et al: Effect of intrathoracic pressure on left ventricular performance, N Engl J Med 301:453-459, 1979.
11. van den Berg PCM., Jansen JRC, Pinsky MR: Effect of positive pressure on venous return in volume-loaded cardiac surgical patients, J Appl Physiol 92:1223-1231, 2002.
12. Takata M, Robatham J: Effects of inspiratory diaphragmatic descent on inferior vena caval venous return, J Appl Physiol 72:597-607, 1992.
13. Felker G, Cuculich P, Gheorghiade M: The Valsalva maneuver: a bedside "biomarker" for heart failure, Am J Med 119:117-122, 2006.
14. McIntyre KMJ, Vita C, Lambrew C et al: A noninvasive method of predicting pulmonary capillary wedge pressure, N Engl J Med 327:1715-1720, 1992.
15. Michard F, Boussat S, Chemla D et al: Relation between respiratory changes in arterial pulse pressure and fluid responsiveness in septic patients with acute circulatory failure, Am J Respir Crit Care Med 162:134-138, 2000.
16. Michard F, Chemla D, Richard C et al: Clinical use of respiratory changes in arterial pulse pressure to monitor the hemodynamic effects of PEEP, Am J Respir Crit Care Med 159:935-939, 1999.
17. Michard F, Teboul JL: Predicting fluid responsiveness in the ICU, Chest 121:2000-2008, 2002.
18. De Baker D, Heenen S, Piagernerelli M et al: Pulse pressure variations to predict fluid responsiveness: influence of tidal volume, Intensive Care Med 31:517-523, 2005.
19. Peters J, Hecker B, Neuser D et al: Regional blood volume distribution during positive and negative airway pressure breathing in supine humans, J Appl Physiol 75:1740-1747, 1993.
20. Fessler HE, Brower RG, Shapiro EP et al: Effects of positive end-expiratory pressure and body position on pressure in the thoracic great veins, Am Rev Respir Dis 148:1657-1664, 1993.
21. Nakhjavan FK, Palmer WHJ, McGregor M: Influence of respiration on venous return in pulmonary emphysema, Circulation 33:8-16, 1966.
22. Masip J, Roque M, Sanchez B et al: Non-invasive ventilation in acute cardiogenic pulmonary edema: systematic review and meta-analysis, JAMA 294:3124-3130, 2005.
23. Bradley TD, Logan AG, Kimoff RJ et al: Continuous positive airway pressure for central sleep apnea and heart failure, N Engl J Med 353:2025-2033, 2005.

24. Wiener C: Ventilatory management of respiratory failure in asthma, JAMA 269:2128-2131, 1993.
25. Tuxen DV, Lane S: The effects of ventilatory pattern on hyperinflation, airway pressures, and circulation in mechanical ventilation of patients with severe air-flow obstruction, Am Rev Respir Dis 136:872-879, 1987.
26. Williams T, Tuxen DV, Scheinkestel C et al: Risk factors for morbidity in mechanically ventilated patients with acute severe asthma, Am Rev Respir Dis 146:607-615, 1992.
27. Ranieri VM, Giuliana R, Cinnella G et al: Physiologic effects of positive end-expiratory pressure in patients with chronic obstructive pulmonary disease during acute ventilatory failure and controlled mechanical ventilation, Am Rev Respir Dis 147:5-13, 1993.
28. Permutt S: Circulatory effects of weaning from mechanical ventilation: the importance of transdiaphragmatic pressure, Anesthesiology 69:157-160, 1988.
29. Lemaire F, Teboul JL, Cinotti L et al: Acute left ventricular dysfunction during unsuccessful weaning from mechanical ventilation, Anesthesiology 69:171-179, 1988.

CHAPTER 10

Ventilator-Induced Lung Injury

Renee D. Stapleton; Kenneth P. Steinberg

OUTLINE

OBJECTIVES

- Explain the concepts of barotrauma, volutrauma, atelectrauma, and biotrauma.
- Describe the mechanisms thought to contribute to the development of ventilator-induced lung injury.
- Discuss the data from clinical human studies that support the concept of ventilator-induced lung injury.
- Recall that low tidal volume ventilation reduces mortality in patients with acute lung injury and is the current standard of care in these patients.
- State the ARDS Network low tidal volume ventilation protocol.

KEY TERMS

atelectrauma
barotrauma
biotrauma
deep sulcus sign
high-frequency oscillatory ventilation (HFOV)
lung-protective ventilation
multiple organ dysfunction syndrome (MODS)
overdistention
permissive hypercapnia
pneumothorax
ventilator-induced lung injury (VILI)
volutrauma

Mechanical ventilation is a fundamental component of care in the intensive care unit (ICU) for most critically ill patients, particularly those with acute lung injury (ALI) and the acute respiratory distress syndrome (ARDS). However, both animal and human studies have found that mechanical ventilation may cause or worsen lung injury, a concept known as **ventilator-induced lung injury (VILI).** The continuum of lung injury associated with mechanical ventilation includes: (1) **barotrauma** manifested as extra-alveolar air from pneumothoraces, pneumomediastinum, and pulmonary interstitial emphysema; (2) **volutrauma** or injury resulting from mechanical stretch, which leads to alveolar-capillary barrier disruption and increases in endothelial and epithelial permeability; (3) **atelectrauma** or injury resulting from mechanical stresses associated with repetitive alveolar collapse and reopening; and (4) **biotrauma** with increases in pulmonary and systemic inflammatory mediators from mechanical lung injury that may further contribute to the development of VILI and **multiple organ dysfunction syndrome (MODS).**

ALVEOLAR RUPTURE AND EXTRA-ALVEOLAR AIR

Patients on mechanical ventilation are predisposed to many complications including the development of extra-alveolar air. One of the most well-recognized clinical manifestations of extra-alveolar air is **pneumothorax,** but extra-alveolar air can also manifest as pneumomediastinum, pulmonary interstitial emphysema (PIE), subcutaneous emphysema, and even pneumoperitoneum and systemic gas embolization. These complications occur not infrequently, with pneumothorax reported to occur in 4% to 15% of patients mechanically ventilated for more than 24 hours.[1-4] Even patients treated with noninvasive positive pressure ventilation (NPPV) can develop pneumothorax though the frequency of this complication is less well documented.[5,6] While any patient on mechanical ventilation is susceptible to these complications, the highest risk groups appear to be patients with severe airflow obstruction (e.g., asthma, chronic obstructive pulmonary disease [COPD]) and those with acute diffuse inflammatory lung disease, such as ALI and ARDS)

There has been debate in the literature over the pathophysiology of mechanical ventilation–induced alveolar rupture and extra-alveolar air. Originally it was believed that high airway pressures were the primary mechanism for alveolar rupture and that peripheral alveoli ruptured directly into the pleural space. Yet in one study, approximately 25 percent of pneumothoraces occurred in patients with right mainstem bronchus intubation, suggesting the importance of alveolar overdistention in the pathogenesis.[1] Macklin and Macklin performed necropsies in a number of patients dying of respiratory failure with clinically recognized pneumomediastinum.[7] They found dissection of air along vascular sheaths passing to the mediastinum, subcutaneous tissue, and retroperitoneum. In other experiments, they were able to determine that the site of air escape was the alveolar base where it contacted the vascular sheaths. A gradient between the alveolus and vascular sheath was postulated to produce alveolar rupture and interstitial emphysema. Studies by Polak and Adams demonstrated that high airway pressure alone was insufficient to cause alveolar rupture.[8] Using a canine model, lungs were inflated with large volumes of air, but expansion of the lungs was limited by thoracic binding. The marked elevation of alveolar pressure was matched by elevation in the supporting pressure on the outside of the chest, thus avoiding a severe gradient between the intra-alveolar and extra-alveolar pressures. Under these conditions, the alveoli did not rupture. Finally, Caldwell and associates likewise showed that the frequency of lesions induced by large alveolar volumes was decreased in animals with restricted chest movement.[9] They concluded that airway pressure itself was not the primary cause of perivascular interstitial emphysema and that excessive alveolar volume was the likely factor leading to alveolar rupture and air dissection. These animal experiments have been corroborated by data in humans that show poor correlation between lung air leaks and airway pressure.[4,10] It is also likely that the severity of the underlying lung injury (e.g., severity of ARDS) plays a role in the development of barotrauma.[3,4,10]

In its most serious form, a pneumothorax can develop very high intrathoracic pressures that can seriously impair both ventilation and cardiac filling (tension pneumothorax) and can cause death if not treated rapidly. Pontoppidan noted that tension pneumothorax occurred more frequently in patients with underlying chronic obstructive lung disease who were on mechanical ventilation.[11] Patients with more severe lung injury and with multiple organ failure are more likely to develop barotrauma and to die, but it is rare for barotrauma to directly contribute to death.[3,4] Despite the danger of tension pneumothorax, barotrauma is generally not associated with a significantly increased mortality.[1,4]

Less commonly, systemic air embolism can occur with disastrous results. Marini and Culver described two critically ill patients in whom recurrent episodes of cerebral infarction, myocardial infarction, and livedo reticularis developed while they were supported by mechanical ventilation.[12] In both patients, preexisting extra-alveolar air collections had enlarged before the catastrophic clinical events took place. The pathophysiology of this event appears to be an extension of processes leading to interstitial emphysema and pneumothorax with air entering the pulmonary venous system.

Abnormal air collections must be recognized on the chest radiograph, especially if the patient is mechanically ventilated, to prevent fatal complications and to improve pulmonary gas exchange. The diagnosis, however, can sometimes be subtle.[13] In a patient without pleural adhesions, air in a pneumothorax rises to the highest part of the pleural space. When the patient is erect, pleural air accumulates at the apex of the thorax. But if the patient is supine when the radiograph is obtained, as in most intubated ICU patients, the highest part of the pleural space is over the anterior surface of the lung, and a small

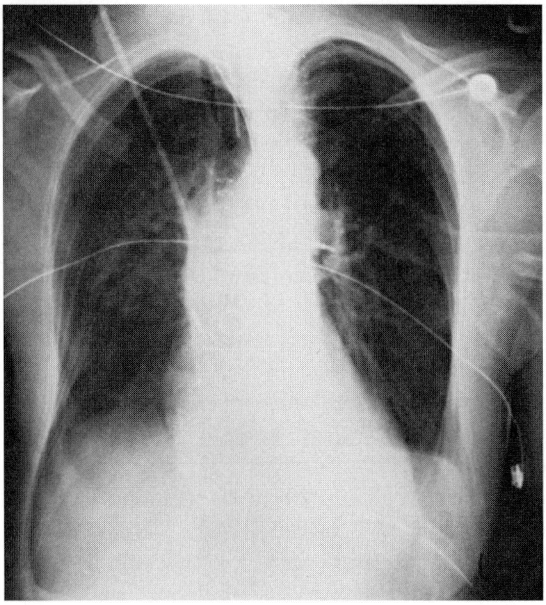

FIGURE 10-1 Supine chest radiograph illustrating the "deep sulcus" sign of a pneumothorax.

pneumothorax may be difficult to detect. A pneumothorax may appear only as a hazy lucency over the lung in this circumstance, but there are associated signs of increased volume in the affected hemithorax as the air collection enlarges. A characteristic finding, the **deep sulcus sign,** may be the only manifestation of an enlarging tension pneumothorax (Figure 10-1). This results from air collecting and expanding over the anterior part of the lower lung field, causing depression of the ipsilateral diaphragm from expanding air under pressure. A high degree of suspicion is necessary and erect or decubitus views of the lung may be helpful to further investigate the possibility of pneumothorax.

Subcutaneous emphysema may be present with or without pneumothorax and is usually most prominent in the head, neck, and anterior chest. Palpable subcutaneous emphysema may also be found at very distal sites, such as the feet and abdomen. Although subcutaneous emphysema is usually not a life-threatening complication, its presence should be interpreted by the clinician to mean that more serious and potentially life-threatening complications are likely unless the course of events is reversed or ventilator management is altered.

Pneumoperitoneum generally follows pneumomediastinum and results from air dissecting into the retroperitoneal space initially.[14] The peritoneum itself may rupture, leading to free intraperitoneal air. Occasionally, this may be painful and almost always presents a diagnostic dilemma that must be differentiated from a rupture of an intra-abdominal viscus. Severe pneumoperitoneum also may interfere with effective mechanical ventilation. Evacuation of a pneumoperitoneum is occasionally attempted, but is rarely successful.

PIE reflects the dissection of air along vascular sheaths after alveolar rupture. Chest radiographic findings are very subtle, often unrecognized, and have been described as multiple small and large parenchymal cysts, linear streaks of air extending to the mediastinum, perivascular "halos" from air collections, intraseptal air, subpleural cysts, or a "salt-and-pepper" appearance of the radiograph. PIE may be mistaken for air bronchograms. On chest computed tomography (CT), air within the interlobular septa and around pulmonary veins is diagnostic.[15] As with other forms of extra-alveolar air, PIE is usually not a life-threatening complication. Altering ventilator management, if possible, and being vigilant for the development of a pneumothorax are the only effective treatments.

STRETCH-INDUCED LUNG INJURY

The significance of VILI has been a recent focus of attention, with publication of clinical trials showing that **lung-protective ventilation** reduce mortality in patients with ARDS[16,17] and result in reduced organ dysfunction[17,18] and decreased lung and serum cytokine levels.[17,18] Despite the proven benefit of lung-protective ventilation, however, the mechanisms of this protective effect and the mechanisms by which mechanical ventilation causes lung injury are only partially understood.

Experimental and Mechanistic Evidence for VILI

Mechanical Stretch and Barrier Disruption: Volutrauma

One well-studied mechanism of VILI is volutrauma. Numerous animal investigations have shown that excessive mechanical stretch during overinflation of the lungs with high inspiratory pressures and large tidal volumes result in increased epithelial and endothelial permeability.[19-27] In their sentinel study, Webb and Tierney were the first to demonstrate this phenomenon[19] when they reported that rats ventilated with high tidal volumes developed pulmonary edema and diffuse alveolar damage that was histologically indistinguishable from ARDS. They also found that

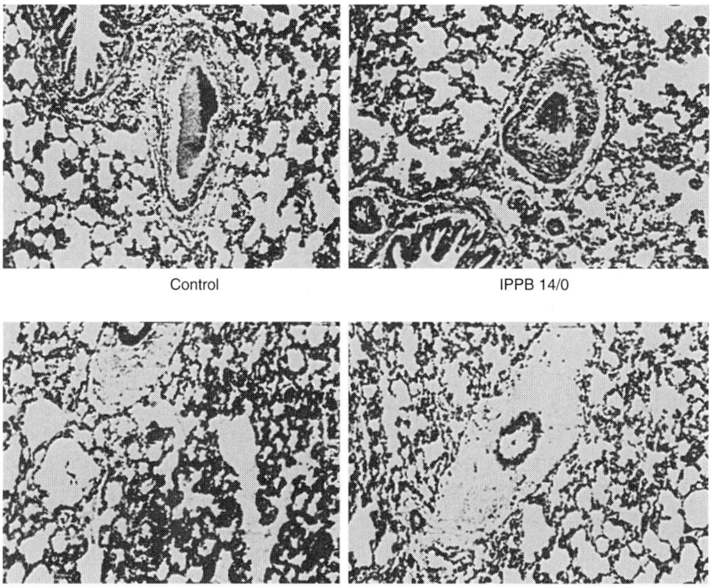

FIGURE 10-2 Lung tissue from rats ventilated with different strategies. Intermittent positive pressure breathing (IPPB) 14/0 delivered a peak pressure of 14 cm H_2O and a positive end-expiratory pressure (PEEP) of 0 cm H_2O; IPPB delivered a peak pressure of 45 cm H_2O and a PEEP of 0 cm H_2O; and IPPB 45/10 delivered a peak pressure of 45 cm H_2O and a PEEP of 10 cm H_2O. Note that IPPB 45/0 has alveolar and perivascular edema, but IPPB 45/10 has only perivascular edema. (From Webb HH, Tierney DF: Experimental pulmonary edema due to intermittent positive pressure ventilation with high inflation pressures: protection by positive end-expiratory pressure. Am Rev Respir Dis 110:556-565, 1974, American Lung Association.)

high volume ventilation caused less injury when positive end-expiratory pressure (PEEP) was added. Rats ventilated with a peak inspiratory pressure (PIP) of 45 cm H_2O and no PEEP developed more pulmonary edema and cellular injury than rats ventilated with PIP of 45 cm H_2O and 10 cm H_2O PEEP (Figure 10-2).

Dreyfuss and associates later published convincing evidence supporting the theory that volume **overdistention** rather than airway pressure is the principal element responsible for tissue injury. By comparing rats who had their chests and abdomens banded to those who did not, they were able to deliver high and low tidal volumes with identical high peak airway pressures.[28,29] Pulmonary edema developed in the high pressure/high tidal volume and low pressure/high tidal volume groups, whereas there was no edema produced in the high pressure/low tidal volume animals (Figure 10-3).

Further data suggest that repeated cyclic opening and closing of alveoli, particularly at low lung volumes, is injurious (atelectrauma). Chu and colleagues, in an *ex vivo* rat lung model, found that bronchoalveolar lavage (BAL) inflammatory mediator concentrations were greater in lungs ventilated at low lung volumes and no PEEP than at low lung volumes and PEEP of 5 cm H_2O or at low volumes while remaining atelectatic.[30] This may explain Webb and Tierney's observation that the addition of PEEP resulted in less lung injury (see Figure 10-2).

Additionally, it also appears that inspiratory flow rate, inspiratory time, and respiratory rate may play a role in development of VILI. Using an *in vivo* rabbit model, Simonson and colleagues[31] found that lung injury, as measured by gas exchange and compliance, was attenuated by reduced inspiratory time (0.45 second) and PEEP of 12 cm H_2O compared with other groups with longer inspiratory times. However, these results are contradicted by another study using tidal volumes of 30 ml/kg, where Maeda and colleagues found that lung injury was most severe in rabbits receiving high peak inspiratory flow rates (20% of cycle time compared with 50% of cycle time).[32] Limited data on respiratory rate are more consistent, with two studies demonstrating that

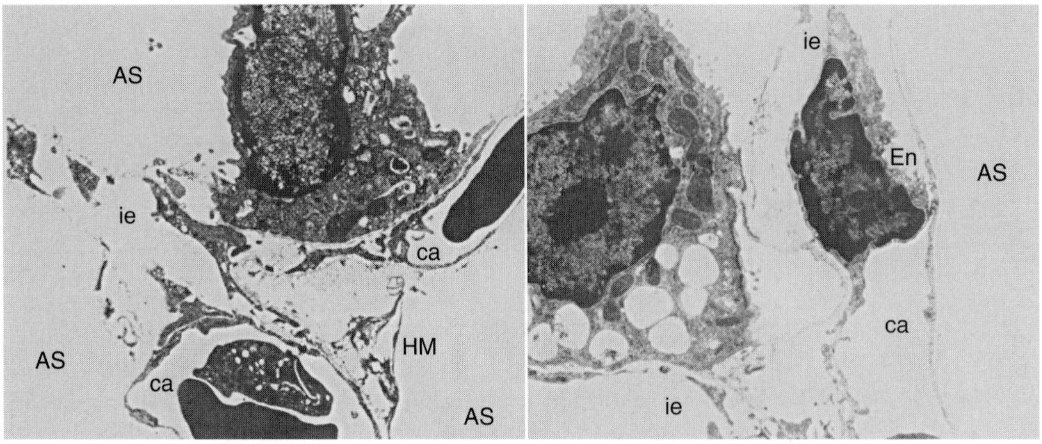

FIGURE 10-3 Ultrastructural aspects of the lungs of intact rats mechanically ventilated at 45 cm H_2O peak airway pressure with and without 10 cm H_2O PEEP. In the left panel, no PEEP was applied, and there is evidence of diffuse alveolar damage. In the right panel, 10 cm H_2O PEEP was applied, and the only abnormality is interstitial edema. *AS*, alveolar space; *ca*, capillary; *En*, endothelial cell; *HM*, hyaline membranes; *ie*, interstitial edema. (From Dreyfuss D, Soler P, Basset G et al: High inflation pressure pulmonary edema: respective effects of high airway pressure, high tidal volume, and positive end-expiratory pressure, Am Rev Respir Dis 137:1159-1164, 1988.)

reduced breath frequency, especially when delivering injuriously high tidal volumes, attenuates development of lung injury.[33,34]

Excessive volume with alveolar overdistention may be the most important mechanism in VILI, and the term volutrauma is appropriate to describe the sequelae. In the setting of ALI, the distribution of ventilation may be uneven because of the heterogeneity of injury.[35] Many years ago, Mead and colleagues suggested that, at a transpulmonary pressure of 30 cm H_2O, the regional distending pressure across an atelectatic or fluid-filled region of lung surrounded by a region of fully expanded lung would be nearly 140 cm H_2O.[36] Thus tidal volumes are preferentially directed to more normal or recruitable lung units, and these areas may be more susceptible to overinflation, overdistention, and tissue injury.

Inflammatory Mediators: Biotrauma

The hypothesis of biotrauma as a mechanism of VILI is a relatively recent development and is controversial.[37,38] Essentially the hypothesis is that the same injurious large tidal volumes causing barrier disruption, as explained above, result in increased release of inflammatory mediators in the lungs, thus perpetuating or worsening lung injury.[39] The hypothesis has been further extended by the proposal that these inflammatory mediators "spill over" into the systemic circulation and contribute to the development of MODS.[40,41] The increase in lung lavage and serum concentrations of inflammatory cytokines and chemokines is well supported by numerous studies, but demonstrating a causal link between these mediators and lung injury or MODS is less clear.

Several studies in intact animals have found that inflammatory mediator concentrations are increased in BAL fluid and serum of animals with lung injury. Using a model of acid-induced lung injury, Chiumello and colleagues found higher levels of tumor necrosis factor-α (TNF-α) and macrophage inflammatory protein-2 (MIP-2) in the serum of rats receiving high tidal volumes and no PEEP versus those with high volumes and PEEP of 5 cm H_2O.[42] Haitsma and colleagues found similar results with regard to TNF-α in a model of lipopolysaccharide-induced lung injury,[43] while Herrera demonstrated increased lung and serum concentrations of TNF-α and interleukin-6 (IL-6) with high tidal volume ventilation in a sepsis-induced model of ALI.[44] Additionally, Imai and colleagues subjected rabbit kidney and small intestine epithelial cells to plasma from other rabbits ventilated with injurious and noninjurious strategies.[45] They found that serum from the rabbits receiving the injurious ventilatory strategy led to increased apoptosis of both kidney and small intestinal cells and increased renal dysfunction in vivo.

Clinical Studies Providing Evidence for VILI

In recent years, several sentinel human studies have been published providing strong evidence for VILI and its potential contribution to the development of MODS. In 1998, Amato and colleagues reported on 53 patients with ARDS randomly assigned to conventional or protective ventilatory strategies.[16] Conventional ventilation was a tidal volume of 12 ml/kg and the least amount of PEEP necessary to improve oxygenation; protective ventilation was a tidal volume of less than 6 ml/kg with PEEP settings determined by the lower inflection point on static pressure-volume curves, and permissive hypercapnia. Patients in the protective ventilation group had significantly decreased mortality (38% versus 71%, $p < 0.001$) at 28 days. Although this study was criticized because mortality in the control group was unexpectedly high, it provided early evidence for the use of low tidal volume ventilation in patients with ALI. However, obtaining static pressure-volume curves to determine potential levels of appropriate PEEP requires heavy sedation or paralysis, may not be reproducible, and must be done repeatedly. Thus the use of pressure-volume curves to limit VILI has not entered routine clinical practice.

Ranieri and associates then published results from a phase II randomized controlled trial of 37 patients with ALI randomized to either conventional (mean tidal volume 11.1 ml/kg and PEEP 6.5 cm H_2O) or protective (mean tidal volume 7.6 ml/kg and PEEP 14.8 cm H_2O) ventilation.[18] BAL and systemic concentrations of the following inflammatory mediators/markers were measured at 36 hours after randomization: IL-1β, IL-6, and IL-1 receptor agonist (IL-1ra), IL-8, TNF-α, and TNF-α receptor, soluble TNF-alpha receptor 55, soluble TNF-alpha receptor 75, and neutrophil count. Most of the lung and serum markers significantly increased over time in the conventional group and decreased over time in the lung-protective group. With the exception of BAL IL-1ra, all inflammatory mediators were significantly decreased at 36 hours in the lung-protective group compared with the conventional ventilation group. This study was the first in humans to find that the inflammatory response induced by injurious mechanical ventilation could be attenuated by a lung-protective ventilation strategy.

Both the Amato[16] and Ranieri[18] studies provided the impetus for the National Institutes of Health/National Heart, Lung, and Blood Institute Acute Respiratory Distress Syndrome Network (ARDS Network) to conduct a large phase III study of lower versus traditional tidal volume ventilation in patients with ALI.[17] Since the first description of ARDS in 1967,[46] this is the only intervention to convincingly demonstrate an improvement in survival. In that trial, 861 patients with ALI were randomized to receive volume-controlled ventilation with either conventional tidal volumes of 12 ml/kg or lower tidal volumes of 6 ml/kg predicted body weight. In the lower tidal volume group, goal plateau pressure was 30 cm H_2O or less, and if the plateau pressure was greater than 30 cm H_2O, tidal volume was decreased to a minimum of 4 ml/kg predicted body weight. Adherence to protocol was excellent, with mean day 3 tidal volume of 6.2 ml/kg in the low-volume group and 11.8 ml/kg in the traditional tidal volume group. Mean plateau pressures were 25 cm H_2O and 33 cm H_2O in the intervention and control groups, respectively. The study was stopped early for efficacy; mortality was reduced from 40% to 31% ($p = 0.007$) with the low tidal volume intervention. Additionally, patients receiving the lower tidal volumes had significantly more ventilator-free days during the first 28 days (12 versus 10, $p = 0.007$). This large study clearly established the benefit of low tidal volume ventilation in patients with ALI and presented compelling evidence in humans for VILI.

Parsons and colleagues recently published data regarding inflammatory mediators from the ARDS Network low versus traditional tidal volume study.[47] During the trial, serum was drawn at baseline and on day 3 and evaluated for IL-6, IL-8, and IL-10. After multivariable analysis controlling for severity of illness, the authors found that low tidal volume ventilation was associated with a significant decrease in the inflammatory response, providing evidence for biotrauma and suggesting a link between circulating inflammatory mediators and mortality.

Subsequently, the ARDS Network went on to conduct a phase III randomized controlled trial of higher versus lower PEEP in ALI patients.[48] In that study, 549 patients were randomly assigned to either higher or lower PEEP levels in combination with fraction of inspired O_2 (FIO_2), according to *a priori* tables. All patients were ventilated with tidal volumes of 6 ml/kg predicted body weight and a goal of limiting plateau pressures to 30 cm H_2O. Mean PEEP during the first 4 days of the study was greater in the high PEEP group (13.2 cm H_2O versus 8.3 cm H_2O). However, neither survival to hospital discharge nor ventilator-free days during the first 28 days were different between the two groups. This study suggests that, when ALI patients receive low tidal volume ventilation, there does not appear to be a systematic benefit to the use of higher levels of PEEP.

Once the therapeutic benefits of low tidal volume ventilation in patients with established ALI became known, researchers began asking whether or not patients at risk for ALI might benefit from a protective ventilation strategy. It has been observed that slightly injured lungs are more susceptible to VILI than normal lungs.[49,50] Thus, if mechanical ventilation can potentiate ALI, the incidence of the syndrome might be decreased if low tidal volumes were used in patients at risk. Two recent observational studies have provided preliminary data on this topic. Gajic and associates reported the results of a retrospective cohort study in which 332 patients without ALI were examined for the development of the syndrome.[51] They found that women were ventilated with higher tidal volumes than men and trended toward greater development of ALI (29% versus 20%, $p = 0.068$). After multivariable analyses controlling for confounders, each milliliter of tidal volume received greater than 6 ml/kg was associated with a 30% increase in the odds of developing ALI. A subsequent prospective cohort study by the same authors analyzed 3261 patients without ALI, 6.2% of whom developed the syndrome.[52] After multivariable regression analysis, tidal volume greater than 700 ml, peak airway pressures greater than 30 cm H_2O, and PEEP greater than 5 cm H_2O were associated with development of ALI. These investigations provide preliminary evidence suggesting that lung-protective ventilation may be beneficial in patients at risk for ALI. This remains unproven, however, and a large randomized controlled trial would be needed to confirm this hypothesis. Such a trial would be an enormous undertaking since several thousand patients would be required to detect a difference in mortality or development of ALI.

Several studies have also examined whether **high-frequency oscillatory ventilation (HFOV)** is useful in patients with ALI, with the idea that HFOV might be the ideal modality to limit VILI. HFOV consists of very low tidal volumes and small pressure fluctuations, thus allowing high mean airway pressures to be used for alveolar recruitment while potentially avoiding alveolar overdistention. These features combine to have the potential to limit volutrauma and cyclic opening and closing of atelectatic areas of the lung.[53] Several observational studies have demonstrated that HFOV improves oxygenation and ventilation in patients with ARDS and suggest that it might be an effective rescue therapy.[54-56] A small randomized controlled trial was then performed; 148 adults with ARDS were randomized to HFOV or conventional ventilation at 6 to 10 ml/kg actual body weight (mean tidal volume for this group was 8 ml/kg).[57] The HFOV group had early improvement in oxygenation, but this difference did not persist. Mortality at 30 days was 37% in the HFOV group and 52% in the conventional ventilation group ($p = 0.102$). This trial was underpowered to detect a survival difference between the two groups, and further randomized trials comparing HFOV to the ARDS Network lung-protective ventilation protocol are needed.

Finally, recent data also suggest that hypercapnic acidosis may have a protective effect against VILI in ALI patients receiving conventional or high tidal volumes. **Permissive hypercapnia** is an accepted consequence of lung-protective ventilation. However, experimental data have provided evidence that hypercapnic acidosis also has favorable anti-inflammatory properties. Broccard and associates demonstrated that respiratory acidosis attenuated the severity of VILI in isolated, perfused rabbit lungs.[58] Sinclair and colleagues then found that hypercapnic acidosis protected against VILI in intact rabbits ventilated at high tidal volumes.[59] Based on these animal data, Kregenow and colleagues performed a secondary analysis of patients participating in the ARDS Network tidal volume trial and defined hypercapnic acidosis as a day 1 pH less than 7.35 with a P_{CO_2} greater than 45 mm Hg.[60] After multivariable analysis, they found significantly decreased odds of death at 28 days for patients with hypercapnic acidosis in the 12 ml/kg tidal volume group (OR = 0.14, 95% confidence interval 0.03-0.70, $p = 0.016$). Acidosis was not associated with decreased mortality in the 6 ml/kg tidal volume group, suggesting that hypercapnia might only be protective when used with injuriously high tidal volumes.

SUMMARY

Current clinical data support the hypotheses that mechanical ventilation contributes to the development of lung injury and MODS. Furthermore, minimizing this VILI with a lung-protective ventilation strategy (tidal volumes of 6 ml/kg predicted body weight or less depending upon plateau pressure) leads to an improvement in survival in patients with ALI and ARDS; therefore low tidal volume ventilation is indicated in patients with ALI and currently represents the standard of care for these patients. A concise description of the protocol is available in a review written by Brower.[61]

Much has been written about implementation of the ARDS Network protocol, and why clinicians might not use lung-protective ventilation as often as indicated. Rubenfeld and colleagues published results from a survey of ICU nurses and respiratory therapists examining barriers to providing lung-protective ventilation.[62] Identified barriers included: physician willingness to relinquish control of ventilator; physician recognition of ALI/ARDS; physician perceptions of patient contraindications to low tidal volumes; concerns over patient discomfort; and concerns over hypercapnia, acidosis, and hypoxemia. Despite these barriers, it has been shown that the protocol can be successfully implemented with ease. Kallet and associates have discussed this implementation and provided specific suggestions for setting up and troubleshooting the protocol.[63] Furthermore, in a single-institution study, Kahn and colleagues found that low tidal volume ventilation was not associated with increased dose or duration of sedatives in patients with ALI, suggesting that concern for oversedation should not be considered a barrier to implementing a lung-protective ventilation strategy.[64]

Other ventilatory strategies and interventions that may reduce VILI include lung-protective ventilation in patients at risk for ALI, HFOV, and the therapeutic use of hypercapnic acidosis. However, although these therapies may provide additional benefit, they need to be examined in appropriate clinical trials before they can be recommended for general use.

KEY POINTS

- Barotrauma, volutrauma, atelectrauma, and biotrauma are all mechanisms that are felt to contribute to VILI.
- Years' worth of animal studies and several recent human clinical studies support the theory that mechanical ventilation can potentiate lung injury and might contribute to the development of MODS.
- Low tidal volume ventilation has been shown to improve survival in patients with ALI.
- Low tidal volume ventilation is the current standard of care in patients with ALI. Tidal volumes should be set at 6 ml/kg predicted body weight, with a goal plateau pressure of 30 cm H_2O or less. If plateau pressure is greater than 30 cm H_2O at 6 ml/kg, the tidal volume should be lowered to a minimum of 4 ml/kg to try to achieve a plateau pressure of 30 cm H_2O or less.
- HFOV, hypercapnic acidosis, and low tidal volume ventilation in patients at risk for ALI are other ventilatory strategies that might be beneficial. However, these therapies are not proven and need to be studied in large randomized trials before recommendation for routine use.

ASSESSMENT QUESTIONS

1. What is the relationship between alveolar volume, airway pressure, and underlying lung pathology in the cause of extra-alveolar air?
2. How does the development of extra-alveolar air affect survival from respiratory failure?
3. Describe the pathophysiology of ventilator-induced extra-alveolar air.
4. The acutely injured lung is not uniform. Some regions are atelectatic or fluid-filled while others are normal. What happens to the normal areas of lungs when high tidal volumes are used?
5. When thinking about VILI, is it ventilating with high volumes or high pressures that is thought to contribute most? How much did this intervention decrease mortality?
6. What is biotrauma? How is it thought to contribute to the development of MODS?
7. What is the only intervention that has ever been convincingly shown to decrease mortality in patients with ALI?
8. To follow the current standard of care in ventilating patients with ALI, what tidal volume should initially be used? What is the goal plateau pressure? If that goal plateau pressure is still exceeded, how low should the tidal volume be decreased?
9. In the ARDS Network trial of higher versus lower PEEP in patients with ALI, was the level of PEEP shown to affect mortality?
10. Given the data we currently have available, should all patients at risk for developing ALI be ventilated with low tidal volumes?

CASE STUDIES

For additional practice, refer to Case Study 10 in the appendix at the back of the book.

REFERENCES

1. Zwilich CW, Pierson DJ, Creagh CE et al: Complications of assisted ventilation. A prospective study of 354 consecutive episodes, Am J Med 57:161-170, 1974.
2. Fleming WH, Bowen JC: Early complications of long-term respiratory support, J Thorac Cardiovasc Surg 54:729-738, 1972.
3. Schnapp LM, Chin DP, Szaflarski N et al: Frequency and importance of barotrauma in 100 patients with acute lung injury, Crit Care Med 23:272-278, 1995.
4. Weg JG, Anzueto A, Balk RA et al: The relation of pneumothorax and other air leaks to mortality in the acute respiratory distress syndrome, N Engl J Med 338:341-346, 1998.
5. Simonds AK: Pneumothorax: an important complication of non-invasive ventilation in neuromuscular disease, Neuromuscul Disord 14:351-352, 2004.
6. Raghavan R, Ellis AK, Wobeser W et al: Hemopneumothorax in a COPD patient treated with noninvasive positive pressure ventilation: the risk of attendant anticoagulation, Can Respir J 11:159-162, 2004.
7. Macklin MT, Macklin CC: Malignant interstitial emphysema of the lungs and mediastinum as an important occult complication in many respiratory diseases and other conditions: an interpretation of the clinical literature in the light of laboratory experiment, Medicine 23:281-358, 1944.
8. Polak B, Adams H: Traumatic air embolism in submarine escape training, US Naval Med Bull 30:165, 1932.
9. Caldwell EJ, Powell RD Jr, Mullooly JP: Interstitial emphysema: a study of physiologic factors involved in experimental induction of the lesion, Am Rev Respir Dis 102:516-525, 1970.
10. Gammon RB, Shin MS, Groves RH Jr et al: Clinical risk factors for pulmonary barotraumas: a multivariate analysis, Am J Respir Crit Care Med 152:1235-1240, 1995.
11. Pontoppidan H: Treatment of respiratory failure in nonthoracic trauma, J Trauma 8:938-951, 1968.
12. Marini JJ, Culver BH: Systemic gas embolism complicating mechanical ventilation in the adult respiratory distress syndrome, Ann Intern Med 110:699-703, 1989.
13. Ball CG, Hameed SM, Evans D et al: Occult pneumothorax in the mechanically ventilated trauma patient, Can J Surg 46:373-379, 2003.
14. Beilin B, Shulman DL, Weiss AT et al: Pneumoperitoneum as the presenting sign of pulmonary barotrauma during artificial ventilation, Intensive Care Med 12:49-51, 1986.
15. Kemper AC, Steinberg KP, Stern EJ: Pulmonary interstitial emphysema: CT findings, AJR Am J Roentgenol 172:1642, 1999.
16. Amato MB, Barbas CS, Medeiros DM et al: Effect of a protective-ventilation strategy on mortality in the acute respiratory distress syndrome, N Engl J Med 338:347-354, 1998.
17. Ventilation with lower tidal volumes as compared with traditional tidal volumes for acute lung injury and the acute respiratory distress syndrome. The Acute Respiratory Distress Syndrome Network, N Engl J Med 342:1301-1308, 2000.
18. Ranieri VM, Suter PM, Tortorella C et al: Effect of mechanical ventilation on inflammatory mediators in patients with acute respiratory distress syndrome: a randomized controlled trial, JAMA 282:54-61, 1999.
19. Webb HH, Tierney DF: Experimental pulmonary edema due to intermittent positive pressure ventilation with high inflation pressures. Protection by positive end-expiratory pressure, Am Rev Respir Dis 110:556-565, 1974.
20. Staub NC, Nagano H, Pearce ML: Pulmonary edema in dogs, especially the sequence of fluid accumulation in lungs, J Appl Physiol 22:227-240, 1967.
21. Parker JC, Hernandez LA, Longenecker GL et al: Lung edema caused by high peak inspiratory pressure in dogs. Role of increased microvascular filtration pressure and permeability, Am Rev Respir Dis 142:321-328, 1990.
22. Kolobow T, Moretti MP, Fumigalli R et al: Severe impairment in lung function induced by high peak airway pressure during mechanical ventilation. An experimental study, Am Rev Respir Dis 135:312-315, 1987.
23. Thornton D, Ponhold H, Butler J et al: Effects of pattern of ventilation on pulmonary metabolism and mechanics, Anesthesiology 42:4-10, 1975.
24. Coalson JJ, King RJ, Winter VT et al: O_2- and pneumonia-induced lung injury. I. Pathological and morphometric studies, J Appl Physiol 67:346-356, 1989.
25. Faridy EE, Permutt S, Riley RL: Effect of ventilation on surface forces in excised dogs' lungs, J Appl Physiol 21:1453-1462, 1996.
26. Dreyfuss D, Basset G, Soler P et al: Intermittent positive-pressure hyperventilation with high inflation pressure produces pulmonary microvascular injury in rats, Am Rev Respir Dis 132:880-884, 1985.
27. Tsuno K, Prato P, Kolobow T: Acute lung injury from mechanical ventilation at moderately high airway pressure, J Appl Physiol 69:956-961, 1990.
28. Dreyfuss D, Soler P, Basset G et al: High inflation pressure pulmonary edema. Respective effects of high airway pressure, high tidal volume, and positive end-expiratory pressure, Am Rev Respir Dis 137:1159-1164, 1988.
29. Dreyfuss D, Saumon G: Ventilator-induced lung injury: lessons from experimental studies, Am J Respir Crit Care Med 157:294-323, 1998.
30. Chu EK, Whitehead T, Slutsky AS: Effects of cyclic opening and closing at low- and high-volume ventilation on bronchoalveolar lavage cytokines, Crit Care Med 32:168-174, 2004.
31. Simonson DA, Adams AB, Wright LA et al: Effects of ventilatory pattern on experimental lung injury caused by high airway pressure, Crit Care Med 32:781-786, 2004.

32. Maeda Y, Fujino Y, Uchiyama A et al: Effects of peak inspiratory flow on development of ventilator-induced lung injury in rabbits, Anesthesiology 101:722-728, 2004.
33. Rich PB, Douillet CD, Hurd H et al: Effect of ventilatory rate on airway cytokine levels and lung injury, J Surg Res 113:139-145, 2003.
34. Hotchkiss JR Jr, Blanch L, Murias G et al: Effects of decreased respiratory frequency on ventilation-induced lung injury, Am J Respir Crit Care Med 161:463-468, 2000.
35. Gattiononi L, Pesenti A, Avalli L et al: Pressure-volume curve of total respiratory system in acute respiratory failure. Computed tomographic scan study, Am Rev Respir Dis 136:730-736, 1987.
36. Mead J, Takishima T, Leith D: Stress distribution in lungs: a model of pulmonary elasticity, J Appl Physiol 28:596-608, 1970.
37. Dreyfuss D, Ricard JD, Saumon G: On the physiologic and clinical relevance of lung-borne cytokines during ventilator-induced lung injury, Am J Respir Crit Care Med 167:1467-1471, 2003.
38. Uhlig S, Ranieri M, Slutsky AS: Biotrauma hypothesis of ventilator-induced lung injury, Am J Respir Crit Care Med 169:314-315, 2004.
39. Plotz FB, Slutsky AS, van Vught AJ et al: Ventilator-induced lung injury and multiple system organ failure: a critical review of facts and hypotheses, Intensive Care Med 30:1865-1872, 2004.
40. Slutsky AS, Tremblay LN: Multiple system organ failure. Is mechanical ventilation a contributing factor? Am J Respir Crit Care Med 157:1721-1725, 1998.
41. Dreyfuss D, Saumon G: From ventilator-induced lung injury to multiple organ dysfunction? Intensive Care Med 24:102-104, 1998.
42. Chiumello D, Pristine G, Slutsky AS: Mechanical ventilation affects local and systemic cytokines in an animal model of acute respiratory distress syndrome, Am J Respir Crit Care Med 160:109-116, 1999.
43. Haitsma JJ, Uhlig S, Goggel R et al: Ventilator-induced lung injury leads to loss of alveolar and system compartmentalization of tumor necrosis factor-alpha, Intensive Care Med 26:1515-1522, 2000.
44. Herrera MT, Toledo C, Valladares F et al: Positive end-expiratory pressure modulates local and systemic inflammatory responses in a sepsis-induced lung injury model, Intensive Care Med 29:1345-1353, 2003.
45. Imai Y, Parodo J, Kajikawa O et al: Injurious mechanical ventilation and end-organ epithelial cell apoptosis and organ dysfunction in an experimental model of acute respiratory distress syndrome, JAMA 289:2104-2112, 2003.
46 Ashbaugh DG, Bigelow DB, Petty TL et al: Acute respiratory distress in adults, Lancet 2:319-323, 1967.
47. Parsons PE, Eisner MD, Thompson BT et al: Lower tidal volume ventilation and plasma cytokine markers of inflammation in patients with acute lung injury, Crit Care Med 33:1-6, 2005, discussion 230-232.
48. Brower RG, Lanken PN, MacIntyre N et al: Higher versus lower positive end-expiratory pressure in patients with the acute respiratory distress syndrome, N Engl J Med 351:327-336, 2004.
49. Hernandez LA, Coker PJ, May S et al: Mechanical ventilation increases microvascular permeability in oleic acid-injured lungs, J Appl Physiol 69:2057-2061, 1990.
50. Dreyfuss D, Soler P, Saumon G: Mechanical ventilation-induced pulmonary edema. Interaction with previous lung alterations, Am J Respir Crit Care Med 151:1568-1575, 1995.
51. Gajic O, Dara SI, Mendez JL et al: Ventilator-associated lung injury in patients without acute lung injury at the onset of mechanical ventilation, Crit Care Med 32:1817-1824, 2004.
52. Gajic O, Frutos-Vivar F, Esteban A et al: Ventilator settings as a risk factor for acute respiratory distress syndrome in mechanically ventilated patients, Intensive Care Med 31:922-926, 2005.
53. Singh JM, Stewart TE: High-frequency mechanical ventilation principles and practices in the era of lung-protective ventilation strategies, Respir Care Clin N Am 8:247-260, 2002.
54. Mehta S, Lapinsky SE, Hallett DC et al: Prospective trial of high-frequency oscillation in adults with acute respiratory distress syndrome, Crit Care Med 29:1360-1369, 2001.
55. David M, Weiler N, Heinrichs W et al: High-frequency oscillatory ventilation in adult acute respiratory distress syndrome, Intensive Care Med 29:1656-1665, 2003.
56. Mehta S, Granton J, MacDonald RJ et al: High-frequency oscillatory ventilation in adults: the Toronto experience, Chest 126:518-527, 2004.
57. Derdak S, Mehta S, Stewart TE et al: High-frequency oscillatory ventilation for acute respiratory distress syndrome in adults: a randomized, controlled trial, Am J Respir Crit Care Med 166:801-808, 2002.
58. Broccard AF, Hotchkiss JR, Vannay C et al: Protective effects of hypercapnic acidosis on ventilator-induced lung injury, Am J Respir Crit Care Med 164:802-806, 2001.
59. Sinclair SE, Kregenow DA, Lamm WJ et al: Hypercapnic acidosis is protective in an in vivo model of ventilator-induced lung injury, Am J Respir Crit Care Med 166:403-408, 2002.
60. Kregenow DA, Rubenfeld GD, Hudson LD et al: Hypercapnic acidosis and mortality in acute lung injury, Crit Care Med 34:1-7, 2006.
61. Brower RG: Mechanical ventilators in acute lung injury and ARDS. Tidal volume reduction, Crit Care Clin 18:1-13, 2002.
62. Rubenfeld GD, Cooper C, Carter G et al: Barriers to providing lung-protective ventilation to patients with acute lung injury, Crit Care Med 32:1289-1293, 2004.
63. Kallet RH, Corral W, Silverman HJ et al: Implementation of a low tidal volume ventilation protocol for patients with acute lung injury or acute respiratory distress syndrome, Respir Care 46:1024-1037, 2001.
64. Kahn JM, Andersson L, Karir V, et al: Low tidal volume ventilation does not increase sedation use in patients with acute lung injury. Crit Care Med 33:766-771, 2005.

SECTION III ADJUNCTIVE THERAPY

CHAPTER 11

Nutrition

Richard D. Branson; Jay A. Johannigman

OUTLINE

OBJECTIVES

- Explain the relationship between nutrition and lung disease.
- List the causes of malnutrition in chronic lung disease.
- Examine the role of nutritional support in care of the mechanically ventilated patient.
- Understand the role of indirect calorimetry in nutritional assessment of the mechanically ventilated patient.
- List the variables that influence the accuracy of indirect calorimetry.
- Describe the use of specific nutritional formulas and respiratory quotient and the inflammatory process.

KEY TERMS

Acute Physiology and Chronic Health Evaluation (APACHE)
Harris-Benedict equation
hypermetabolism
indirect calorimetry
respiratory quotient (RQ)
resting energy expenditure (REE)
steady state

Patients on mechanical ventilation are under significant physiologic stress and are at risk for deterioration of nutritional status. The patient's nutritional state is vitally important to outcome because it is fundamentally associated with overall pulmonary status, immune competence, and the patient's ability to mount an overall stress response.[1] Caloric requirements and nutritional needs are not easily anticipated clinically or accurately predicted by conventional equations. Complications occur from both underfeeding and overfeeding, and the clinical consequences of inappropriate feeding are not always readily discernible at the bedside by the health care practitioner.[2] **Indirect calorimetry** therefore becomes a useful tool for designing nutrition support regimens that precisely meet caloric requirements.

In this chapter, the effects of inappropriate feeding in the patient with respiratory failure requiring mechanical ventilation are enumerated. A clinically useful nutritional assessment with the means for determining nutritional requirements is discussed. Performance of indirect calorimetry, design of an appropriate nutritional support regimen, and monitoring the patient for response and tolerance to the nutritional support regimen are outlined.

MALNUTRTION IN THE MECHANICALLY VENTILATED PATIENT

Critical illness requiring endotracheal intubation and mechanical ventilation predisposes the patient to the consequences of malnutrition. Hypermetabolism, inability to provide oral intake, inflammation, and preexisting conditions all contribute to this predisposition. Generally speaking, the patient requiring more than 3 to 5 days of mechanical ventilation is at high risk for malnutrition and should be evaluated for nutritional supplementation.

The patient with chronic obstructive pulmonary disease (COPD) is at particular risk for malnutrition. This is further complicated by the requirement for mechanical ventilation. Malnutrition in the COPD patient is common and weight loss is directly related to worsening lung function and mortality.[3] The causes of malnutrition in COPD include hypermetabolism, infection, medications, and reduced intake. Box 11-1 lists these in detail.

EFFECT OF UNDERFEEDING

An important perspective is obtained by reviewing the effects of underfeeding as they relate to the underlying mechanisms of respiratory failure. A traditional way of viewing respiratory failure is to separate the disease process into hypercapnic and hypoxemic varieties. Both categories include patients who may require mechanical ventilatory support. In considering the effects of nutrition on patients, the mechanisms responsible for producing the respiratory failure should be kept in mind. Hypercapnia is caused by hypoventilation, which results from one or more of the following: (1) inadequate respiratory center drive; (2) inadequate transmission of the respiratory center drive to the myoneural junction; (3) interference with transmission of the signal across the myoneural junction; and (4) muscle weakness. Hypoxemic respiratory failure typically results from ventilation-perfusion abnormalities ranging from dead space to shunt. It is pertinent to assess any effects of nutrition on lung anatomy and host defense mechanisms. The findings as they relate to these underlying mechanisms are briefly summarized.

There are no known studies directly evaluating respiratory center drive or conduction of the signal to the muscle (by diaphragmatic electromyogram [EMG] or phrenic nerve conduction studies) in the setting of underfeeding. Weissman and colleagues[4] looked at an indirect measure of this in subjects deprived of protein for 7 days. A 26% decrease in the ratio of tidal volume/inspiratory time (V_T/T_I or mean inspiratory flow rate) was found. Intravenous administration of an amino acid solution for 24 hours resulted in reversal. Because ventilatory response to chemical stimuli as measured by minute ventilation could be impaired by decreased respiratory drive or impaired muscle function, studies measuring only this parameter do not differentiate effects produced by one or another of these mechanisms. A study by Doekel and associates[5] involved this methodology and found that a semistarvation diet for 10 days resulted in a 58% reduction in hypoxemic ventilatory response. Refeeding with a normal diet reversed this effect.

A number of studies have addressed the effects of underfeeding on respiratory muscle function. In a group of patients dying after a chronic illness, patients whose body weight was normal had minimal loss of diaphragmatic muscle mass compared with a control group of individuals who had experienced sudden death. A second group of patients dying after a chronic illness who had sustained loss of body weight (down to a mean 71% of ideal body weight) had a 43% reduction in diaphragmatic muscle mass compared with the control group experiencing sudden death.[6] In a study of healthy volunteers placed on modest

BOX 11-1 *Factors Contributing to Malnutrition in the Patient With COPD*

- Hypermetabolism
- Chronic inflammatory state
- Increased O_2 cost of breathing due to hyperinflation and airway obstruction
- Increased energy requirements associated with β-agonist therapy
- Greater activity-related thermogenesis
- Cumulative effects of the above during exacerbations
- Corticosteroids leading to protein loss
- Decreased intake
- Dental and peptic ulcer disease
- Early satiety
- Dyspnea on exertion limiting intake after food preparation
- Reduced intake during exacerbation

caloric restriction for almost 6 months, Keys and associates[7] found a mean reduction in vital capacity of 8%. This improved to near baseline following 12 weeks of refeeding.[7] In another group of patients who had sustained substantial weight loss, respiratory muscle strength appeared to be affected, as evidenced by maximal inspiratory pressures that were 35% and maximal expiratory pressures that were 59% of normal values. On the average, vital capacity was 63% and respiratory muscle strength was 37% of those values seen in healthy controls.[8] Similarly, Grant found that malnourished patients had reductions to 59% of predicted for maximum expiratory pressures and 43% of predicted for maximal inspiratory pressures.[1] Two weeks of total parenteral nutrition (TPN) therapy produced significant but not complete normalization of these parameters. As a frame of reference, in normal lungs of patients who had proximal myopathies, reductions in vital capacity to less than 55% of predicted or respiratory muscle strength to less than 30% of normal was associated with hypoventilation.[9] Further evidence that nutritional support may improve respiratory muscle strength was provided by Whitaker and colleagues,[10] who found increases in maximal inspiratory pressure and mean sustained inspiratory pressure in chronically ill malnourished patients with COPD given dietary supplements, compared with a control group not receiving the supplement.

Deterioration of nutritional status has been shown in other studies to result in physiologic and anatomic changes in the lung. Patients who were nutritionally depleted showed evidence of higher tracheal colonization and greater tracheal cell adherence by bacteria[11,12] when compared with well-nourished controls. When nutritionally depleted patients undergoing elective gastrointestinal (GI) surgery were compared with well-nourished controls undergoing the same operation, these changes corresponded to a higher rate of pneumonia and longer hospital stays.[13] Morphologic changes and structural damage to the lung have been demonstrated in response to underfeeding. In an animal model in which rats were exposed to 3 weeks of semistarvation, decreases in alveolar wall surface tension, surfactant production, and overall elastic compliance were seen.[14] Adequate refeeding corrected the changes in surfactant, but the morphologic emphysematous changes in the lungs were not corrected.[14] Similar evidence has been shown in humans where world famines have resulted in emphysematous changes even in young adults.[1,15]

These deleterious changes in the respiratory response to nutritional deterioration correlate with adverse effects on patient outcome. In patients with COPD with severe nutritional deficits, there were less frequent hospitalizations for those patients who successfully ingested a high-calorie diet compared with those patients who refused to eat.[16] Weaning capability in patients on mechanical ventilation improved with adequate nutritional support. Combining the results of two studies, successful weaning occurred in 88% of patients (22 of 25) who received adequate feeding but in only 32% (10 of 31) who failed to receive an adequate regimen.[17,18] Despite these anecdotal reports and a common sense approach that nourished patients may be withdrawn from ventilatory support quicker than those who are malnourished, no direct evidence relating nutritional support and weaning is available.

EFFECT OF OVERFEEDING

A number of clinical problems arise from overfeeding patients in respiratory failure on mechanical ventilation. At the outset, overfeeding may promote fluid overload, hyperlipidemia, hyperglycemia, and azotemia.[2] Overfeeding actually may increase the overall stress response and raise energy expenditure for the critically ill patient on mechanical ventilation. The increased energy response is caused by increases in diet-induced thermogenesis related to overfeeding. The degree to which energy expenditure is increased is related to the degree to which the fixed rate of carbohydrate metabolism is exceeded.[19,20] Once the fixed rate of carbohydrate metabolism is exceeded, the additional calories must be converted to either glycogen or fat. Lipogenesis to a greater extent than glycogenesis accounts for the dramatic increase in energy expenditure, with increases in diet-induced thermogenesis of up to 25% to 26%.[21] The hypermetabolic response is accompanied by increases in catecholamine secretion.[22,23]

Overfeeding, which results in lipogenesis, promotes excessive carbon dioxide (CO_2) production, which may overwhelm respiratory function in individuals with reduced ventilatory capacity. In one study using parenteral nutrition, significant elevation in CO_2 production was seen as total caloric provision and was increased from 1.0 to 1.5 to 2.0 times the **resting energy expenditure (REE).**[24] In case series, high-caloric loads provided through parenteral nutrition actually precipitated hypercapnia, respiratory acidosis, and respiratory failure, requiring placement on mechanical ventilation.[25-27] Increases in CO_2 production and minute ventilation were greater in patients who were adequately nourished before injury compared with those with evidence of depleted nutritional status.[26] Patients with mild to moderate injury showed greater increases in minute ventilation in response to overfeeding than patients with a greater severity of injury.[26] In studies with indirect calorimetry, the effects of overfeeding on substrate use are seen, as is the evidence of increased load to the pulmonary system. In a retrospective review of 78 patients on mechanical ventilation receiving TPN, those patients with a **respiratory quotient (RQ)** of greater than 1.0 (suggesting lipogenesis from overfeeding) showed that they received carbohydrate infusions that were 31.6% higher, had a minute ventilation that was 27.5% higher, and required intermittent minute ventilation (IMV) settings that were 210% greater than patients whose measured RQ was less than 1.0.[28] Even in those patients on mechanical ventilation who received enteral tube feedings, a direct correlation was seen between overfeeding (percentage calories provided/required) and increasing RQ.[29] When the RQ increased in response to overfeeding, patients developed shallow, rapid respirations.[29] In general, these changes in response to overfeeding result in effects on minute ventilation, increase dead-space ventilation, promote respiratory failure, and delay weaning from mechanical ventilation. It is important to note that the changes in CO_2 production are most often observed in patients who receive calories in excess of needs. Isocaloric feedings with high carbohydrate concentrations slightly alter CO_2 production and generally only have negative consequences in patients with chronic hypercapnic respiratory failure.

NUTRITIONAL ASSESSMENT

Nutritional assessment in the patient on mechanical ventilation should focus on three main areas: (1) a determination of level of physiologic stress, as measured by the **Acute Physiology and Chronic Health Evaluation (APACHE)** scoring system; (2) a brief clinical examination of current nutritional status and respiratory muscle function; and (3) a thorough evaluation of the status of the GI tract in anticipation of use for enteral access. More traditional markers of nutritional assessment (i.e., anthropometry, immune markers, and visceral protein levels) have very little value in the stressed critically ill patient on mechanical ventilation.[30,31] Anthropometric measures (such as midarm circumference and triceps skin-fold thickness) and immune markers (i.e., total lymphocyte count and anergy panel) tend to be inaccurate and poorly reproducible, rarely reflect true nutritional status, and almost never affect the design of the nutrition support regimen.[31] Decreases in visceral protein levels (albumin, prealbumin, and transferrin) in the critically ill patient reflect the stress response and are related not only to decreased production of these proteins by the liver but also to extravasation of the proteins out of the vascular space.[32] Use of the visceral proteins as a marker of nutritional status in the critically ill patient is fallacious.[32] In theory, bioelectric impedance should be helpful in determining body composition and in differentiating lean body mass from fat mass, but it has diminished usefulness in the critical care setting because of the significant error introduced by volume shifts and the presence of edema.

Level of stress is the single greatest factor affecting risk of nutritional deterioration and ultimate patient outcome. The more critically ill the patient, the more likely that even subtle aspects of nutritional support (such as route of nutrient administration[33] and control of hyperglycemia[34]) would have an impact on patient outcome.[34,35] The APACHE scoring systems are the most carefully researched and commonly used marker for degree of critical illness and overall physiologic stress.[36-38] Whether the more convenient APACHE II system[37] or the more comprehensive (and possibly more reliable for serial use) APACHE III system is used,[38] these scores correlate with increased energy expenditure, overall stress response, development of nosocomial infection and multiple-organ failure, and ultimately, mortality.[36-39] These scoring systems indicate the degree of risk of nutritional deterioration and the urgency with which nutritional support should be instigated.

A brief clinical examination with attention to actual body weight (ABW) as a percentage of ideal body weight (IBW) and simple bedside tests for respiratory muscle function provide valuable clues as to the patient's current nutritional status. ABW as a percentage of IBW or usual body weight should be determined because weight loss correlates with acuity of respiratory failure and partial pressure of carbon dioxide (P_{CO_2}) levels.[40] Patients with COPD with acute respiratory failure have been shown to have significantly lower percent IBW than stable patients with COPD.[41] In a large group of patients with acute respiratory failure, 56% were shown to have ABWs less than 80% of IBW.[30] Muscle atrophy tends to parallel weight loss. Patients who had profound nutritional depletion at a mean 71% of IBW were shown to have 43% less diaphragmatic muscle mass than healthy controls.[6] A simple bedside measure of respiratory muscle function is the maximal inspiratory and expiratory pressure. Absolute values reflect respiratory muscle strength, whereas sustaining pressures indicate endurance. In patients with COPD, respiratory endurance usually is affected more than the absolute inspiratory/expiratory pressures.[42] Serial inspiratory pressure measurements are one parameter reflecting response of muscle strength to nutritional support.

The need to obtain enteral access to maintain gut integrity and to contain the stress response with enteral feeding makes assessment of the GI tract imperative. The enteral route of nutrition support has been shown to reduce cost, nosocomial infection, multiple-organ failure, length of hospitalization, and mortality when compared with the parenteral route.[35] The term "ileus" and the axiom "If the gut works, use it" are outdated, misleading, and inaccurate, and should be avoided in the nutritional assessment of the patient on mechanical ventilation. The gut is always "working"; it never stops absorbing nutrients that are infused into its lumen. At times, it may not be safe for the gut to absorb luminal nutrients, particularly in the patient with systemic hypotension on pressor agents, such as norepinephrine, dopamine, and dobutamine. Feeding through the enteral route in these circumstances may promote a shift of blood flow to the splanchnic circulation and may promote even further deterioration into clinical shock. It may be more appropriate to wait until these patients are no longer being given pressor agents or are at least being given renal perfusion doses of dopamine to initiate enteral feeding.

The more important factor to be addressed by nutritional assessment relates to which segments of the GI tract have adequate contractility. With an acute physiologic insult, the small bowel is the last segment of the GI tract to stop contracting and the first to return to contractility as the acute event abates. Residual volumes and nasogastric output from a saline sump tube are good clinical markers of gastric contractibility. Passage of stool and gas per rectum are good measures for colonic contractility. Although the presence of bowel sounds indicates small bowel contractility, bowel sounds are not required to initiate feeding into the jejunum. Assessment of contractility of the various segments of the GI tract helps determine which feeding tube is required and at what level feedings need to be infused. Significant gastric atony often is accompanied by duodenal atony and often requires feeding into the jejunum with or without simultaneous aspiration and decompression of the stomach. Finally, some assessment of the degree of gut disuse and villous atrophy (estimated by the time period in which there are no luminal nutrients) should be made to determine the need for a specialized small peptide hydrolyzed formula (over a more standard formula).

NUTRITIONAL REQUIREMENTS

A number of factors in the critical care setting lead to **hypermetabolism** and increased energy expenditure in the respiratory failure patient on mechanical ventilation.[43] The disease process itself, with its concomitant stress response, may increase energy expenditure through stimulation of the sympathetic nervous system and the release of catecholamines. Other factors contributing to the increase in energy expenditure include fever, futile substrate cycling, medications (aspirin, pressor agents, catecholamines), release of counter-regulatory hormones (glucagon, cortisol, adrenocorticotropic hormone), inflammatory cytokines, shivering thermogenesis, and increased work of breathing.[43] The work of breathing, which may represent only 2% to 3% of energy expenditure in a healthy person, may increase up to 25% to 26% of energy expenditure in a patient in respiratory failure before placement on mechanical ventilation.[44,45] Weight loss and nutritional deterioration of the patient with COPD may increase energy expenditure further compared with similar patients with COPD who remain well nourished at a stable weight.[46-48] COPD by itself may cause defects in diet-induced thermogenesis (DIT). Increased DIT was shown in patients with COPD compared with undernourished (non-COPD) controls,[49] indicating that greater energy expenditure was required to metabolize the same amount of nutrients (and thus fewer calories were available as fuel for muscles and lean body mass). Additionally, patients with COPD may have defects of certain adaptive mechanisms, lacking the ability to become hypometabolic during periods of fasting or caloric deprivation.[47] A misconception for some clinicians is that providing mechanical ventilation to a patient in respiratory failure greatly increases REE,[30] but it is really the underlying respiratory failure that causes the increase in energy expenditure. A patient on mechanical ventilation who is weaned successfully usually demonstrates an increase in energy expenditure as the patient assumes the work of breathing done previously by the machine.[44,45]

Not all patients who are critically ill on mechanical ventilation manifest a hypermetabolic response. In multiple studies in the critical care setting, only 35% to 62% of patients were shown to be hypermetabolic (>110% of the Harris-Benedict predicted REE).[44,50-52]

The rest were normometabolic (within 10%) or even hypometabolic (<90% of the Harris-Benedict value). This seemingly inappropriate hypometabolic response may be explained by a number of factitious reasons,[43] such as pharmacologic treatment, choice of predictive formula, inaccurate weights, timing of the study, issues related to nutritional support, and even level of consciousness. However, progressive, inappropriate low metabolism may imply impending septic shock, and patients should be evaluated for underlying infection.[43,53,54]

More than 200 equations have been published in the literature, using a variety of clinical factors, to predict REE.[55] Surprisingly, none of these equations are more accurate than the time-honored **Harris-Benedict equation**,[55] despite modification of the equation for patient activity,[29] disease process,[56,57] level of stress,[58] and even ventilatory status.[59] Use of the Harris-Benedict equation alone (which was developed in healthy volunteers) tends to underpredict measured REE,[51] but correcting the equation by a metabolic injury factor, such as those derived by Grant[56] or Elwyn and colleagues,[57] results in overprediction of measured REE.[51] Patients on mechanical ventilation have been shown in one study to have a mean measured REE greater than 105% of predicted, the range being 70% to 140% of predicted.[44] Box 11-2 lists commonly used equations for predicting caloric requirements.

Use of predictive equations in the individual patient is inherently inaccurate because these equations are based on faulty clinical presumptions. Patients do not respond identically to a single disease process. Owen and associates have described the concept of a "metabolic signature" or "fingerprint," whereby patients inherit their own unique metabolic machinery, which causes them to respond differently to the same disease process or similar extent of injury.[60] In large studies of patients with the same disease process, the standard deviation for measured REE can range from 19% to 40% about a mean value, with variability from one patient to the next by up to 30% to 40%.[61-63] In an individual patient, energy expenditure is not constant, consistent, or easily predictable, with variation even in controls (without a disease process) of 12% to 25% when tested over several days to weeks.[64-66] The metabolic response to an injury is not the same throughout the disease process.[44] Early in the course of the critically ill patient, daily energy expenditure may vary by up to 46% about a mean REE, whereas later in the patient's recovery process REE may vary up to only 12% about the mean.[44] Additional disease processes may complicate the "usual" metabolic response to respiratory failure. Organ failure, development of sepsis, or repeated surgical procedures may lead to increases in energy expenditure. Typically, recommendations based on predictive equations or tables for these various disease states tend to break down in the face of multiple concomitant disease processes.

BOX 11-2 *Common Equations Used for the Prediction of Caloric Requirements in Hospitalized Patients*

Harris-Benedict

Men

BEE = 5 (height in cm) + 13.7 (weight in kg) − 6.8 (age in years) + 66

Women

BEE = 1.9 (height in cm) + 9.6 (weight in kg) − 4.7 (age in years) + 655

Ireton-Jones Equation for the Mechanically Ventilated Patient

RMR = 5 (weight in kg) − 10 (age in years) + 281 (for men, 0 for women) + 292 (for trauma) + 851 (for burns) + 1925

Ireton-Jones Equation for the Spontaneously Breathing Patient

RMR = 629 − 11 (age in years) + 25 (weight in kg) − 609 (if obesity is present)

Mifflin-St. Jeor Equation

Men RMR = 9.99 (weight in kg) + 6.25 (height in cm) − 5 (age in years)

Women RMR = 9.99 (weight in kg) + 6.25 (height in cm) − 4.92 (age in years) − 161

Where BEE = basal energy expenditure and RMR = resting metabolic rate

PERFORMANCE OF INDIRECT CALORIMETRY

The best means to determine nutritional requirements is to measure energy expenditure by indirect calorimetry. Indirect calorimetry uses measurements of gas exchange parameters (oxygen [O_2] consumption and CO_2 production) to indirectly, but accurately, predict energy expenditure. The physiologic principles that underlie conventional respiratory indirect calorimetry relate to the abbreviated Weir equation (REE = [3.94 × O_2 consumption] + [1.11 × CO_2 production]).[67] Indirect calorimetry has been shown to be as accurate as the large-chamber direct calorimeters, with the mean difference between the two methods for measuring REE at less than 3%.[66] Modern computerized portable instruments that are relatively inexpensive have facilitated the performance of indirect calorimetry in the critical care setting.

A slight modification of the principles of respiratory indirect calorimetry has led to the use and development of circulatory indirect calorimetry, in which the reverse Fick equation is used to derive O_2 consumption from cardiac output and arteriovenous O_2 difference using a Swan-Ganz catheter. A standard default RQ then is used with the O_2 consumption to calculate the REE. Multiple studies have shown that although measurements from both methods correlate significantly, the REE value obtained from the circulatory indirect calorimetry may underestimate the value obtained by respiratory indirect calorimetry by as much as 15%.[68-73] (The difference reflects the fact that the circulatory indirect calorimetry does not measure or account for the O_2 consumption by the pulmonary system.)

A number of routine steps should be taken to optimize test conditions at the time of an indirect calorimetric study.[74,75] Patients should be tested in a quiet thermoneutral environment, and interruptions should be avoided. Patients receiving an oral diet should be fasted after midnight the night before, and patients not receiving continuous enteral or parenteral feedings should be switched to continuous infusion (which is maintained through the time of the testing). Standard physician orders are helpful and should alert staff and support personnel to the time of testing. Ventilator settings should not be changed for 90 minutes before the test, and any sedatives or analgesics should be administered 1 hour before the test. Patients with end-stage renal disease should not be tested on the day of hemodialysis. During hemodialysis, CO_2 is lost across the dialysate membrane, rendering REE and RQ measurements inaccurate. A multidisciplinary team that can be assembled to interpret results is a key factor in the success of an indirect calorimetry program.

The respiratory therapist must pay attention to a number of details when the patient on mechanical ventilation undergoes indirect calorimetry.[74,75] The patient should be prepared by carefully suctioning the tracheostomy tube and ensuring a good seal on the cuff. Stability of the inspired O_2 is essential for success of the measurement. This can be accomplished in two ways. In the first, the source of O_2 from the wall is attached to an external O_2 blender. This, however. requires interruption of ventilation and may unsettle the patient. A simpler method of achieving FIO_2 stability is placing an inspiratory mixing chamber (usually an empty humidifier chamber) between the ventilator and the patient's humidifier. This can be connected at the same time that an inspiratory sample line is placed, eliminating the need to disrupt ventilation. This system is shown in Figure 11-1.[76] The requirements for successful measurement of energy expenditure using indirect calorimetry are shown in Box 11-3.

BOX 11-3 *Requirements for Successful Measurement of Energy Expenditure Using Indirect Calorimetry*

Technical

- Stable FIO_2
- $FIO_2 < 0.60$ (FIO_2 0.60-0.80 is less reliable, >0.80 should be avoided)
- No leaks in the system (ventilator circuit, tracheal tube cuff, chest tubes)
- No changes in minute ventilation or FIO_2 over the last 4 hours

Patient Related

- Patient awake and aware of his or her surroundings
- If bolus feeding is used, measure 1 hour after feeding
- If feeding is continuous, it should remain on during the measurement
- Study should not be performed during hemodialysis
- Routine nursing procedures should be avoided during measurement
- A period of 4-6 hours after surgery should be allowed before measurement (elimination of anesthetic gases)

Indirect calorimeters should be calibrated carefully before testing with regard to the gas analyzers and volume transducers. Gas analyzers may be tested against reference tanks of known gas concentrations, and volume transducers usually are tested with a standard 3-L syringe. Further validation of instrument results may be done by using the indirect calorimeters to measure the RQ from a methanol-burning kit (which can be performed only on certain models) or by placing the indirect calorimeter on an artificial lung machine (which simulates O_2 consumption and CO_2 production).

Once indirect calorimetry is initiated, the end point of testing is achievement of **steady state**, defined by variation of the O_2 consumption and CO_2

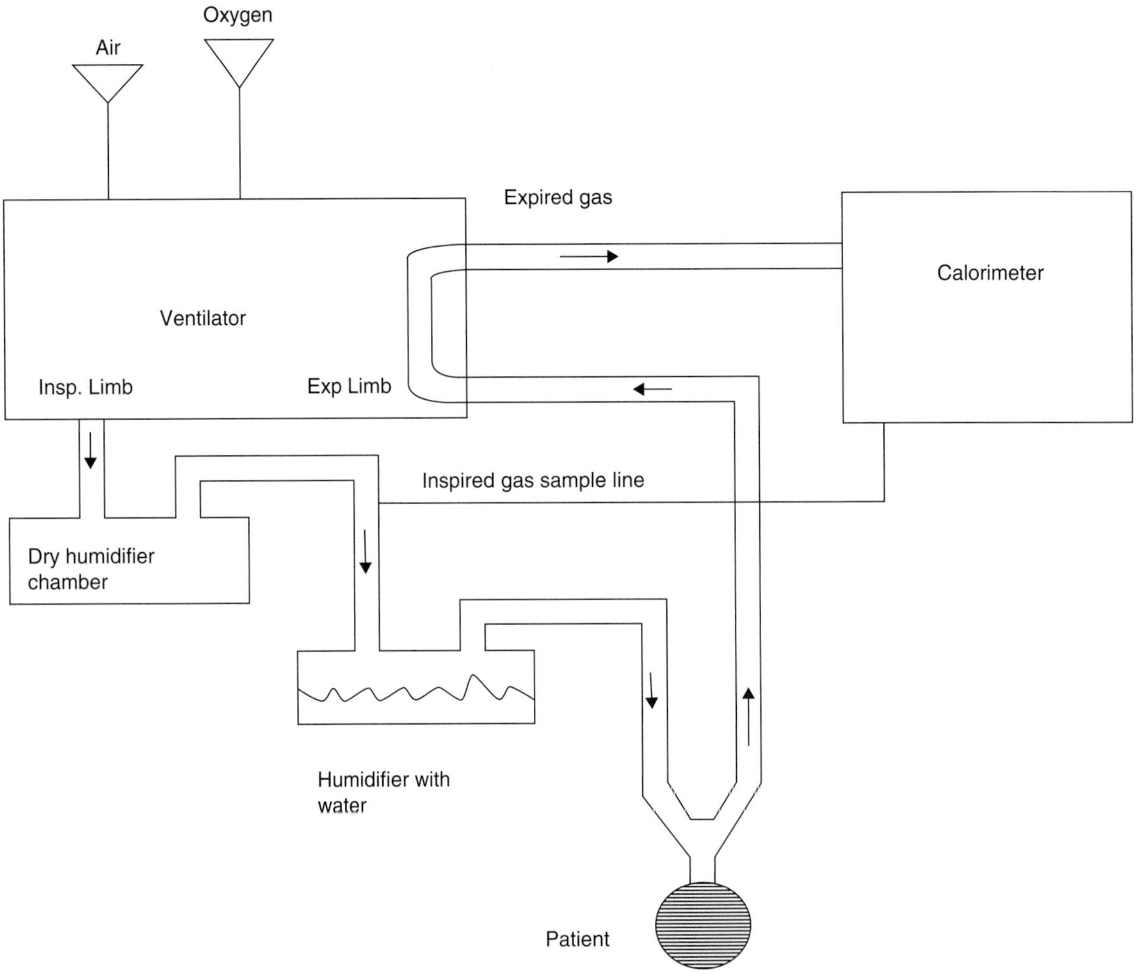

FIGURE 11-1 Setup of an indirect calorimeter and mechanical ventilator for the measurement of energy expenditure. The dry humidifier chamber acts as an inspiratory mixing chamber to stabilize the delivered O_2 concentration.

production by less than 10%, and RQ by less than 5% over a consecutive 5-minute interval.[50,51,77-81] Extrapolating test results from this brief steady-state period out over 24 hours provides an adequate measure of caloric expenditure.[78] However, when the critically ill patient is tested, it may be more difficult to obtain or achieve steady state. The achievement of steady state ensures a greater degree of validity of measurements. In those patients who fail to achieve steady state, however, it may be more appropriate to take a mean value for REE over the entire testing period. This value obtained still provides a valuable reference point for clinicians in determining caloric requirements.

A number of modifications may need to be made for proper interpretation of test results (Figure 11-2).[74,75] Overall validity of the test should be evaluated by confirming that none of the values for RQ fall outside the physiologic range from 0.67 to 1.3.[82] Measured RQ values outside this range are nonphysiologic, represent significant error, and indicate an invalid test. In the presence of fever, the value obtained for measured REE should be reduced by 7% for each degree above 100° F.[56] The measured REE may be compared with the Harris-Benedict predicted value to provide the clinician with a sense of the metabolic response and the degree to which the patient is hypermetabolic or hypometabolic.[44,50,52] Total energy expenditure (TEE) is calculated by adding an activity factor to the measured REE—10% for bedridden patients and 15% for ambulatory patients.[83] Most importantly, the number of calories provided by the nutrition support regimen should be compared with the caloric requirements measured by

Name________________ MR#________________
Room#____________ Study Date_________
Ordering M.D.________

We appreciate the opportunity to perform Indirect Calorimetry on ____________. Pertinent clinical information reveals a ____ year old (Male/Female) with a medical history of

____
____
____

□ Mechanical Ventilation □ Spontaneously breathing / Room air

Pertinent physical findings show that the patient's height is ____inches, ideal body weight (IBW) is ____Kg, actual body weight (ABW) is ____Kg (____% of IBW), and BMI is____. The patient was receiving ____ at the time of testing.

A. An oral diet with no indication of additional supplements and NPO at time of testing.

B. Enteral tube feedings with________________________________

C. TPN with________________________________

D. NPO for__________

Significant laboratories include:

Sodium	____mEq/L	BUN	____ml/dL	Hgb	____g/dL
Potassium	____mEq/L	Creatinine	____mg/dL	MCV	____mg/dL
Chloride	____mEq/L	Albumin	____mg/dL	PCO_2	____
Glucose	____mg/dL	WBC	____mg/dL	Triglyceride	____g/dL

Steady state was: □ Achieved during minutes ____through____ □ Not achieved during the test.

Thus the overall validity of the test was:

A. Excellent. (Steady state, as indicated by CV for VO_2 and $VCO_2 \leq 5$, or variation in VO_2 and $VCO_2 \leq$ 10%)
B. Adequate. (Steady state not reached. Though this measured REE can reliably be used to direct current nutritional therapy, retesting is recommended at a later date when patient is clinically more stable.)
C. Reduced. Results may be unreliable for the following reasons:
 □ RQ out of physiologic range
 □ VE abnormalities
 □ Drift if FIO_2
Therefore, simplistic equations to estimate needs would be recommended until test can be repeated:
25-30 Kcal/Kg actual body weight with BMI ≤ 30

FIGURE 11-2 Typical report for results of a nutritional assessment, including indirect calorimetry in a ventilated patient. *Continued*

the metabolic cart (TEE) to determine the appropriateness of current feeding.

DESIGN OF THE NUTRITION SUPPORT REGIMEN

An appropriate nutrition support regimen should meet basic requirements to fulfill the needs of the patient in respiratory failure on mechanical ventilation. The design of the nutrition support regimen and the speed with which it is initiated are determined by the level of stress and status of the gut. Measurement of caloric requirements is important to establish the goal of nutrition support with rapid advancement of the infusion rate to meet that goal. The nutrition support regimen should provide a mixed fuel regimen, should be infused through the enteral route, and must be adequate to enhance the weaning process. Finally, patients should be monitored throughout their infusion period for tolerance.

In designing the nutrition support regimen, the clinician must be aware that all three of the basic fuel substrates (carbohydrate, fat, and protein) individually can have deleterious effects on respiratory function. The individual effects of each substrate are probably much more pronounced when given by the parenteral route. With the enteral infusion of nutrients, formulas are more standardized, problems with absorption and assimilation may override theoretical problems with individual substrates, and the gut may act as its own governor, failing to absorb excesses of any one individual substrate.

The most pronounced effect on pulmonary function may come from excess caloric intake and carbohydrate infusion. The metabolism of carbohydrate is associated with a higher RQ than fat, which results

Determination of Energy Requirements Based on Indirect Calorimetry Results

Measured Respiratory Quotient (RQ): ____________

Measured Resting Energy Expenditure (REE): [ ]

Temperature at Time of Testing: ____________

REE Adjusted for Fever: ____________

Total Caloric Requirements [ ]

Kilocalories/Kg ABW: ____________

Estimated Protein Requirements
Based on: [ ]

☐ UUN Based Protein Requirements (as available)

☐ Simplistic Equations

☐ 0.8-1.1g/Kg (Non stressed) ☐ 1.2-1.5g/Kg (Moderately stressed) ☐ 1.6-2.0g/Kg (Severely stressed) ☐ other ____g/Kg

The patient was receiving ________ calories and _____g of protein from feeding at the time of indirect calorimetry assessment meeting ________% of energy requirements for weight maintenance and ________% of protein requirements.
Current Caloric Balance Based on Nutrient Provision and IC Results____________

Clinical Nutrition Recommendations:

In order to meet nutritional requirements based on the indirect calorimetry study and the goal of nutrition therapy to promote weight (maintenance/loss/gain), we would recommend:

____________ Total Calories
____________ Grams Protein Providing ____g Protein/ Kg ABW/day
Providing ____g Protein/ Kg IBW/day
____________ Estimated fluid requirements (25-35mL/Kg/day)
____________ Amount provided by formula

Therefore current nutrition therapy should be_____.

A. Maintained
B. Reduced to ____________
C. Increased to ____________
D. Adjusted by switching to ____________

Recommended water flushes: ____________

Additional comments:

Medical Nutrition Team Attending Physician ____________ Dietitian ____________ Pager:____________

FIGURE 11-2, cont'd

from greater CO_2 production. High-carbohydrate load given through the parenteral route has been shown to raise the RQ, CO_2 production, and minute ventilation to the point of actually precipitating hypercapnia, respiratory failure, and need for mechanical ventilation.[26] In one study, switching from 100% carbohydrate meal to a mixed fuel regimen (50 : 50 carbohydrate : fat ratio), CO_2 production was shown to decrease by 20% and minute ventilation by 26%.[84] Excess protein stimulates ventilatory drive and may increase the work of breathing because of its effect on increasing mean inspiratory flow, minute ventilation, and O_2 consumption.[85,86] Use of branched-chain amino acids may have an even greater effect on ventilatory drive than standard protein.[86] Theoretically, increasing protein provision may be used to stimulate ventilatory drive in weaning efforts, but pushing too hard with protein infusion in a patient with COPD (who already has an increased ventilatory drive) actually may precipitate fatigue and dyspnea.[30]

Excess infusion of fat—particularly over a short period of time—can also have a deleterious effect on respiratory function. High fat infusion actually may clog the reticuloendothelial system (RES) with deposition of fat in leukocytes and macrophages,[87-89] an effect that suppresses phagocytosis and bacterial killing. The rate of clearance of fat from the RES decreases as patient stress increases.[90,91] There may be a cumulative dose response effect on the RES over several days of fat infusion.[30] Infusion of fat may lead to increased mean pulmonary artery pressure, increased shunting, increased pulmonary vascular resistance, increased vasoconstrictive response, and decreased arterial partial pressure of O_2 (PaO_2).[92] Lipid-induced hyperlipemia actually can decrease pulmonary diffusion capacity.[93] Hyperlipemia may cause ventilation/perfusion inequalities, with decreases in the ratio of $PaO_2 : FIO_2$, increases in the O_2 gradient, and pulmonary shunting.[94] A key concept in the infusion of lipids, particularly through the parenteral route, is to feed "low and slow." Many of these effects on the respiratory system can be prevented by using lower concentrations of fat infused over the entire 24-hour period.[95] Prolonged infusion of low concentrations of fat avoids lipemia, reduces clogging of the RES, and may enhance clearance and use.[30]

The basic principles by which to design the nutritional regimen partly depend on the type of pulmonary disease process that necessitated the mechanical ventilation.[1] Patients maintained on mechanical ventilation because of respiratory muscle dysfunction or patients with hypoxemic respiratory failure may tolerate a fairly standard enteral formula or a parenteral regimen.[1] In these patients, a standard substrate profile is appropriate, with fat making up 20% to 30% of the calories, carbohydrates 40% to 50%, and protein the remainder. In patients with hypercapnic respiratory failure, however, the problems with excess carbohydrate infusion and consequent increases in CO_2 production must be avoided. In these patients, fat should make up a greater percentage of the nonprotein calories such that an overall profile with 40% fat, 40% carbohydrate, and 20% protein calories is more appropriate.[1]

The route of feeding is extremely important in the critical care setting. When compared with the parenteral route of feeding, early enteral feeding has been shown to decrease the overall stress response, hyperglycemia, and REE, and actually increase visceral protein levels.[33,35] Early enteral feeding decreases the cost of nutrition support and is associated with decreases in nosocomial infection, multiple-organ failure, length of hospitalization, and mortality when compared with the parenteral route.[33,35,96] Enteral feeding may provide the added benefit of stress ulcer prophylaxis in the patient on mechanical ventilation.[30] In an older retrospective study, Pingleton and Hadzima demonstrated significantly less evidence of GI bleeding in patients placed on enteral feeding when compared with patients placed on acid-reducing therapy or sucralfate (Carafate).[93] In a group of patients in the intensive care unit (ICU), the duodenal infusion of an enteral formula was shown to increase gastric pH with no change in serum gastrin levels when compared with the duodenal infusion of saline, an effect that was interpreted as providing some degree of stress prophylaxis.[97,98]

Standardization of enteral formulas avoids some of the problems seen with the infinite variations that occurred in the past with parenteral regimens. Specific pulmonary formulas are characterized by having increased protein and a lower carbohydrate : fat ratio (in which the ratio of carbohydrate : fat is decreased from 70:30 to 50:50). In one prospective randomized trial, patients treated with Pulmocare were shown to require an average of 62 fewer hours on mechanical ventilation and demonstrated a decrease of 16% in their $PaCO_2$ when compared with controls.[99] Use of pulmonary formulas has been criticized because of failure to show any impact on actual patient outcome. This criticism may not be warranted because these formulas are inexpensive (costing less than 20% more than standard formulas) and have a substrate profile that makes physiologic sense for use in the patient on mechanical ventilation. High-fat enteral formulas are sometimes associated with bloating, abdominal cramping, and diarrhea in some patients.

More recently a specific enteral formula for the mechanically ventilated patient with acute respiratory distress syndrome (ARDS) has been introduced.[100-105] This formula (Oxepa, Ross Laboratories, Columbus, Ohio) relies on the use of anti-inflammatory specific fatty acids to modulate the inflammatory response. Fatty acids such as eicosapentaenoic acid (EPA; omega-3 fatty acid, 20 : 5n3) have been used successfully to dampen inflammation in several chronic diseases (e.g., Crohn's disease, ulcerative colitis, coronary artery disease, and rheumatoid arthritis). Arachidonic acid (AA) (omega-6 fatty acid, 20 : 4n-6) and its metabolites are central in inflammation. AA is an integral component of immune cell membranes and, once mobilized by phospholipase A2 during inflammation, is metabolized by cyclooxygenase to proinflammatory mediators, such as prostaglandin E2 and thromboxane A2 (Figure 11-3). These prostanoids cause inflammation, immune suppression, and chemotaxis and promote platelet aggregation, microvascular thrombosis, and the production of proinflammatory cytokines, all factors identified as playing a role in the development of ARDS.

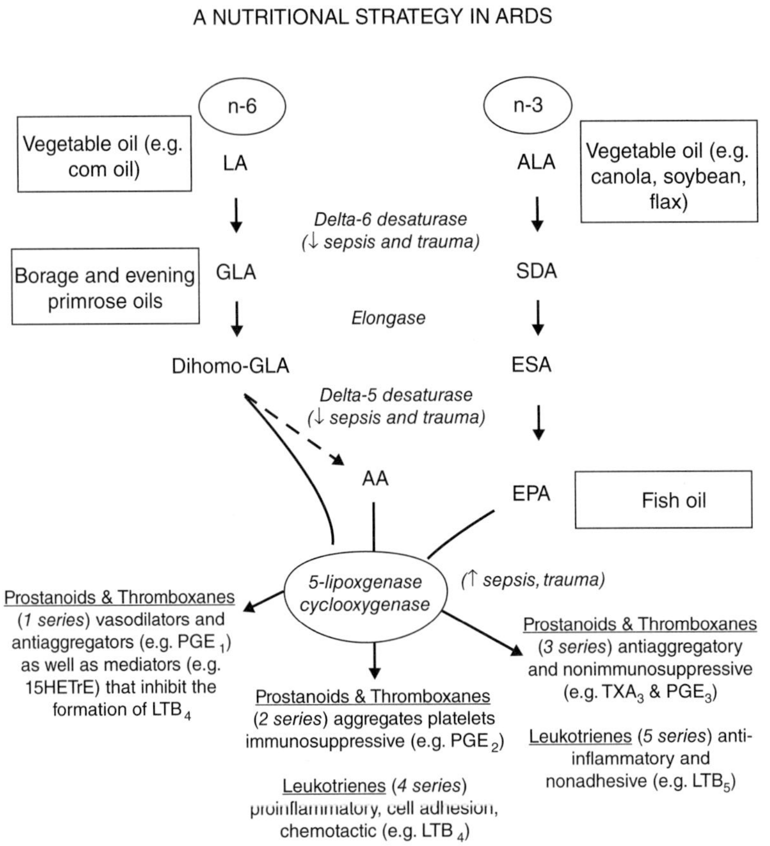

FIGURE 11-3 Pathways and enzymes of n-6 and n-3 polyunsaturated acid families. *AA,* Arachidonic acid; *ALA,* α-linolenic acid; *SDA,* stearidonic acid; *EPA,* eicosapentaenoic acid; *ES,* eicosatetraenoic acid; *GLA,* linolenic acid; *LA,* linoleic acid; *LTB_4,* leukotriene B_4; *PG,* prostaglandin; *TXA_3,* thromboxane A_3; *15HETrE,* 15-hydroxyeicosatrienoic acid.

Similarly, AA can be metabolized by 5-lipoxygenase to produce proinflammatory leukotriene B_4 (LTB_4), which increases cell adhesion and chemoattractive factors (see Figure 11-3). EPA can displace AA in immune cell membranes, and its metabolites (through cyclooxygenase and 5-lipoxygenase) have primarily anti-inflammatory activity and inhibit platelet aggregation (e.g., prostaglandin E_3, thromboxane A3, and LTB_5). Furthermore, prostaglandins from EPA (e.g., prostaglandin E_3) that is derived from AA also lack the immunosuppressive activity of prostaglandin E_2.

Gadek and colleagues[100] performed the first trial assessing the effects of EPA plus linoleic acid (GLA) on clinical pathophysiology and outcomes in patients who had ARDS. Patients receiving the EPA-plus-GLA diet for at least 4 to 7 days had reduced pulmonary inflammation as evidenced by a drop in the number of neutrophils in bronchoalveolar lavage (BAL) fluid compared with control patients fed a standard diet. Arterial oxygenation was also improved. The important clinical benefits observed in patients given EPA plus GLA were a significant reduction in ventilator days and ICU days and a decrease in supplemental O_2 days, as compared with controls. In addition, patients fed EPA plus GLA had significantly fewer new organ failures during the study period, suggesting that this diet had the ability to modulate systemic inflammation that contributes to organ failure.

Follow-up studies have also shown improved oxygenation and ICU-free days compared with patients fed the control standard diet. In young, critically ill burn victims who had respiratory failure, Oxepa was found to be safe, well tolerated and facilitated recovery with improvements in oxygenation and pulmonary compliance. Improvements in survival were noted in patients receiving EPA plus GLA when compared with National Burn Repository statistics.

One of the most consistent findings in the clinical studies of the EPA-plus-GLA diet is the significant improvements in gas exchange and the resultant improvements in ventilatory and oxygenation variables. These studies suggest that a specialized diet containing EPA plus GLA and elevated antioxidants can modulate pulmonary and systemic inflammation in a heterogeneous (ALI, ARDS, severe sepsis, and septic shock) collection of ICU patients. The use of a specialized nutritional formula containing EPA plus GLA and elevated antioxidants offers physiologic and anti-inflammatory benefits over standard formulas.

These findings are limited by the relatively small numbers of patients and are often criticized for use of an inappropriate control. Additionally, it has been suggested that the changes in inflammation may be solely derived from the additional antioxidants (vitamins A and E). Further large randomized trials using an isocaloric regimen are needed before considering Oxepa a standard formula for ARDS.

MONITORING RESPONSE AND PATIENT TOLERANCE

Fear of aspiration is often the greatest concern for clinicians when feeding patients through the enteral route in the critical care setting. The actual risk of aspiration, however, is overemphasized and should never limit the use of early enteral feeding in the ICU. Evidence of subclinical aspiration, in which gastric contents pass up into the esophagus or into the tracheal secretions, has been shown to occur in 36% to 44% of patients.[106,107] However, the actual development of pneumonia with an infiltrate on chest radiograph, fever, and need for antibiotics occurs in only 1% to 4% of patients.[106,107] The true risk of significant aspiration pneumonia is related more to misplacement of an enteral feeding tube into the lungs than it is to aspiration of gastric contents from a tube placed properly in the GI tract. Specific risk factors, which have been identified as increasing the risk of aspiration, include age older than 70 years, decreasing level of consciousness, location in the hospital (transfer from the ICU to a general ward), supine patient position, bolus style of infusion, increasing diameter of the feeding tube, and position of the feeding tube in the GI tract. Patients determined to be at high risk for aspiration on the basis of these factors should be managed by using the reverse Trendelenburg position, switching from bolus to continuous infusion of nutrients, placing the tube at or below the ligament of Treitz, adding metoclopramide monohydrochloride monohydrate (Reglan) or cisapride (Propulsid) to promote gastric emptying, and even switching to a combination tube that allows simultaneous aspiration and decompression of the stomach while feeding distally into the jejunum.

A number of clinical parameters should be followed in treating the patient on enteral feeding. Although it is important to monitor residual volumes, they are an imprecise measure of gastric emptying. High residual volumes are often a single isolated event in patients otherwise tolerating their enteral feeding. Residual volumes have been shown to correlate poorly with physical examinations and abdominal radiographs.[106] The value of concern should be no less than 200 to 400 ml. The management of patients who demonstrate high residual volumes should be to hold feedings, if concerned, only after the second residual volume above 200 ml. Feedings should be held for 2 hours before rechecking. If the patient demonstrates persistently high residual volumes over 8 to 12 hours, efforts should be made to place the tube at or below the ligament of Treitz. Above all, clinical judgment should be used in interpreting residual volumes. Low residual volumes do not always guarantee adequate tolerance, and high residual volumes in the patient who is passing gas and stool with no nausea or vomiting may be of little concern.[107]

Diarrhea is a frequent problem in the ICU, but it is only rarely directly related to the tube feedings. Prospective studies evaluating the cause of diarrhea in this setting reveal that the diarrhea is related to sorbitol in medications in 51% of cases, related to pseudomembranous colitis and *Clostridium difficile* in 17%, and only directly related to the feeding formula in 21% of cases.[107] Low-volume diarrhea in the ICU setting is often more a problem with incontinence, and rectal tubes or ostomy bags should be used readily. All patients should be evaluated to determine the cause of the diarrhea. Stool studies should be obtained to rule out *C. difficile* infection, and medications should be reviewed to eliminate ingestion of sorbitol. Switching from standard formula to a small peptide formula may enhance assimilation and reduce the volume of stool output.

In general, the greatest problem to avoid is cessation of tube feedings.[108] "Down time" from enteral feeding may be reduced by avoiding placement of patients NPO after midnight for routine procedures and diagnostic testing. Feedings often can be continued up to within 4 hours of a procedure without a deleterious affect.[109] Tube displacement can be prevented by securing the tubes by bridling or placing a hemoclip on a string on the distal end of the feeding tube. Attention to hydration is warranted because adequate hydration promotes clearance of pulmonary secretions.[110] Indirect calorimetry can be used as a measure of respiratory tolerance of feeding, particularly in those patients intentionally being overfed to make up deficits. The patient whose RQ rises above 1.0 as feeding is initiated may be showing signs of pulmonary compromise and poor tolerance of the caloric load.[111]

CONCLUSIONS

Patients on mechanical ventilation allowed to experience compromise of nutritional status have fairly well-documented consequences, with respiratory muscle dysfunction, atrophy of respiratory muscle mass, and even structural changes of emphysema.[1] Providing adequate calories to meet requirements, especially through the enteric route, should be expected to help contain the stress response and promote weaning from the ventilator, and may help to reduce in-hospital complications, overall cost, and length of hospitalization.[33,35] Indirect calorimetry is the most accurate means to determine the caloric goal, and careful attention to technique is important. The efforts of the nutritionist in managing the patient with respiratory failure on mechanical ventilation should be to assess the level of stress and status of the gut, to achieve enteral access and maintain gut integrity, to determine caloric requirements by indirect calorimetry, to establish the goal of nutrition support, to monitor feedings closely, and to anticipate problems before they occur.

KEY POINTS

- Malnutrition is a common finding in patients with chronic lung disease.
- Malnutrition in chronic lung disease is associated with worsening lung function and mortality.
- Elevated energy requirements, co-morbid conditions, and decreased intake all contribute to malnutrition in chronic lung disease.
- Overfeeding is associated with an increase in CO_2 production and required minute ventilation.
- Indirect calorimetry is one tool in the nutritional assessment of the mechanically ventilated patient.
- High-fat, low-carbohydrate diets are effective at reducing ventilatory requirements in patients with hypercapnia.
- Manipulation of fatty acids may reduce inflammation and speed recovery from acute respiratory failure.

ASSESSMENT QUESTIONS

1. What variables are measured by an indirect calorimeter to determine resting energy expenditure?

I. O_2 consumption
II. Inspired and expired O_2 concentration
III. Inspired and expired CO_2 concentration
IV. Minute volume
V. Inspired and expired nitrogen concentration

A. II, III, and IV
B. II, III, and V
C. I and IV
D. All of the above

2. True or False. The accuracy of indirect calorimetry increases as FIO_2 increases.

3. Calories in excess of needs result in lipogenesis and an increase in:

A. O_2 consumption.
B. CO_2 production.
C. minute ventilation.
D. all of the above.

4. Malnutrition is associated with what changes in lung function?

I. Reduced muscle strength
II. Increased response to hypoxemia and hypercapnia
III. Increased surfactant production
IV. Increased risk of infection

A. I and IV
B. I and III
C. I, III, and IV
D. All of the above

ASSESSMENT QUESTIONS—cont'd

5. Malnutrition in chronic lung disease may result from which of the following?
- **A.** Increased energy requirement due to the O_2 cost of breathing
- **B.** Decreased intake owing to dental and gastrointestinal disease
- **C.** A chronic inflammatory state
- **D.** The effect of β-agonists
- **E.** All of the above

6. Which of the following variables render measurement of energy expenditure with indirect calorimetry inaccurate?
- **I.** Air leak through a chest tube
- **II.** Unstable FIO_2
- **III.** Minute ventilation <10 L/min
- **IV.** Peak airway pressure of >30 cm H_2O
  - **A.** I, II, and III
  - **B.** I, III, and IV
  - **C.** I and II
  - **D.** All of the above

7. High carbohydrate intake is associated with excess CO_2 production when
- **A.** isocaloric calories are provided.
- **B.** calories in lieu of patient needs are provided.
- **C.** calories in excess of patient demand are provided.
- **D.** Always

8. High-fat formulas in patients with chronic lung disease have been shown to decrease CO_2 production and reduce minute ventilation requirements under the following conditions:
- **A.** Patients with baseline hypoxemia
- **B.** Patients with baseline hypocarbia
- **C.** Patients with normal blood gases
- **D.** Patients with baseline hypercarbia

REFERENCES

1. Grant JP: Nutrition care of patients with acute and chronic respiratory failure, Nutr Clin Pract 9:11-17, 1994.
2. McClave SA: The consequences of overfeeding and underfeeding: indirect calorimetry plays a key role in designing nutrition regimens for mechanically ventilated patients, J Respir Care Pract Apr/May:57-64, 1997.
3. Cote CG: Surrogates of mortality in chronic obstructive pulmonary disease, Am J Med 119(10 Suppl 1): 54-62, 2006.
4. Weissman C, Askanazi J, Rosenbaum S et al: Amino acids and respiration, Ann Intern Med 98:41-44, 1983.
5. Doekel RC Jr, Zwillich CW, Scoggin CH et al: Clinical semi-starvation: depression of hypoxic ventilatory response, N Engl J Med 295:358-361, 1976.
6. Arora NS, Rochester DF: Effect of body weight and muscularity on human diaphragm muscle mass, thickness, and area, J Appl Physiol 52:64-70, 1982.
7. Keys A, Brozek J, Henschel A et al: The biology of human starvation, Minneapolis: University of Minnesota Press, 1950.
8. Arora NS, Rochester DF: Respiratory muscle strength and maximal voluntary ventilation in undernourished patients, Am Rev Respir Dis 126:5-8, 1982.
9. Braun NM, Arora NS, Rochester DF: Respiratory muscle and pulmonary function in polymyositis and other proximal myopathies, Thorax 38:616-623, 1983.
10. Whittaker JC, Ryan CF, Buckley PA et al: The effects of refeeding on peripheral and respiratory muscle function in malnourished chronic obstructive pulmonary disease patients, Am Rev Respir Dis 142:283-288, 1990.
11. Niederman MS, Merrill WW, Ferranti RD et al: Nutritional status and bacterial binding in the lower respiratory tract in patients with chronic tracheostomy, Ann Intern Med 100:795-800, 1984.
12. Niderman MS, Mantovani R, Schoch P et al: Patterns and routes of tracheobronchial colonization in mechanically ventilated patients: the role of nutritional status in colonization of the lower airway by *Pseudomonas* species, Chest 95:155-161, 1989.
13. Windsor JA, Hill GL: Risk factors for postoperative pneumonia: the importance of protein depletion, Ann Surg 208:209-214, 1988.
14. Sahebjami H, Wirman JA: Emphysema-like changes in the lungs of starved rats, Am Rev Respir Dis 124:619-624, 1981.
15. Stein J, Fenigstein H: Anatomic pathologique de la maladie de famine. In: Apfelbaum E, editor: Maladie de famine. Rescherches cliniques sur la famine executees dans le ghetto de Varsovie en 1942. Warsaw: American Joint Distribution Committee, 1946, pp 21-77.
16. Braun SR, Dixon RM, Keim NL et al: Predictive clinical value of nutritional assessment factors in COPD, Chest 85:353-357, 1984.
17. Bassili HR, Deitel M: Effect of nutritional support on weaning patients off mechanical ventilators, JPEN J Parenter Enteral Nutr 5:161-163, 1981.
18. Mattar JA, Velasco IT, Esgalb AS: Parenteral nutrition as a useful method of weaning patients from

mechanical ventilation, JPEN J Parenter Enteral Nutr 2:50, 1978.
19. Elwyn DH, Kinney JM, Malayappa J et al: Influence of increasing carbohydrate intake on glucose kinetics in injured patients, Ann Surg 190:117-127, 1979.
20. Burke JF, Wolfe RR, Mullany CJ et al: Glucose requirements following burn injury: parameters of optimal glucose infusion and possible hepatic and respiratory abnormalities following excessive glucose intake, Ann Surg 190:274-285, 1969.
21. Heymsfield SB, Hill JO, Evert M et al: Energy expenditure during continuous intragastric infusion of fuel, Am J Clin Nutr 45:526-533, 1987.
22. Askanazi J, Carpentier YA, Elwyn DH et al: Influence of total parenteral nutrition on fuel utilization in injury and sepsis, Ann Surg 191:40-46, 1980.
23. Swinamer DL, Grace MG, Hamilton SM et al: Predictive equation for assessing energy expenditure in mechanically ventilated critically ill patients, Crit Care Med 18:657-661, 1990.
24. Talpers SS, Romberger DJ, Bunce SB et al: Nutritionally associated increased carbon dioxide production: excess total calories vs high proportion of carbohydrate calories, Chest 102:551-555, 1992.
25. Covelli HD, Black JW, Olsen MS, Beekman JF: Respiratory failure precipitated by high carbohydrate loads, Ann Intern Med 95:579-581, 1981.
26. Askanazi J, Rosenbaum SH, Hyman AI et al: Respiratory changes induced by the large glucose loads of total parenteral nutrition, JAMA 243:1444-1447, 1980.
27. Amene P, Sladen R, Feeley T et al: Hypercapnia during total parenteral nutrition with hypertonic dextrose, Crit Care Med 15:171-172, 1987.
28. Liposkey JM, Nelson LD: Ventilatory response to high caloric loads in critically ill patients, Crit Care Med 22:796-802, 1994.
29. McClave SA, Lowen CC, Kleber MJ et al: Is the respiratory quotient a useful indicator of over- or underfeeding? JPEN J Parenter Enteral Nutr 21:S113, 1997.
30. Mowatt-Larssen CA, Brown RO: Specialized nutritional support in respiratory disease, Clin Pharm 12:276-292, 1993.
31. Grant JP: Nutritional assessment in clinical practice, Nutr Clin Pract 1:3-11, 1986.
32. Fleck A: Acute phase response: implications for nutrition and recovery, Nutrition 4:109-117, 1988.
33. Kudsk KA, Croce MA, Fabian RC et al: Enteral versus parenteral feeding—effects on septic morbidity after blunt and penetrating abdominal trauma, Ann Surg 215:503-511, 1992.
34. Baxter JK, Babineau TJ, Apovian CM et al: Perioperative glucose control predicts increased nosocomial infection in diabetics, Crit Care Med 18:S207, 1990.
35. Zaloga GP, MacGregory DA: What to consider when choosing enteral or parenteral nutrition, J Crit Illness 5:1180-1200, 1990.
36. Knaus WA, Zimmerman JE, Wagner DP et al: APACHE—Acute Physiology and Chronic Health Evaluation: a physiologically based classification system, Crit Care Med 9:591-597, 1981.
37. Knaus WA, Draper EA, Wagner DP et al: APACHE II: a severity of disease classification system, Crit Care Med 13:818-829, 1985.
38. Knaus WA, Wagner DP, Draper EA et al: The APACHE III prognostic system: risk prediction of hospital mortality for critically ill hospitalized adults, Chest 100:1619-1636, 1991.
39. Brown PE, McClave SA, Hoy NW et al: The Acute Physiology and Chronic Health Evaluation II classification system is a valid marker for physiologic stress in the critically ill patient, Crit Care Med 21:363-367, 1993.
40. Fiaccadori E, Del Canale S, Coffrini E et al: Hypercapnic-hypoxemic chronic obstructive pulmonary disease (COPD): influence of severity of COPD on nutritional status, Am J Clin Nutr 48:680-685, 1988.
41. Driver AG, McAlevy MT, Smith JL: Nutritional assessment of patients with chronic obstructive pulmonary disease and acute respiratory failure, Chest 82:568-571, 1982.
42. Morrison NJ, Richardson J, Dunn L et al: Respiratory muscle performance in normal elderly subjects and patients with COPD, Chest 95:90-94, 1989.
43. McClave SA, Snider HL: Understanding the metabolic response to critical illness: factors that cause patients to deviate from the expected pattern of hypermetabolism, New Horiz 2:139-146, 1994.
44. Weissman C, Kemper M, Askanazi J et al: Resting metabolic rate of the critically ill patient: measured versus predicted, J Anesthesiol 64:673-679, 1986.
45. Weissman C, Kemper M, Damask MC et al: Effect of routine intensive care interactions on metabolic rate, Chest 86:815-818, 1984.
46. Schols AM, Fredrix E, Soeters PB et al: Resting energy expenditure in patients with chronic obstructive pulmonary disease, Am J Clin Nutr 54:983-987, 1991.
47. Schols AM, Soeters PB, Mostert R et al: Energy balance in chronic obstructive pulmonary disease, Am Rev Respir Dis 413:1246-1252, 1991.
48. Goldstein SA, Thomashow BM, Kvetan V et al: Nitrogen and energy relationships in malnourished patients with emphysema, Am Rev Respir Dis 138:636-644, 1988.
49. Goldstein S, Askanazi J, Weissman C et al: Energy expenditure in patients with chronic obstructive pulmonary disease, Chest 91:222-224, 1987.
50. Feurer ID, Crosby LO, Mullen JL: Measured and predicted resting energy expenditure in clinically stable patients, Clin Nutr 3:27-34, 1984.
51. Makk LJK, McClave SA, Creech PW et al: Clinical application of the metabolic cart to the delivery of total parenteral nutrition, Crit Care Med 18:1320-1327, 1990.
52. Van Lanschot JJB, Feenstra BWA, Vermeij CG et al: Calculation versus measurement of total energy expenditure, Crit Care Med 14:981-985, 1986.
53. Kreymann G, Grosser S, Buggisch P et al: Oxygen consumption and resting metabolic rate in sepsis,

sepsis syndrome, and septic shock, Crit Care Med 21:1012-1019, 1993.
54. Abraham E, Bland RD, Cobo JC et al: Sequential cardiorespiratory patterns associated with outcome in septic shock, Chest 85:75-80, 1984.
55. Foster GD, Knox LS, Dempsey DT et al: Caloric requirements in total parenteral nutrition, J Am Coll Nutr 6:231-253, 1987.
56. Grant JP: Handbook of Total Parenteral Nutrition, Philadelphia: Saunders, 1975, pp 12-26.
57. Elwyn DH, Kinney JM, Askanazi J: Energy expenditure in surgical patients, Surg Clin North Am 61:545-556, 1981.
58. Long CL, Schaffel N, Geiger JW et al: Metabolic response to injury and illness: estimation of energy and protein needs from indirect calorimetry and nitrogen balance, JPEN J Parenter Enteral Nutr 3:452-456, 1979.
59. Ireton-Jones CS, Turner WW Jr, Liepa GU et al: Equations for the estimation of energy expenditures in patients with burns with special reference to ventilatory status, J Burn Care Rehabil 13:330-333, 1992.
60. Owen OE, Colliver JA, Schrage JP: Adult human energy requirements, Front Clin Nutr 2:1-8, 1993.
61. Swinamer DL, Grace MG, Hamilton SM et al: Predictive equation for assessing energy expenditure in mechanically ventilated critically ill patients, Crit Care Med 18:657-661, 1990.
62. Baker JP, Detsky AS, Stewart S et al: Randomized trial of total parenteral nutrition in critically ill patients: metabolic effects of varying glucose-lipid ratios as the energy source, Gastroenterology 87:53, 1984.
63. Cunningham JJ: Factors contributing to increased energy expenditure in thermal injury: a review of studies employing indirect calorimetry, JPEN J Parenter Enteral Nutr 14:649-656, 1990.
64. Leff ML, Hill JO, Yates AA et al: Resting metabolic rate: measurement reliability, JPEN J Parenter Enteral Nutr 11:354-359, 1987.
65. McClave SA, Kaiser SC, Olash BM et al: Variation in resting energy expenditure for normals over a two year period of study, Gastroenterology 100: A536, 1991.
66. Daly JM, Heymsfield SB, Head CA et al: Human energy requirements: overestimation by widely used prediction equation, Am J Clin Nutr 42:1170-1174, 1985.
67. Weir JB: New methods for calculating metabolic rate with special reference to protein metabolism, J Physiol 109:1-9, 1949.
68. Williams RR, Fuenning CR: Circulatory indirect calorimetry in the critically ill, JPEN J Parenter Enteral Nutr 15:509-512, 1991.
69. Smithies MN, Royston B, Makita K et al: Comparison of oxygen consumption measurements: indirect calorimetry versus the reversed Fick method, Crit Care Med 19:1401-1406, 1991.
70. Takala J, Keinanen O, Vaisanen P et al: Measurement of gas exchange in intensive care: laboratory and clinical validation of a new device, Crit Care Med 17:1041-1047, 1989.
71. Liggett SB, St. John RE, Lefrak SS: Determination of resting energy expenditure utilizing the thermodilution pulmonary artery catheter, Chest 91:562-566, 1987.
72. Walsh BJ, Murley TF: Comparison of three methods of determining oxygen consumption and resting energy expenditure, J Am Osteopath Assoc 89:43-46, 1989.
73. Levinson MR, Groeger JS, Miodownik S et al: Indirect calorimetry in mechanically ventilated patients, Crit Care Med 154:144-147, 1987.
74. McClave SA, Snider HL: Use of indirect calorimetry in clinical nutrition, Nutr Clin Pract 7:207-221, 1992.
75. McClave SA, Snider HL, Greene L et al: Effective utilization of indirect calorimetry during critical care, Intensive Care World 9:194-200, 1992.
76. Branson RD, Johannigman JA: The measurement of energy expenditure, Nutr Clin Pract 19:622-636, 2004.
77. Zavala DC: In: Nutritional Assessment in Critical Care: A Training Handbook. Iowa City, 1989, University of Iowa Press, pp 41-59.
78. Frankenfield DC, Sarson GY, Blosser SA et al: Validation of a 5-minute steady state indirect calorimetry protocol for resting energy expenditure in critically ill patients, J Am Coll Nutr 15:397-402, 1996.
79. Cunningham KF, Aeberhardt LE, Wiggs BR et al: Appropriate interpretation of indirect calorimetry for determining energy expenditure in intensive care units, Am J Surg 167:54-57, 1994.
80. Smyrnios NA, Curley FJ, Shaker KG: Accuracy of 30-minute indirect calorimetry studies in predicting 24-hour energy expenditure in mechanically ventilated, critically ill patients, JPEN J Parenter Enteral Nutr 21:168-174, 1997.
81. Isbell TR, Klesges RC, Meyers AW et al: Measurement reliability and reactivity using repeated measurements of resting energy expenditure with a face mask, mouthpiece, and ventilated canopy, JPEN J Parenter Enteral Nutr 15:165-168, 1991.
82. Branson RD: The measurement of energy expenditure: instrumentation, practical considerations, and clinical application, Respir Care 35:640-659, 1990.
83. Weissman C, Kemper M, Elwyn DH et al: The energy expenditure of the mechanically ventilated critically ill patient—an analysis, Chest 89:254-259, 1989.
84. Askanazi J, Nordenstrom J, Rosenbaum SH et al: Nutrition for the patient with respiratory failure: glucose vs. fat, Anesthesiology 54:373-377, 1981.
85. Askanazi J, Weissman C, LaSala PA et al: Effect of protein intake on ventilatory drive, Anesthesiology 60:106-110, 1984.
86. Takala J, Askanazi J, Weissman C et al: Changes in respiratory control induced by amino acid infusions, Crit Care Med 16:465-469, 1988.
87. Hamawy KJ, Moldawer LL, Georgieff M et al: The effect of lipid emulsions on reticuloendothelial system function in the injured animal, JPEN J Parenter Enteral Nutr 9:559-565, 1985.
88. Seidner DL, Mascioli EA, Istfan NW et al: Effects of long-chain triglyceride emulsions on reticuloendo-

thelial system function in humans, JPEN J Parenter Enteral Nutr 13:614-619, 1989.
89. Salo M: Inhibition of immunoglobulin synthesis in vitro by intravenous lipid emulsion (Intralipid), JPEN J Parenter Enteral Nutr 14:459-462, 1990.
90. Cerra FB, Siegel JH, Border JR et al: The hepatic failure of sepsis: cellular versus substrate, Surgery 86:409-422, 1979.
91. Lundholm M, Rossner S: Rate of elimination of the Intralipid fat emulsion from the circulation in ICU patients, Crit Care Med 10:740-746, 1982.
92. Venus B, Smith RA, Patel CB et al: Hemodynamic and gas exchange alterations during Intralipid infusion in patients with adult respiratory distress syndrome, Chest 95:1278-1281, 1989.
93. Greene HL, Hazlett D, Demaree R: Relationship between Intralipid-induced hyperlipemia and pulmonary function, Am J Clin Nutr 29:127-135, 1976.
94. Hwang TL, Huang SL, Chen MF: Effects of intravenous fat emulsion on respiratory failure, Chest 97:934-938, 1990.
95. Ota DM, Jessup JM, Babcock GF et al: Immune function during intravenous administration of a soybean oil emulsion, JPEN J Parenter Enteral Nutr 9:23-27, 1985.
96. Charash WE, Kearney PA, Annis KA et al: Early enteral feeding is associated with an attenuation of the acute phase/cytokine response following multiple trauma [abstract], J Trauma 37:1015, 1994.
97. Pingleton SK, Hadzima SK: Enteral alimentation and gastrointestinal bleeding in mechanically ventilated patients, Crit Care Med 11:13-16, 1983.
98. Layon AJ, Florete OG, Day AL et al: The effect of duodenojejunal alimentation on gastric pH and hormones in intensive care unit patients, Chest 99:695-702, 1991.
99. Al-Saady N, Blackmore C, Bennett ED: High fat, low carbohydrate enteral feeding reduced $PaCO_2$ and the period of ventilation in ventilated patients, Intensive Care Med 15:290-295, 1989.
100. Gadek JE, DeMichele SJ, Karlstad MD et al: Effect of enteral feeding with eicosapentaenoic acid, gamma-linolenic acid, and antioxidants in patients with acute respiratory distress syndrome. Enteral Nutrition in ARDS Study Group, Crit Care Med 27:1409-1420, 1999.
101. Pacht ER, DeMichele SJ, Nelson JL et al: Enteral nutrition with eicosapentaenoic acid, gamma-linolenic acid, and antioxidants reduces alveolar inflammatory mediators and protein influx in patients with acute respiratory distress syndrome, Crit Care Med 31:491-500, 2003.
102. Singer P, Theilla M, Fisher H et al: Benefit of an enteral diet enriched with eicosapentaenoic acid and gamma-linolenic acid in ventilated patients with acute lung injury, Crit Care Med 34:1033-1038, 2006.
103. Pontes-Arruda A: The effects of enteral feeding with eicosapentaenoic acid, gamma-linolenic acid and antioxidants in patients with sepsis, Crit Care 9:363, 2005.
104. Elamin E, Hughes L, Drew D: Effect of enteral nutrition with eicosapentaenoic acid (EPA), gamma-linolenic acid (GLA), and antioxidants reduces alveolar inflammatory mediators and protein influx in patients with acute respiratory distress syndrome (ARDS), Chest 128:225S, 2005.
105. Mayes T, Gottschlich M, Carman B et al: An evaluation of the safety and efficacy of an antiinflammatory, pulmonary enteral formula in the treatment of pediatric burn patients with respiratory failure, Nutr Clin Prac 20:30-31, 2005.
106. Metheny N: Minimizing respiratory complications of nasoenteric tube feedings: state of the science, Heart Lung 22:213-223, 1993.
107. Metheny N: Preventing pulmonary complications during enteral feeding in the critically ill. Program Manual, ASPEN 18th Clinical Congress, Jan 30-Feb 2, 1994, San Antonio, Tex, pp 318-322.
108. McClave SA, Snider HL, Lowen CC et al: Use of residual volume as a marker for enteral feeding intolerance: prospective blinded comparison with physical examination and radiographic findings, JPEN J Parenter Enteral Nutr 16:99-105, 1992.
109. Edes TE, Walk BE, Austin JL: Diarrhea in tube-fed patients: feeding formula not necessarily the cause, Am J Med 88:91-94, 1990.
110. McClave SA, Sexton LK, Adams JL et al: Enteral tube feeding in the intensive care unit: factors impeding adequate delivery, Gastroenterology 112:A892, 1997.
111. Chapman KM, Winter L: COPD: using nutrition to prevent respiratory function decline. Geriatrics 51:37-42, 1996.

CHAPTER

12

Sedation, Analgesia, and Neuromuscular Blockade

BRYAN A. FISK*; LISA K MOORES*

OUTLINE

OBJECTIVES

- List the reasons for patient discomfort and anxiety while on mechanical ventilation.
- Explain the importance of managing pain in the patient on mechanical ventilation.
- Discuss the importance of the management of delirium in a patient on a mechanical ventilator.
- State the indications for neuromuscular blockade in a patient on mechanical ventilation.

KEY TERMS

agitation
analgesics
anxiety
benzodiazepines
delirium
dexmedetomidine
end points
myopathy
neuromuscular blockade
nonsteroidal antiinflammatory drugs (NSAIDs)
opioids
propofol
sedation
titration
torsades de pointes
train-of-four (TOF)

*The opinions contained herein are solely those of the authors, and do not represent the opinions or policy of the United States Army or the Department of Defense.

The development of neuropsychiatric disturbances is a common problem for critically ill patients in the intensive care unit (ICU). These unpleasant sensations can have a significant impact on patient care and management when left unaddressed or undertreated. Problems that may arise include patient-ventilator dys-synchrony, self-extubation, and overaggressive behavior that may pose a threat to both the patient and health care providers. Without proper treatment, these disturbances may give rise to additional sequelae, including decreased immune responsiveness and posttraumatic stress disorder.

Various forms of neuropsychiatric disturbances are encountered in the ICU and include anxiety, delirium, pain, and agitation. **Anxiety** is a sustained

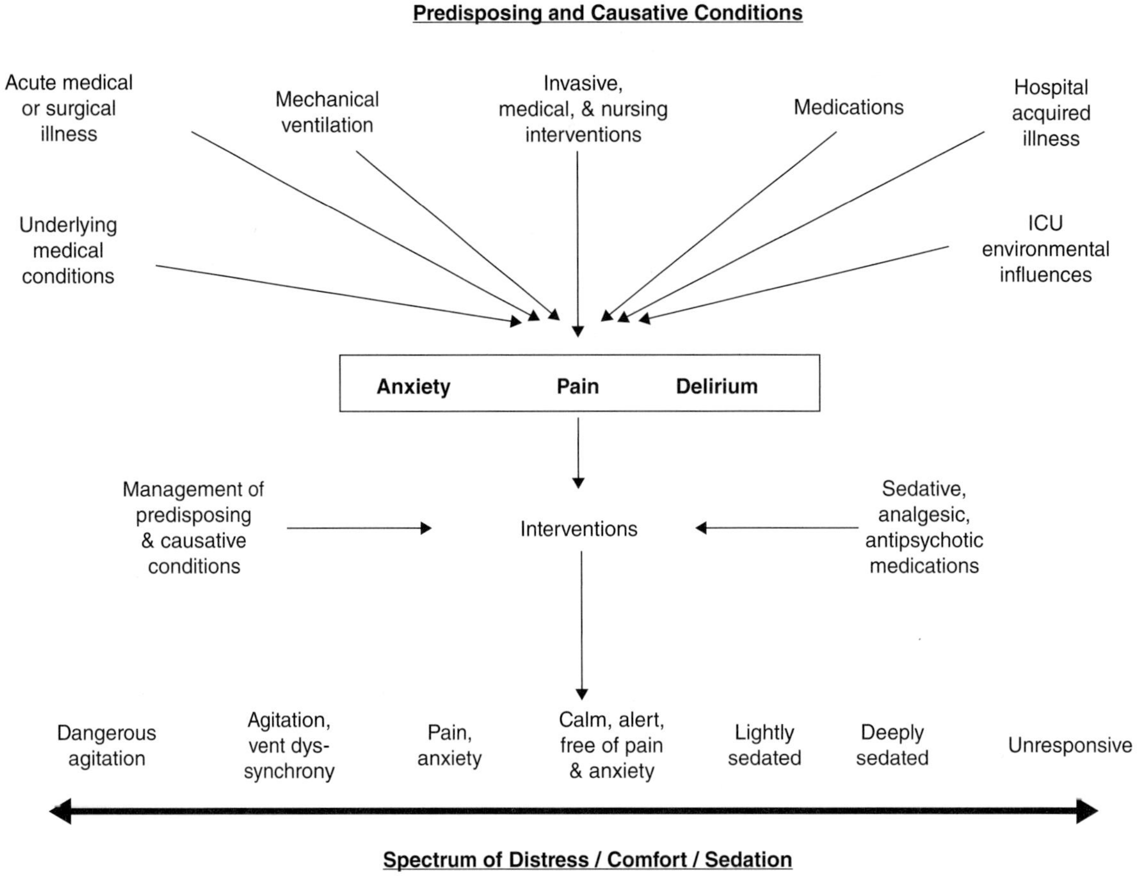

FIGURE 12-1 Overview of factors related to anxiety, pain, and delirium in ICU patients, along with management that can lead to sensations ranging from dangerous agitation to unresponsiveness. (Modified from Sessler CN, Grap MJ, Brophy GM: Multidisciplinary management of sedation and analgesia in critical care, Semin Respir Crit Care Med 22:211-226, 2001.)

state of apprehension in response to new or perceived threats. Critical illness and medications may also lead to **delirium,** which is an acute, potentially reversible impairment of consciousness and cognitive function that waxes and wanes. Physical pain or discomfort is also common, either due directly to underlying disease, trauma, surgery, or from the monitoring, diagnostic, and therapeutic interventions that are common in the ICU. Anxiety, delirium, and pain perception may all give rise to **agitation**, which is excessive motor activity associated with internal tension (Figure 12-1).

Patients who require mechanical ventilation are at particular risk of experiencing neuropsychiatric disturbances. When investigators evaluated the psychological status in a series of intubated patients, they found that 13 out of 43 patients reported intolerable pain.[1] Thus 30% of intubated patients did not receive adequate analgesics. A significant proportion also reported distress from excessive stimulation: 42% were bothered by noise and 35% by light. Additionally, 39% reported disordered sleep during their ICU stay. Anxiety and frustration were also prevalent. Fifty-eight percent expressed frustration due to the inability to communicate effectively. Fifty percent expressed having diffuse anxiety, and 40% suffered from an intense fear of dying. All of these disturbances can lead to increased agitation and may contribute to worsening of delirium. These data suggest that the recent standards of care for recognizing pain and anxiety, and initiation and monitoring effectiveness of therapy are inadequate.

The first step in the management of patient distress is to rule out any life-threatening abnormalities, particularly of the cardiac, pulmonary, and central nervous systems. Acute onset of patient distress may be a sign of myocardial ischemia, hypoxia, hypercarbia, pneumothorax, cerebral hemorrhage or infarction, an acute abdomen, or hypoglycemia. Once life-threatening causes are excluded, the next step should be the determination of the underlying cause for the neuropsychiatric disturbance, as the optimal management of pain, delirium, and anxiety is not typically the same. Attempting to simply medicate for agitation can potentially aggravate the problem if the wrong therapy is administered. Or, it may merely mask the signs without providing effective treatment, which can lead to further complications.

PAIN

Per one published report, pain was noted in 71% of patients in the ICU, with 63% reporting moderate to severe pain.[2] Given the high incidence and the ethical and humane considerations involved in the alleviation of patient suffering, a high vigilance for the recognition and treatment of pain is always warranted. However, there are many ways that pain can also affect patient outcomes. Some of the complications that may arise from uncontrolled pain are immune system dysfunction, increased myocardial O_2 demand, acute restrictive ventilatory defects, altered bowel motility, hypercoagulability, and persistent catabolism.[3,4,5]

Rationale for Pain Management

Untreated pain is associated with sustained stress responses, including increased catecholamine, cortisol, and glucagon release. The majority of the deleterious effects of pain are related to the host responses that are elicited by these mediators. The stress response is not only associated with a generalized catabolic state, but also with immune system dysfunction as a result of increased levels of numerous cytokines (i.e., IL-1, IL-6, IL-8, TNF-α). These derangements can result in a decrease in levels of interleukin-2 (IL-2), a cytokine that is central to the function and proliferation of T lymphocytes. Diminished levels of IL-2 adversely affect the ability to mount effective T-cell-mediated immune responses and may result in decreased delayed hypersensitivity responses to recall antigens, diminished antibody production due to ineffectual T-helper function, and decreased T-cell proliferation.[3] Stress responses also lead to hyperglycemia secondary to increased hepatic gluconeogenesis and increased peripheral insulin resistance. Hyperglycemia can also have many effects on the immune system, including decreased chemotaxis and phagocytosis by neutrophils.[6] Thus uncontrolled pain may significantly increase the risk for developing nosocomial infections, particularly ventilator associated pneumonia.

The pain-induced stress response may also lead to a hypercoagulable state and increased risks for development of thrombotic events. Stress hormones increase circulating fibrinogen concentrations and platelet reactivity,[7] factors involved in thrombosis. The same hormones increase levels of plasminogen activator inhibitor (PAI),[3] with subsequent decreased conversion of plasminogen to plasmin. This leads to a decrease in fibrinolysis, with a net effect of tilting the thrombotic-fibrinolytic balance in favor of thrombosis.[8]

Pain also has direct effects on the cardiovascular system. The stress response results in increased sympathetic tone and increased myocardial O_2 demand due to increased heart rate and afterload. This can lead to myocardial ischemia and decreased contractility, particularly in patients with limited coronary perfusion due to the presence of significant coronary artery atherosclerosis. O_2 delivery may be further impaired in the presence of increased sympathetic tone by vasospasm of the coronary arteries at atherosclerotic sites.[9] The hyperdynamic state induced by the stress response also increases the degree of shear forces present in the coronary arteries, increasing the risk for endothelial damage and plaque disruption. This increases the risk for coronary thrombosis and myocardial infarction, particularly when coupled with the aforementioned stress response–induced hypercoagulable state.

Furthermore, unrelieved pain can result in an acute restrictive ventilatory defect. This may result from localized guarding of muscles due to chest wall pain, or from generalized muscle rigidity that restricts chest wall and diaphragm movement.[10]

Uncontrolled pain may also result in complications of the gastrointestinal tract. Bowel motility is a function of the balance of sympathetic and parasympathetic tone. A result of increased sympathetic tone associated with stress responses is decreased gastric and colonic motility leading to elevated gastric residual volumes, ileus, constipation, and nausea. As a consequence, the risk of aspiration is increased and the success of enteral feeding is decreased. Lack of enteral feeding results in suboptimal nutrition and increased bacterial translocation.

Recognition of Pain

It is important to determine if a patient is in pain before institution of sedative medications. Otherwise, patients may continue to experience significant pain, expressed as continued agitation that may require excessive amounts of **sedation** and unchecked stress responses. The detection of pain is most reliable and straightforward in patients who are alert and oriented. In these instances, various subjective pain scales are useful to quantify the degree of pain that is present. These include visual analog scales, verbal rating scales, and numeric rating scales. Both numeric rating and visual analog scales have been validated in patient studies.[11,12] However, elderly patients may experience difficulty with the visual analog scale.[13] Since the numeric rating scale is applicable to patients in many age groups and may be completed by writing or speaking, it is recommended as the tool of choice for pain assessment by the American College of Critical Care Medicine of the Society of Critical Care Medicine's (ACCM/SCCM) Sedation and Analgesia Task Force.[14]

The detection of pain in patients with an altered level of consciousness is more difficult because they cannot reliably convey subjective assessments. This includes patients who are sedated, intubated, receiving **neuromuscular blockade,** have head injuries, or are encephalopathic as a result of sepsis, drugs, etc. For these cases, subjective observation of behavioral responses and objective physical findings may provide clues to the presence of pain. Behavioral signs of pain include writhing, posturing, and facial expression, whereas physiologic findings include tachycardia, hypertension, and tachypnea. There is moderate agreement between visual analog scales and the observer reported FACES scale (a scale that relates facial expressions showing more and more discomfort to a standard 1-10 numeric scale), though this agreement was mostly seen at lesser degrees of pain intensity.[15] A combined behavioral-physiologic scale was found to have a moderate-to-strong correlation with a numeric rating scale.[13] Thus patients who are not able to communicate should have pain assessed via a combination of subjective observations of pain-related behaviors and physiologic indicators.[14]

Management of Pain

The goal of pain management is the attainment of adequate analgesia, which refers to the attenuation or abrogation of painful or noxious stimuli. Before instituting pharmacologic interventions, any removable sources of noxious stimuli should be identified and corrected. This includes proper patient positioning, stabilization of fractures, and elimination of unnecessary physical irritants, such as endotracheal tube malposition. If pain relief is not achieved, then pharmacologic intervention is warranted. Pharmacologic therapies include **opioids,** anesthetics (i.e., ketamine), **nonsteroidal antiinflammatory drugs (NSAIDs),** acetaminophen, and neural blockade.

Opioids

In the ICU, administration of opioids remains the most common method of analgesia. These drugs are agonists of central and peripheral nervous system opioid receptors, with μ-receptors and κ-receptors being the most important for producing analgesia. Administration is most commonly via continuous intravenous infusion. An intravenous route is preferred because it tends to be more potent and more easily titratable to patient response than longer acting intramuscular, transdermal, or enteral dosing. The shorter half-life of the intravenous route also allows for daily wake-ups, which has been shown to result in shorter times to extubation and ICU length of stays.[16] Continuous administration is preferred over intermittent, "as needed" dosing because the prevention of pain is easier to achieve than the treatment of established pain. Other options are patient-controlled analgesia (PCA) and transdermal administration of fentanyl. Use of a PCA device requires that a patient understand the purpose and use of the device, and as such, is limited to less ill patients.

Opioids, however, have potentially significant adverse effects in critically ill patients. These drugs can cause respiratory depression, raising the risk for apnea and respiratory arrest in spontaneously breathing patients. Opioid use may also result in hypotension. This is most likely to occur in patients who are hypovolemic and often responds to the administration of intravenous fluids. However, hypotension is also possible in euvolemic patients due to sympatholysis, vagally mediated bradycardia, and histamine release.[17] While stress responses in critically ill patients can cause gastric retention and ileus, opioids can further decrease gastrointestinal motility and lead to the complications discussed above. Laxatives are useful in prevention of constipation, and placement of a small bowel feeding tube can bypass gastric retention. Other effects include sedation, confusion, and urinary retention. Although sedation is a side effect of opioids, they are weak sedatives and have no amnestic properties and should not be used for the sole purpose of patient sedation. Pain in the ICU is frequently undertreated due to concerns of these adverse effects and/or fears regarding addiction. While these may be legitimate concerns, adequate analgesia should remain one of the primary goals of ICU care.

A variety of opioids are available for intravenous use and the selection of the most appropriate agent

TABLE 12-1 *Analgesics Used in the ICU*

DRUG	BOLUS DOSE	INFUSION RATE	HALF-LIFE	ELIMINATION	COMMENTS
Fentanyl	25-100 μg	1-30 μg/kg/hr	1.5-5 hr	Hepatic	Drug of choice in hemodynamically unstable patients; accumulation with time and large doses
Morphine	1-10 mg	0.03-0.15 mg/kg/hr	2-6 hr	Hepatic/renal	Histamine release; sphincter of Oddi contractions; accumulation in renal insufficiency
Hydromorphone	0.5-2 mg	7-15 μg/kg/hr	2-5 hr	Hepatic	

is dependent upon the presence of desirable pharmacologic attributes and the risk of adverse side effects. Desirable attributes include rapid onset and lack of accumulation of the parent compound or its metabolites. The onset of action and duration of effect will vary based on the drug's lipid solubility. Additionally, the presence of renal or hepatic insufficiency can decrease the elimination of opioids and their metabolites, prolonging the half-life of both desired and undesired effects. The pharmacologic properties of the most commonly used **analgesics** can be found in Table 12-1.

Among the opioids, fentanyl is the preferred agent for the relief of acute pain due to its more rapid onset of action. This is a function of its increased lipid solubility. However, peripheral accumulation of fentanyl can occur with continued use, resulting in prolonged sedation. When intermittent dosing is used, either morphine or hydromorphone is preferred owing to their longer duration of effect.

Morphine should be used with caution, though, in patients with renal insufficiency as the clearance of active metabolites will be delayed and sedation can be prolonged. This can make daily wake-ups problematic and may result in unnecessary neurologic evaluations, such computed tomography (CT) scans to assess for neurologic catastrophe. The lack of active metabolites and histamine release make hydromorphone and fentanyl more attractive choices in the setting of renal failure and in patients with hemodynamic instability.

Meperidine is not commonly used in the ICU owing to its neuroexcitatory characteristics and increased risk of seizure, especially in the setting of renal failure. Codeine is also not commonly used in the ICU because of its weaker analgesic properties. Newer agents, such as sufentanil and remifentanil, have been developed with rapid onset and shorter half-lives and may prove to be useful agents in the future. Remifentanil appears promising for patients with hepatic and renal failure because it is metabolized by tissue and plasma esterases.[18]

Nonopioid Analgesia

Ketamine is an IV anesthetic that has intense analgesic properties doses below its anesthetic threshold. This drug is an attractive analgesic choice for nonintubated patients since it does not typically cause airway compromise at subanesthetic doses. It has found particular use in the ICU for providing pain control during dressing changes. It is associated with sympathetic stimulation, which may result in tachycardia, hypertension, and elevations in intracranial pressure. Thus it should be avoided in the head-injured patient. It may also cause hallucinations, but the incidence is significantly reduced with the coadministration of benzodiazepines.[3]

Ketorolac is an intravenous NSAID that is particularly effective against somatic pain. The analgesic effects are synergistic with opioids and may allow for reduced opioid use. However, the inhibition of cyclooxygenase that is responsible for ketorolac's analgesic properties also results in numerous side effects including bleeding due to platelet dysfunction, gastrointestinal bleeding caused by erosive gastritis, and renal insufficiency, particularly with preexisting renal disease. The adverse side effects have limited the use of ketorolac in the ICU.

Acetaminophen is useful for the treatment of mild pain or discomfort. However, caution is required because of the risk for hepatotoxicity, particularly in patients who are more likely to have depleted glutathione stores. This includes patients with a significant alcohol history, poor nutritional status, or preexisting hepatic dysfunction.

Various techniques are available to block afferent neural stimuli with local anesthetics. These include neuraxial anesthetics and opioids and peripheral nerve blocks. Anesthetic neural blockade appears to be more effective at reduction of stress responses than use of systemic opioids or NSAIDS.[19-21] Paravertebral nerve blocks are useful for allowing pulmonary toilet in postthoracotomy patients and decreasing the incidence of atelectasis, mucus plugs, and risk for nosocomial pneumonia. Hypotension is a possible complication of epidural neural blockade because anesthetics inhibit conduction in sympathetic and sensory fibers. There is also a risk of respiratory depression with epidural opioids, particularly with rostral spread to the medulla. Coagulopathy and infection at the site of intended catheter placement are absolute contraindications to placement of epidural catheters. Coagulopathy is also a contraindication to catheter removal.

DELIRIUM

The development of delirium in hospitalized patients is common and occurs in up to 60% of older hospitalized patients. This number increases to greater than 80% in ICU patients.[22] The higher incidence in the ICU results from a combination of more severe illness and location in the more stressful ICU environment, and more frequent use of psycho-active medications. Identification of this disorder is of importance because it has been associated with increased morbidity and mortality, along with length of stay and functional decline.[23-25] Furthermore, symptoms of delirium may be exacerbated by inappropriate use of sedation or analgesia. Obtundation and confusion may be increased in delirious patients treated with sedatives, and this may lead to increased agitation.[26]

Delirium is manifested as an acutely changing or fluctuating mental status, inattention, disorganized thought, and altered level of consciousness. Patients with delirium will usually experience fluctuating levels of arousal and alertness throughout the day, accompanied by disruption of the normal sleep-wake cycle. This may or may not be accompanied by agitation (hyperactive form versus hypoactive form). The hyperactive form is easily recognized because of the presence of agitation and combative behaviors. The hypoactive form is manifested by psychomotor retardation and is more likely to be overlooked by caregivers. However, the hypoactive form is more common and may be associated with a worse prognosis.[22]

Recognition of Delirium

The standard for the diagnosis of delirium is the classification by a psychiatrist, in accordance with the Diagnostic and Statistical Manual of Mental Disorders, 4th edition (DSM-IV), and guided by history and examination. Many scales and diagnostic tools have been developed to aid the nonpsychiatrist in identifying patients with delirium, but the majority of these were developed with the exclusion of ICU patients because of the difficulty of these patients to communicate.

One such tool, the confusion assessment method (CAM), has been modified specifically for use in the ICU (CAM-ICU). It comprises four features: the acute onset of mental status changes, inattention, disorganized thinking, and an altered level of consciousness. The diagnosis of delirium is made with the presence of both of the first two features and either of the last two. This assessment tool was validated in ICU patients when compared with a reference standard of diagnoses made by psychiatrists with expertise in delirium. The sensitivity and specificity of the tool were high (95% to 100% and 89% to 93%, respectively).[22]

Treatment of Delirium

Neuroleptic drugs are the agents most frequently used to treat delirium. Their mechanism of action is antagonism of dopamine in the brain, particularly in the basal ganglia. The effect is to inhibit many of the symptoms of delirium, such as delusions, hallucinations, and unstructured thought. Among the neuroleptics, haloperidol is considered the agent of choice per ACCM/SCCM guidelines.[14] In the ICU, this agent is typically administered as intermittent IV boluses. Initial doses of 2 to 5 mg may be repeated every 15 to 20 minutes until agitation abates. However, total daily doses should be limited to less than 300 mg total dose per 24 hours because of the increased risk of **torsades de pointes.**[27,28]

The risk of torsades is a class effect shared among neuroleptics and is secondary to the ability of these agents to cause dose-dependent QT-interval prolongation. As such, it is important that patients receiving neuroleptic agents in the ICU be monitored for electrocardiographic changes, and that they receive adequate electrolyte repletion. ECG evaluation should not be limited to patients receiving very high doses, as arrhythmias have been reported at substantially lower doses.[27] Further caution is warranted in patients with a history of cardiac disease as this may increase the risk for torsades.[28]

Patients who are treated with neuroleptic agents should also be monitored for the development of extrapyramidal symptoms (EPS) and neuroleptic malignant syndrome. The offending agent should be discontinued if either of these complications is suspected. In addition, patients with EPS should be treated with either diphenhydramine or benztropine.

Besides pharmacologic therapy, patients with delirium should also be treated with behavioral modification interventions. This is most important in nonintubated patients who are not receiving continuous intravenous sedation. Simple interventions such as reorientation may be helpful. This includes frequent verbal orientation to location and situation, and verbal and visual orientation to time (such as prominent placement of a calendar). Attention to sleep hygiene and resetting the sleep-wake cycle may also be beneficial in the delirious patient. This includes limiting the degree of interruptions, noise, and light during nighttime sleep periods. Finally, oral hypnotics may help by decreasing sleep latency and increasing sleep duration.[29]

SEDATION

Rationale for Sedation Management

Sedation should be considered for patients who remain agitated after appropriately identifying and treating underlying physiologic precipitants, pain, and delirium. Anxiety is a common problem in the ICU, especially in the intubated and mechanically ventilated patient. Patients' fears, excessive stimulation, and frustrations in regard to ineffective communication can precipitate and exacerbate patient anxiety. Also the possibility of drug or alcohol withdrawal should be considered as a cause of anxiety and agitation in hospitalized patients.

As with pain, unalleviated anxiety is a stimulus for the stress response, with the potential for the same sequelae as previously discussed in regard to uncontrolled pain. Furthermore, anxious patients may become agitated and endanger the welfare of themselves (i.e., self-extubation, removal of catheters, ventilator dys-synchrony) or caregivers (i.e., aggressive behaviors). Patients who are agitated have excessive O_2 requirements, which may be detrimental in the setting of respiratory failure or shock. In these patients, sedation may be important for favorable O_2 delivery/O_2 consumption balance (DO_2/VO_2) and improved cardiopulmonary stability.[30] Further indications for sedation are the potentiation of analgesia, facilitation of procedures, and as a mandatory adjunct to neuromuscular blockade.

Attainment of amnesia is another indication for sedation of critically ill patients. Patients who are not treated with amnestic sedatives may recall unpleasant or frightening memories of their ICU stay, which may contribute to the development of posttraumatic stress disorder (PTSD).[31] However, amnesia as an indication is not without debate because there is evidence to suggest that sedation may actually be associated with development of PTSD.[32,33] It is hypothesized that sedatives impair explicit memory to the degree that the only memories retained from the patient's time spent in the ICU are of the delusions and hallucinations experienced there.[34] Furthermore, the duration of sedative use in the ICU has also been linked to depression.[33]

Titration and End Points

When initiating sedation therapy, it is important to establish defined goals of therapy, and then titrate the drug to effectively meet those goals without causing oversedation. While inadequate sedation has serious consequences for the reasons previously discussed, excessive sedation is also detrimental to patient outcome, particularly as a result of delayed weaning from mechanical ventilation.[35] Prolonged mechanical ventilation subsequently leads to increased risks for ventilator-associated pneumonia[36] and ventilator-induced lung injury.[37]

Once the goals are met, frequent assessment is required to ensure a continued appropriate level of sedation. Thus it is beneficial to optimize therapy by **titration** of sedatives as guided by a sedation scoring system. One study has shown that using a sedation scale (the Ramsay Scale in this case) to define goals and determine sedation status resulted in decreased duration of mechanical ventilation and length of stay.[38] A valid sedation scale should accurately describe a patient's current level of sedation and allow comparison with the desired level of sedation. An acceptable scoring system should be simple, user-friendly, reliable, validated by rigorous testing, and responsive (defined as the ability to detect important changes in sedation).[39] Sedation scales are also valuable in providing an objective method of communication between providers.

Numerous instruments have been developed and evaluated for assessing sedation in critically ill patients. These include the Ramsay Scale,[40] the Sedation-Agitation Scale,[41] the Motor Activity Assessment Scale,[42] and the Richmond Agitation-Sedation Scale.[43] While these scales have been evaluated by clinical testing, a significant limitation has been the lack of an accepted gold standard for comparison.[39] As such, validity has been assessed by comparison with other sedation scales, which are in turn further validated against different sedation scales. So there may be a high degree of correlation found between investigated scales, but the true relation to levels of sedation is still incompletely defined.

Sedation scales are of limited utility when deep sedation or neuromuscular blockade is required. Monitoring objective data, such as heart rate and blood pressure, can provide clues of inadequate sedation, but vital signs are neither sensitive nor specific to the level of sedation. Evaluation of an electroencephalogram (EEG) is another means of objectively assessing sedation levels. The Bispectral index (BIS) is one tool that converts raw EEG signals into a digital scale that ranges from 0 (absence of waves) to 100 (fully awake patient).[44] While BIS shows promise as a tool for monitoring sedation in deeply sedated or paralyzed patients, it is of limited utility in the evaluation of the remainder of ICU patients. Most patients require only light sedation and, at these levels, subjective scales may be more reliable.[45]

Drugs Used for Sedation

The choice of medication to use for sedation should be individualized on the basis of the patient's characteristics and comorbidities to determine the pharmacokinetics of the selected medication. The anticipated duration of mechanical ventilation may affect the choice based on the half-lives of different agents, where shorter-acting drugs are preferred if the duration of mechanical ventilation is expected to be relatively short. The costs of different medications also factor into choice, particularly when duration is expected to be prolonged. Regardless of the agent selected, the lowest effective dose to achieve sedation goals should be used. This allows for more efficient daily "wake-ups," and decreasing expense due to lower total drug dosages.

Benzodiazepines

Benzodiazepines are the drugs most commonly used in the ICU for sedation therapy. In addition to providing sedation, these agents also result in antegrade amnesia. They also have the effect of potentiating analgesia and result in lower dosage requirements for opioids.[46] All of the benzodiazepines can result in hypotension, so caution must be used during initiation, particularly with hemodynamically tenuous patients. All patients should have adequate intravenous access and be volume replete before administration. Vasopressive agents should also be available if required for hypotension after administration of a benzodiazepine.

Multiple factors affect the duration and intensity of action of benzodiazepines and necessitate individualized titration to desired **end points.** Patients with a history of alcohol abuse may exhibit increased drug metabolism and therefore require higher dosages. On the other hand, elderly patients and those with hepatic or renal impairments may have decreased clearance, resulting in a prolonged duration of activity. An increased volume of drug distribution contributes to delayed clearance in the elderly.[47]

Diazepam has a rapid onset of action but a long half-life (greater than 20 hours). It also has active metabolites, so duration of effect may be even greater with prolonged administration. Lorazepam has a shorter half-life, but somewhat slower onset of action, so it is not useful when rapid sedation is required. A possible benefit over diazepam is the decrease in drug interactions with lorazepam as a result of its metabolism via the glucuronidation pathway.[48] A potential complication associated with the use of either diazepam or lorazepam is the development of an osmolar gap and lactic acidosis.[49] This is due to the presence of propylene glycol as a carrier for these medications. Consequently, these agents should not be used in very high doses or for prolonged periods.

Midazolam is a benzodiazepine with both a rapid onset and a relatively short half-life. The short half-life is a favorable property for the facilitation of daily wake-ups and treatment of acute agitation. However, the duration of effect may be increased in patients who are obese or in renal failure. The prolonged effect in renal failure is secondary to the accumulation of an active metabolite, alpha-hydroxy midazolam.[50] Midazolam is not carried by propylene glycol so it does not have the same risks for metabolic acidosis as diazepam and lorazepam.

A useful characteristic of benzodiazepines is the ability to reverse sedation with the use of flumazenil. This is of greatest utility in the management of oversedation in the unintubated patient. It is occasionally used to evaluate whether continued unresponsiveness is caused by unintended prolonged sedative effects. However, care should be used because of the risk of precipitating withdrawal symptoms, including seizure. If flumazenil is used for this purpose, it is recommended that a single low dose be used.[14]

Propofol

Propofol is an intravenous anesthetic agent that is useful for sedation when titrated at lower doses. Like benzodiazepines, it can provide antegrade amnesia, though not as effectively or reliably as benzodiazepines. It also has anticonvulsant properties and has been used in the treatment of refractory status epilepticus. Another neurologic use for the drug is the reduction of elevated intracranial pressures.[51] The most significant advantage of propofol is its rapid onset and offset of action, making it an attractive agent for those patients expected to undergo a short course of mechanical ventilation or for whom rapid emergence from sedation is required. Continuous intravenous administration is required for sedation because of the rapid offset of action. However, if use is expected to be greater than 48 hours, some of the benefit from the short duration of action may be lost because there is a tendency towards drug accumulation.

Costs may be prohibitive with prolonged administration as well. An assessment of the total cost of propofol usage should also take into account the need for ancillary testing. In particular, prolonged usage and high dose requirements are associated with hypertriglyceridemia, for which there have been reports of associated pancreatitis.[52] Therefore lipid levels should be monitored with high dosages and prolonged use. Also the contribution of propofol to total caloric intake should be considered when assessing nutritional requirements. It is provided as an emulsion in a phospholipid vehicle that provides 1.1 kcal/ml. Similar to parenteral nutrition, continuous propofol requires the use of a dedicated IV catheter and the manufacturer recommends that bottles of propofol and the associated IV tubings hang for no longer than 12 hours.

It should be noted that there is a risk for lactic acidosis and cardiac arrhythmias with propofol, particularly with doses greater than 100 μg/kg/min.[53] The risks for these complications may be even higher in children and the FDA has warned against the prolonged use of propofol in the pediatric population. Also, despite its use in status epilepticus, there have been reports of myoclonus associated with its use.

Dexmedetomidine

Dexmedetomidine is a drug that is finding increased usage in ICUs. It exhibits sedative, analgesic, and sympatholytic properties (due to its high affinity for α_2-adrenoreceptors). Small studies in operating room and ICU patients have shown that use of dexmedetomidine can reduce the requirements for other sedatives and analgesics. Despite causing sedation, patients remained easily arousable. Perhaps most importantly, this drug can provide anxiolysis with little or no respiratory suppression or hemodynamic instability. This property is useful in patients in whom spontaneous breathing trials are hampered by severe anxiety and agitation after other means of sedation have been weaned. To date, however, there have been no large randomized trials in critically ill patients.[54] A comparison of the characteristics of frequently used sedative medications is listed in Table 12-2.

Approach to Management

When initiating sedation therapy, consideration should be given whether to use continuous or intermittent IV dosing. An obvious benefit of continuous therapy is the provision of smoother levels of sedation. Also, continuous sedation is easier to administer by the nursing staff, as opposed to intermittent boluses via IV pushes. However, continuous sedation may result in prolonged mechanical ventilation, longer hospital stays, complications, and increased cost.

Kollef et al compared the use of intermittent versus continuous sedation in a prospective, observational cohort study of 242 mechanically ventilated patients.[35] Thirty-eight percent of the patients received continuous sedation, and the rest received intermittent sedation. Both arms were sedated with commonly used agents (i.e., lorazepam, fentanyl, propofol). The patients in the intermittent arm had significantly decreased duration of mechanical ventilation and length of stays, both in the ICU and in the hospital. However, another study demonstrated that similar improvements in these same variables could be achieved by instituting a nursing-driven, sedation scale–directed, sedation protocol when compared with usual care without a protocol.[38]

Another important study evaluated whether the performance of daily interruptions in sedation would decrease mechanical ventilation and length of stays.[16] The study population included 128 medical ICU (MICU) patients on continuous IV sedation who were titrated to a Ramsay Score of 3 to 4. Patients were randomized either to continuous, uninterupted sedation or to daily interruption until either awake or agitated. Each arm was further randomized to use of either midazolam or propofol. Again, the investigators found a significant decrease in the duration of mechanical ventilation and length of ICU stay when daily interruptions were employed.

The potential development of withdrawal symptoms after prolonged sedation should always be considered after the discontinuation of sedatives. The incidence of acute withdrawal syndrome has been estimated to be as high as 32% in ICU patients.[55]

TABLE 12-2 *Sedatives Used in the ICU*

DRUG	BOLUS DOSE	ONSET	INFUSION RATE	HALF-LIFE	ELIMINATION	COMMENTS
Propofol	1-2 mg/kg	1-2 min	5-75 μg/kg/min		Hepatic	Hypertriglyceridemia; cardiovascular depressant; not significantly altered by hepatic or renal failure, but accumulation in peripheral tissue with prolonged administration
Midazolam	2-5 mg	2-5 min	0.5-10 mg/hr	3-5 hr	Hepatic/renal	Good agent for short-duration sedation
Lorazepam	1-4 mg	5-20 min	0.5-10 mg/hr	10-20 hr	Hepatic/renal	Metabolic acidosis; useful for prolonged sedation
Diazepam	2-20 mg	2-5 min	N/A*	20-40 hr	Hepatic/renal	Metabolic acidosis; accumulation with prolonged use
Dexmedetomidine	1 μg/kg†		0.2-1 μg/kg/hr	2 hr	Hepatic	α_2-adrenoreceptor agonist; lack of respiratory depression
Haloperidol	2-10 mg	3-20 min	2-10 mg/hr	10-24 hr	Hepatic/renal	QT prolongation, torsades de pointes; watch for extrapyramidal symptoms

*Not generally administered as a continuous infusion.
†Load over 10 minutes.

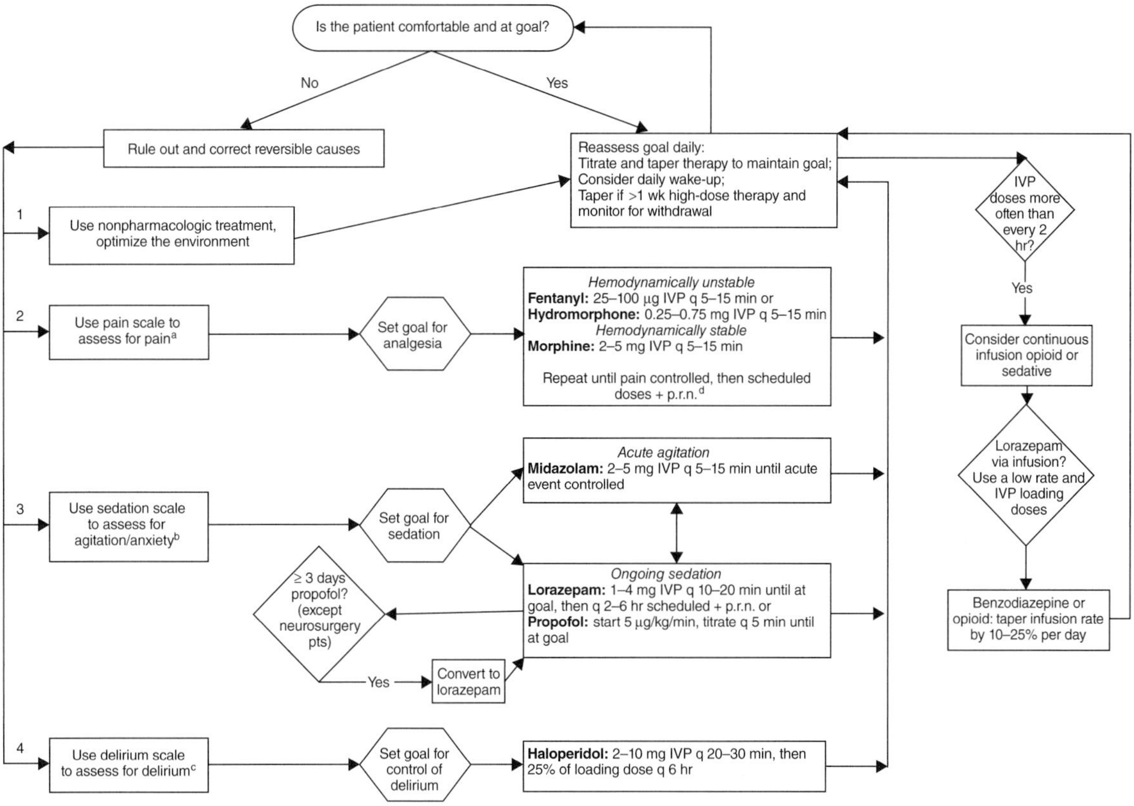

[a]Numeric rating scale or other pain scale.
[b]Riker Sedation-Agitation Scale or other sedation scale
[c]Confusion Assessment Method for ICU.
[d]See Table 1 for intermittent dosing for specific agents.

FIGURE 12-2 Algorithm for sedation and analgesia for mechanically ventilated patients. (Modified from Jacobi J, Fraser GL, Coursin DB et al: Clinical practice guidelines for the sustained use of sedatives and analgesics in the critically ill adult, Crit Care Med 30:119-141, 2002.)

Symptoms include tremor, nausea, headache, agitation, myoclonus, delirium, and seizures. It is associated with high doses, longer duration, rapid weaning, and concomitant use of neuromuscular blocking agents (NMBAs). The mode of delivery (i.e. continuous versus intermittent), however, does not appear to be a factor. A recommended algorithm for the overall approach to management is shown in Figure 12-2.

NEUROMUSCULAR BLOCKADE

While the overall use of NMBAs in the ICU, outside of initial intubation, has substantially decreased, there are still occasional instances in which they may be indicated. However, before opting for the use of NMBAs, all other possible modalities should be used. NMBAs should only be used as a last resort if these other measures fail to improve the patient's clinical status. An often cited indication is the facilitation of mechanical ventilation in patients who are difficult to ventilate or synchronize with the ventilator. However, appropriate sedation, trials of various modes of ventilation, and adjustments in flow rate and inspiratory and expiratory times should always be attempted before advancing to the use of neuromuscular blockade therapy.[56] Other indications include control of elevated intracranial pressures, management of status epilepticus, and tetanus. Neuromuscular blockade may also be beneficial in reducing O_2 demand for patients in septic shock.

Drugs Used for Neuromuscular Blockade

Agents for neuromuscular blockade are divided into either depolarizing or nondepolarizing agents. Depolarizing agents are similar to the neurotransmitter acetylcholine and exert their effects by binding to and activating nicotinic acetylcholine receptors. Drug administration causes initial skeletal muscle stimulation that is manifested by fasciculations. This is followed by flaccid paralysis due to continued depolarization and accommodation. The only clinically relevant depolarizing agent is succinylcholine and it is not used in the ICU for long-term blockade.

Nondepolarizing NMBAs also bind to acetylcholine receptors, but do not cause activation. Drugs in this class include aminosteroids and benzylisoquinolinium drugs. Pancuronium and pipecuronium are long-acting aminosteroids, whereas vecuronium and rocuronium are intermediate acting. Rocuronium also has a very rapid onset, with onset of neuromuscular blockade within 2 minutes (R*apid*O*nset*curonium).

In the benzylisoquinolinium group, D-tubocurarine and doxacurium are long acting, atracurium and cisatracurium are intermediate, and mivacurium is short-acting. D-tubocurarine may induce histamine release, and rapid administration must be avoided to limit hypotension. Both atracurium and its isomer, cisatracurium, are unique in that they are inactivated in the plasma by ester hydrolysis and Hoffman elimination. Thus clearance is not directly dependent upon renal or hepatic function. As for mivacurium, it has a very short half-life (2 minutes) but is not generally used as a continuous infusion in the ICU. The characteristics of common NMBAs are shown in Table 12-3.

As with other agents, choices of paralytics should be individualized as dictated by patient characteristics and circumstances. For tracheal intubation, succinylcholine is preferred if there is concern for residual gastric contents. However, succinylcholine should not be used if there is known or suspected hyperkalemia or neuromuscular disease, or in burn patients, because it may lead to rapid life-threatening hyperkalemia. For short surgical procedures, atracurium or vecuronium is preferred. A suggested algorithmic approach is shown in Figure 12-3.

In patients with renal disease, caution is warranted in the use of aminosteroids because clearance can be

TABLE 12-3 *Neuromuscular Blocking Agents in the ICU*

DRUG	BOLUS DOSE	ONSET	DURATION OF ACTION	ELIMINATION	COMMENTS
AMINOSTEROIDS					
Pancuronium	0.1 mg/kg	3-4 min	74-116 min	Kidney/liver	Tachycardia secondary to vagolysis
Vecuronium	0.1 mg/kg	2-3 min	32-44 min	Renal/bile	Minimal cardiac/ vagolytic effects; active metabolite may prolong effects; avoid in cirrhosis/hepatic failure
Rocuronium	1.5 mg/kg	1-2 min	20-40 min	Renal/bile	Rapid onset, attractive for intubation if succinylcholine contraindicated
BENZYLISOQUINOLINIUMS					
Atracurium	0.5 mg/kg	2.0-2.5 min	35-45 min	Hoffman/Ester hydrolysis	Watch for hypotension due to histamine release; good choice in hepatic and/or renal failure
Cisatracurium	0.1 mg/kg	4-7 min	40-60 min	Hoffman	Good choice in hepatic and/or renal failure
Mivacurium	0.2 mg/kg	1.8-2.5 min	15-20 min	Plasma cholinesterase	Shortest half-life among nondepolarizing agents

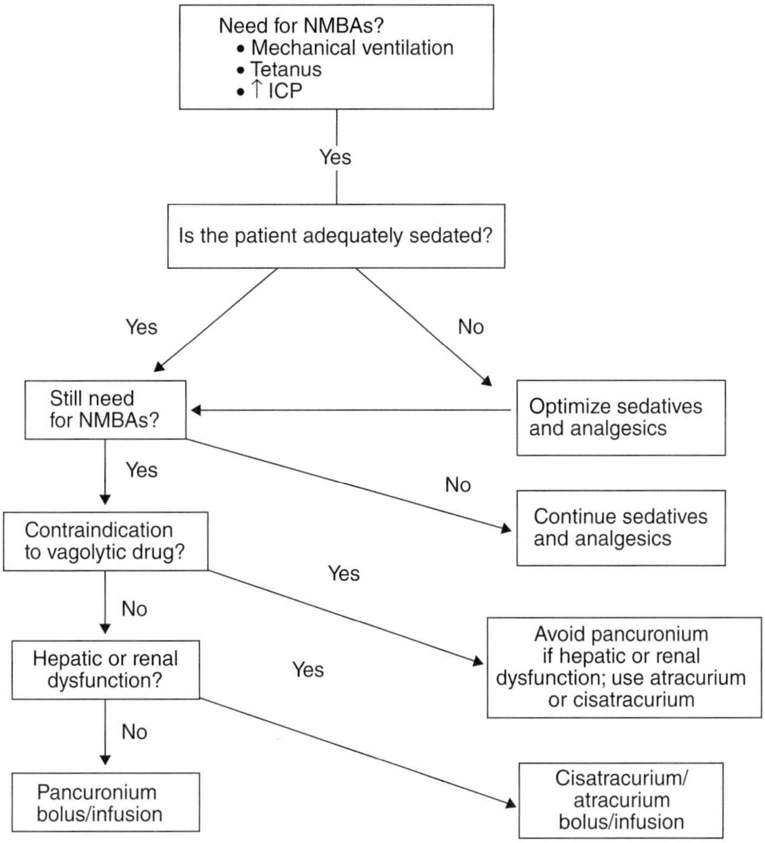

FIGURE 12-3 Algorithm for the use of NMBA's in the ICU. (Modified from Murray MJ, Cowen J, DeBlock H et al: Clinical practice guidelines for sustained neuromuscular blockade in the adult critically ill patient, Crit Care Med 30:142-156, 2002.)

greatly reduced and duration prolonged. Similar caution for this class is indicated in patients with cirrhosis. Vecuronium has been reported to be most associated with prolonged duration of action after discontinuation and should be avoided in these patients.[56] D-tubocurarine clearance is also decreased with renal and hepatic dysfunction. Atracurium and cisatracurium are the preferred agents in these patients because their clearance is not affected by renal or hepatic dysfunction.

For patients with cardiovascular disease who cannot tolerate an increase in heart rate, pancuronium should be avoided because it is vagolytic and typically results in an increase of greater than 10 beats/min.[57] Vecuronium may be preferred in these patients because it is a structural analogue of pancuronium without vagolytic effects. Alternatively, cisatracurium also has little cardiovascular effect and has lesser effect on histamine release than atracurium. Doxacurium is another agent that is free of cardiovascular effects.

In elderly patients, poor circulation may result in slow onset and prolonged duration of paralysis. Atracurium may be preferred in these patients because it is not affected due to its unique means of elimination.

A theoretical concern exists for use of atracurium in patients at risk for seizures. This is because Hoffman elimination of the drug produces laudanosine, a breakdown product associated with CNS excitation. The risk is mainly in patients who receive high doses, though there is some concern in patients with hepatic failure because laudanosine is metabolized in the liver. However, it has been used in patients with end-stage liver disease without deleterious effect.[56]

Monitoring Use of NMBAs

As with sedatives and analgesics, paralytics must be titrated to effect to avoid excessive dosing, which can lead to prolonged duration of effect and subsequent complications. While there is no rigorous data that reduced doses of NMBAs decreases the incidence of persistent weakness, it is recommended that the lowest effective dose be used.[56]

An evaluation of the depth of neuromuscular blockade may be performed by subjective observation of muscle activity, objective grading of muscle responses to stimuli, or electronic measurement of muscle effort. Clinical assessment typically entails observation of skeletal and respiratory muscle activity. This is limited by its subjective nature and low sensitivity because of the lack of stimulus to elicit responses. A more objective assessment is provided by ventilator software that allows detection and quantification of spontaneous ventilatory efforts.

Perhaps the must common means of objective assessment of the degree of neuromuscular blockade in the ICU is peripheral nerve stimulation or "twitch monitoring." One of the most reliable means of performing this assessment is by the **train-of-four (TOF).** Four electrical impulses are delivered to a muscle group, in series, and the number of muscle contractions is observed. The degree of muscle blockade is related to the number of contractions elicited, with complete blockade resulting in no contractions and the absence of blockade allowing four contractions. There is not an ideal number of contractions desired. Rather, the choice is influenced by the patient's status and goals of therapy from blockade.

It is essential that paralyzed patients be closely monitored to ensure that they are receiving adequate analgesia and sedation, generally to a level deeper than that required without paralysis to provide amnesia for the period of use. Undersedation can result in tremendous fear and anxiety and the risk for development of PTSD is significantly elevated. However, undersedated patients will be unable to display many signs and symptoms of pain, anxiety, and agitation while in a paralyzed state (e.g., grimace, motor activity, withdrawal from noxious stimuli, tachypnea). Therefore, the onset of tachycardia and hypertension must be evaluated as potential signs of undersedation or lack of analgesia. For patients with seizures who are treated with NMBAs, EEG monitoring should be performed to ensure that they are not continuing to seize.

Patients who are treated with continuous neuromuscular blockade must be monitored for potential complications. There is risk for corneal desiccation and abrasion in patients with eyelids that remain persistently open. The corneas should be lubricated and the eyelids possibly taped shut to prevent this. Also, rapid development of decubitus ulcers is a concern with paralysis and therefore patients should be turned on a routine schedule.

Acute **myopathy** is another potential complication associated with the use of continuous neuromuscular blockade.[56] Development of this serious complication is often manifested as an inability to wean the patient from the ventilator. It may be related to reduced synthesis of muscle proteins during administration of NMBAs. Besides difficulty weaning from the ventilator, acute myopathy is manifested as symmetric weakness of proximal and distal muscle groups after withdrawal of NMBAs. There is an increased risk for developing this complication when corticosteroids are used concomitantly, as is the concomitant use of aminoglycosides. There also appears to be an increased incidence with the use of aminosteroid compounds compared with benzylisoquinoliniums, though it is unclear whether this simply reflects practice patterns of preferential use of these agents.[58] The diagnosis may be confused with critical illness polyneuropathy, another cause of severe weakness in critically ill patients. The mechanisms of these disorders are different and the diagnosis should be differentiated. An electromyogram nerve conduction study (EMG/NCS) is often useful in confirming the diagnosis, as the pattern will be consistent with myopathy as opposed to axonal denervation.

To minimize the occurrence of acute myopathy, neuromuscular blockade should be used as a last resort, and only after optimizing sedation. Extreme caution is warranted if the patient is also receiving corticosteroids because the combination of these drugs is associated with an increase in incidence of myopathy and should be limited to less than 1 or 2 days. Monitoring responses by use of TOF will aid in limiting total exposure, as will the intermittent use of short-acting agents. The need for continued use should be frequently assessed and the drug should be discontinued as soon as possible. Periodic measurement of serum creatine kinase may be useful in early detection of myopathy.

SUMMARY

It is important to make patients as comfortable as medically feasible during their ICU stay. The presence of pain should be continually assessed and treated. Also, delirium should always be considered in the agitated patient, and treated appropriately (i.e., haloperidol). Once pain and delirium have been ruled out or treated appropriately, if the patient is still agitated then intravenous sedation is warranted. This should be titrated to a predetermined goal. Patients should receive daily interruption in sedation to allow for assessment of neurologic function and performance of a spontaneous breathing trial, if ventilatory goals have been met. Neuromuscular blockade may be required in rare instances. However, use requires a deeper level of sedation to provide amnesia. Development of complications must be monitored for and the drug discontinued as soon as feasible.

KEY POINTS

- Pain, anxiety, and delirium are conditions that frequently affect ICU patients but the presence or severity is often unrecognized.
- Ineffective treatment of these conditions can adversely affect patient care and worsen clinical outcomes.
- Agitation may be a sign of uncontrolled pain, anxiety, or delirium. However, a newly agitated patient must be assessed for possibly life-threatening disorders of the cardiopulmonary and central nervous systems.
- Treatment of agitation should be targeted to the underlying cause and not simply masked by heavy sedation. Otherwise, this can lead to suboptimal treatment, excessive medication usage, and further clinical complications.
- Intubated patients who are in pain or suspected to be in pain should receive a titrated analgesic (usually either morphine or fentanyl).
- Agitated patients with fluctuating mental status should receive neuroleptics for treatment of delirium (most often haloperidol).
- Agitated patients who have had life-threatening abnormalities ruled out and who have been evaluated and, if indicated, treated for pain and delirium should subsequently receive sedation therapy. Currently, this is most often achieved with titrated benzodiazepines (i.e., midazolam or lorazepam) or propofol. Dexmedetomidine is a newer agent that provides anxiolysis without excessive sedation or respiratory depression.
- Sedatives should be titrated to an appropriate sedation scale to minimize dosages and exposure. Daily cessation of sedatives is also warranted to allow better neurologic and respiratory assessment of intubated patients.
- Neuromuscular blockade should only be considered after other measures have failed or are contraindicated. When neuromuscular blockade is used, therapy should be guided by monitoring of responses (such as train-of-four stimulation) to minimize exposure and therapy discontinued as soon as feasible.

ASSESSMENT QUESTIONS

1. True or False. Pain is a common consequence of mechanical ventilation.
2. True or False. Altered sleep patterns contribute to the neuropsychiatric disturbances of patients on mechanical ventilators.
3. True or False. Opioids are the pain medication of last resort.
4. True or False. Haloperidol is considered the agent of course for the treatment of delirium.
5. True or False. Sedation scales do not do a good job of facilitating communication.
6. True or False. Benzodiazepines are the most commonly used drugs in the ICU for sedation therapy.
7. True or False. A disadvantage to propofol is its very slow onset of action.
8. True or False. Daily assessment of sedation needs can help reduce sedation dosage and shorten the stay on mechanical ventilation.
9. True or False. Neuromuscular blockade can lead to long-term myopathies.
10. True or False. When using neuromuscular blocking agents, it is recommended to use the highest dose that the patient can tolerate.

CASE STUDIES

For additional practice, refer to Case Study 12 in the appendix at the back of the book.

REFERENCES

1. Pochard F, Lanore JJ, Ferrand I et al: Subjective psychological status of severely ill patients discharged from mechanical ventilation, Clin Intensive Care 6:57-61, 1995.
2. Desbiens N, Wu A, Broste S et al: Pain and satisfaction with pain control in seriously ill hospitalized adults: findings from the SUPPORT research investigations, Crit Care Med 24:1953-1961, 1996.
3. Sanders KD, McArdle P, Lang JD: Pain in the intensive care unit: Recognition, measurement, and management, Semin Respir Crit Care Med 22:127-135, 2001.

4. Lewis KS, Whipple JK, Michael KA et al: Effect of analgesic treatment on the physiologic consequences of acute pain, Am J Hosp Pharm 51:1539-1554, 1994.
5. Epstein J, Breslow MJ: The stress response of critical illness, Crit Care Clin 15:17-33. 1999.
6. Turina M, Fry DE, Polk HC Jr: Acute hyperglycemia and the innate immune system: clinical, cellular, and molecular aspects, Crit Care Med 33(7):1624-1633, 2005.
7. Rosenfeld BA, Faraday N, Campbell D et al: Hemostatic effects of stress hormone infusion, Anesthesiology 81(5):1116-1126, 1994.
8. Kehlet H: Multimodal approach to control postoperative pathophysiology and rehabilitation, Br J Anaesth 78:606-617, 1997.
9. Vanhoutte PM, Shimokawa H: Endothelium-derived relaxing factor and coronary vasospasm, Circulation 80:1-9, 1989.
10. Desai PM: Pain management and pulmonary dysfunction, Crit Care Clin 15:151-166. 1999.
11. Meehan DA, McRae ME, Rourke DA et al: Analgesia administration, pain intensity, and patient satisfaction in cardiac surgical patients, Am J Crit Care 4:435-442, 1995.
12. Ho K, Spence J, Murphy MF: Review of pain management tools, Ann Emerg Med 27:427-432, 1996.
13. Puntillo KA: Dimensions of procedural pain and its analgesic management in critically ill surgical patients, Am J Crit Care 3:116-128, 1994.
14. Jacobi J, Fraser GL, Coursin DB et al: Clinical practice guidelines for the sustained use of sedatives and analgesics in the critically ill adult, Crit Care Med 30:119-141, 2002.
15. Terai T, Yukioka H, Asada A: Pain evaluation in the intensive care unit: Observer-reported FACES scale compared with self-reported visual analog scale, Reg Anesth Pain Med 23:147-151, 1998.
16. Kress JP, Pohlman AS, O'Connor MF et al: Daily interruption of sedative infusions in critically ill patients undergoing mechanical ventilation, N Engl J Med 342:1471-1477, 2000.
17. Grossman M, Abiose A, Tangphao O et al: Morphine-induced venodilation in humans, Clin Pharm Ther 60:554-560, 1996.
18. Thompson JP, Rowbotham DJ: Remifentanil—an opioid for the 21st century, Br J Anaesth 76:341-343, 1996.
19. Kehlet M: Modifications of responses to surgery by neural blockade: Clinical implications. In: Cousins MJ, Bridenbaugh PO, eds. Neural Blockade in Clinical Anesthesia and Management of Pain, Philadelphia: 1997, Lippincott.
20. Liu SS, Carpenter RL, Neal JM: Epidural anesthesia and analgesia. Their role in post-operative outcome, Anesthesiology 82:1474-1506, 1995.
21. Desborough JP, Hall GM: Modification of the hormone and metabolic response to surgery by narcotics and general anesthesia, Clin Anesthesiol 3:317-335, 1989.
22. Ely EW, Margolin R, Francis J et al: Evaluation of delirium in critically ill patients: Validation of the confusion assessment method for the intensive care unit (CAM-ICU), Crit Care Med 29:1370-1379, 2001.
23. Francis J, Martin D, Kapoor EN: A prospective study of delirium in hospitalized elderly, JAMA 263:1097-1101, 1990.
24. Inouye SK, Rushing JT, Foreman MD et al: Does delirium contribute to poor hospital outcomes? A three-site epidemiologic study, J Gen Int Med 13:234-242, 1998.
25. Hebert PC, Drummond AJ, Singer J et al: A simple multiple system organ failure scoring system predicts mortality of patients who have sepsis syndrome, Chest 104:230-235, 1993.
26. Breitbart W, Marotta R, Platt MM et al: A double-blind trial of haloperidol, chlorpromazine, and lorazepam in the treatment of delirium in hospitalized AIDS patients, Am J Psychiatr 153:231-237, 1996.
27. Sharma ND, Rosman HS, Pdhi D et al: Torsades de pointes associated with intravenous haloperidol in critically ill patients, Am J Cardiol 81:238-240, 1998.
28. Lawrence KR, Nasraway SA: Conduction disturbances associated with administration of butyrophenone antipsychotics in the critically ill: a review of the literature, Pharmacotherapy 17:531-537, 1997.
29. Krachman SL, D'Alonzo GE, Criner GJ: Sleep in the intensive care unit, Chest 107:1713-1720, 1995.
30. Kress JP, Pohlman AS, Hall JB: Sedation and analgesia in the intensive care unit, Am J Resp Crit Care Med 166:1024-1028, 2002.
31. Schelling G, Stoll C, Meier M et al: Health-related quality of life and post-traumatic stress disorder in survivors of adult respiratory stress syndrome, Crit Care Med 26:651-659, 1998.
32. Jones C, Griffiths RD: Disturbed memory and amnesia related to intensive care, Memory 8:79-94, 2000.
33. Nelson BJ, Weinert CR, Bury CL et al: Intensive care unit drug use and subsequent quality of life in acute lung injury patients, Crit Care Med 28:3626-3630, 2000.
34. Jones C, Griffiths RD, Humpris G et al: Memory, delusions, and the development of acute post-traumatic stress disorder-related symptoms after intensive care, Crit Care Med 29:573-580, 2001.
35. Kollef MH, Levy NT, Ahrens TS et al: The continuous use of i.v. sedation is associated with prolongation of mechanical ventilation, Chest 114:541-548, 1998.
36. Cook DJ, Walter SD, Cook RJ et al: Incidence of and risk factors for ventilator-associated pneumonia in critically ill patients, Ann Intern Med 129:433-440, 1998.
37. Meade MO, Cook DJ, Kernerman P et al: How to use articles about harm: the relationship between high tidal volumes, ventilating pressures, and ventilator-induced lung injury, Crit Care Med 25:1915-1922, 1997.
38. Brook AD, Ahrens TS, Schaiff R et al: Effect of a nursing-implemented sedation protocol on the duration of mechanical ventilation, Crit Care Med 27:2609-2615, 1999.
39. De Jonghe B, Cook D, Appere-De-Vecchi C et al: Using and understanding sedation scoring systems: a systematic review, Intensive Care Med 26:275-285, 2000.

40. Ramsay M, Savage T, Simpson B et al: Controlled sedation with alphaxalone-alphadolone, BMJ ii:656-659, 1974.
41. Riker RR, Fraser GL, Cox PM: Continuous infusion of haloperidol controls agitation in critically ill patients, Crit Care Med 22:433-440, 1994.
42. Devlin JW, Boleski G, Mlynarek M et al: Motor activity assessment scale: a valid and reliable sedation scale for use with mechanically ventilated patients in an adult surgical intensive care unit, Crit Care Med 27:1271-1275, 1999.
43. Sessler CN, Gosnell MS, Grap MJ et al: The Richmond agitation-sedation scale: validity and reliability in adult intensive care unit patients, Am J Respir Crit Care Med 166:1338-1344, 2002.
44. Rosow C, Manberg PJ: Bispectral index monitoring, Anesthesiol Clin North Am 2:89-107, 1998.
45. Simmons LE, Riker RR, Prato BS et al: Assessing sedation levels in mechanically ventilated ICU patients with the bispectral index and the sedation-agitation scale, Crit Care Med 27:1499-1504, 1999.
46. Gilliland HE, Prashad BK, Mirakhur RK et al: An investigation of the potential morphine sparing effect of midazolam, Anesthesiology 51:808-811, 1996.
47. Hammerlein A, Derendorf H, Lowenthal DT: Pharmacokinetic and pharmacodynamic changes in the elderly, Clin Pharmacokinet 35:49-64, 1998.
48. Greenblatt DJ, Ehrenberg BL, Gunderman J et al: Kinetic and dynamic study of intravenous lorazepam: comparison with intravenous diazepam, J Pharmacol Exp Ther 250:134-139, 1989.
49. Wilson KC, Reardon C, Theodore AC et al: Propylene glycol toxicity: a severe iatrogenic illness in ICU patients receiving IV benzodiazepines, Chest 128:1674-1681, 2005.
50. Bauer TM, Ritz R, Haberthur C et al: Prolonged sedation due to conjugated metabolites of midazolam, Lancet 346:145-147, 1995.
51. Kelly DF, Goodale DB, Williams J et al: Propofol in the treatment of moderate and severe head injury: a randomized, prospective double-blinded pilot trial, J Neurosurg 90:1042-1052, 1999.
52. Kumar AN, Schwartz DE, Lim KG: Propofol-induced pancreatitis; recurrence after rechallenge, Chest 115:1198-1199, 1999.
53. Cremer OL, Moons KGM, Bouman EAC et al: Long-term propofol infusion and cardiac failure in adult head-injured patients, Lancet 357:117-118, 2001.
54. Hogarth DK, Hall J: Management of sedation in mechanically ventilated patients, Curr Opinion Crit Care 10:40-46, 2004.
55. Cammarano WB, Pittet JF, Weistz S et al: Acute withdrawal syndrome related to the administration of analgesic and sedative medications in adult intensive care patients, Crit Care Med 26:676-684, 1998.
56. Murray MJ, Cowen J, DeBlock H et al: Clinical practice guidelines for sustained neuromuscular blockade in the adult critically ill patient, Crit Care Med 30:142-156, 2002.
57. Murray MJ, Coursin DB, Scuderi PE et al: Double-blind, randomized, multicenter study of doxacurium vs. pancurium in intensive care patients who require neuromuscular blocking agents, Crit Care Med 23:450-458, 1995.
58. Gehr LC, Sessler CN: Neuromuscular blockade in the intensive care unit, Semin Respir Crit Care Med 22:175-188, 2001.

CHAPTER

13 Patient Positioning

Joseph A. Govert

OUTLINE

OBJECTIVES

- Explain the effects of gravity on ventilation and perfusion distribution.
- Explain the effects of gravity on regional pleural pressure.
- Describe how these effects translate into gas exchange in various disease states.
- Discuss the outcome effects of various positioning strategies.

KEY TERMS

abdominal pressure
compliance
elastance
lateral decubitus
pleural pressure (P_{pl})
prone
shunting
supine

Frequent changes in body position and posture are universal in healthy animals and human beings even during sleep. Many practitioners believe that repositioning is also important during illness. They believe that frequent patient repositioning and early mobilization during illness and after surgical procedures help prevent complications such as pressure sores, musculoskeletal wasting, atelectasis, pneumonia, and thromboembolism. Despite these benefits, patients with respiratory failure requiring mechanical ventilation commonly remain in a supine horizontal position for days, weeks, or even months.

Both clinical experience and experimental evidence in animals and humans indicate that changes in position and posture alter the regional forces in the airways, alveoli, and pulmonary vasculature. Profound differences are noted in healthy patients mechanically ventilated for elective surgery and in patients with cardiopulmonary disease. Perhaps the most common clinical example of the effect of posture is the increased dyspnea and worsened oxygenation in patients with obstructive lung disease or heart failure when **supine.** Consequently, these patients often strongly prefer to remain upright, or sleep on a number of pillows. Mechanically ventilated patients often cannot express any sort of preference for certain body positions. As a consequence, they usually remain supine because it is almost always the most convenient for the caregiver.

Recently there has been increased interest in the physiologic and clinical effects of body position in mechanically ventilated patients. It is likely that a combination of mechanisms is responsible for the changes in the distribution of ventilation and perfusion that occur in these patients when body position is altered. This chapter reviews several mechanisms including improved regional lung inflation, alterations in lung **compliance,** regional variation in **pleural pressure (P_{pl}),** redistribution of lung water, changes in functional residual capacity (FRC), and positional effects on diaphragmatic function. A number of clinical series demonstrating changes in oxygenation in mechanically ventilated patients who are placed in the **lateral decubitus** or **prone** positions will also be described.

EFFECTS OF POSTURE AND POSITION ON HEALTHY PATIENTS

Lung Volumes

In healthy patients, moving from the sitting to the supine position reduces FRC by approximately 25%.[1] This is mainly due to the abdominal contents exerting greater pressure on the diaphragm. During mechanical ventilation and anesthesia, decreased inspiratory muscle tone further reduces FRC. General anesthetics and mechanical ventilation also impact diaphragmatic mechanics, which in turn affects FRC. Froese and Bryan found that actively breathing nonmechanically ventilated supine patients had more diaphragmatic movement in the posterior, or dependent, regions of the diaphragm. They suggest that the cause of this is the posterior diaphragm's decreased radius of curvature and the increased stretch of the muscle fibers in that region.[2] However, when patients in that series were mechanically ventilated under anesthesia, the diaphragm moved passively with motion predominantly in the anterior, or nondependent, regions because of the decreased **abdominal pressure** in these regions.[2] This led to worsened ventilation-perfusion ($\dot{V}/\dot{Q}$) relationships and mild deterioration in oxygenation.[2]

In spontaneously breathing patients, moving from the horizontal supine position to the prone or lateral decubitus position increases FRC by 15% to 20%.[1,3] This improvement is even more dramatic in mechanically ventilated patients. In a study of 17 normal, anesthetized and paralyzed patients undergoing elective surgery, Pelosi et al found that FRC improved by approximately 50% when patients were shifted from the supine to the prone position.[4] At this time, the effects of body position on vital capacity and total lung capacity are less well studied than the effects on FRC. However, both vital capacity and total lung capacity appear to decrease somewhat in recumbent, supine spontaneously breathing individuals, probably because of the accumulation of intrathoracic blood.[3,5] There are no data available on the effect of the prone position on vital capacity.

Regional Pleural Pressures

The P_{pl} surrounding the lung varies regionally mainly because of the effect of gravity on the lung and, to a lesser extent, on the structures of the mediastinum, chest wall, and abdomen.[6] The weight of the lung at any vertical height produces hydrostatic pressure, which significantly influences the P_{pl} at that height. For example, in healthy upright individuals, P_{pl} increases linearly from the lung apex to the diaphragm. The P_{pl} gradient in normal individuals is approximately 0.2 to 0.3 cm H_2O/cm, which is very close to normal lung density, suggesting that lung weight is the main determinant of the P_{pl} gradient.[6,7] As a consequence of the P_{pl} gradient, lung alveoli are more distended in the apical, or nondependent, portions and less distended in the basilar, dependent portions of the normal upright lung. While P_{pl} gradients have not been measured in humans in the prone, supine, or lateral decubitus positions they have been measured experimentally in animals.[8,9] In all instances, regardless of position, regional P_{pl} is less and alveolar distention is greater in the nondependent portions of the lung.

The position of the lung's surrounding structures also influences regional P_{pl}. For example, the heart rests primarily on the lungs during ventilation in the supine position, whereas it rests primarily on the sternum in the prone position. As a result, the weight of the heart exerts less effect on P_{pl} in the region of the left lower lobe when patients are in the prone position. This partially explains the decreased P_{pl} gradients in both healthy and diseased animals in the prone position as compared with the supine position.[9,10] Similarly, in the lateral decubitus position, the weight of the abdominal contents and mediastinum is preferentially distributed toward the dependent lung, causing decreased FRC and atelectasis in the dependent lung relative to the nondependent lung (Figure 13-1).[11]

The effect of general anesthetic or mechanical ventilation on regional P_{pl} in humans is not well described, though it is known that muscle tone decreases during anesthesia, increasing chest wall

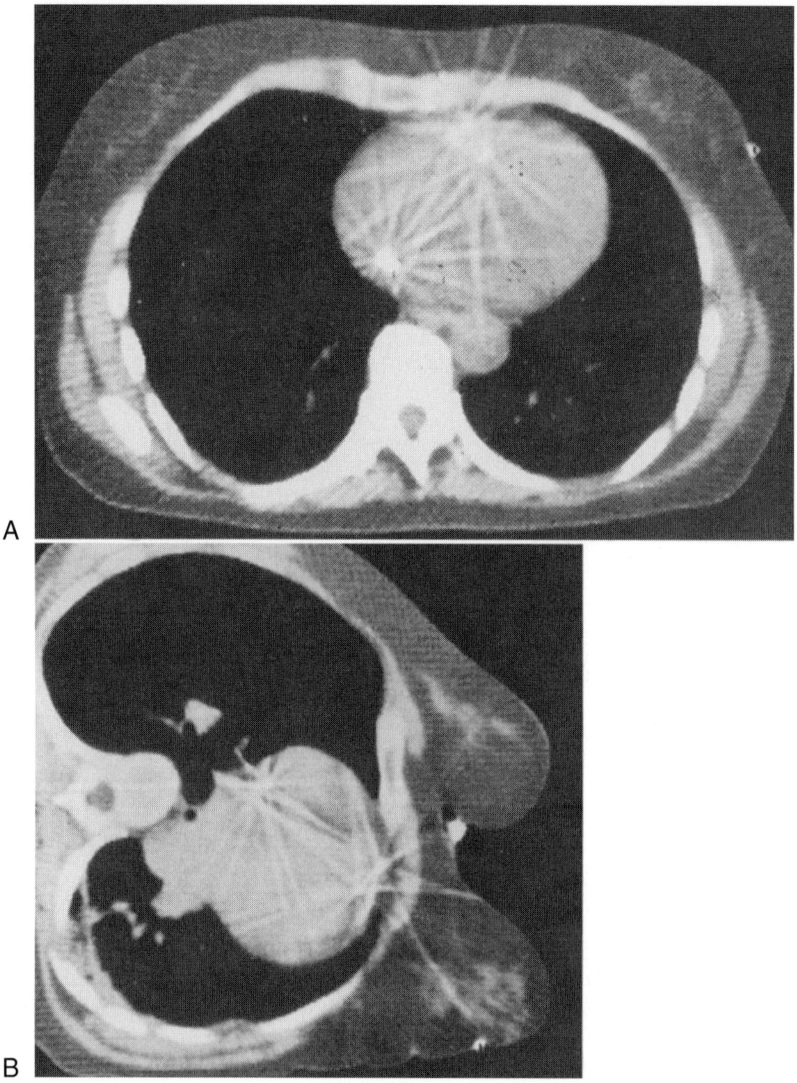

FIGURE 13-1 Computed tomographic images of the chest in supine and lateral decubitus positions. A, Supine position before anesthesia. B, Lateral decubitus position during anesthesia. Note the downward shift of mediastinal structures and loss of lung volume in the dependent lung in the lower panel. (From Klingstedt C, Hedenstierna G, Lundquist H et al: The influence of body position and differential ventilation on lung dimensions and atelectasis formation in anaesthetized man, Acta Anaesthesiol Scand 34:315-322, 1990.)

elastance and thus increasing P_{pl}.[4] This helps explain the diminished FRC and eventual development of atelectasis in the dependent regions of normal subjects undergoing prolonged mechanical ventilation for elective surgery (Figure 13-2).[4,11]

Regional Lung Inflation

Regional lung inflation depends on the local transpulmonary pressure, which is the difference between the pressure in the alveoli and pressure at the pleural surface ($P_{transpulmonary} = P_{pl} - P_{alveolar}$). At FRC, alveolar pressure equals atmospheric pressure so transpulmonary pressure is equal to P_{pl}, making any differences in regional transpulmonary pressures due to differences in regional P_{pl}. Therefore any gradient in regional P_{pl} results in a regional lung inflation gradient.

Over the last decade, Gattinoni and Pelosi et al have used computed tomography to measure regional lung inflation.[11-13] By quantitative analysis of computed tomography (CT) density, they defined a gas/tissue ratio to describe regional lung density for a

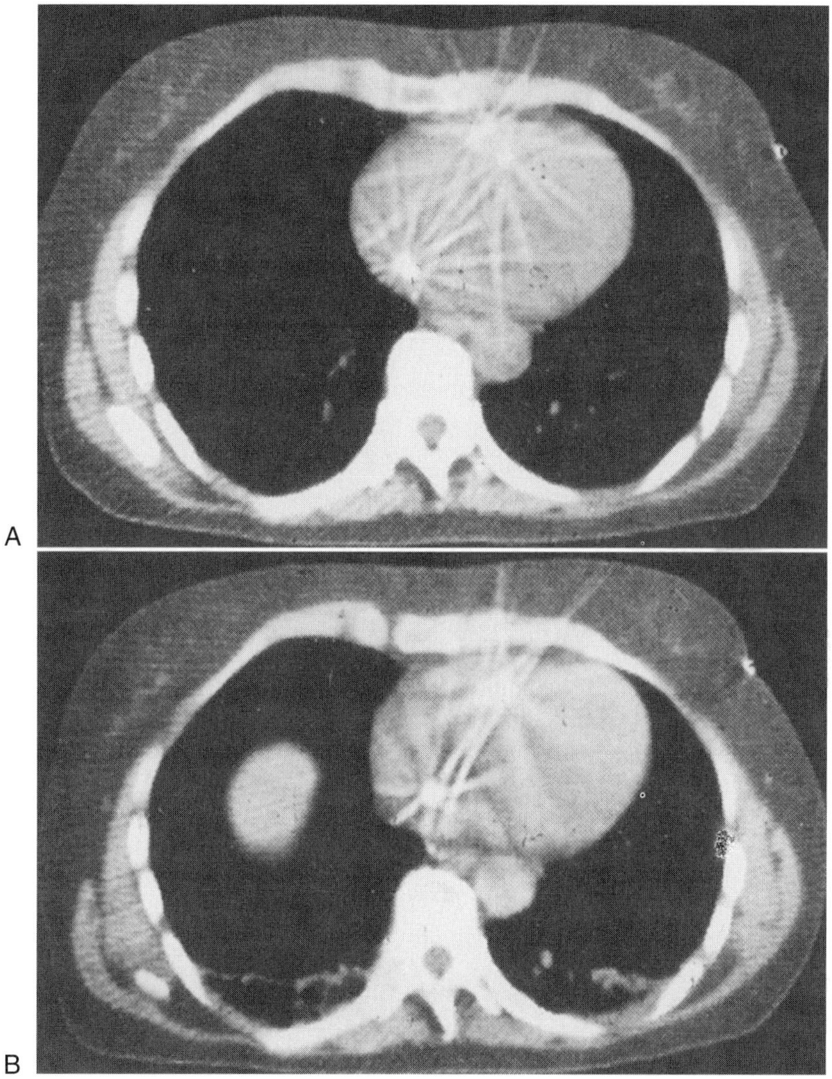

FIGURE 13-2 Computed tomographic image of the chest following anesthesia and mechanical ventilation. **A,** Supine position before anesthesia. **B,** Supine position after anesthesia. Note the development of atelectasis in the dependent, dorsal lung regions. (From Klingstedt C, Hedenstierna G, Lundquist H et al: The influence of body position and differential ventilation on lung dimensions and atelectasis formation in anaesthetized man, Acta Anaesthesiol Scand 34:315-322, 1990.)

single CT section, usually at the base of the lung. This gas/tissue ratio also acts as an index of regional lung inflation. In normal supine subjects, regional lung inflation decreases along the vertical gravitational axis with a constant exponential rate of change (13.9 ± 2.5 cm).[13] Consequently the alveolar dimensions in the posterior or dorsal regions of the lung are only one third those of the ventral surface.

When normal subjects are turned into the prone position, regional inflation again decreases exponentially along the vertical axis, but more slowly (decay constant = 26.2 ± 2.2 cm) than when the subjects are supine.[13] These studies suggest that positional changes in FRC are related to regional lung inflation gradients, which in turn, are a result of varying regional P_{pl}.[11-13]

Pulmonary Mechanics

Position and posture affect lung and chest wall compliance (inverse of elastance) and airway resistance.[14,15] In normal subjects, moving from a sitting to a supine position reduces lung compliance.[15] Although the mechanism remains unclear, some speculate that the P_{pl} and regional lung inflation gradients change when subjects are supine due to a combination of increased pulmonary blood volume, atelectasis, and small airway closure.[16] Moving from a supine to a lateral decubitus position improves lung compliance.[16] The effects of the prone position on lung compliance in normal subjects are unknown; however, a recent study suggests that in patients with acute lung injury lung compliance does not change greatly when the position is altered. Unfortunately, this study was not designed to detect small differences in lung compliance.[17]

The effect of position on chest wall compliance is more difficult to ascertain. In the supine position, the stiffening of the ribcage is offset by the softened resting tone of the abdominal muscles making the abdomen/diaphragm compartment more compliant. Consequently, chest wall compliance in normal upright subjects is similar to that in supine subjects.[18] This finding may vary greatly according to the individual's body habitus. Again there are few data regarding the effects of prone positioning on chest wall compliance in normal subjects, although a recent study suggests that chest wall compliance may decrease in prone patients with acute lung injury.[17]

Airflow resistance increases by 30% to 40% in healthy spontaneously breathing subjects in the supine as compared with the upright position.[14,16] Although the underlying cause of this change is not completely understood, diminished airway caliber related to decreased lung volumes is thought to play a significant role. Generally, changes in pulmonary mechanics are of little consequence to healthy individuals; however, increased airway resistance in the supine position contributes to the orthopnea seen in patients with flares of obstructive lung disease and may explain the prominence of nocturnal symptoms in asthmatics. Currently the effects of prone positioning on airway mechanics are not known.

Distribution of Ventilation

For healthy spontaneously breathing adults, regardless of position, ventilation is predominantly distributed to the dependent lung as a result of at least two factors.[6] First, regional lung inflation and alveolar inflation are greater in the nondependent portions of the lung, distending those alveoli and thereby placing them on the flatter, or less compliant, portion of the pressure-volume curve. This preferentially directs ventilation to the less distended, dependent alveoli.[18-19] Second, Froese and Bryan found that the greater displacement of the dependent hemidiaphragm shifted ventilation to the dependent lung, which is maintained in the upright, supine, prone, and lateral decubitus positions.[2,6,20]

However, there are three conditions under which ventilation increases in the nondependent lung relative to the dependent lung. First, ventilation at low lung volumes shifts the pressure-volume relationships between the dependent and nondependent alveoli so as to favor alveoli in the nondependent lung.[19] Additionally, under these conditions there is increased atelectasis in the dependent regions, driving ventilation preferentially towards the nondependent lung regions. Second, a high inspiratory flow rate or the use of accessory respiratory muscles preferentially distributes ventilation to the nondependent regions.[20] Third, in mechanically ventilated patients, especially those anesthetized or sedated, the abdominal contents restrict the dependent diaphragm, increasing the movement of the nondependent diaphragm and the nondependent portions of the lung.[2,21] Unfortunately, the distribution of ventilation in mechanically ventilated prone patients is controversial, with greatly differing results among studies.[6,21]

Distribution of Perfusion

The classic model of pulmonary perfusion in healthy lungs proposed by West in 1960 describes lung vasculature using three main compartments according to the relationships between pulmonary arterial (P_{art}), alveolar (P_{alv}), and pulmonary venous (P_{ven}) pressures (Figure 13-3).[22,23] In zone 1, vessels are held closed and there is no flow (P_{alv} greater than P_{art}). In zone 2 (P_{art} greater than P_{alv} greater than P_{ven}), the pressure gradient causing flow is arterial-alveolar, which increases linearly with gravity, therefore so does flow. In zone 3 (P_{ven} greater than P_{alv}), venous pressure exceeds alveolar pressure. Now the pressure gradient is arterial-venous, which is relatively constant, although there is some increase in blood flow according to a gravitational gradient due to changes in transmural pressure.[23]

Many authors now agree that zone 1 conditions do not exist in normal subjects.[24-27] Zone 2 conditions occur in the upright and lateral positions; however, there remains significant debate regarding the presence of zone 2 conditions in supine or prone positions because of the lung's greatly reduced vertical lung dimension in these positions compared with upright or lateral patients.[24-27] These same investigators suggest that zone 3 conditions occur throughout the supine lung with relatively homogeneous perfusion, though small gravitational gradients do exist.[24-27] Little is known about the distribution of lung perfusion in prone humans; however, one dog model of acute lung injury identified no significant gravitational perfusion gradient.[28] That study positively correlated regional blood flow in the supine and prone

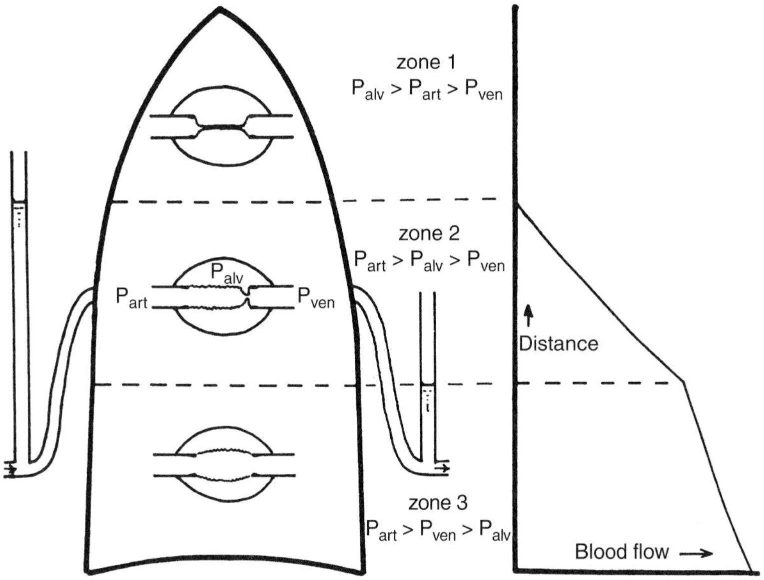

FIGURE 13-3 **Classic three zone model of pulmonary perfusion. The lung is divided into three zones according to the relative magnitudes of the pulmonary arterial (P_{art}), pulmonary venous (P_{ven}), and pulmonary alveolar (P_{alv}) pressures. In zone 1 alveolar pressure exceeds arterial pressure. In zone 2 arterial pressure exceeds alveolar pressure but alveolar pressure exceeds venous pressure. In zone 3 venous pressure exceeds alveolar pressure.** (Modified from West JB, Dollery CT, Naimark A: Distribution of blood flow in isolated lung: Relation to vascular and alveolar pressures, J Appl Physiol 19:713-724, 1964.)

positions with blood flow preferentially distributed to the dorsal regions, rather than negatively as would be expected with a purely gravitational model.[28]

Ventilation-Perfusion ($\dot{V}/\dot{Q}$) Relationships

In healthy spontaneously breathing subjects, both ventilation and perfusion are highest in the dependent lung regions. Interestingly, $\dot{V}/\dot{Q}$ ratios tend to decrease along the vertical gradient in upright and prone positions, but increase in the supine position.[24] During mechanical ventilation of healthy subjects, the distribution of perfusion remains unchanged; however, the overall $\dot{V}/\dot{Q}$ relationship is less favorable due to the tendency of ventilation to be distributed to the nondependent lung in these patients.[22,29]

EFFECTS OF POSTURE AND POSITION ON PATIENTS WITH RESPIRATORY DISEASE

Neuromuscular Disease

Orthopnea is a common symptom in patients with diaphragmatic weakness or paralysis, with the degree of orthopnea correlating with the severity of disease.[30] When the patient is supine, the weight of the abdominal contents increases the inspiratory load on the already weakened diaphragm. With complete diaphragmatic paralysis, accessory inspiratory muscle contractions reduce P_{pl}, displacing the diaphragm paradoxically into the chest during inspiration. In the upright position, this displacement is opposed by the weight of the abdomen. However, in the supine position, it is enhanced by pressure from the abdominal contents.[30] As a result, the normal reduction in vital capacity associated with the supine position is greatly accentuated by diaphragmatic weakness, with vital capacity decreasing by more than 25% when going from upright to supine.[3] In contrast, patients who have quadriplegia, but intact diaphragmatic function, may significantly increase vital capacity by shifting from upright to supine.[31] This is due to the increased residual volume in the upright position created by the outward bulging of the abdominal contents and consequent drop in the diaphragm.[31]

Atelectasis and secretion retention cause significant morbidity in patients with neuromuscular weakness. Multiple studies in both normal and diseased subjects indicate that, in the supine position, atelectasis tends to occur in the dorsal lung regions where elevated pleural pressures cause decreased regional lung inflation. Prone positioning tends to expand the dorsal lung regions and may facilitate secretion drainage from dependent portions of the lungs.[32] In a study of patients with acute quadriplegia, a respiratory care program that included deep breathing, chest percussion, and prone positioning decreased both the need for mechanical ventilation and the mortality rate when compared with historical controls.[32] Consequently, frequent position changes are recommended for patients with neuromuscular weakness.[32]

Obstructive Airway Disease

Position and posture may have important effects in patients with airway disease. In the upright position, there is a decrease in airway resistance. Conversely in the supine position, the increase in airway resistance results in air trapping, which may explain why stable chronic obstructive pulmonary disease (COPD) patients experience less of a decrease in FRC when supine compared with control patients.[1] In patients with severe COPD, hyperinflation flattens the diaphragm. Dyspnea is sometimes improved by leaning forward and contracting the abdominal muscles at expiration. Researchers hypothesize that the pressure from the abdominal contents generated by contracting the abdominal muscles causes a cephalad shift in the diaphragm, enhancing the length-tension relationship of the diaphragm. [33]

During acute crisis, COPD and asthma patients tend to avoid lying flat.[33,34] In one study of patients in acute asthmatic flare, no asthmatic with a peak expiratory flow of less than 150 L/min chose to be recumbent. [34] The many reasons for this include the increase in airway resistance while supine, and recruitment and optimization of accessory inspiratory and expiratory muscles in the upright position.[33]

In the absence of specific data for mechanically ventilated patients, practitioners extrapolate what is known in nonventilated patients with airflow obstruction to ventilated patients. As a result, it is generally recommended that actively weaning COPD patients be placed in the upright position. Unfortunately, there are no data describing the effects of the prone as compared with the supine position in these patients.

Unilateral Lung Injury

As described above, both perfusion and ventilation are normally preferentially distributed to the dependent portions of the lung. Extending this principle to patients with unilateral lung disease, a number of case series (Table 13-1) demonstrate that placing these patients in a "good lung down" lateral decubitus position significantly improves oxygenation in both spontaneously breathing and mechanically ventilated patients.[35-40] As is apparent from the table there is a wide range of clinical responses to decubitus positioning.

Most, but not all, patients with unilateral lung disease benefit from placing the healthy lung in the dependent position. Occasionally, critically ill patients require prompt return to the supine position due to arrhythmia, hypotension, or desaturation.[41] In COPD patients and in patients who are paralyzed, the benefit is suspect since ventilation is preferentially distributed to the nondependent lung. When these patients are positioned with the "good lung down," the greater perfusion in the dependent lung may create shunt in the dependent lung and increase dead space in the nondependent lung, effectively worsening $\dot{V}/\dot{Q}$ matching.[42] Another exception to the "good lung down" rule involves patients with unilateral pleural effusion, where lateral decubitus positioning does not appear to affect $\dot{V}/\dot{Q}$ matching or oxygenation.[43] Interestingly, in acute unilateral pulmonary embolism requiring mechanical ventilation, gas exchange improves when the affected lung is dependent.[44] Finally, "good lung down" positioning is also contraindicated in pulmonary hemorrhage and lung

TABLE 13-1 *Clinical Series Describing the Effect of "Good Side Down" Positioning in Unilateral Lung Disease*

AUTHOR	YEAR	NO. OF PATIENTS	NO. RESPONDING	Po_2 SUPINE, (mm Hg)	Po_2—"GOOD SIDE DOWN" (mm Hg)	Po_2—"GOOD SIDE UP" (mm Hg)
Zack et al.[35]	1974	19	13	–	86	77
Dhainaut et al.[36]	1980	4	4	–	–	–
Remolina et al.[37]	1981	9	6	66 ± 3	106 ± 13	58 ± 3
Ibanez et al.[38]	1981	10	8	102 ± 23	144 ± 25	86 ± 15
Gillespie et al.[39]	1987	4	4	–	101 ± 29	61 ± 10
Dreyfus et al.[40]	1992	8	7	100 ± 14	156 ± 23	–

abscess because of the risk of spillage of blood or pus into the uninvolved lung.

Acute Respiratory Distress Syndrome

Physiologic Mechanism of Prone Positioning

In 1974, Bryan first proposed using prone positioning in the treatment of acute respiratory distress syndrome (ARDS) patients, speculating that the prone position improved diaphragmatic excursion in the dorsal aspect of the lung, improving FRC, $\dot{V}/\dot{Q}$ matching and oxygenation.[45] In 1976, Piehl and Brown improved oxygenation in five ARDS patients by shifting them from the supine to the prone position.[46] In their patients the mean Po_2 improved from 72 to 106, lasting for at least 4 hours. In 1977, Douglas et al reported a similar series of six patients in which five showed improved oxygenation, with a mean Po_2 increase of 69 mm Hg (range 2-178 mm Hg).[47] They speculated that the improved oxygenation might be due to a combination of causes including better $\dot{V}/\dot{Q}$ matching, larger FRC, improved regional diaphragmatic movement, and enhanced secretion removal.[47]

Research on delineation of the mechanisms leading to improved oxygenation was not published until 1987 when Albert et al found dramatic, reproducible improvement in oxygenation due to prone positioning in a study of mongrel dogs with oleic acid–induced acute lung injury.[48] To explain the mechanism for the improved oxygenation they studied regional diaphragm movement, $\dot{V}/\dot{Q}$ relationships, changes in FRC, and hemodynamics. As predicted by Bryan, diaphragmatic motion in the nondependent portions of the lung increased, regardless of whether the animals were supine or prone. However, turning initially prone animals to a supine position did not enhance oxygenation as would be predicted if diaphragmatic motion was the sole mechanism causing improved oxygenation[48] Using the multiple inert gas method they noted dramatic decreases in the shunt fraction of prone animals, suggesting that the improved oxygenation in the prone position was due to improved $\dot{V}/\dot{Q}$ matching.[48] They found no significant change in FRC or hemodynamic variables.[48]

To study regional lung perfusion, Wiener, Kirk and Albert performed experiments in oleic acid–induced acute lung injury in dogs using radio-labeled microspheres.[49] Before injury, perfusion increased along a gravitational gradient in supine animals, but was more evenly distributed in prone animals. After oleic acid injury lung water increased dramatically, and perfusion, once again, increased gravitationally in supine animals with maximal perfusion in the dorsal region of the lung. However, in prone animals, perfusion was preferentially distributed to the nondependent dorsal regions, suggesting that the West model does not adequately explain perfusion in acute lung injury. Extravascular lung water was evenly distributed to all regions for both supine and prone animals, suggesting identical injury patterns.[49] In subsequent experiments this group of researchers found gravity to be a minor determinant of regional perfusion under West zone 3 conditions, the condition presumably present in most if not all of the ARDS lung.[28]

It appears that prone positioning does not significantly affect the distribution of regional perfusion, i.e., perfusion remains preferentially distributed to the dorsal lung regardless of position. If this is true then improvements in $\dot{V}/\dot{Q}$ must be due to changes in the distribution of ventilation. As was discussed earlier, regional pleural pressure gradients (P_{pl}) are in fact lower in prone animals than in supine animals.[8,9] Mutoh et al demonstrated that the P_{pl} in the dependent lung regions of animals with acute lung injury becomes positive, presumably leading to airway collapse and atelectasis in those regions.[10] When compared with supine animals, prone animals had a much smaller gravitational gradient and a much less positive P_{pl} in the dependent portions of the lung. Therefore, when injured animals are turned prone, the dorsal (nondependent) regions are exposed to a lower P_{pl}, resulting in the opening of previously atelectatic lung. Because perfusion remains greatest in the dorsal lung, even in the prone position, intrapulmonary **shunting** decreases, leading to improved oxygenation.[49] Additional experimental evidence in oleic acid–injured dogs revealed that supine dogs had greatly diminished ventilation in the dorsal lung regions while maintaining perfusion to these areas, creating areas of shunt and low $\dot{V}/\dot{Q}$.[50] In contrast, prone animals demonstrated significantly improved ventilation in the well-perfused dorsal regions, with no great effects on $\dot{V}/\dot{Q}$ in the ventral regions.[50]

Although there are no detailed physiologic studies of humans in the prone position, Gattinoni et al used CT densitometry to demonstrate changes in ARDS subjects that are consistent with those measured in experimental animals.[11-13] They measured regional lung density using a gas/tissue ratio for single CT sections, usually taken at the base of the lung. For supine ARDS patients, the regional inflation gradient

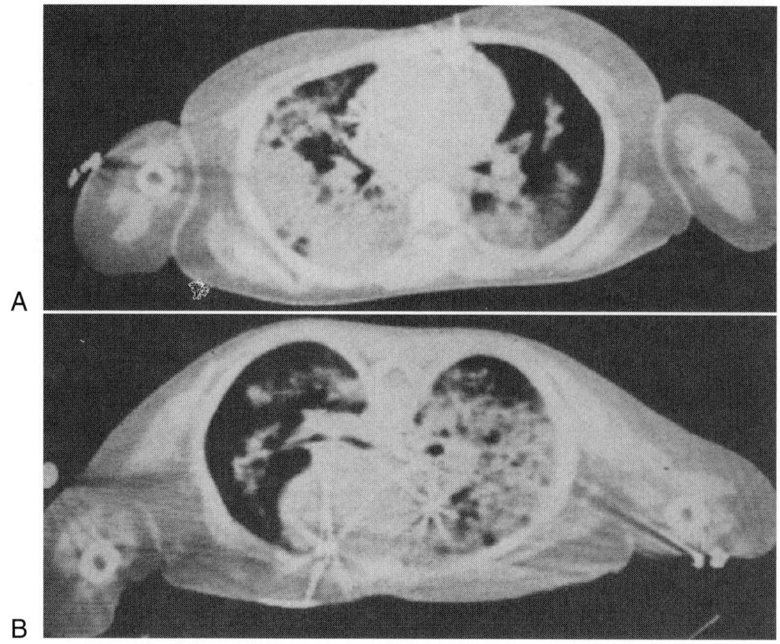

FIGURE 13-4 **Chest tomographic images of prone and supine patient with ARDS. Chest tomographic images of a patient with ARDS in the supine (A) and prone (B) positions. In the supine position, tissue densities predominate in the dorsal regions. After 15 minutes in the prone position, tissue densities are redistributed to the ventral lung regions.** (Modified from Langer M, Mascheroni MD, Marcolin R: The prone position in ARDS patients. Chest 94:103-107, 1988.)

decreased along the gravitational axis at a rate double that in the normal lung.[11] They theorized that the decreased regional inflation gradient is due to increased P_{pl} gradients in patients with ARDS caused by increased lung weight due to edema. These results suggest that in supine patients with 0 positive end-expiratory pressure (PEEP), the increased P_{pl} gradient should result in complete collapse of the posterior half of the lungs. In prone patients, the gradient of regional inflation was more heterogeneous, but reversed, leading to some collapse in the ventral lung zones with improved regional aeration in the dorsal lung (Figure 13-4). The collapse in the ventral lung zones of prone positions was generally less than the dorsal collapse seen when the patients were prone.[11] Additional mechanisms to explain the improved regional alveolar inflation and oxygenation include decreased effects of the cardiac mass on the lung, improved regional diaphragmatic movement, and reduced chest wall compliance.[17,51-53]

Clinical Effects of Prone Positioning

Many clinical series describe the use of prone positioning beginning with Bryan in 1974.[17,45-47,54-62] Based on the early available published data outlined in Table 13-2, it appears that prone positioning results in improved oxygenation for a majority of patients in whom it is tried. While the magnitude of the response varies widely from marginal to dramatic, there is no adequate model predicting where a particular ARDS patient will fall in the spectrum. Furthermore, the patients' response times vary from immediate to several hours. Based on these early results a number of randomized controlled trials of prone positioning were undertaken and have now been published. As described in the case series, these trials consistently confirm that the prone position improves oxygenation when compared with the supine position; however, the prone position appears to offer no mortality benefit compared with supine in patients with acute lung injury (Table 13-3).[63-66] The two largest trials in adults included 304 and 791 patients, respectively.[63,64] Although there were some differences in patient population (the smaller trial included only those patients with ARDS, whereas the larger trial also included those with acute lung injury) the proning regimens were similar. Both trials demonstrated that prone positioning improved oxygenation but in neither trial was there a difference in

TABLE 13-2 *Clinical Series Describing the Effect of Prone Positioning in ARDS*

AUTHOR	YEAR	NO. OF PATIENTS	NO. RESPONDING	Po_2 SUPINE (mm Hg)	Po_2 PRONE (mm Hg)	DURATION, hr	POSITION REPEATED
Phiehl et al.[46]	1976	5	5	72 ± 13	106 ± 9	4-8	Yes
Douglas et al.[47]	1977	6	6	63 ± 10	138 ± 69	4-33	Yes
Faller et al.[51]	1988	3	3	103 ± 25	197 ± 29	6	Yes
Langer et al.[52]	1988	13	8	69 ± 8	111 ± 20	2	Yes
DuBois et al.[53]	1992	4	4	92 ± 37*	153 ± 5*	–	Yes
Brussel et al.[54]	1993	10	–	114 ± 47*	241 ± 92*	2	No
Albert[55]	1993	9	7	63 ± 15	123 ± 121	–	Yes
Pappert et al.[56]	1994	12	7	98 ± 50	146 ± 95	2	Yes
Vollman et al.[57]	1996	15	9	86 ± 14	102 ± 33	0.5	Yes
Fridrich et al.[58]	1996	20	–	126 ± 9*	204 ± 19*	96	Yes
Chatte et al.[59]	1997	32	25	103 ± 28*	159 ± 59*	4	Yes
Pelosi et al.[17]	1998	16	12	103 ± 24	130 ± 33	2	No

*Po_2 / Fio_2 ratio.

mortality.[63,64] The smaller trial was underpowered to show a mortality difference; however, even if the results of the trials are pooled there was no mortality benefit from application of prone positioning (prone mortality 45.3%, supine mortality 43.8%; $p > 0.20$). Additionally both of these trials demonstrated an increased risk of pressure sores in the prone group[63,64] and the larger trial also demonstrated increased risk of selective bronchial intubation and endotracheal tube obstruction in the prone group.[64] A third trial, exclusively in children, demonstrated no benefit of prone position.[65]

It is unclear why prone positioning improves oxygenation but fails to improve mortality. Part of the reason may be that improvements in oxygenation, while persistent in the prone position, decrease in magnitude over time. Patients respond to a return to a supine position after a trial of prone positioning in one of three ways. Some "prone dependent" patients revert to their original supine oxygenation when returned to supine.[59,61,67] Others display reduced oxygenation compared with the prone position, but still better than their original supine levels,[17,54-57] whereas some patients have even greater oxygenation levels than either previous supine or prone values.[68] Unfortunately, it is our experience that the latter response is quite rare. To further cloud this issue, when the same patient is turned several times, the response to turning usually varies.[47,61]

The mechanisms underlying the variable oxygenation response to proning are not well understood. It appears that position-induced differences in regional pleural pressures cause a steeper decrease in regional lung inflation in the supine position compared with the prone position. However regional inflation patterns may be quite variable for individual patients.[61] It is also likely that changes in oxygenation in individual patients have more to do with the natural history of the patients' disease than with body position.

The failure of prone positioning to improve mortality may in part relate to an increase in complications related to either the prone positioning maneuver or the prone position itself. These range from skin breakdown to loss of airway.[46,47,57,60-62] The exact rate of complications is unknown; however, in the largest randomized trial to date, there was an increased incidence of selective bronchial intubation, airway obstruction, and pressure sores in the prone group.

Institutions use various methods for turning patients prone including commercial devices.[60] It may not be necessary to use these devices. One simple proning technique employs five individuals for the turning procedure. One individual is assigned to the head of the bed to maintain the airway, while four others, two on each side of the bed, move the patient to the edge of the bed and "logroll" the patient into the prone position. Additional people may be required for patients with multiple intravascular lines or chest tubes. Using this technique, the entire turning process is generally accomplished within a few minutes.

TABLE 13-3 *Randomized Controlled Trials of Prone Positioning in Acute Lung Injury*

AUTHOR, YEAR	NUMBER OF PATIENTS	AGE (MEAN OR RANGE)	DURATION OF PRONE POSITION	OXYGENATION (CHANGE IN Po_2/Fio_2)	DURATION OF MECHANICAL VENTILATION	MORTALITY (%)	COMPLICATION RATES
Gattinoni et al.,[63] 2001	Supine 152 Prone 152	58 yr	>6 hr for 10 days	Prone 63 Supine 44 ($p = 0.02$)		Prone 77/152 (51%) Supine 73/152 (48%) ($p > 0.05$)	Prone 2.7 pressure sores/pt Supine 1.9 pressure sores/pt ($p = 0.004$)
Guerin et al.,[64] 2004	Supine 413 Prone 378	62 yr	>8 hr/day	Prone 39 Supine 24 ($p < 0.001$)	Prone 13.7 Supine 14.1 (p = NS)	Prone 179/413 (43%) Supine 159/377 (42%) ($p = 0.74$)	Prone pts. with increased rate of pressure sores, ETT obstruction, selective intubation
Curley et al.,[65] 2005	Prone 51 Supine 51	2 wk-18 yr	>20 hr/day for maximum 7 days	Prone 30 Supine 29 ($p > 0.05$)	Prone 12.2 Supine 12.4 ($p = 0.91$)	Prone 4/51 (8%) Supine 4/51 (8%) ($p > 0.99$)	Prone: 4 serious events Supine: 1 serious event ($p = 0.36$)
Voggenriter et al.,[66] 2005	Prone 21 Supine 19	18-80 yr	8-23 hr/day	Prone 71.8 Supine 27.7 ($p = 0.03$)	Prone 30 days Supine 33 days (p = NS)	Prone 1/21 Supine 3/19 ($p = 0.27$)	No difference

KEY POINTS

- Body position has multiple effects on respiratory physiology and mechanics. These effects are important in the treatment of some conditions requiring mechanical ventilation.
- There is intriguing evidence that changes in body position may represent a supportive therapy for unilateral lung disease and some airway disease.
- For patients with acute lung injury/ARDS, it appears that while placing patients in the prone position offers a reasonable chance of improving $\dot{V}/\dot{Q}$ matching and oxygenation, randomized controlled trials have demonstrated no mortality benefit of intermittent prone position therapy.
- Future studies may seek to combine prone positioning with other experimental therapies, such as nitric oxide or high frequency ventilation; however, at this time, because prone position therapy has not demonstrated a mortality benefit in patients with ARDS, its use should not be considered as part of standard care.

ASSESSMENT QUESTIONS

1. True or False. In healthy subjects, moving from the sitting to the supine position increases FRC.
2. True or False. In supine patients receiving controlled mechanical ventilation, ventilation is preferentially distributed to the ventral or anterior regions of the lung.
3. True or False. Compared with the controlled mechanically ventilated patients, the spontaneously breathing supine patient will have a greater distribution of gas flow to the basal or dorsal regions of the lung.
4. True or False. Rotating a patient to the lateral decubitus or prone position will help aerate formerly dependent lung regions.
5. True or False. Airway resistance is lower in patients in the supine position.
6. True or False. In weaning a COPD patient from mechanical ventilation, the upright position facilitates respiratory muscle function.
7. True or False. In unilateral lung disease generally the healthy lung should be in the dependent position.
8. True or False. The prone position has been shown in several studies to improve gas exchange in many ARDS patients.
9. True or False. Randomized controlled trials have shown that prone positioning improves outcomes (length of stay and mortality) in patients with ARDS.
10. True or False. A complication of being in the prone position is pressure injury to the face.

REFERENCES

1. Marini JJ, Tyler ML, Hudson LD et al: Influence of head-dependent positions on lung voume and oxygen saturation in chronic airflow obstruction, Am Rev Respir Dis 128:101-105, 1984.
2. Froese AB, Bryan AC: Effects of anesthesia and paralysis on diaphragmatic mechanics in man, Anesth 41:242-255, 1974.
3. Lumb AB, Nunn JF: Respiratory function and ribcage contribution to ventilation in body positions commonly used during anesthesia, Anesth Analg 73:422-426, 1991.
4. Pelosi P, Croci M, Calappi E et al: The prone positioning during general anesthesia minimally affects respiratory mechanics while improving functional residual capacity and increasing oxygen tension, Anesth Analg 80:955-960, 1995.
5. Cambell GS, Harvey RB: Postural changes in vital capacity with differential cuff pressures at the bases of the extremities, Am J Physiol 152:671-673, 1948.
6. Kaneko K, Milic-Emili J, Dolovich MD et al: Regional distribution of ventilation and perfusion as a function of body position, J Appl Physiol 21:767-777, 1966.
7. Krugger JJ, Bain T, Patterson JL: Elevation gradient of intrathoracic pressure, J Appl Physiol 16:465-468, 1961.
8. Olson LE, Wardle RL: Pleural pressure as a function of body position in rabbits, J Appl Physiol 69:336-344, 1990.
9. Wiener-Kronish JP, Gropper M, Lai-Fook SJ: Pleural liquid pressure in dogs measured using a rib capsule, J Appl Physiol 59:597-602, 1985.
10. Mutoh T, Guest RJ, Lamm WJE et al: Prone position alters the effect of volume overload on regional pleural

pressures and improves hypoxemia in pigs in vivo, Am Rev Respir Dis 146:300-306, 1992.
11. Gattinoni L, Pelosi P, Vitale G et al: Body position changes redistribute lung computed-tomographic density in patients with acute respiratory failure, Anesthesiology 74:15-23, 1991.
12. Gattinoni L, D'Andrea L, Pelosi P et al: Regional effects and mechanism of positive end-expiratory pressure in early adult respiratory distress syndrome, JAMA 269:2122-2127, 1993.
13. Pelosi P, D'Andrea L, Vitale G et al: Vertical gradient of regional lung inflation in adult respiratory distress syndrome, Am J Respir Crit Care 149:8-13, 1994.
14. Navajas D, Farre R, Rotger M et al: Effect of body position on respiratory impedence, J Appl Physiol 64:194-199, 1988.
15. Berger R, Burki NK: The effects of posture on total respiratory system compliance, Am Rev Respir Dis 125:262-263, 1982.
16. Behrakis PK, Baydur A, Jaeger MJ et al: Lung mechanics in the sitting and horizontal positions, Chest 83:643-646, 1983.
17. Pelosi P, Tubiolo D, Mascheroni D et al: Effects of prone position on respiratory mechanics and gas exchange during acute lung injury, Am J Respir Crit Care Med 157:387-393, 1998.
18. Mead J, Lindgren I, Gaenser EA: Mechanical properties of the lungs in emphysema, J Clin Invest 34:1005-1016, 1955.
19. Pedley TJ, Sudlow MF, Milic-Emili J: A non linear theory of the distribution of pulmonary ventilation, Respir Physiol 15:1-38, 1972.
20. Roussos CS, Fixley M, Genest J et al: Voluntary factors influencing the distribution of inspired gas, Am Rev Respir Dis 116:457-467, 1977.
21. Rheder K, Knopp JJ, Sessler AD: Regional intrapulmonary gas in awake and anesthetized-paralyzed prone man, J Appl Physiol 45:528-535, 1978.
22. West JB, Dollery CT: Distribution of blood flow and ventilation perfusion ratio in the lung, measured with radioactive CO_2.[15] J Appl Physiol 15:405-410, 1960.
23. West JB, Dollery CT, Naimark A: Distribution of blood flow in isolated lung relation to vascular and alveolar pressures, J Appl Physiol 19:713-724, 1964.
24. Amis TC, Jones HA, Hughes JMB: Effect of posture on interregional distribution of pulmonary perfusion and V_A/Q ratios in man, Respir Physiol 56:169-182, 1984.
25. Orphanidou D, Hughes JMB, Myers MJ et al: Tomography of regional ventilation and perfusion using krypton 81m in normal subjects and asthmatic patients, Thorax 41:542-551, 1986.
26. Reed JH, Wood EH: Effect of body position on vertical distribution of pulmonary blood flow, J Appl Physiol 28:303-311, 1970.
27. Glenny RW, Robertson HT: Fractal properties of pulmonary blood flow: characterization of spacial heterogeneity, J Appl Physiol 69:532-545. 1990.
28. Glenny RW, Lamm WJE, Albert RK et al: Gravity is a minor determinant of pulmonary blood flow distribution, J Appl Physiol 71:620-629, 1991.
29. Chevrolet JC, Martin JG, Flood R et al: Topographical ventilation and perfusion during IPPB in the lateral position, Am Rev Respir Dis 118:847-854, 1978.
30. Mier-Jedrzejowicz, Brophy C, Moxham J et al: Assessment of diaphragmatic weakness, Am Rev Respir Dis 137:877-883, 1988.
31. Estenne M, DeTroyer A: Mechanism of the postural dependence in vital capacity in tetraplegic subjects, Am Rev Respir Dis 135:367-371, 1987.
32. McMichan JC, Michel L, Westbrook PR: Pulmonary dysfunction following traumatic tetraplegia. Recognition, prevention and treatment, JAMA 243:528-531, 1980.
33. Sharp JT, Drutz WS, Moisan T et al: Postural relief of dyspnea in severe chronic obstructive pulmonary disease, Am Rev Respir Dis 122:201-211, 1980.
34. Brenner BE, Abraham E, Simon RR: Position and diaphoresis in acute asthma, Am J Med 74:1005-1009, 1983.
35. Zack MB, Pontoppidan H, Kazemi H et al: The effect of lateral positions on gas exchange in pulmonary disease. A prospective evaluation, Am Rev Respir Dis 110:49-55. 1974.
36. Dhainaut JF, Bons J, Bricard C et al: Improved oxygenation in patients with extensive unilateral pneumonia using the lateral decubitus position, Thorax 35:792-793, 1980.
37. Remolina C, Khan AU, Santiago TV et al: Positional hypoxemia in unilateral lung disease, New Engl J Med 304:523-525, 1981.
38. Ibanez J, Raurich JM, Abizanda R et al: The effect of lateral positions on gas exchange in patients with unilateral lung disease during mechanical ventilation, Intensive Care Med 7:231-234, 1981.
39. Gillespie DJ, Rehder K: Body position and ventilation-perfusion relationships in unilateral pulmonary disease, Chest 91:75-79, 1987.
40. Dreyfuss D, Djedaini K, Lanore JJ et al: A comparative study of the effects of almitrine bismesylate and lateral position during unilateral pneumonia with severe hypoxemia, Am Rev Respir Dis 146:295-299, 1992.
41. Winslow EH, Clark AP, White KM et al: Effects of a lateral turn on mixed venous oxygen saturation and heart rate in critically ill adults, Heart Lung 19:557-561, 1990.
42. Shim C, Chun KJ, Williams MHJ et al: Positional effects on the distribution of ventilation in chronic obstructive pulmonary disease, Ann Intern Med 105:346-350, 1986.
43. Gilespie DJ, Rehder K: Effect of positional change on ventilation-perfusion distribution in unilateral pleural effusion, Intensive Care Med 15:266-268, 1989.
44. Badr MS, Grossman JE: Positional changes in gas exchange after unilateral pulmonary embolism, Chest 98:1514-1516, 1990.
45. Bryan AC: Comments of a devil's advocate, Am Rev Respir Dis 110(suppl):143-144, 1974.
46. Phiel MA, Brown RS: Use of extreme position changes in acute respiratory failure, Crit Care Med 4:13-14, 1976.
47. Douglas WW, Rehder K, Beynen FM et al: Improved oxygenation in patients with acute respiratory failure:

the prone position, Am Rev Respir Dis 115:559-565, 1977.
48. Albert RK, Leasa D, Sanderson M et al: The prone position improves arterial oxygenation and reduces shunt in oleic-acid-induced acute lung injury, Am Rev Respir Dis 135:628-633, 1987.
49. Wiener CM, Kirk W, Albert RK: Prone position reverses gravitational distribution of perfusion in dog lungs with oleic acid-induced injury, J Appl Phys 68:1386-1392, 1990.
50. Lamm WJE, Graham MM, Albert RK: Mechanism by which the prone position improves oxygenation in acute lung injury, Am J Respir Crit Care Med 150:184-193, 1994.
51. Krayer S, Rehder K, Vettermann J et al: Position and motion of the human diaphragm during anesthesia-paralysis, Anesthesiology 70:891-898, 1989.
52. Richter T, Bellani G, Scott Harris R et al: Effect of prone position on regional shunt, aeration, and perfusion in experimental acute lung injury, Am J Respir Crit Care Med 172:480-487, 2005.
53. Albert RK, Hubmayr RD: The prone position eliminates compression of the lungs by the heart, Am J Respir Crit Care Med 161:1660-1665, 2000.
54. Faller JP, Feissel M, Kara A et al: La ventilation en procubitus dans les syndromes de detresse respoiratoire aigue d'evolution severe, Presse Med 22:1154, 1988.
55. Langer M, Mascheroni MD, Marcolin R: The prone position in ARDS patients, Chest 94:103-107, 1988.
56. DuBois JM, Gaussorgues PH, Sirodot M et al: Prone position dependency in severely hypoxic patients, Intensive Care Med 18(suppl):A18, 1992.
57. Brussel T, Hachenberg T, Roos N et al: Mechanical ventilation in the prone position for acute respiratory failure after cardiac surgery, J Cardio Vasc Anesth 7:541-546, 1993.
58. Albert RK: New ideas in the treatment of ARDS. In: Vincent JL, editor: Yearbook of Intensive Care and Emergency Medicine, Berlin: 1993, Springer-Verlag, 1993, pp 135-447.
59. Pappert D, Rossaint R, Slama K et al: Influence of positioning on ventilation perfusion relationships in severe adult respiratory distress syndrome, Chest 106:1511-1516, 1994.
60. Vollman KM, Bander JJ: Improved oxygenation utilizing a prone positioner in patients with acute respiratory distress syndrome, Intensive Care Med 22:1105-1111, 1996.
61. Fridrich P, Krafft P, Hochleuthner H et al: The effects of long-term prone positioning in patients with trauma-induced adult respiratory distress syndrome, Anesth Analg 83:1206-1211, 1996.
62. Chatte G, Sab JM, Dubois JM et al: Prone position in mechanically ventilated patients with severe acute respiratory failure, Am J Respir Crit Care Med 155:473-478, 1997.
63. Gattinoni L, Tognoni G, Pesenti A et al: Effect of prone positioning on the survival of patients with acute respiratory failure, New Engl J Med 345:568-573, 2001.
64. Guerin C, Gaillard S, Lemasson S et al: Effects of systematic prone positioning in hypoxemic acute respiratory failure: a randomized controlled trial, JAMA 292:2379-2387, 2004.
65. Curley MA, Hibberd PL, Fineman LD et al: Effect of prone positioning on clinical outcomes in children with acute lung injury: a randomized controlled trial, JAMA 294:229-237, 2005.
66. Voggenreiter G, Aufmkolk M, Stiletto RJ et al: Prone positioning improves oxygenation in post-traumatic lung injury—a prospective randomized trial, J Trauma 59:333-343, 2005.
67. Marik PE, Iglesias J: A "prone dependent" patient with severe adult respiratory distress syndrome, Crit Care Med 25:1085-1086, 1997.
68. Gattinoni L, Pelosi P, Valenza F et al: Patient positioning in acute respiratory failure. In: Tobin M, editor: Principles and Practice of Mechanical Ventilation, ed 1, New York: 1994, McGraw-Hill.

CHAPTER 14

Ventilator-Associated Pneumonia

Mohammed Hijazi; Mariam Al-Ansari

OUTLINE

OBJECTIVES

- Explain the importance of ventilator-associated pneumonia as a cause of morbidity and mortality in mechanically ventilated patients.
- Describe methods for ventilator-associated pneumonia prevention and management.
- List the various risk factors for the development of ventilator-associated pneumonia.
- Identify techniques used to diagnose ventilator-associated pneumonia.
- Explain ways to prevent ventilator-associated pneumonia.

KEY TERMS

The 100,000 Lives Campaign
aspiration
bronchoalveolar lavage (BAL)
bronchoscopy
bundles
clinical pneumonia infection score (CPIS)
de-escalation
heat and moisture exchangers (HMEs)
nosocomial infection
pneumonia
protected specimen brush (PSB)
suction catheters

Pneumonia is a common complication of mechanical ventilation, affecting 10% to 48% of patients requiring mechanical ventilation via an artificial airway.[1-5] It is an important cause of morbidity and mortality in the intensive care unit (ICU).[5-7] Despite current advances in diagnostic and therapeutic modalities, inappropriate therapy has been shown to cause increased mortality.[8-11] In the face of increasing resistance to antimicrobials, timely appropriate therapy is an important and challenging aspect in managing patients with ventilator-associated pneumonia (VAP).

INCIDENCE AND RISK FACTORS

The rate of nosocomial pneumonia, pneumonia acquired in the hospital, is 6 to 21 times higher in patients requiring mechanical ventilation compared with nonventilated hospitalized patients.[12] The reported incidence of VAP varies according to the diagnostic method used, ICU type, duration of mechanical ventilation, and patient's risk factors. It is the most common **nosocomial infection** in the ICU, with an incidence rate ranging from 1 to more than 20/1000 ventilator days.[13] Based on the most recent National Nosocomial Infections Surveillance (NNIS) report, the mean rates of VAP (episode/1000 ventilation days) in the United States between January 2002 and June 2004 were higher in neurosurgical, surgical, and burn ICUs compared with medical, coronary, and respiratory ICUs (Table 14-1).[14]

Certain patients are at increased risk of developing VAP. The cumulative risk of developing VAP is about 1% to 3% per day of mechanical ventilation, being highest during the first 2 weeks of mechanical ventilation.[3,15,16] Common risk factors are listed in Box 14-1 and analyzed in Table 14-2. More recently, blood transfusion has been found to be an independent risk factor for developing VAP.[17,18]

MORBIDITY, MORTALITY, AND COST

VAP is the leading cause of mortality from nosocomial infections and is an important drain on hospital resources.[1] The crude mortality of patients who develop VAP ranges from 24% to 76%.[1,4,32] While several studies reported higher mortality in patients

TABLE 14-1 *NNIS VAP Rates by ICU Type (January 2002-June 2004)*

TYPE OF ICU	NUMBER OF UNITS	VENTILATOR DAYS	POOLED MEAN RATE*
Coronary	59	76,145	4.4
Cardiothoracic	47	98,358	7.2
Medical	92	268,518	4.9
Medical-surgical			
Major teaching	99	320,916	5.4
All others	109	351,705	5.1
Neurosurgical	29	45,073	11.2
Pediatric	52	133,995	2.9
Surgical	98	253,900	9.3
Trauma	22	63,137	15.2
Burn	14	23,117	12.0
Respiratory	6	18,838	4.9

National Nosocomial Infections Surveillance (NNIS) System Report, data summary from January 1992 through June 2004, issued October 2004, Am J Infect Control 32:470-485, 2004.
*Number of VAP/1000 ventilator days.

TABLE 14-2 *Selected Risk Factors for VAP Using Multivariate Analysis*

AUTHOR	RISK FACTORS	ADJUSTED ODDS RATIO
Rello[20]	Male gender	1.58
	Trauma admission	1.75
	Underlying illness severity at time of hospital admission	1.47 to 1.70
Ibrahim[21]	Tracheostomy	6.71
	Multiple central venous line insertions	4.20
	Reintubation	2.88
	Use of antacids	2.81
Apostolopoulou[15]	Tracheostomy	3.56
	Bronchoscopy	2.95
	Tube thoracostomy	2.78
	APACHE II greater than 18	2.33
	Enteral feeding	2.89
Cavalcant[29]	Severity of head and neck injury in trauma patients	11.9
Shorr[18]	Blood transfusion	1.89-2.16
Leone[30]	Nondepolarizing neuromuscular blocking agents	3.4
Bercault[31]	Transport outside ICU	2.9

who develop VAP with an attributable mortality of 5% to 30%,[1,6,7,23,33] others reported no difference in mortality rates between patients with and without VAP (Table 14-3).[4,20,22,35-39]

In a recent systematic review, VAP was found to increase the mortality of critically ill patients by twofold.[5] The variability in the reported attributable mortality might be related to variability in ICU type, a patient's characteristics, diagnostic methods, adequacy of therapy, and pathogens involved. Nevertheless, the development of VAP has been shown to increase ICU stay (26 vs. 4 days; $p < 0.001$), hospital stay (38 vs. 13 days; $p < 0.001$), and hospital costs ($70,568 vs. $21,620, $p < 0.001$).[1]

In another retrospective matched cohort study in the United States, the occurrence of VAP increased ventilator days by 9.6 days, ICU stay by 6.1 days, hospital stay by 11.5 days, and cost by more than $40,000.[20] However, after adjusting for the severity of underlying illness, the attributable cost of VAP is estimated to be $11,897.[1] Similar findings were found in a recent systematic review of the economic impact of VAP (mean increase in ICU length of stay by 6.1 days and attributable cost of more than or equal to $10,019).[5]

Time of onset is an important epidemiologic variable and risk factor for specific pathogens in patients with VAP. Early-onset VAP, onset within the first 4 days of hospitalization, usually carries a better prognosis and is more likely to be caused by antibiotic-sensitive bacteria. Late-onset VAP, onset after 4 days of hospitalization, is more likely to be caused by multidrug-resistant (MDR) pathogens and is associated with increased patient mortality and morbidity.[40] Factors associated with higher mortality in patients with VAP are listed in Box 14-2. Patients with early-onset VAP and prior hospitalization or antibiotic use are at greater risk for colonization and infection with MDR pathogens.[40]

BOX 14-1 *Risk Factors for Developing VAP*

- Male gender
- Age greater than 59 yr
- Supine head position
- Prior antibiotic exposure (late-onset VAP)
- Transport out of the ICU
- Reintubation
- Duration of mechanical ventilation
- Bronchoscopy
- Tracheostomy
- Higher APACHE II score
- Enteral feeding
- Nasogastric tube
- Trauma
- Cardiothoracic surgery
- Central nervous system disorders
- Use of antacids
- ARDS
- Chronic pulmonary disorders
- Corticosteroid use
- Paralytic agent use
- Blood transfusion

Data compiled from references 4, 15, 17-28.
APACHE, Acute Physiologic and Chronic Health Evaluation Score; *ARDS,* acute respiratory distress syndrome.

PATHOGENESIS

For lower respiratory tract infections to occur, the delicate balance between host defenses and microbial propensity for invasion must be shifted in favor of developing pneumonia. The majority of these infections appear to result from **aspiration** of potential pathogens that have colonized the oropharyngeal airways. Once an adequate concentration of pathogens is present in distal lung tissue and is able to overcome host defenses, pneumonia develops.[46,47]

TABLE 14-3 *Mortality in Patients With and Without VAP*

AUTHOR	% MORTALITY IN PATIENTS WITH VAP	% MORTALITY IN PATIENTS WITHOUT VAP	p VALUE
Rello[20]	30.5	30.4	0.713
Tejerina[4]	38.1	37.9	0.95
Fagon[33]	54.2	27.1	<0.01
Apostolopoulou[15]	39.3	36	0.464
Markowicz[22]	57	59	0.8
Ibrahim[21]	45.5	32.2	0.004
Bercault[34]	41	14	<0.0001
Heyland[6]	23.7	17.9	0.19

BOX 14-2 *Factors Associated With High Mortality in Patients With VAP*

- Supine head position
- Inappropriate antibiotic therapy
- Infection with high-risk pathogens, such as:
  - *Pseudomonas aeruginosa*
  - *Acinetobacter* species*
  - *Stenotrophomonas maltophilia*
  - Methicillin-resistant *Staphylococcus aureas*
- Premorbid lifestyle
- Higher organ system failure
- Antacid use
- Histamine-H_2 receptor antagonists
- Nonsurgical diagnosis

Data compiled from references 6, 7, 11, 41-44.
*Other studies showed that *Acinetobacter baumannii* was not associated with higher mortality or morbidity.[45]

Factors that increase the source of pathogens, facilitate entrance to distal lung, and impair host defenses increase the risk of developing VAP. The oropharynx, subglottic area, maxillary sinuses, and less importantly, stomach, respiratory therapy equipment, ICU environment, and ICU personnel are potential reservoirs from which pathogens can reach the distal lung by microaspiration (main route), and less commonly by macroaspiration, or inhalation of aerosols.[32,47] Other less likely routes of infection are contagious and hematogenous spread.[48]

Colonization

Colonization of the oropharynx and trachea with the causative pathogen has been shown to be important in the pathogenesis of VAP.[49,50] In ventilated patients, the normal oropharyngeal flora changes from facultative anaerobes and gram-positive cocci to potentially pathogenic gram-negative microorganisms.[49,51] Endogenous sources (intestine and stomach) are believed to be more important sources of colonizing pathogens compared with exogenous ones (contaminated equipment and hands of health workers in contact with other patients in the ICU).[52,53] Endogenous bacteria can reach the oropharynx after colonizing the skin or via a vector, such as hands of the ICU team, or by gastroesophageal reflux. Attachment of gram-negative bacteria to the oropharyngeal epithelium is facilitated by low cellular fibronectin and altered cell surface carbohydrate. Trauma to the surface epithelium by instrumentation, azotemia, critical illness, malnutrition, and prior antibiotic therapy may facilitate colonization. Dental plaque colonization may play a role in the pathogenesis of pneumonia.[54,55] It has been shown that 57% of the ICU patients had colonization of their dental plaque by potential pathogens commonly causing pneumonia.[55]

Colonization of the stomach plays a role in the pathogenesis of VAP.[28,51,56] While the stomach is normally sterile because of a low pH, colonization can occur in critically ill patients with an increase in the pH. H_2 blockers, antacids, and enteral feeding increase gastric pH and can lead to gastric colonization.[15,28,56-58] Once colonized, the stomach acts as a reservoir from which pathogenic bacteria can colonize the oropharynx and trachea or get aspirated directly into the lungs (gastropulmonary route). Factors that facilitate aspiration, such as the supine position, nasogastric tube, and transport out of the ICU (possibly via supine position), are independent risk factors for VAP.[28,31,59] Although bacteria colonizing the stomach can eventually colonize the respiratory tract and cause VAP, microaspiration of colonized oropharyngeal secretions has been shown to be more important in the pathogenesis of VAP.[40,50,51,53]

Respiratory Therapy Equipment

Endotracheal Tubes

The endotracheal tube increases the risk of developing pneumonia. It bypasses the upper airways, prevents closure of the vocal cords, and facilitates accumulation of secretions above the cuff (subglottic area). Moreover, it causes injury to the respiratory epithelium, which promotes colonization, impairs the mucociliary clearance, and makes performing oral hygiene suboptimal. Nasal intubation predisposes to sinusitis, which has been shown to be associated with VAP.[60,61] Despite the cuff of the endotracheal tube, aspiration has been detected in 20% to 77% of intubated patients.[62,63] Factors that facilitate aspiration are supine position, low cuff pressure (<20 to 25 cm H_2O), heavy sedation, large size feeding tubes, and muscle relaxants.[28,64]

In a study of 15 mechanically ventilated patients with nasogastric tubes, radioactive material was placed in the stomach and radioactivity was measured in the bronchial and oropharyngeal secretions every hour for 5 hours in two different body positions (supine and semirecumbent).[65] Gastroesophageal reflux occurred in all patients irrespective of the body position, but pulmonary aspiration was less in the semirecumbent position.[28] The use of small-bore feeding tubes has been shown to prevent reflux and aspiration.[66] Once aspiration occurs, the development of VAP depends on the balance between the burden and virulence of pathogens and host defense mechanisms.

Other Equipment

Ventilator tubing, humidifiers, in-line medication nebulizers, and suction catheters may play a role in the pathogenesis of VAP.

Ventilator Tubing Colonization of ventilator tubing occurs within hours of tubing change. Although aspiration of colonized tubing condensate may lead to VAP, patients are more likely to develop VAP from secretions aspirated past the cuff of the endotracheal tube than through the endotracheal tube.[67]

Humidifiers The use of heated tubing or **heat and moisture exchangers (HMEs)** decreases the formation of condensate, with no difference in VAP rate between them.[68,69] Current humidifiers are unlikely to be a source of pathogens causing VAP because the temperature of the water kills most bacteria, and they do not produce aerosols (no means for transporting bacteria if present). They generate humidity in the form of single molecules of water that are too small to transport bacteria.

In-Line Medication Nebulizers In-line medication nebulizers can produce aerosol particles that are ideal for deposition into patient terminal bronchioles and alveoli (0.5 to 4 μm) and may become contaminated by reflux of tubing condensate or use of contaminated solutions, acting as a potential source of infection.[70]

Suction Catheters Tracheal **suction catheters** may facilitate entrance of bacteria into the lungs. Although closed suction systems conceptually might reduce this risk, a recent study showed no difference between closed multiuse systems and conventional systems.[71,72]

Host Defenses

The gas exchange function of the lungs requires a constant exposure to the environment. Although aspiration of oropharyngeal secretions is common in healthy individuals during sleep, they do not develop pneumonia.[73] Normally, once microbial agents bypass the upper airway and reach the distal lung tissue, pulmonary defenses are able to overcome the inoculum most of the time via effective cough, mucociliary clearance, secretory IgA, IgG, surfactant, complements, phagocytic function, circulating neutrophils, and specific cellular and humoral responses.[74] Impaired pulmonary defenses, because of critical illness and interventional devices used, facilitate colonization by pathogenic bacteria and impair cough, mucociliary clearance, phagocytosis, and cellular and humoral responses, favoring the occurrence of pneumonia.

MICROBIOLOGY

The distribution of pathogens causing VAP (Table 14-4) varies based on ICU type, diagnostic methods used, prior antibiotic exposure, and the time of onset. VAP may be monomicrobial (52%) or polymicrobial (48%).[76] Gram-negative bacilli are the most commonly associated organisms (50% to 64%) followed by *Staphylococcus aureus*.[76-79] The most common pathogen among gram-negative bacilli is *Pseudomonas aeruginosa* (14% to 23%).[76,79] Early-onset VAP in patients without other risk factors for MDR pathogens is usually caused by sensitive community organisms (*Streptococcus pneumoniae*, methicillin-sensitive *Staphylococcus aureus* [MSSA], *Haemophilus influenzae*, and sensitive gram-negative bacilli).[40] Late-onset VAP or VAP in patients with risk factors for MDR (Box 14-3) is usually caused by resistant hospital organisms (*Pseudomonas aeruginosa*, *Acinetobacter* sp., *Stenotrophomonas maltophilia*, and methicillin-resistant *Staphylococcus aureus* [MRSA]).[40,76,78,80] *Staphylococcus aureus* is becoming the most common organism in many ICUs.[83] Patients with traumatic, neurologic, or neurosurgical disorders are at increased risk of *Staphylococcus aureus*.[84] While involved in community-acquired and aspiration pneumonia, anaerobes are rarely (0.7% to 3.1%) associated with VAP.[40,76,85] *Legionella* species, *Pneumocystis jiroveci*, cytomegalovirus, or other viruses are rarely associated with VAP.[32,40]

BOX 14-3 *Factors That Increase the Risk of MDR Pathogens*[40,42,81,82]

- Late-onset VAP
- Prior antibiotic within 90 days
- Prior hospitalization for more than 2 days within 90 days
- Chronic dialysis
- Residence in nursing homes and long-term facilities

TABLE 14-4 *Distribution of Organisms Associated With VAP*

PATHOGEN	HEYLAND[6] 173 PATIENTS %	FAGON[16] 52 VAP PSB %	CHASTRE[32] 1689 VAP BAL, PSB PUBLISHED IN 24 STUDIES %	KOLLEF[41] 87 PATIENTS LATE VAP %	CHASTRE[74] 402 PATIENTS BAL, PSB %
P. aeruginosa	22	31	24	26	19
E. coli	9.8	8	12	3.3	9.1
Klebsiella	8.7	4		8.2	3.1
Acinetobacter	3.5	15	8	6.5	1.7
S. maltophilia			2	3.3	0.75
Proteus	5.2	15			3.8
Enterobacter	12.1 (and Citrobacter)			14.8	3.8
Serratia	2.9	2			2.5
Haemophilus	2.6	10	10	6.5	7.2
MSSA	34.7	16	20	14.8	13.2
MRSA	2.3	17		14.8	7.1
Streptococcus	8.1	15	8	3.3	13.2
Enterococcus					1.4
CNS			1		3.4
Anaerobes	0.6	2	1		
Fungi	15		1		1.2

VAP, Ventilator-associated pneumonia; *BAL*, bronchoalveolar lavage; *PSB*, protected specimen brush; *BPSB*, blinded protected specimen brush; *MRSA*, methicillin-resistant *Staphylococcus aureus*; *MSSA*, methicillin-sensitive *Staphylococcus aureus*; *CNS*, coagulase-negative staphylococci.

Pneumonia caused by fungal infections is known to occur in immunocompromised patients. Its occurrence in immunocompetent ventilated patients is rare.[40] *Candida* is a common colonizer in ventilated patients, making it difficult to determine the significance of isolating it in critically ill patients.[86,87]

In a multicenter study of 803 immunocompetent critically ill patients receiving mechanical ventilation for more than 2 days, 214 patients (26.6%) had respiratory tract *Candida* colonization. *Candida albicans* was the most common species (68.7%), followed by *Candida glabrata* (20.1%) and *Candida tropicalis* (13.1%). The study identified bronchial *Candida* colonization as an independent risk factor for *Pseudomonas* pneumonia (9% compared with 4.8%; adjusted odds ratio of 2.22; $p = 0.049$).[86] In a retrospective review of 37 non-neutropenic patients with *Candida* isolated by culture of bronchoscopic samples, no cases of pulmonary candidiasis could be identified, although 23 patients had **protected specimen brush (PSB)** samples with greater than 10^3 colony-forming units (CFU)/ml.[88] Similarly, *Candida* sp. isolates from **bronchoalveolar lavage (BAL)** cultures in immunocompetent trauma patients were found to be contaminants rather than pathogens.[87] Out of 1077 BAL cultures, 85 (8%) grew *Candida* but no colony counts exceeded the diagnostic threshold for bacterial VAP. Only 2 of 64 episodes (3%) were treated with systemic antifungals. The majority of episodes were not treated with antifungals and were considered contaminants (59/64, 92%). No patients developed candidemia, and most follow-up BALs (74%) were negative for *Candida*.[87] Antifungal therapy in ventilated patients is not part of the routine empiric therapy unless there are risk factors for systemic fungal infection or tissue evidence of infection.[87,89]

An important feature of most organisms isolated in the ICU is the increasing resistance to antimicrobials. The latest NNIS report in 2004 shows an alarming increase in resistance (Table 14-5).[90] Because of the wide variability in the distribution of pathogens and its impact on the selection of appropriate therapy, it is important to consider the local pattern of pathogen distribution in each ICU.[40,91,92] In 753 cases of VAP at different hospitals, the most common organisms at all hospitals were *Staphylococcus aureus* (28.4%) followed by *Pseudomonas aeruginosa* (25.2%). The same study showed higher *Acinetobacter baumannii* rates in surgical ICUs (10.2% vs. 1.7%; $p < 0.001$).[83] Other factors associated with risk of *Acinetobacter baumannii* are neurosurgery, head trauma, acute respiratory distress syndrome (ARDS), and large volume

TABLE 14-5 *NNIS Reports Showing Antimicrobial Resistance Rates in ICUs January Through December 2002 and 2003 as Compared to Resistance Rates 1997 Through 2001 and 1998 Through 2002*

PATHOGENS	ANTIBIOTICS	% RESISTANCE RATES JAN-DEC 2002	% INCREASE IN RESISTANCE RATES JAN-DEC 2002 COMPARED TO 1997-2001	% RESISTANCE RATES JAN-DEC 2003	% INCREASE IN RESISTANCE RATES JAN-DEC 2003 COMPARED TO 1998-2002
Pseudomonas aeruginosa	Quinolone	32.8	37	29.5	9
	Imipenem	22.3	32	21.1	15
	Third generation cephalosporins	30.2	22	31.9	20
Escherichia coli	Third generation cephalosporins and aztreonam	6.3	14	5.8	0
Staphylococcus aureus	Methicillin	57.1	13	59.5	11
Enterococci	Vancomycin	27.5	11	28.5	12

aspiration.[82] Factors associated with imipenem-resistant *Acinetobacter baumannii* are ICU stay and treatment with imipenem.[93]

In summary, MDR pathogens should be anticipated in patients with risk factors. The local distribution of pathogens is important in selecting empiric therapy.

DIAGNOSIS

A high index of suspicion is needed in mechanically ventilated patients not to miss or delay the diagnosis. VAP should be suspected in intubated patients if two or more of the following clinical features are present:

- Purulent respiratory secretions
- Temperature greater than 38° C or less than 36° C
- Leukocytosis or leukopenia
- Hypoxemia[40,94]

Once VAP is suspected, radiologic studies should be done. If a newer or persistent chest radiologic abnormality is found, bacteriologic studies should be performed (qualitative or quantitative) and empiric therapy should be started.[40,94] The presence of a cavity by radiology or positive blood culture with the same pathogen isolated from respiratory secretions confirms the diagnosis. If no abnormality is detected by imaging, evaluate for an extrapulmonary source of an infectious or noninfectious nature.

Clinical Features and Chest X-ray

Many conditions can mimic VAP. Radiologic abnormalities can be caused by atelectasis, collapse, pulmonary edema, pulmonary embolism, lung contusion, and alveolar hemorrhage. On the other hand, a new infiltrate is easily missed in patients with abnormal baseline chest radiograph, such as those with ARDS. Purulent respiratory secretions can be caused by tracheobronchitis, whereas systemic inflammatory response can be due to other infectious (catheter-related infections, sinusitis) or noninfectious (trauma, medications, thromboembolic disorders) causes. Moreover, most critically ill patients are colonized by pathogens similar to those involved in VAP, which makes the interpretation of microbiologic studies difficult.

The lack of an easily performed, widely accepted gold standard makes it difficult to evaluate diagnostic modalities. Kirtland et al showed no correlation between any of the clinical features and autopsy evidence of VAP in 39 patients who died after a mean of 14 days of mechanical ventilation.[95] Torres et al performed postmortem pulmonary biopsies in 30 patients who died in the ICU (all were on antibiotics before death). VAP was diagnosed by postmortem lung biopsy in 18 patients. The sensitivities and specificities were 55% and 58% for fever, 78% and 33% for purulent secretions, and 78% and 42% for radiographic density, respectively. The combination of purulent secretions, leukocytosis, and radiographic signs was 70% sensitive and 45% specific.[96]

Portable chest x-rays are used routinely in most ICUs to assess for VAP. The accuracy of portable chest x-ray was evaluated in 69 patients based on autopsy findings.[97] Twenty-four patients had evidence of VAP by autopsy. The most sensitive findings were alveolar infiltrate and any air bronchogram (88% and 83%, respectively) with low specificity at less than 50%. The most specific sign was single air bronchogram and fissure abatement (95%), although sensitivity was less than 20%.[97] In patients with ARDS, no radiologic sign correlated with pneumonia and alveolar hemorrhage was present in 38% of autopsies.[97] A recent evidence-based assessment of the usefulness of the radiologic diagnosis of VAP concluded that while the specificity is unknown, the sensitivity of chest radiographic signs is as follows: 87% to 100% for alveolar infiltrate, 58% to 83% for air bronchogram, and 50% to 78% for new or worsening infiltrate.[98]

In summary, the presence of abnormal x-ray and clinical features of VAP is the most accurate clinical strategy to initiate performing cultures and empiric therapy.[40,48,99]

Qualitative Culture Techniques

Qualitative studies (Gram stain and culture) of endotracheal aspirate are widely used in managing patients with suspected VAP because they are easy to perform. Despite high sensitivity, they are unable to differentiate colonization from infection (lack specificity).[94] For example, in an autopsy study of 39 patients who died while mechanically ventilated, endotracheal aspirate had 87% sensitivity and 31% specificity compared with lung parenchymal culture.[95] Moreover, there was a significant correlation between qualitative and quantitative microbiologic results obtained by **bronchoscopy.** The high sensitivity of tracheal aspirate qualitative studies (usually identified organisms through bronchoscopic techniques) makes VAP unlikely if the cultures are negative in patients receiving no antibiotics.[100] On the other hand, the low specificity causes overtreatment of patients with colonization, missing the correct diagnosis, and might increase the emergence of resistant pathogens.[99]

The combination of clinical features, radiologic abnormalities, volume and character of tracheal secretions, hypoxemia, and tracheal aspirate culture into the **clinical pneumonia infection score (CPIS)** might be more useful to predict the probability of VAP and follow its course.[99,101,102] In an autopsy study of 38 patients, a CPIS score of six or more was found to have a sensitivity of 72% and specificity of 85%.[103] A persistently low score (less than six) for 3 days in a patient with suspected nosocomial pneumonia makes the diagnosis unlikely and might guide the decision to stop antibiotics.[104] One disadvantage of the score is the fact that the complete score can be calculated only in retrospect when the tracheal aspirate culture is available. A modified CPIS overcomes this shortcoming. More studies are needed before it is routine in practice.

Quantitative Culture Techniques

To improve the accuracy of diagnosing VAP, several quantitative methods (bronchoscopic BAL, bronchoscopic PSB, and nonbronchoscopic techniques) have been studied. The results of an extensive evidence-based review of the accuracy of diagnostic tests for the diagnosis of VAP are summarized in the following sections.[105-107]

Bronchoscopic BAL

Bronchoscopic BAL is one of the most widely used quantitative diagnostic techniques in patients with suspected VAP. For bronchoscopic BAL, 23 studies were reviewed (957 patients), 5 of which were postmortem.[105] Most of the studies used a cut-off point of quantitative culture of 10^4 CFU/ml. The sensitivity of BAL ranged from 42% to 93% (mean of 73%) and the specificity ranged from 45% to 100% (mean of 82%). The finding of intracellular organisms equal to or greater than 2% to 5% in BAL was found to have a higher positive predictive value for VAP (sensitivity of 37% to 100% and specificity of 89% to 100%). Assessment of the quality of BAL (less than 1% epithelial cells/low power field) was assessed in 2 of the 23 studies. The most important risk associated with BAL was hypoxemia.

Bronchoscopic PSB

Evaluating the less widely used bronchoscopic PSB, 18 studies were reviewed (846 patients), 5 of which compared PSB with samples obtained postmortem.[106] The recommended cut-off point of quantitative culture was 10^3 CFU/ml. The sensitivity ranged from 33% to 100% and specificity ranged from 50% to 100% (more specific than sensitive). The reproducibility of the results for PSB is not optimal, as 25% of the results were discordant in one study.[108]

Nonbronchoscopic Techniques

The accuracy of nonbronchoscopic techniques (blinded bronchial sampling = BBS; mini-BAL; blinded protected specimen brush = BPSB) was assessed by reviewing 15 studies (654 patients). The sensitivities (74% to 97% for BBS, 63% to 100% for mini-BAL, and 58% to 86% for BPSB) and specificities (74% to 100% for BBS, 66% to 96% for mini-BAL, and 71% to 100% for BPSB) were compared with the bronchoscopic techniques despite the lack of standardization.[107]

In summary, VAP is difficult to diagnose. Once suspected based on clinical and radiologic criteria, either qualitative or quantitative diagnostic testing should be done.[40] There is no strong evidence to favor one approach over the other and the choice depends on the clinical expertise available.[40,94] While several nonrandomized studies showed that patient outcome is similar for both methods, Fagon et al showed in a randomized trial of 413 patients with suspected VAP that mortality was less in the group that was managed based on quantitative diagnostic testing.[109] Moreover, the use of quantitative testing was associated with less antibiotic use. The use of BAL before introduction of new antibiotics helps physicians to de-escalate or optimize treatment. The use of clinical and quantitative bacteriologic evaluation is safe and helps to optimize the use of antimicrobials and may result in minimizing the emergence of resistant flora.[40,110]

THERAPY

Timely appropriate antimicrobial therapy that is modified based on lower respiratory cultures is the cornerstone of VAP therapy.[40] Inappropriate therapy for VAP (delay in initiation or inappropriate choice) is associated with increased mortality.[111] The risk of inappropriate therapy is increased by the difficulty in predicting the organism associated with VAP because of the variable distribution of pathogens between patients, and between ICUs within the same hospital.[91,92] Rello et al showed that the mortality of patients who received inappropriate initial therapy was 37% compared with 15.4% in patients who received appropriate therapy from the beginning.[112] Similar findings were reported by Luna, Iregui, and Kollef.[8,10,11] Inappropriate therapy and delayed initiation of appropriate therapy (DIAT) were prospectively evaluated in 76 mechanically ventilated patients with confirmed VAP.[111] Mortality was 29% in 24 patients who received adequate therapy, while it was 63.5% in the remaining 52 patients who received either inappropriate therapy (number = 16) or DIAT (number = 36).[111] Moreover, mortality remains high despite changing to appropriate therapy based on cultures.

The therapeutic strategy should be based on an updated unit-specific distribution of pathogens and patients' risk factors assessment.[48,89,92,113] The American Thoracic Society (ATS) Guidelines published in 2005 provide evidence-based recommendations for the management of immunocompetent patients with VAP.[40] Timing, adequate initial empiric regimen, **de-escalation,** duration of therapy, and pharmacologic consideration are important in managing patients with VAP.[40]

Empiric Therapy

Therapy should be started promptly once VAP is suspected based on clinical and radiologic features.[40,89,113] Patients with VAP who received delayed therapy had higher mortality compared with patients who received adequate timely therapy (58.3% compared with 29.3%).[111] Diagnostic testing should be started at the same time, but should not delay the initiation of therapy.[40,113] The initial antimicrobial regimen should be broad and based on an updated local distribution of pathogens, duration of hospitalization, prior antibiotic treatment, patients' risk factors, and antimicrobial characteristics.[40,113-115] Gram stain of respiratory secretions might be helpful in guiding such choice when positive.[89]

Immunocompetent patients with early-onset VAP, none of the factors listed in Box 14-3, and Gram stains that are not suggestive of high-risk pathogens can be treated with agents that cover *Streptococcus pneumoniae*, *Haemophilus influenzae*, MSSA, and antibiotic-sensitive gram-negative bacilli (Table 14-6).[40,76,78,80,89] Monotherapy with a second or third generation cephalosporin, a beta-lactam/beta-lactamase inhibitor combination, or a quinolone is recommended based on the latest ATS guidelines.[40]

On the other hand, the ATS guidelines for patients with risk factors for MDR pathogens (see Box 14-3) recommend the initial use of combination therapy (see Table 14-6) against resistant gram-negative pathogens (*Pseudomonas aeruginosa*, *Acinetobacter* spp., extended spectrum beta-lactamase producing *Klebsiella pneumoniae*), and antibiotics against MRSA.[40,42,89,116-118] The choice of antibiotics should take into consideration prior antibiotics received. Using agents from different classes will increase the chance of covering pathogens that are resistant to the class of antimicrobial the patient received. An antipseudomonal cephalosporin, beta-lactam/beta-lactamase inhibitor, or carbapenems plus an aminoglycoside or antipseudomonal fluoroquinolone plus anti-MRSA antibiotic (linezolid or vancomycin) is the recommended initial combination for late-onset VAP and for VAP in high-

TABLE 14-6 *Initial Empiric Therapy for VAP*

	POTENTIAL PATHOGENS	ANTIBIOTIC THERAPY
Early onset and no risk factors for MDR	*Streptococcus pneumoniae,* methicillin-sensitive *Staphylococcus aureus, Haemophilus influenzae,* sensitive gram-negative bacilli	Ceftriaxone OR Levofloxacin, moxifloxacin, or ciprofloxacin OR Ampicillin/sulbactam OR Ertapenem
VAP with risk factors for MDR*	Early-onset pathogens plus *Pseudomonas aeruginosa, Acinetobacter* spp., *Klebsiella* (ESBL)† MRSA	Antipseudomonal cephalosporin OR Beta-lactam/beta-lactamase inhibitor OR Carbapenems plus aminoglycoside OR Antipseudomonal fluoroquinolone plus anti-MRSA antibiotic (linezolid or vancomycin)

Data from Guidelines for the management of adults with hospital-acquired, ventilator-associated, and healthcare-associated pneumonia, Am J Respir Crit Care Med 171:388-416, 2005.
MDR, Multidrug resistant; *VAP,* ventilator-associated pneumonia; *ESBL,* extended spectrum beta-lactamase producing; *MRSA,* methicillin-resistant *Staphylococcus aureus.*
*Hospitalization of 5 days or more, prior antibiotic use within 90 days, prior hospitalization for 2 days or more within 90 days, nursing home, chronic dialysis.
†Carbapenems should be used.

risk patients.[40] Once culture results are available, consolidation to monotherapy that is specific against the causative pathogen is recommended unless *Pseudomonas aeruginosa* is isolated.[40] *Acinetobacter baumannii* is frequently resistant to multiple antibiotics and should be targeted (with carbapenems) if known to be prevalent in the ICU and in patients with late-onset VAP, prior antibiotic treatment, ARDS, neurosurgery, head trauma, or large volume aspiration.[40,82,89] Monotherapy for *Acinetobacter* based on culture results is adequate.[40] Similarly, monotherapy with carbapenems is adequate against extended spectrum beta-lactamase producing *Klebsiella pneumoniae.* The combination of two antibiotics from the same class should be avoided to prevent antagonism. Patients allergic to beta-lactams can be treated with aztreonam in combination with a quinolone or an aminoglycoside when combination therapy is indicated. A strategy that promotes the rotation of antibiotics has been shown to decrease the emergence of resistant organisms, both short and long term.[40,119,120]

Pharmacologic Consideration

Choosing the right antibiotic at the right dose is important. Adequate antibiotic dosing and penetration into lung tissue to achieve adequate concentration are crucial for effective therapy.[40] Adequate dosing of antibiotics should take into consideration antibiotic characteristics, host factors, and the minimal inhibitory concentration (MIC) for the pathogen isolated. Aminoglycosides and fluoroquinolones are bactericidal in a concentration-dependent fashion (more rapid killing at higher concentration) with postdose effect, whereas beta-lactams and vancomycin are bactericidal in time-dependent fashion (killing is dependent on the time concentration is above MIC) with no postantibiotic effect.[40] Beta-lactams and vancomycin need to be dosed in a way to maintain concentration above MIC as long as possible, requiring frequent dosing or constant infusion. On the other hand, aminoglycosides and fluoroquinolones require less frequent dosing. The latest ATS guidelines recommending dosing of some of the antibiotics used for VAP in patients with normal renal function are listed in Table 14-7. All patients should receive intravenous therapy and doses need to be adjusted in patients with renal dysfunction.

The use of antibiotics with poor penetration (aminoglycosides, vancomycin) might lead to poor response to therapy and needs to be considered when selecting a therapeutic regimen.[40] Antibiotics with poor penetration should be used in combination with other agents.[32] While direct delivery of aminoglycosides to the distal lung tissue via nebulization can be

TABLE 14-7 *American Thoracic Society Guidelines for Some Recommended Antibiotic Dosages for VAP Patients With Normal Renal Function*

DRUG	DOSAGE
Cefepime	1 g every 8 to 12 hr
Ceftazidime	2 g every 8 hr
Imipenem	500 mg every 6 hr or 1 g every 8 hr
Piperacillin-tazobactam	4.5 g every 6 hr
Gentamicin	7 mg/kg per day
Tobramycin	7 mg/kg per day
Amikacin	20 mg/kg per day
Levofloxacin	750 mg every day
Ciprofloxacin	400 mg every 8 hr
Vancomycin	15 mg/kg every 12 hr
Linezolid	600 mg every 12 hr

Data from Guidelines for the management of adults with hospital-acquired, ventilator-associated, and healthcare-associated pneumonia, Am J Respir Crit Care Med 171:388-416, 2005.

used as adjunctive therapy in patients with MDR gram-negative VAP with poor response to systemic therapy, more studies are needed before one can recommend it for routine clinical use.[40]

The use of vancomycin to treat suspected or confirmed MRSA is a common practice in most ICUs. However, recent studies suggested poor outcome in patients with both MRSA and MSSA pneumonia when treated with vancomycin (compared with MSSA pneumonia treated with cloxacillin), possibly because of poor penetration to the alveolar space.[40,89] Moreover, in 160 patients with MRSA VAP, the mortality was 36.5% in patients treated with vancomycin compared with 20% in patients treated with linezolid.[121] Based on this, it has been suggested that vancomycin should not be considered the agent of choice for the treatment of MRSA VAP, and when used, it should be combined with another agent that is active against MRSA and dosed to maintain high serum concentration (trough level more than 15 μg/ml).[89] Other agents like linezolid, teicoplanin, or trimethoprim-sulfamethoxazole should be considered for the treatment of MRSA.[40,48,122]

In an effort to maintain high antibiotic concentration in the patient with gram-negative VAP, the use of tobramycin plus continuous infusion of meropenem (1 g over 360 minutes every 6 hours) compared with tobramycin plus intermittent infusion (1 g over 30 minutes every 6 hours) of meropenem resulted in superior cure rates (38 of 42, 90.47%, and 28 of 47, 59.57%, respectively).[123] It is important to achieve adequate antibiotic concentrations in plasma and lung tissue that is above MIC to optimize VAP therapy.

De-escalation and Specific Therapy

It is important to reassess the therapeutic regimen in 2 to 3 days once the results of the cultures are available.[40,114,115,124] The initial broad-spectrum therapy should be modified according to the sensitivity of the organism isolated.[114,115,125] The antibiotic that is specific for the isolated organism should be used. Shorter (5 days) courses of aminoglycosides should be considered in cases of combination therapy against *Pseudomonas aeruginosa*.[40] If no MRSA is isolated, gram-positive coverage is not needed.

De-escalation is thought to reduce the incidence of resistant organisms by reducing the unnecessary use of antibiotics without adversely affecting outcome.[40,89,125] In 413 patients, Fagon et al showed that an invasive management strategy using bronchoscopy to guide therapy resulted in less antibiotic use and less 14 days mortality compared with clinical management strategy.[109] As it is important to start with a broad-spectrum antibiotic regimen to cover for all possible resistant organisms, it is important as well to de-escalate therapy on days two to three once more clinical and culture results are available.[40,125,126] Once the cultures are known, the use of combination therapy in the absence of resistant pathogens is not superior to effective monotherapy, and might result in the emergence of resistant pathogens and higher cost and more medication side effects.[40]

In a recent systematic review, the use of a combination of beta-lactam and aminoglycosides compared with monotherapy with beta-lactams did not provide any survival benefit in patients with severe gram-negative infections (1835 patients) or *Pseudomonas aeruginosa* infections (426 patients) while it increased the occurrence of renal dysfunction.[127] There was no difference in the emergence of resistance, and failure rates were higher in the combination group.[127] If cultures show resistant organism or *Pseudomonas aeruginosa*, combination therapy is recommended by the ATS 2005 guidelines to overcome the problem of inappropriate therapy caused by the emergence of resistance while on therapy.[40]

Duration of Therapy

The optimal duration of therapy is not well known.[114,115,128,129] The previous ATS guidelines recommend a 1- to 2-week course for gram-positive and *Haemophilus influenzae* pneumonia, and a 2- to

3-week course for *Pseudomonas aeruginosa, Acinetobacter* spp., or gram-negative necrotizing pneumonia.[118] Based on current evidence, the most recent ATS guidelines recommend 7 days of antibiotic therapy in patients with good response to therapy in the absence of *Pseudomonas aeruginosa.*[40]

A recent prospective multicenter clinical trial by Chastre et al randomly assigned 401 patients with VAP (based on quantitative testing) who received appropriate initial treatment to an 8-day versus 15-day course of antibiotic therapy.[75] Mortality was the same for both groups. Although the mortality was the same in patients with nonfermenting gram-negative bacilli, including *Pseudomonas aeruginosa*, recurrence was 40.6% in the 8-day group compared with 25.4% in the 15-day group. Based on this well-conducted study, with the exception of VAP due to nonfermenting gram-negative bacilli, an 8-day course is as effective as a 15-day course and results in less antibiotic use and less cost, and might decrease the emergence of resistant organisms.

Another approach is to stop antibiotics 3 days after defervescence and change in respiratory secretion.[89] In one study of patients with low CPIS (less than six) at day one and day three of empiric therapy with a quinolone, stopping the antibiotics at day three was associated with less antibiotic use and no adverse outcomes.[104] In patients with negative lower respiratory cultures while not receiving antibiotics over the past 72 hours, empiric therapy can be stopped once culture results are known.[40] Shorter duration of therapy (7 days compared with the traditional 14 to 21 days) is safe and may decrease the emergence of resistance.

Response to Therapy

The clinical response to therapy is slow. Two to three days may elapse before starting to see some clinical response.[118] Therapy should not be changed during the first 3 days unless there are signs of deterioration.[40] Improvement is commonly gradual—up to 1 week or more. Dennesen showed that the mean time to resolution of clinical futures of VAP is 6 days.[130] Colonization with gram-negative bacilli commonly persists despite clinical improvement.[130] Moreover, chest x-ray abnormalities usually lag behind clinical improvement. Failure to respond to therapy or deterioration while on therapy can be due to complicated pneumonia (empyema), resistant organisms, abscess, extrapulmonary infections, or noninfectious causes and should prompt a complete clinical re-evaluation, septic work-up, and possibly a change in the antibiotic regimen based on the clinical situation.[40]

PREVENTION

The high incidence, morbidity, and mortality associated with VAP make applying effective preventive measures essential. In addition to general infection control measures, such as handwashing and regular surveillance, specific preventive measures for VAP are available. The latest Centers for Disease Control and Prevention (CDC) Guidelines published in 2004 provide an evidence-based recommendation for the prevention of VAP.[131] Recommendations are categorized as follow:

- Category IA: Strongly recommended for implementation and strongly supported by experimental, clinical, or epidemiologic studies.
- Category IB: Strongly recommended for implementation and supported by some experimental, clinical, or strong theoretical rationale.
- Category IC: Required for implementation based on federal regulations.
- Category II: Suggested for implementation and supported by suggestive experimental, clinical, or strong theoretical rational.
- No recommendation; unresolved: practice for which no evidence or no consensus exists about efficacy.

The recommendations are summarized in Table 14-8.[131]

Compliance with simple proven preventive measures has been shown to be low.[132-134] Developing evidence-based guidelines and protocols that are unit specific and educating the staff on who to use such measures is essential to improve compliance. The use of an educational program has been shown to reduce the occurrence of VAP by more than 50%.[135] It is important to develop a global approach based on the latest published guidelines (see Table 14-8) for the prevention of VAP rather than applying individual preventive methods.

The use of **bundles,** a group of effective evidence-based interventions applied at the same time, has been shown to be an effective preventive strategy.[136,137] The bundle is recommended by the Institute for Healthcare Improvement as part of **The 100,000 Lives Campaign** and consists of protocols for prophylaxis against peptic ulceration, prophylaxis against deep vein thrombosis, daily cessation of sedation, and elevation of the patient's head and chest to at least 30 degrees.[138]

Oral care has been shown to decrease the occurrence of VAP.[139] In a prospective randomized placebo-controlled trial, oral decontamination with either chlorhexidine (CHX, 2%) or chlorhexidine-colistin

TABLE 14-8 *Summary of VAP Preventive Measures*

IA	IB	II	NO RECOMMENDATION; UNRESOLVED ISSUE
Staff education and involvement in infection control	Infection and microbiologic surveillance	Do not routinely sterilize internals of ventilators	Place a trap at the distal end of the expiratory tubing
Clean and sterilize certain equipment	Periodically drain condensate	Sterile water to fill humidifiers	The use of HME or heated humidifiers
Do not routinely change ventilator circuits unless soiled	Clean, sterilize, and rinse in-line and hand-held nebulizers in-between use	Change HMEs if they malfunction or become soiled	Frequency of changing the filter placed on resuscitation bags
Only use sterile water for nebulization	Use single-vial aerosolized medications	Use sterile single-use suction catheter only	Single-use versus multiuse in-line suction catheters
Decontaminate hands before and after contact with patients	Sterilize or disinfect resuscitation bags between patients	Use sterile fluid to remove suction catheter secretions	Sterile rather than clean gloves during suctioning
Pneumococcal vaccine for patient at risk	Use gloves when in contact with patients or equipment	Use noninvasive ventilation if not contraindicated	Frequency of changing in-line suction catheters
	Wear a gown when soiling is anticipated	Avoid reintubation	Enteral glutamine administration
	Remove devices once possible	Subglottic secretion suctioning	Small-bore feeding tubes, acidification
	Use oral route for tube insertion	Suction above tube cuff before deflation	Continuous versus intermittent feeding
	Confirm feeding tube placement	Semirecumbent position	Postpyloric feeding tube placement
		Regular oral hygiene	Chlorhexidine oral rinse routinely
		Chlorhexidine oral rinse for cardiac surgery patients	Oral and gastric decontamination with antibiotics
			Sucralfate or H_2 blockers used to prevent stress ulcers
			Systemic antibiotic prophylaxis
			Antibiotic rotation
			Chest physiotherapy
			Rotational bed therapy

Data from Tablan OC, Anderson LJ, Bessar R et al: Guidelines for preventing health-care associated pneumonia, 2003: recommendations of CDC and the Healthcare Infection Control Practices Advisory Committee, MMWR Recomm Rep 53:1-36, 2004.

(CHX/COL, 2%/2%) every 6 hours reduced the occurrence of VAP.[140] On the other hand, the use of oral iseganan (an antimicrobial peptide, active against aerobic and anaerobic gram-positive and gram-negative bacteria and fungi and yeasts) for the prevention of VAP was not effective.[141]

Supine position should be avoided. Despite the recommendation to maintain a semirecumbent position, it is not achieved in routine practice nor in a research setting.[142] Noninvasive positive pressure ventilation (NPPV) should be considered in all eligible patients with no contraindication because it has been shown to reduce the need for intubation, prevent VAP, and improve outcome.[143-145] In addition, avoiding unnecessary blood transfusion, the use of a lung-protective mechanical ventilation strategy, timely weaning and extubation, and sedation vacations are strategies that may directly or indirectly decrease the occurrence of VAP.[17,18,137,146-148]

While more research is needed to assess the efficacy of new preventive methods, more efforts are needed to improve the implementation of currently available and effective preventive measures (see Table 14-8).

KEY POINTS

- VAP is the most common nosocomial infection in the ICU, causing significant morbidity and mortality.
- Poor outcomes have been associated with inappropriate therapy despite switching to appropriate therapy.
- The increase in MDR pathogens and the variability in the distribution of pathogens based on patient and ICU characteristics make selecting the appropriate empiric therapy challenging.
- High index of suspicion and aggressive empiric broad-spectrum antibiotics are essential to improve survival.
- Review of culture results to modify and focus the initial empiric (de-escalation) regimen will help to reduce the cost of therapy and minimize the emergence of resistance.
- Shorter antibiotic courses are effective, are less costly, and reduce the emergence of resistance.
- Despite the availability of effective preventive measures, full implementation is yet to be seen.
- Every effort should be made to improve compliance with effective preventive and therapeutic measures.

ASSESSMENT QUESTIONS

1. The most common nosocomial infection in the ICU is:
   A. Urinary tract infection
   B. Central line–related infection
   C. VAP

2. The risk of developing VAP is highest during:
   A. First week of mechanical ventilation
   B. Second week of mechanical ventilation
   C. Third week of mechanical ventilation

3. Which of the following factors is associated with increased risk of developing VAP?
   A. Blood transfusion
   B. Admission to medical versus neurosurgical ICU
   C. Endotracheal cuff pressure of 25 cm H_2O

4. Which of the following is associated with higher mortality in patients with VAP?
   A. Prior antibiotic therapy
   B. Hypoxemia
   C. Use of peptic ulcer prophylaxis

5. Which of the following is true regarding the microbiology of VAP?
   A. About 10% to 15% of cases are caused by fungal infection.
   B. Anaerobic pathogens are isolated in 10% of cases.
   C. Polymicrobial infection is present in about 50% of cases.

6. The most common mode of infection in VAP is:
   A. Inhalation of contaminated aerosols
   B. Microaspiration of oropharyngeal secretions
   C. Aspiration of gastric contents

Continued

ASSESSMENT QUESTIONS—cont'd

7. Multidrug resistant pathogens causing VAP are more likely in which of the following:

A. A patient admitted to the hospital three days ago with history of antibiotic use 1 month back

B. A patient admitted to the hospital 3 days ago with a history of hospital admission 6 months back

C. A patient admitted to the hospital 3 days ago with history of aspiration

8. Which of the following management strategies has been shown to be associated with better outcomes in patients with VAP?

A. Combination antibiotic therapy compared with monotherapy

B. Therapy based on clinical features, chest x-ray, and qualitative cultures

C. Therapy based on clinical features, chest x-ray, and quantitative cultures

9. Which of the following is true regarding the duration of therapy for VAP?

A. All patients should be treated for at least 14 days.

B. Antibiotic therapy for 8 days is safe and effective.

C. It should be based on clinical and chest x-ray improvement.

10. Which of the following is an effective preventive measure against VAP?

A. The use of VAP prevention bundle

B. The use of HMEs rather than bubble humidifiers

C. The use of closed in-line rather than open single-use suction catheters

REFERENCES

1. Warren DK, Shukla SJ, Olsen MA et al: Outcome and attributable cost of ventilator-associated pneumonia among intensive care unit patients in a suburban medical center, Crit Care Med 31:1312-1317, 2003.
2. Woske HJ, Roding T, Shultz I et al: Ventilator-associated pneumonia in a surgical intensive care unit: epidemiology, etiology and comparison of three bronchoscopic methods for microbiological specimen sampling, Crit Care 5:167-173, 2001.
3. Cook DJ, Walter SD, Cook RJ et al: Incidence of and risk factors for ventilator-associated pneumonia in critically ill patients, Ann Intern Med 129:443-440, 1998.
4. Tejerina E, Frutos-Vivar F, Restrepo MI et al: Incidence, risk factors, and outcome of ventilator-associated pneumonia, J Crit Care 21:56-65, 2006.
5. Safdar N, Dezfulian C, Collard HR et al: Clinical and economic consequences of ventilator-associated pneumonia: a systematic review, Crit Care Med 33:2184-2193, 2005.
6. Heyland DK, Cook DJ, Griffith L et al: The attributable morbidity and mortality of ventilator-associated pneumonia in the critically ill patient. The Canadian Critical Trials Group, Am J Respir Crit Care Med 159:1249-1256, 1999.
7. Kollef MH: Ventilator-associated pneumonia. A multivariate analysis, JAMA 270:1965-1970, 1993.
8. Luna CM, Vujacich P, Niederman MS et al: Impact of BAL data on the therapy and outcome of ventilator-associated pneumonia, Chest 111:676-685, 1997.
9. Dupont H, Mentec H, Sollet JP et al: Impact of appropriateness of initial antibiotic therapy on the outcome of ventilator-associated pneumonia, Intensive Care Med 27:355-362, 2001.
10. Iregui M, Ward S, Sherman G et al: Clinical importance of delays in the initiation of appropriate antibiotic treatment for ventilator-associated pneumonia, Chest 122:262-268, 2002.
11. Kollef MH, Ward S: The influence of mini-BAL cultures on patient outcomes: implications for the antibiotic management of ventilator-associated pneumonia, Chest 113:412-420, 1998.
12. Craven DE, Steger KA: Nosocomial pneumonia in mechanically ventilated adult patients: epidemiology and prevention in 1996, Semin Respir Infect 11:32-53, 1996.
13. Hubmayr RD, Burchardi H, Elliot M et al: Statement of the 4th International Consensus Conference in Critical Care on ICU-Acquired Pneumonia-Chicago, Illinois, May 2002, Intensive Care Med 28:1521-1536, 2002.
14. National Nosocomial Infections Surveillance (NNIS) System Report, data summary from January 1992 through June 2004, issued October 2004, Am J Infect Control 32:470-485, 2004.
15. Apostolopoulou E, Bakakos P, Katostaras T et al: Incidence and risk factors for ventilator-associated pneumonia in 4 multidisciplinary intensive care units in Athens, Greece, Respir Care 48:681-688, 2003.
16. Fagon JY, Chastre J, Dormart Y et al: Nosocomial pneumonia in patients receiving continuous mechanical ventilation. Prospective analysis of 52 episodes with use of a protected specimen brush and quantitative culture techniques, Am Rev Respir Dis 139:877-884, 1989.
17. Croce MA, Tolley EA, Claridge JA et al: Transfusions result in pulmonary morbidity and death after a

moderate degree of injury, J Trauma 59:19-23, 2005.
18. Shorr AF, Duh MS, Kelly KM et al: Red blood cell transfusion and ventilator-associated pneumonia: A potential link? Crit Care Med 32:666-674, 2004.
19. Bouza E, Perez A, Munoz P et al: Ventilator-associated pneumonia after heart surgery: a prospective analysis and the value of surveillance, Crit Care Med 31:1964-1970, 2003.
20. Rello J, Ollendorf DA, Oster G et al: Epidemiology and outcomes of ventilator-associated pneumonia in a large US database, Chest 122:2115-2121, 2002.
21. Ibrahim EH, Tracy L, Hill C et al: The occurrence of ventilator-associated pneumonia in a community hospital: risk factors and clinical outcomes, Chest 120:555-561, 2001.
22. Markowicz P, Wolff M, Djedaini K et al: Multicenter prospective study of ventilator-associated pneumonia during acute respiratory distress syndrome. Incidence, prognosis, and risk factors. ARDS Study Group, Am J Respir Crit Care Med 161:1942-1948, 2000.
23. Cook D: Ventilator associated pneumonia: perspectives on the burden of illness, Intensive Care Med 26: S31-37, 2000.
24. Memish ZA, Cunningham G, Oni GA et al: The incidence and risk factors of ventilator-associated pneumonia in a Riyadh hospital, Infect Control Hosp Epidemiol 21:271-273, 2000.
25. Kollef MH, Von Harz B, Prentice D et al: Patient transport from intensive care increases the risk of developing ventilator-associated pneumonia, Chest 112:765-773, 1997.
26. Pawar M, Mehta Y, Khurana P et al: Ventilator-associated pneumonia: Incidence, risk factors, outcome, and microbiology, J Cardiothorac Vasc Anesth 17:22-28, 2003.
27. Joshi N, Localio AR, Hamory BH: A predictive risk index for nosocomial pneumonia in the intensive care unit, Am J Med 93:135-142, 1992.
28. Metheny NA, Clouse RE, Chang YH et al: Tracheobronchial aspiration of gastric contents in critically ill tube-fed patients: frequency, outcomes, and risk factors, Crit Care Med 34:1007-1015, 2006.
29. Cavalcant M, Ferrer M, Ferrer R et al: Risk and prognostic factors of ventilator-associated pneumonia in trauma patients, Crit Care Med 34:1067-1072, 2006.
30. Leone M, Delliaux S, Bourgoin A et al: Risk factors for late-onset ventilator-associated pneumonia in trauma patients receiving selective digestive decontamination, Intensive Care Med 31:64-70, 2005.
31. Bercault N, Wolf M, Runge I et al: Intrahospital transport of critically ill ventilated patients: a risk factor for ventilator-associated pneumonia—a matched cohort study, Crit Care Med 33:2471-2478, 2005.
32. Chastre J, Fagon JY: Ventilator-associated pneumonia, Am J Respir Crit Care Med 165:867-903, 2002.
33. Fagon JY, Chastre J, Hance AJ et al: Nosocomial pneumonia in ventilated patients: a cohort study evaluating attributable mortality and hospital stay, Am J Med 94:281-288, 1993.
34. Bercault N, Boulain T: Mortality rate attributable to ventilator-associated nosocomial pneumonia in an adult intensive care unit: a prospective case-control study, Crit Care Med 29:2303-2309, 2001.
35. Rello J, Lorente C, Diaz E et al: Incidence, etiology, and outcome of nosocomial pneumonia in ICU patients requiring percutaneous tracheotomy for mechanical ventilation, Chest 124:2239-2243, 2003.
36. Rello J, Quintana E, Ausina V et al: Incidence, etiology, and outcomes of nosocomial pneumonia in mechanically ventilated patients, Chest 100:439-444, 1991.
37. Sofianou DC, Constandinidis TC, Yannacou M et al: Analysis of risk factors for ventilator-associated pneumonia in a multidisciplinary intensive care unit, Eur J Clin Microbiol Infect Dis 19:460-463, 2000.
38. Papazian L, Bregeon F, Thirion X et al: Effect of ventilator-associated pneumonia on mortality and morbidity, Am J Respir Crit Care Med 154:91-97, 1996.
39. Bregeon F, Ciais V, Carret V et al: Is ventilator-associated pneumonia an independent risk factor for death? Anesthesiology 94:554-560, 2001.
40. Guidelines for the management of adults with hospital-acquired, ventilator-associated, and healthcare-associated pneumonia, Am J Respir Crit Care Med 171:388-416, 2005.
41. Kollef MH, Silver P, Murphy DM et al: The effect of late-onset ventilator-associated pneumonia in determining patient mortality, Chest 108:1655-1662, 1995.
42. Rello J, Torres A, Ricart M et al: Ventilator-associated pneumonia by *Staphylococcus aureus*. Comparison of methicillin-resistant and methicillin-sensitive episodes, Am J Respir Crit Care Med 150:1545-1549, 1994.
43. Fagon JY, Chastre J, Dormart Y et al: Mortality due to ventilator-associated pneumonia or colonization with Pseudomonas or Acinetobacter species: assessment by quantitative culture of samples obtained by a protected specimen brush, Clin Infect Dis 23:538-542, 1996.
44. Mueller EW, Hanes SD, Croce MA et al: Effect from multiple episodes of inadequate empiric antibiotic therapy for ventilator-associated pneumonia on morbidity and mortality among critically ill trauma patients, J Trauma 58:94-101, 2005.
45. Garnacho J, Sole-Violan J, Sa-Borges M et al: Clinical impact of pneumonia caused by *Acinetobacter baumannii* in intubated patients: a matched cohort study, Crit Care Med 31:2478-2482, 2003.
46. Hijazi M, Al-Ansari M: Therapy for ventilator-associated pneumonia: what works, what doesn't, Respir Care Clin N Am 10:341-358, 2004.
47. Hijazi M, MacIntyre NR: Advances in infection control: ventilator-associated pneumonia. Semin Respir Crit Care Med 21:245-262, 2000.
48. Rello J, Diaz E: Pneumonia in the intensive care unit, Crit Care Med 31:2544-2551, 2003.
49. Johanson WG Jr, Pierce AK, Sanford JP et al: Nosocomial respiratory infections with gram-negative bacilli. The significance of colonization of

the respiratory tract, Ann Intern Med 77:701-706, 1972.
50. Bonten MJ, Bergmans DC, Ambergen AW et al: Risk factors for pneumonia, and colonization of respiratory tract and stomach in mechanically ventilated ICU patients, Am J Respir Crit Care Med 154:1339-1346, 1996.
51. Torres A, el-Ebiary M, Gonzalez J et al: Gastric and pharyngeal flora in nosocomial pneumonia acquired during mechanical ventilation, Am Rev Respir Dis 148:352-357, 1993.
52. Bonten MJ, Gaillard CA, de Leeuw PW et al: Role of colonization of the upper intestinal tract in the pathogenesis of ventilator-associated pneumonia, Clin Infect Dis 24:309-319, 1997.
53. Garrouste-Orgeas M, Chevret S, Arlet G et al: Oropharyngeal or gastric colonization and nosocomial pneumonia in adult intensive care unit patients. A prospective study based on genomic DNA analysis, Am J Respir Crit Care Med 156:1647-1655, 1997.
54. Pesola GR: Ventilator-associated pneumonia in institutionalized elders: are teeth a reservoir for respiratory pathogens? Chest 126:1401-1403, 2004.
55. El-Solh AA, Pietrantoni C, Bhat A et al: Colonization of dental plaques: a reservoir of respiratory pathogens for hospital-acquired pneumonia in institutionalized elders, Chest 126:1575-1582, 2004.
56. Torres A, el-Ebiary M, Soler N et al: The role of the gastric reservoir in ventilator-associated pneumonia, Clin Intensive Care 6:174-180, 1995.
57. Beck-Sague CM, Sinkowitz RL, Chinn RY et al: Risk factors for ventilator-associated pneumonia in surgical intensive-care-unit patients, Infect Control Hosp Epidemiol 17:374-376, 1996.
58. Craven DE, Kunches LM, Kilinsky V et al: Risk factors for pneumonia and fatality in patients receiving continuous mechanical ventilation, Am Rev Respir Dis 133:792-796, 1986.
59. Noor A, Hussain SF: Risk factors associated with development of ventilator associated pneumonia, J Coll Physicians Surg Pak 15:92-95, 2005.
60. Souweine B, Mom T, Traore O et al: Ventilator-associated sinusitis: microbiological results of sinus aspirates in patients on antibiotics, Anesthesiology 93:1255-1260, 2000.
61. Holzapfel L, Chastang C, Demingeon G et al: A randomized study assessing the systematic search for maxillary sinusitis in nasotracheally mechanically ventilated patients. Influence of nosocomial maxillary sinusitis on the occurrence of ventilator-associated pneumonia, Am J Respir Crit Care Med 159:695-701, 1999.
62. Spray SB, Zuidema GD, Cameron JL: Aspiration pneumonia; incidence of aspiration with endotracheal tubes, Am J Surg 131:701-703, 1976.
63. Elpern EH, Jacobs ER, Bone RC: Incidence of aspiration in tracheally intubated adults, Heart Lung 16:527-531, 1987.
64. Diaz E, Rodriguez AH, Rello J: Ventilator-associated pneumonia: issues related to the artificial airway, Respir Care 50:900-906, 2005.
65. Orozco-Levi M, Torres A, Ferrer M et al: Semirecumbent position protects from pulmonary aspiration but not completely from gastroesophageal reflux in mechanically ventilated patients, Am J Respir Crit Care Med 152:1387-1390, 1995.
66. Ibanez J, Penafiel A, Marse P et al: Incidence of gastroesophageal reflux and aspiration in mechanically ventilated patients using small-bore nasogastric tubes, JPEN J Parenter Enteral Nutr 24:103-106, 2000.
67. Hess D: Infection control in the intensive care unit. The role of the ventilator circuit, Minerva Anesthesiol 68:356-359, 2002.
68. Boots RJ, George N, Faoagali JL et al: Double-heater-wire circuits and heat-and-moisture exchangers and the risk of ventilator-associated pneumonia, Crit Care Med 34:687-693, 2006.
69. Lacherade JC, Auburtin M, Cerf C et al: Impact of humidification systems on ventilator-associated pneumonia: a randomized multicenter trial, Am J Respir Crit Care Med 172:1276-1282, 2005.
70. Craven DE, Lictenberg DA, Goularte TA et al: Contaminated medication nebulizers in mechanical ventilator circuits. Source of bacterial aerosols, Am J Med 77:834-838, 1984.
71. Topeli A, Harmanci A, Cetinkaya Y et al: Comparison of the effect of closed versus open endotracheal suction systems on the development of ventilator-associated pneumonia, J Hosp Infect 58:14-19, 2004.
72. Cook D, De Jonghe B, Brochard L et al: Influence of airway management on ventilator-associated pneumonia: evidence from randomized trials, JAMA 279:781-787, 1998.
73. Huxley EJ VJ, Gray WR: Pharyngeal aspiration in normal subjects in patients with depressed consciousness, Am J Med 64:564-568, 1978.
74. Fishman AP: Pulmonary Diseases and Disorders, ed 3, New York: 1998, McGraw-Hill.
75. Chastre J, Wolff M, Fagon JY et al: Comparison of 8 vs 15 days of antibiotic therapy for ventilator-associated pneumonia in adults: a randomized trial, JAMA 290:2588-2598, 2003.
76. Combes A, Figliolini C, Trouillet JL et al: Incidence and outcome of polymicrobial ventilator-associated pneumonia, Chest 121:1618-1623, 2002.
77. Richards MJ, Edwards JR, Culver DH et al: Nosocomial infections in medical intensive care units in the United States. National Nosocomial Infections Surveillance System, Crit Care Med 27:887-892, 1999.
78. Rello J, Torres A: Microbial causes of ventilator-associated pneumonia, Semin Respir Infect 11:24-31, 1996.
79. Heyland DK, Cook DJ, Marshall J et al: The clinical utility of invasive diagnostic techniques in the setting of ventilator-associated pneumonia. Canadian Critical Care Trials Group, Chest 115:1076-1084, 1999.
80. Rello J, Ricart M, Ausina V et al: Pneumonia due to *Haemophilus influenzae* among mechanically ventilated patients. Incidence, outcome, and risk factors, Chest 102:1562-1565, 1992.
81. Rello J, Ausina V, Ricart M et al: Risk factors for infection by *Pseudomonas aeruginosa* in patients with ventilator-associated pneumonia, Intensive Care Med 20:193-198, 1994.

82. Baraibar J, Correa H, Mariscal D et al: Risk factors for infection by *Acinetobacter baumannii* in intubated patients with nosocomial pneumonia, Chest 112:1050-1054, 1997.
83. Babcock HM, Zack JE, Garrison T et al: Ventilator-associated pneumonia in a multi-hospital system: difference in microbiology by location, Infect Control Hosp Epidemiol 24:853-858, 2003.
84. Bergmans D, Bonten M, Gaillard C et al: Clinical spectrum of ventilator-associated pneumonia caused by methicillin-sensitive *Staphylococcus aureus*, Eur J Clin Microbiol Infect Dis 15:437-445, 1996.
85. Marik PE, Careau P: The role of anaerobes in patients with ventilator-associated pneumonia and aspiration pneumonia: a prospective study, Chest 115:178-183, 1999.
86. Azoulay E, Timsit JF, Tafflet M et al: Candida colonization of the respiratory tract and subsequent Pseudomonas ventilator-associated pneumonia, Chest 129:110-117, 2006.
87. Wood GC, Mueller EW, Croce MA et al: Candida sp. isolated from bronchoalveolar lavage: clinical significance in critically ill trauma patients, Intensive Care Med 32:599-603, 2006.
88. Rello J, Esandi ME, Diaz E et al: The role of Candida sp isolated from bronchoscopic samples in nonneutropenic patients, Chest 114:146-149, 1998.
89. Sandiumenge A, Diaz E, Bodi M et al: Therapy of ventilator-associated pneumonia. A patient-based approach based on the ten rules of "The Tarragona Strategy," Intensive Care Med 29:876-883, 2003.
90. National Nosocomial Infections Surveillance (NNIS) System Report, data summary from January 1992 through June 2003, issued August 2003, Am J Infect Control 31:481-498, 2003.
91. Namias N, Samiian L, Nino D et al: Incidence and susceptibility of pathogenic bacteria vary between intensive care units within a single hospital: implications for empiric antibiotic strategies, J Trauma 49:638-645, 2000.
92. Rello J, Sa-Borges M, Correa H et al: Variations in etiology of ventilator-associated pneumonia across four treatment sites: implications for antimicrobial prescribing practices, Am J Respir Crit Care Med 160:608-613, 1999.
93. Lee SO, Kim NJ, Choi SH et al: Risk factors for acquisition of imipenem-resistant *Acinetobacter baumannii*: a case-control study, Antimicrob Agents Chemother 48:224-228, 2004.
94. Grossman RF, Fein A: Evidence-based assessment of diagnostic tests for ventilator-associated pneumonia. Executive summary, Chest 117:177S-181S, 2000.
95. Kirtland SH, Corley DE, Winterbauer RH et al: The diagnosis of ventilator-associated pneumonia: a comparison of histologic, microbiologic, and clinical criteria, Chest 112:445-457, 1997.
96. Torres A, el-Ebiary M, Padro L et al: Validation of different techniques for the diagnosis of ventilator-associated pneumonia. Comparison with immediate post-mortem biopsy, Am J Respir Crit Care Med 149:324-331, 1994.
97. Wunderink RG, Woldenberg LS, Zeiss J et al: The radiologic diagnosis of autopsy-proven ventilator-associated pneumonia, Chest 101:458-463, 1992.
98. Wunderink RG: Radiologic diagnosis of ventilator-associated pneumonia, Chest 117:188S-190S, 2000.
99. Wunderink RG: Clinical criteria in the diagnosis of ventilator-associated pneumonia, Chest 117:191S-194S, 2000.
100. Cook D, Mandell L: Endotracheal aspiration in the diagnosis of ventilator-associated pneumonia, Chest 117:195S-197S, 2000.
101. Pugin J: Clinical signs and scores for the diagnosis of ventilator-associated pneumonia, Minerva Anestesiol 68:261-265, 2002.
102. Luna CM, Blanzaco D, Niederman MS et al: Resolution of ventilator-associated pneumonia: prospective evaluation of the clinical pulmonary infection score as an early clinical predictor of outcome, Crit Care Med 31:676-682, 2003.
103. Papazian L, Thomas P, Garbe L et al: Bronchoscopic or blind sampling techniques for the diagnosis of ventilator-associated pneumonia, Am J Respir Crit Care Med 152:1982-1991, 1995.
104. Singh N, Rogers P, Atwood CW et al: Short-course empiric antibiotic therapy for patients with pulmonary infiltrates in the intensive care unit. A proposed solution for indiscriminate antibiotic prescription, Am J Respir Crit Care Med 162:505-511, 2000.
105. Torres A, el-Ebiary M: Bronchoscopic BAL in the diagnosis of ventilator-associated pneumonia, Chest 117:198S-202S, 2000.
106. Baughman RP: Protected-specimen brush technique in the diagnosis of ventilator-associated pneumonia, Chest 117:203S-206S, 2000.
107. Campbell GD Jr: Blinded invasive diagnostic procedures in ventilator-associated pneumonia, Chest 117:207S-211S, 2000.
108. Torres A, Martos A, Puig de la Bellacasa J et al: Specificity of endotracheal aspiration, protected specimen brush, and bronchoalveolar lavage in mechanically ventilated patients, Am Rev Respir Dis 147:952-957, 1993.
109. Fagon JY, Chastre J, Wolff M et al: Invasive and noninvasive strategies for management of suspected ventilator-associated pneumonia. A randomized trial, Ann Intern Med 132:621-630, 2000.
110. Fagon JY: Diagnosis and treatment of ventilator-associated pneumonia: fiberoptic bronchoscopy with bronchoalveolar lavage is essential, Semin Respir Crit Care Med 27:34-44, 2006.
111. Luna CM, Aruj P, Niederman MS et al: Appropriateness and delay to initiate therapy in ventilator-associated pneumonia, Eur Respir J 27:158-164, 2006.
112. Rello J, Gallego M, Mariscal D et al: The value of routine microbial investigation in ventilator-associated pneumonia, Am J Respir Crit Care Med 156:196-200, 1997.
113. Rello J, Paiva JA, Baraibar J et al: International conference for the development of consensus on the diagnosis and treatment of ventilator-associated pneumonia, Chest 120:955-970, 2001.

114. Vincent JL, Jacobs F: Initial empirical antibacterial therapy of ventilator-associated pneumonia, Treat Respir Med 5:85-91, 2006.
115. Niederman MS: Use of broad-spectrum antimicrobials for the treatment of pneumonia in seriously ill patients: maximizing clinical outcomes and minimizing selection of resistant organisms, Clin Infect Dis 42:S72-81, 2006.
116. Pujol M, Corbella X, Pena C et al: Clinical and epidemiological findings in mechanically-ventilated patients with methicillin-resistant *Staphylococcus aureus* pneumonia, Eur J Clin Microbiol Infect Dis 17:622-628, 1998.
117. Fagon JY, Maillet JM, Novara A: Hospital-acquired pneumonia: methicillin resistance and intensive care unit admission, Am J Med 104:17S-23S, 1998.
118. Hospital-acquired pneumonia in adults: diagnosis, assessment of severity, initial antimicrobial therapy, and preventive strategies. A consensus statement, American Thoracic Society, November 1995, Am J Respir Crit Care Med 153:1711-1725, 1996.
119. Gruson D, Hilbert G, Vargas F et al: Strategy of antibiotic rotation: long-term effect on incidence and susceptibilities of Gram-negative bacilli responsible for ventilator-associated pneumonia, Crit Care Med 31:1908-1914, 2003.
120. Gruson D, Hilbert G, Vargas F et al: Rotation and restricted use of antibiotics in a medical intensive care unit. Impact on the incidence of ventilator-associated pneumonia caused by antibiotic-resistant gram-negative bacteria, Am J Respir Crit Care Med 162:837-843, 2000.
121. Wunderink RG, Rello J, Cammarata SK et al: Linezolid vs vancomycin: analysis of two double-blind studies of patient with methicillin-resistant *Staphylococcus aureus* nosocomial pneumonia, Chest 124:1789-1797, 2003.
122. Lam AP, Wunderink RG: Methicillin-resistant *S. aureus* ventilator-associated pneumonia: strategies to prevent and treat, Semin Respir Crit Care Med 27:92-203, 2006.
123. Lorente L, Lorenzo L, Martin MM et al: Meropenem by continuous versus intermittent infusion in ventilator-associated pneumonia due to gram-negative bacilli, Ann Pharmacother 40:219-223, 2006.
124. Craven DE: What is healthcare-associated pneumonia, and how should it be treated? Curr Opin Infect Dis 19:153-160, 2006.
125. Hoffken G, Niederman MS: Nosocomial pneumonia: the importance of a de-escalating strategy for antibiotic treatment of pneumonia in the ICU, Chest 122:2183-2196, 2002.
126. Niederman MS: The importance of de-escalating antimicrobial therapy in patients with ventilator-associated pneumonia, Semin Respir Crit Care Med 27:45-50, 2006.
127. Paul M, Benuri-Silbiger I, Soares-Weiser K et al: Beta lactam monotherapy versus beta lactam-aminoglycoside combination therapy for sepsis in immunocompetent patients: systematic review and meta-analysis of randomised trials, BMJ 328:668, 2004.
128. de Jesus Chua T, File TM Jr: Ventilator-associated pneumonia: gearing towards shorter-course therapy, Curr Opin Infect Dis 19:185-188, 2006.
129. Koulenti D, Rello J: Gram-negative bacterial pneumonia: aetiology and management, Curr Opin Pulm Med 12:198-204, 2006.
130. Dennesen PJ, van der Ven AJ, Kessels AG et al: Resolution of infectious parameters after antimicrobial therapy in patients with ventilator-associated pneumonia, Am J Respir Crit Care Med 163:1371-1375, 2001.
131. Tablan OC, Anderson LJ, Besser R et al: Guidelines for preventing health-care associated pneumonia, 2003: recommendations of CDC and the Healthcare Infection Control Practices Advisory Committee, MMWR Recomm Rep 53:1-36, 2004.
132. Rello J, Lorente C, Bodi M et al: Why do physicians not follow evidence-based guidelines for preventing ventilator-associated pneumonia? A survey based on the opinions of an international panel of intensivists, Chest 122:656-661, 2002.
133. Heyland DK, Cook DJ, Dodek PM: Prevention of ventilator-associated pneumonia: current practice in Canadian intensive care units, J Crit Care 17:161-167, 2002.
134. Ricart M, Lorente C, Diaz E et al: Nursing adherence with evidence-based guidelines for preventing ventilator-associated pneumonia, Crit Care Med 31:2693-2696, 2003.
135. Zack JE, Garrison T, Trovillion E et al: Effect of an education program aimed at reducing the occurrence of ventilator-associated pneumonia, Crit Care Med 30:2407-2412, 2002.
136. Crunden E, Boyce C, Woodman H et al: An evaluation of the impact of the ventilator care bundle, Nurs Crit Care 10:242-246, 2005.
137. Resar R, Pronovost P, Haraden C et al: Using a bundle approach to improve ventilator care processes and reduce ventilator-associated pneumonia, Jt Comm J Qual Patient Saf 31:243-248, 2005.
138. IHI proposes six patient safety goals to prevent 100,000 annual deaths, Qual Lett Healthcare Lead 17:11-12, 2005.
139. Mori H, Hirasawa H, Oda S et al: Oral care reduces incidence of ventilator-associated pneumonia in ICU populations, Intensive Care Med 32:230-236, 2006.
140. Koeman M, van der Ven AJ, Hak E et al: Oral decontamination with chlorhexidine reduces incidence of ventilator-associated pneumonia, Am J Respir Crit Care Med 173:1348-1355, 2006.
141. Kollef M, Pittet D, Sanchez Garcia M et al: A randomized double-blind trial of iseganan in prevention of ventilator-associated pneumonia, Am J Respir Crit Care Med 173:91-97, 2006.
142. van Nieuwenhoven CA, Vanderbroucke-Grauls C, van Tiel FH et al: Feasibility and effects of the semi-recumbent position to prevent ventilator-associated pneumonia: a randomized study, Crit Care Med 34:396-402, 2006.
143. Lightowler JV, Wedzicha JA, Elliot MW et al: Non-invasive positive pressure ventilation to treat respira-

tory failure resulting from exacerbations of chronic obstructive pulmonary disease. Cochrane systematic review and meta-analysis, BMJ 326:185, 2003.
144. Peter JV, Moran JL, Philips-Hughes J et al: Noninvasive ventilation in acute respiratory failure—a meta-analysis update, Crit Care Med 30:555-562, 2002.
145. Hess DR: Noninvasive positive-pressure ventilation and ventilator-associated pneumonia, Respir Care 50:924-929, 2005.
146. Shorr AF, Jackson WL: Transfusion practice and nosocomial infection: assessing the evidence, Curr Opin Crit Care 11:468-472, 2005.
147. MacIntyre NR: Ventilator-associated pneumonia: the role of ventilator management strategies, Respir Care 50:766-772, 2005.
148. Schweickert WD, Gehlbach BK, Pohlman AS et al: Daily interruption of sedative infusions and complications of critical illness in mechanically ventilated patients, Crit Care Med 32:1272-1276, 2004.

SECTION IV CLINICAL APPLICATIONS

CHAPTER 15

Management of Parenchymal Lung Injury

Neil R. MacIntyre

OUTLINE

OBJECTIVES

- Describe the causes of respiratory failure from parenchymal lung injury.
- Explain the concept of ventilator-induced lung injury in parenchymal lung disease.
- Discuss the tradeoffs involved in balancing gas exchange support with lung injury.
- Compare and contrast current evidence-based approaches to managing parenchymal lung disease.

KEY TERMS

acute lung injury (ALI)
acute respiratory distress syndrome (ARDS)
airway pressure release ventilation (APRV)
ARDS Network
assist-control (A-C) mode
high frequency ventilation (HFV)
lung protective strategies
parenchymal lung injury
pressure-regulated volume control (PRVC)

Parenchymal lung injury describes disease processes that involve the air spaces and the interstitium of the lung. Examples range from focal infections to multilobe contusions to diffuse alveolar damage. Although not technically an injury, cardiogenic edema produces alveolar flooding and gas exchange abnormalities similar to those seen in a parenchymal injury.

The **acute respiratory distress syndrome (ARDS)** and **acute lung injury (ALI)** syndrome are parenchymal injuries that have specific diagnostic criteria[1] (Box 15-1). ARDS and ALI can be divided further into lung-specific injuries, such as massive aspiration, bilateral pneumonias, and drowning and lung injuries as part of a systemic process, such as sepsis or pancreatitis (i.e., the lung is one of many organs affected by a diffuse inflammatory response, the systemic inflammatory response syndrome [SIRS]).

BOX 15-1 *Acute Respiratory Distress Syndrome and Acute Lung Injury Diagnostic Criteria*

Acute-onset disease consistent with ALI/ARDS
$PaO_2/FIO_2 < 200$ (ARDS) <300 (ALI)
Bilateral lung infiltrates on chest radiograph
Injury not reflecting cardiogenic edema (PCWP < 18 if measured)

FIO_2, Inspired O_2 concentration; *PaO_2*, arterial O_2 pressure; *PCWP*, pulmonary capillary wedge pressure.

PATHOPHYSIOLOGY OF PARENCHYMAL LUNG INJURY

Although the disease processes involved in parenchymal lung injury are clearly different, there are a number of important pathophysiologic similarities that relate to the management of mechanical ventilation. Specifically, all these disease processes have varying degrees of interstitial edema, alveolar flooding, surfactant dysfunction, and small airway dysfunction. These produce stiff, low compliance lungs with atelectasis and reduced lung volumes.[2,3]

It is important to remember that many seemingly diffuse parenchymal injuries actually have notable regional differences in the degree of inflammation present and thus the degree of mechanical abnormalities that exist. This heterogeneity can have significant impact on the effects of a particular mechanical ventilation strategy. This is because delivered gases preferentially go to the regions with the highest compliance and the lowest resistance (i.e., the more normal regions) rather than to more affected regions. A normal-sized tidal volume (V_T) thus will be distributed preferentially to the healthier regions and may result in a much higher regional V_T with the potential for regional overstretching and ventilator-induced lung injury (VILI)[4-6] (Figure 15-1).

Parenchymal injury also can affect the airways, especially the bronchioles and alveolar ducts.[7] Injured small airways are narrowed and collapsible and thus can contribute to reduced regional ventilation to injured lung units. These airway abnormalities also can lead to regions of air trapping, and may be a factor in subsequent cyst formation during the healing phase.[8]

Gas exchange abnormalities in parenchymal lung injury are a consequence of ventilation-perfusion ($\dot{V}/\dot{Q}$) mismatching and shunts.[9] Of note is that the

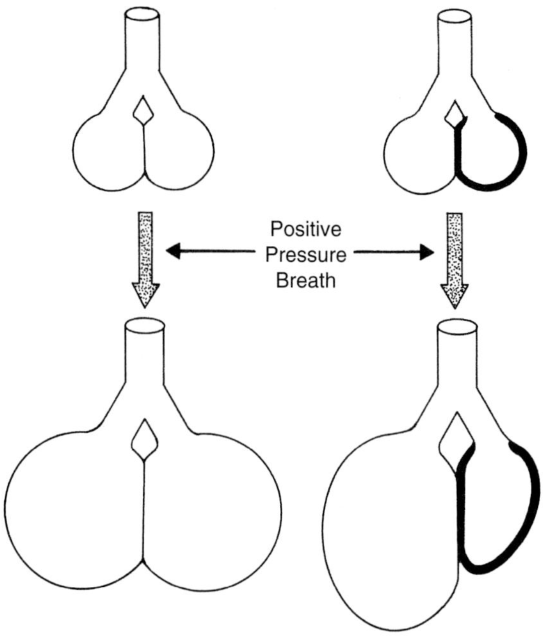

FIGURE 15-1 Effects of a regional compliance abnormality on the distribution of a tidal breath. Note that in a lung with compliance inhomogeneities, a delivered tidal volume distributes to the region with the highest compliance. The resulting regional tidal volume may be sufficiently large to produce regional overdistention. *C_L*, Calculated compliance.

degree of $\dot{V}/\dot{Q}$ mismatch often changes during the ventilatory cycle. For example, a low $\dot{V}/\dot{Q}$ relationship at end inspiration could become a shunt at end expiration if cyclical alveolar collapse occurs. Because dead space ($\dot{V}/\dot{Q} = \infty$) is not a major manifestation of parenchymal lung disease unless there is very severe or end-stage injury, hypoxemia tends to be more of a problem than CO_2 clearance in parenchymal lung disease.

Finally, in parenchymal injury, severe hypoxemia coupled with direct vascular injury often leads to high pulmonary artery pressures. This can compound an O_2 delivery problem by overloading the right ventricle and reducing perfusion through the lung. The need for adequate right heart filling pressures must be balanced against the risk of worsening lung edema when fluid therapy and ventilator pressures are adjusted.[10]

GOALS OF VENTILATORY SUPPORT

The overarching goal of mechanical ventilatory support is to provide adequate gas exchange while avoiding lung injury. Achieving this goal, however, often involves tradeoffs.[11] It is now well understood that VILI is a potentially fatal consequence of lung overdistention and repetitive opening and closing of atelectatic lung units. Importantly, these injuries are often regional and are a consequence of aggressive ventilator strategies aimed at the sicker regions, inadvertently causing VILI in healthier regions as noted above[4-6,12-15] (see Figure 15-1). Thus the need for potentially injurious pressures, volumes, and supplemental O_2 must be weighed against the benefits of gas exchange support. To this end, a rethinking of gas exchange goals has occurred over the last 2 decades and now pH goals as low as 7.15 and PO_2 goals as low as 55 mm Hg are often considered acceptable if the lung can be protected from VILI.[11,16-18] Ventilator settings are thus selected to provide at least this level of gas exchange support while at the same time meeting two mechanical goals:

1. Provision of enough positive end-expiratory pressure (PEEP) to recruit the "recruitable" alveoli.
2. Avoidance of a PEEP-V_T combination that unnecessarily overdistends lung regions.

These gas exchange and mechanical goals embody the concept of a **lung protective strategy** and these principles guide current recommendations for the specific management of parenchymal and most other forms of mechanical ventilatory support.[11,18-20]

In practical terms, balancing four clinical parameters (pH, SaO_2, lung stretch, and FIO_2) constitutes the art of mechanical ventilation in parenchymal lung injury.[11] Unfortunately, few data exist on the relative importance of the critical thresholds for these four parameters (Table 15-1) and thus balancing the tradeoffs is usually based on experience, opinion, and clinical judgment. Management of the very ill patient who is near or at all of these critical thresholds thus constitutes one of the greatest challenges of intensive care unit (ICU) medicine.

MECHANICAL VENTILATION STRATEGIES

Mode Selection

Generally, severe respiratory failure is managed during the acute phases with an **assist-control (A-C) mode** of ventilation. This ensures that all breaths have positive pressure supplied by the ventilator to provide virtually all the work of breathing and unload the acutely overloaded ventilatory muscles.

Choosing flow-volume versus pressure-targeted ventilation for A-C modes depends largely on clinician experience, as the two approaches are far more similar (i.e., both can provide similar frequency-V_T patterns) than they are different and clinical data showing outcome benefits to one over the other are lacking. Flow-volume targeted A-C ventilation (volume assist-control ventilation [VACV]) guarantees a certain V_T. This in turn gives the clinician substantial control over minute ventilation and CO_2 clearance. Under these conditions, however, airway and alveolar pressures are dependent variables and increase or decrease depending on changes in lung mechanics or patient effort. Thus sudden worsening of compliance or resistance can cause abrupt increases in airway and alveolar pressures to preserve minute ventilation. The set flow of VACV during assisted breaths may also produce discomfort in patients with vigorous inspiratory efforts.

In contrast, pressure-targeted ventilation (pressure assist-control ventilation [PACV]), does not guarantee a volume but rather controls inspiratory airway pressure. Volume is thus a dependent variable and will change as lung mechanics or patient efforts change. Changes in compliance or resistance with pressure-targeted ventilation result in changes in volume (i.e., V_T decreases with worsening mechanics and increases with improving mechanics), but maximal airway pressures remain constant. Pressure-targeted ventilation also has a variable decelerating flow waveform, which may improve gas mixing[21] and

TABLE 15-1 *Goals of Mechanical Ventilatory Support*

GOALS	KEY PARAMETER	KEY THRESHOLD
Ventilation	pH	7.15
Oxygenation	SaO_2 (PaO_2)	88%-95% (55-80 mm Hg)
Avoid iatrogenic stretch injury	P_{PLAT}* (V_T)	<30 cm H_2O (4-8 ml/kg IBW)
Oxidant injury	FIO_2	<0.6

CO_2, Carbon dioxide; *FIO_2*, inspired O_2 concentration; *P_{PLAT}*, plateau pressure, *V_T*, tidal volume.
*Lower and upper inflection points on a pressure–volume plot may be more appropriate future parameters.

may interact with any patient efforts more synchronously.[22]

On many modern ventilators, a hybrid form of ventilation mode exists that incorporates features of both pressure and flow-volume targeting. Commonly referred to as **pressure-regulated volume control (PRVC),** this mode is basically a pressure targeted mode with a volume feedback feature. Specifically, with PRVC the clinician selects a tidal volume and the machine then adjusts the inspiratory pressure to assure this volume. On one hand, this preserves the decelerating variable flow features of pressure-targeted breaths while also providing a more constant V_T in the setting of changing mechanics. On the other hand, the inspiratory pressure limit will vary with PRVC and thus potentially expose healthier lung units to higher pressures and regional volumes[6] should overall mechanics worsen. Clinical data exist showing that PRVC behaves as designed but outcome benefits have not been demonstrated to date.[23]

In patients with less severe lung injury (e.g., those not in florid respiratory failure or those recovering from an episode of acute respiratory failure), non–A-C modes, such as pressure support or pressure assist (PACV with a set rate of zero), can be used. The dual control hybrid mode, volume support (VS), is functionally pressure support with a feedback control on the inspiratory pressure to assure a target volume (similar to PRVC). VS attempts to combine some of the synchrony features of pressure targeting with the volume guarantee of flow-volume targeting. These modes, if properly applied, encourage muscle activity to prevent atrophy and allow significant patient control over the ventilatory pattern, which may reduce discomfort.

Frequency-Tidal Volume Settings

Because the rationale behind lung protective ventilatory strategies is to limit tidal and end inspiratory stretch, the delivered V_T should be restricted as much as possible. Accordingly, at the present time it seems reasonable to recommend that the initial V_T setting should be 6 ml/kg ideal body weight (IBW),[18,19,23-25] the V_T shown by the **ARDS Network** to be associated with improved survival when compared with 12 ml/kg IBW.[18] Importantly, this lower V_T in this trial was associated with less lung recruitment and a lower PaO_2/FIO_2 ratio. Nevertheless, the ultimate reduction in lung stretch on outcome was worth this physiologic compromise.

Other features of the ARDS Network V_T strategy include: (1) further reduction in V_T if airway plateau pressure (P_{PLAT}) is greater than 30 cm H_2O; and (2) increases in V_T up to 8 ml/kg IBW if severe respiratory acidosis (see later discussion) or severe patient-ventilator dys-synchrony is present provided that the P_{PLAT} remains below 30 cm H_2O. Note that the use of only P_{PLAT} in this strategy to estimate end inspiratory lung stretching pressure ignores the potential effects of chest wall compliance.[26] If a severely reduced chest wall compliance (e.g., from obesity or ascites) is present, its effects on P_{PLAT} need to be considered either empirically (i.e., arbitrarily assume that an increased pleural pressure is contributing to the P_{PLAT} and increase ventilator pressures accordingly) or else directly measure true transpulmonary pressure using an esophageal pressure monitor.

The set ventilator frequency generally is used to control the CO_2. A reasonable starting point is a normal frequency of between 12 and 20 breaths per minute. Increasing the frequency increases minute ventilation and generally increases CO_2 clearance. At some point, however, air trapping (intrinsic PEEP or PEEPi) develops because of inadequate expiratory times.[27] Under these conditions, either minute ventilation starts to decrease (pressure-targeted ventilation) or airway pressures start to increase (flow-volume targeted ventilation). In general, this begins to happen in parenchymal lung injuries at breathing frequencies exceeding 30 to 35 breaths per minute, although it can occur at much lower frequencies if the inspiratory : expiratory (I:E) ratio is high or the time constant for lung emptying (resistance × compliance) is very high.[27]

The assist capabilities of A-C ventilation allow the patient to trigger breaths. This may help in controlling CO_2 and improving patient comfort. It may also forestall the development of respiratory muscle atrophy—often described as ventilator induced diaphragmatic dysfunction (VIDD).[28] If an inappropriate respiratory drive exists or if patient triggering of assisted breaths is uncomfortable, sedation or paralysis or both may be needed such that only the control breaths of A-C ventilation are provided. However, unless the patient is grossly dys-synchronous with the ventilator despite every effort to make the assisted breaths comfortable, paralysis to eliminate muscle activity should be avoided.[29] Similarly, strategies that routinely employ paralysis and controlled ventilation to reduce O_2 consumption ($\dot{V}O_2$) also should be avoided because the potential decrease in $\dot{V}O_2$ is generally small and the risk of long-term myopathy from neuromuscular blockers is substantial.[30]

The inspiratory flow pattern is generally set to provide synchronous interactions during assisted

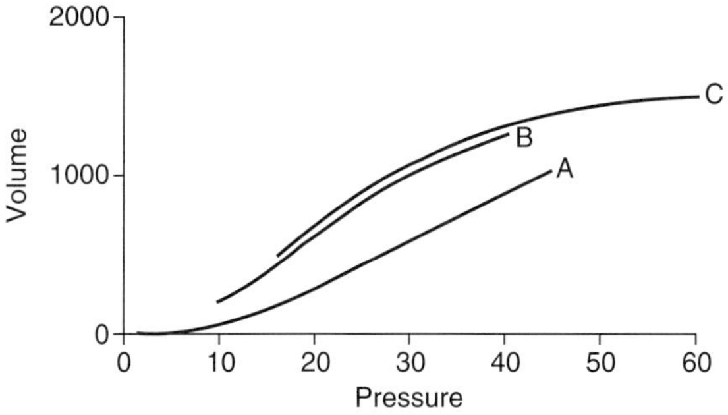

FIGURE 15-2 Pressure-volume plot depicting effects of PEEP in parenchymal lung injury with atelectasis. Curve *A* represents a lung unit with no PEEP and 1 L inflation. Note that at end expiration, this unit is gasless, that it takes 8 cm H_2O of positive pressure to open this lung unit, and that the end inspiratory pressure is 45 cm H_2O. In Curve *B*, 10 cm H_2O PEEP is present. The unit is no longer gasless at end expiration (and thus $\dot{V}/\dot{Q}$ is better), and the end inspiratory pressure following the 1 L inflation is reduced to 40 cm H_2O (reflecting better compliance from intact surfactant). In Curve *C*, 15 cm H_2O PEEP is present. This PEEP level is higher than that needed to maintain recruitment and, when coupled with the 1 L inflation volume, takes the lung unit to excessive end inspiratory pressure and volume ("stretch"). (From MacIntyre NR: Oxygenation support. In Dantzker D, MacIntyre NR, Bakow E, editors: Comprehensive respiratory care, Philadelphia, 1995, Saunders.)

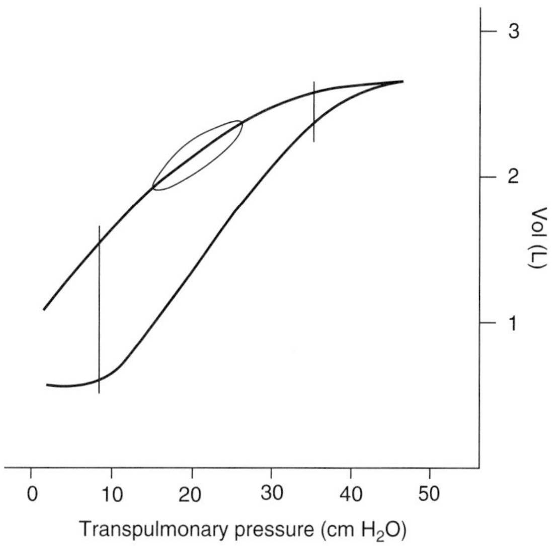

FIGURE 15-3 Pressure-volume plot indicating the ideal place to have the lung during positive pressure ventilation. The lower curve is during inflation, the upper during deflation. The tidal loops on the deflation limb are below the overdistention threshold and above the derecruitment threshold.

breaths and to provide an adequate expiratory time to prevent air trapping (PEEPi). This generally results in I:E of 1:1 to 1:4. An exception to this is when using **airway pressure release ventilation (APRV)**, where long lung inflation periods are interspersed with brief deflation periods. APRV is discussed in more detail below.

Positive End-Expiratory Pressure and Inspired Oxygen Concentration

The goal of PEEP therapy is to engage *recruitable* alveoli while not overdistending already patent alveoli (Figure 15-2). As noted in Chapter 7, PEEP performs its recruitment action primarily by preventing the deflation and collapse of an alveolus opened during inspiration.[14,30-32] To optimize this effect while using the least amount of pressure, PEEP settings can be integrated with a recruitment maneuver, which takes the lung to full inflation and maximally recruits all the recruitable alveoli.[33] The resultant PEEP setting then occurs on the deflation portion of the pressure volume relationship, which requires less pressure for a given volume (Figure 15-3). The actual PEEP setting is usually guided by either mechanical or gas exchange criteria.

Mechanical Criteria

Mechanical criteria involve usually one of two approaches:

1. **Pressure-volume curves**. This approach sets the PEEP/V_T combination to place the lung between upper and lower inflection points[34-36] of a pressure-volume plot in an attempt to minimize overdistention and collapse-reopening injury (see Figure 15-3). Although much of the published literature refers to the inflection points on the inflation limb, it makes more physiologic sense to determine these points on the deflation limb after a recruitment maneuver. As noted previously and in Chapter 6, using an esophageal pressure to account for chest wall mechanical effects on inflection points enhances these techniques.
2. **Best compliance determinations.** This approach uses step changes in PEEP to determine the PEEP level that gives the best compliance.[32] As with the pressure-volume curve approach, best PEEP is probably best determined after a recruitment maneuver has placed the lung on the deflation limb of the curve.

With mechanical approaches to setting PEEP, the F_{IO_2} is adjusted after the PEEP is set to provide the lowest O_2 exposure compatible with P_{O_2} goals (generally P_{O_2} values above 55 to 60 mm Hg). Studies on mechanically targeted PEEP suggest that the operational PEEP in parenchymal lung disease is 8 to 25 cm H_2O, with average first-day requirements in the 10- to 20-cm H_2O range.[11,30]

Gas Exchange Criteria

Gas exchange approaches are the traditional ways to set PEEP.[18,30,37] When using gas exchange goals, the idea is to use F_{IO_2} requirements, Pa_{O_2}, or the calculated shunt fraction as the target. In general the goal is to provide an adequate Pa_{O_2} with a minimal F_{IO_2} requirement. A more aggressive approach would be to normalize (or at least minimize) shunt fraction. This, however, may require very high levels of PEEP and has lost popularity in recent years because it has become apparent that overdistending healthier lung regions is an unacceptable trade-off for aggressive shunt reduction.[11,40] Moreover, some of the apparent shunt reduction that occurs with high PEEP levels may be a consequence of reduced cardiac output from the high intrathoracic pressures.[10]

Two current approaches to using gas exchange criteria to set PEEP are:

1. **PEEP titration curve.** Like the mechanical best PEEP determination above, this approach generally follows a volume recruitment maneuver. Step changes in PEEP are then used to determine the lowest F_{IO_2} that can be achieved for the desired Pa_{O_2} goal.
2. **PEEP-F_{IO_2} Table.** This is an empirical approach that attempts to balance a Sa_{O_2} goal with the harmful effects of pressure and F_{IO_2}. These tables describe step changes in both PEEP and F_{IO_2} to maintain a target Pa_{O_2} (or Sp_{O_2}). The relationship of PEEP and F_{IO_2} in these step changes depends on the clinician's perception of the relative "toxicities" of distending pressures versus high F_{IO_2}—an aggressive PEEP strategy would favor PEEP increases over F_{IO_2} increases; a less aggressive PEEP strategy would do the opposite. A number of recent trials have evaluated PEEP-F_{IO_2} tables with varying degrees of PEEP aggressiveness using small V_T ventilation.[37,38,39] Interestingly, all of these trials showed that more modest PEEP approaches give equivalent outcomes compared with more aggressive PEEP approaches. These results would suggest that as long as opening-closing stresses are reduced by a low V_T strategy, aggressive recruitment strategies with PEEP add little to patient outcomes. Two practical examples of easy to use PEEP-F_{IO_2} tables come from the ARDS Network, which used a Pa_{O_2} goal of 55 to 80 mm Hg (Sp_{O_2} goal of 88 to 95); they are given in Table 15-2.[18,37]

NOVEL APPROACHES TO LUNG PROTECTION IN PARENCHYMAL LUNG INJURY

Two interesting approaches to providing lung protective ventilatory support in adult patients with parenchymal lung injury have been reported over the last two decades: APRV and **high frequency ventilation (HFV).** Interestingly, both strategies attempt to increase lung recruitment with higher mean airway pressures while limiting maximal and tidal airway pressures.

TABLE 15-2 *PEEP/F_{IO_2} Tables Used During the NIH ARDS Network Studies*

The clinical target is a P_{O_2} of 55-80 mm Hg or Sp_{O_2} of 88%-95%. If the patient is below these target values, move up the table to the right. If the patient is above these targets, move down the table to the left.

LOW PEEP APPROACH[17,36]

F_{IO_2}	0.30	0.40	0.40	0.50	0.50	0.60	0.70	0.70	0.70	0.80	0.90	0.90	0.90	1.0	1.0	1.0
PEEP	5	5	8	8	10	10	10	12	14	14	16	18	18	20	22	24

HIGH PEEP APPROACH[36]

F_{IO_2}	0.30	0.30	0.40	0.40	0.50	0.50	0.60	0.60	0.70	0.80	0.80	0.90	1.0	1.0
PEEP	12	14	14	16	16	18	18	20	20	20	22	22	22	24

From National Heart, Lung, and Blood Institute ARDS Clinical Trials Network: Ventilation with lower tidal volumes as compared with traditional tidal volumes for acute lung injury and the acute respiratory distress syndrome, N Engl J Med 342:1301-1308, 2000; and National Heart, Lung, and Blood Institute ARDS Clinical Trials Network: Higher versus lower positive end-expiratory pressures in patients with the acute respiratory distress syndrome, N Engl J Med 351:327-336, 2004.

Airway Pressure Release Ventilation

APRV is a pressure-targeted mode of ventilatory support that is similar to PACV in that it supplies patient- or machine-triggered, pressure-targeted, time-cycled breaths.[41-43] APRV differs from PACV in that a pressure release feature is present, which allows spontaneous breaths to occur during the inflation phase. This capability allows for the use of long inflation times to recruit alveoli while allowing patients to continue to breathe spontaneously. Intermittent short deflation periods provide for ventilatory support. Taken together, the long inflation times (and often resulting PEEPi) can be considered an alternative way to raise mean pressures and maintain recruitment without applying additional PEEP or V_T. Moreover, the spontaneous breaths during APRV may contribute to better $\dot{V}/\dot{Q}$ matching and cardiac function.[41,43] Indeed, APRV can be weaned by reducing the inflation pressure as spontaneous breathing increases.

APRV has been shown to provide generally better lung recruitment at higher mean pressures than conventional strategies with similar maximal applied pressures.[41-43] It is important to remember, however, that spontaneous breaths during the inflation period will *add* to the end-inspiratory stretching pressure on the lung. Thus unlike conventional ventilation, the set inflation pressure with APRV is a gross underestimate of end-inspiratory transpulmonary pressure. Moreover, the prolonged high pressure inflations and the periodic rapid deflation-reinflations may have their own injury potential.

Two randomized controlled trials have been conducted using APRV. In one, however, the control group strategy required paralysis and was associated with significant worsening in gas exchange.[43] It is thus difficult to judge the effects of APRV from these data. In the other trial, no difference in sedation, gas exchange, or outcome could be demonstrated using APRV.[44] The role of APRV in parenchymal lung injury thus remains speculative.[45] APRV is discussed in more detail in Chapter 22.

High Frequency Ventilation

HFV is a strategy to also raise mean airway pressures (and thus maintain better recruitment) that avoids large tidal pressure swings and thus theoretically could reduce overdistention injury.[46-50] HFV uses V_Ts notably less than anatomic dead space along with frequencies of 100 to 300 (or even up to 900) breaths per minute. Gas transport between the airways and the alveoli under these circumstances involves a number of nonconvective mechanisms that are not well understood. Importantly, at the alveolar level, V_T and pressure swings are so small that some have labeled HFV as "CPAP with a wiggle."

HFV has been shown to improve outcomes in numerous studies of infants with respiratory failure.[48] The adult HFV literature is much smaller, but has shown HFV to safely provide adequate gas exchange.[50] The only true randomized trial of HFV in ARDS showed only a promising trend towards improved outcomes with HFV.[51] As a consequence HFV is generally used only when lung protection is judged inadequate using conventional techniques. HFV is discussed in much more detail in Chapter 23.

OTHER CONSIDERATIONS IN MANAGING PARENCHYMAL LUNG INJURY

Although beyond the scope of this chapter to discuss in detail, it is always important for clinicians to realize that other supportive strategies can have significant impact on mechanical ventilation outcomes. One recent example is the importance of fluid management on the duration of mechanical ventilation. Specifically, a fluid management strategy focused on keeping the lungs "dry" by maintaining balanced intake (output and low central venous pressures significantly shortened the duration of mechanical ventilation).[52] Additional considerations include nutrition (Chapter 11), positioning (Chapter 13), infection control (Chapter 14) and other intensive care unit protocols focused on minimizing complications (e.g., deep venous thrombosis prophylaxis, stress ulcer prophylaxis, airway care, wound care, etc.).

OUTCOME OF PARENCHYMAL LUNG INJURY

The outcome of patients with parenchymal lung injury requiring mechanical ventilation depends heavily on the cause of the injury and the severity of the injury.[53,54] The cause of the lung injury is of particular importance. Specifically, in ARDS, the highest mortality is associated with lung injury as a manifestation of systemic injury. Depending on the numbers of other organs involved, mortality rates can approach 100% under these circumstances. Conversely, lung injury from a lung-only process may be associated with a mortality rate of less than 30%. Initial oxygenation impairment is not a good predictor of mortality in ARDS, although persistence of lung injury is. There is some evidence that short-term survival statistics of patients with ARDS have been improving over the last 2 decades,[54] probably a reflection of better overall ICU management than any single new treatment modality. The most impressive reported mortality reduction to date in ARDS was the result of reducing V_T from 12 to 6 ml/kg IBW in the ARDS Network trial.[18]

Long-term outcomes from parenchymal lung injury requiring mechanical ventilation are mixed in survivors with ARDS. Long-term pulmonary function testing often reveals good function, with near normal recovery in many of these patients.[55] On the other hand, significant neuro-psychiatric sequelae may persist for years.[56] Patients with chronic underlying lung disease, such as fibrosis or other significant co-morbidities, can have extended recovery periods and often never return to baseline function.

KEY POINTS

- The pathophysiologic consequences of parenchymal lung injury include a heterogeneous distribution of stiff, low-compliance lung units with impaired gas exchange.
- Current approaches to positive pressure ventilation focus not only on recruiting and ventilating diseased units but also on avoiding injuring healthy units.
- The goals of mechanical ventilatory support of parenchymal lung injury have shifted over the last decade to providing smaller (and thus less injurious) V_Ts and accepting consequently lower arterial values for PO_2 and the development of respiratory acidosis. This has resulted in significant improvements in outcomes.
- Future developments will need to further refine this lung protective concept.

ASSESSMENT QUESTIONS

1. True or False. In the ARDS Network trial, the small V_T strategy improved both the PO_2 and the mortality rate in ARDS.
2. True or False. In several recent trials using small V_T ventilation, adding an aggressive PEEP strategy further improved outcomes.
3. True or False. VILI can be reduced by limiting P_{PLAT} to less than 30 cm H_2O.
4. True or False. Parenchymal lung disease refers to injury to the alveolar spaces and interstitium.
5. True or False. Parenchymal lung injury is characterized by high-compliance, high-resistance lung units.
6. True or False. PEEP is primarily used to prevent alveolar derecruitment.
7. True or False. The P_{PLAT} is largely determined by the pressures required to drive flow into atelectatic lung units.
8. True or False. The ARDS Network recommendation is to start with V_Ts of 6 ml/kg of actual body weight.
9. True or False. Repetitive opening and closing of alveolar units has little effect on VILI.
10. True or False. APRV has been shown in well-designed randomized clinical trials to improve outcome in ARDS.

CASE STUDIES

For additional practice, refer to Case Studies 1, 2, 7, 8, and 10 in the appendix at the back of this book.

REFERENCES

1. Bernard GR, Artigas A, Brigham KL et al: American-European consensus conference on ARDS, Am J Respir Crit Care Med 149:818-824, 1994.
2. Petty TL, Ashbaugh DG: The adult respiratory distress syndrome: clinical features, factors influencing prognosis, and principles of management, Chest 60:233-239, 1971.
3. Fulkerson WJ, MacIntyre NR: Pathogenesis and treatment of the adult respiratory distress syndrome, Arch Intern Med 156:29-38, 1996.
4. Gattinoni L, Pesenti A, Torresin A et al: Adult respiratory distress syndrome profiles by computed tomography, J Thorac Imaging 3:25-30, 1988.

5. Gattinoni L, Pesenti A, Baglioni S et al: Inflammatory pulmonary edema and PEEP: correlation between imaging and physiologic studies, J Thorac Imaging 3:59-64, 1988.
6. Terragni PP, Rosboch G, Tealdi A et al: Tidal hyperinflation during low tidal volume ventilation in ARDS, Am J Respir Crit Care Med 175:160-166, 2007.
7. Pratt PC: Pathology of the adult respiratory distress syndrome. In: Thurlbeck WM, Abel MR, editors: The lung: structure, function and disease, Baltimore, 1978, Williams and Wilkins, pp 43-57.
8. Pratt P, Vollmer R, Shelburne J et al: Pulmonary morphology in a multihospital collaborative extracorporeal membrane oxygenation project: I, light microscopy, Am J Pathol 95:191-214, 1979.
9. Wagner PD: Ventilation-perfusion relationships, Annu Rev Physiol 42:235-247, 1980.
10. Pinsky MR, Guimond JG: The effects of positive end-expiratory pressure on heart-lung interactions, J Crit Care 6:1-15, 1991.
11. Slutsky AS: ACCP consensus conference: mechanical ventilation, Chest 104:1833-1859, 1993.
12. Dreyfus D, Soler P, Bassett G et al: High inflation pressure pulmonary edema, Am Rev Respir Dis 137:1159-1164, 1988.
13. Plotz FB, Slutsky AS, van Vught AJ et al: Ventilator-induced lung injury and multiple system organ failure: a critical review of facts and hypotheses, Intensive Care Med 30:1865-1872, 2004.
14. Webb HJH, Tierney DF: Experimental pulmonary edema due to intermittent positive pressure ventilation with high inflation pressures: Protection by positive end-expiratory pressure, Am Rev Respir Dis 110:556-565, 1974.
15. Dreyfuss D, Savmon G: Ventilator induced lung injury: lessons from experimental studies Am J Respir Crit Care Med 157:294-323, 1998.
16. Fiehl F, Perret C: Permissive hypercapnia—how permissive should we be? Am J Respir Crit Care Med 150:1722-1737, 1994.
17. Hickling KG, Walsh J, Henderson S et al: Low mortality rate in adult respiratory distress syndrome using low-volume, pressure-limited ventilation with permissive hypercapnia: a prospective study, Crit Care Med 22:1568-1578, 1994.
18. NIH ARDS Network: Ventilation with lower tidal volumes as compared with traditional tidal volumes for acute lung injury and the acute respiratory distress syndrome, N Engl J Med 342:1301-1308, 2000.
19. Villar J, Kacmarek R, Peres-Mendez L et al: A high positive end expiratory pressure low tidal volume strategy improves outcome in persistent ARDS, Crit Care Med 34:1311-1318, 2006.
20. Amato MB, Barbas CSV, Medeivos DM et al: Effect of a protective-ventilation strategy on mortality in the acute respiratory distress syndrome, N Engl J Med 338:347-354, 1998.
21. Abraham E, Yoshihara G: Cardiorespiratory effects of pressure controlled ventilation in severe respiratory failure, Chest 98:1445-1449, 1990.
22. MacIntyre NR, McConnell R, Cheng KC et al: Pressure limited breaths improve flow dyssynchrony during assisted ventilation, Crit Care Med 25:1671-1677, 1997.
23. MacIntyre NR, Branson RD: Feedback enhancements on ventilator breaths. In Tobin M, editor: Principles and practice of mechanical ventilation, ed 2, New York, 2006, McGraw-Hill.
24. Gajic O, Frutos-Vivar F, Esteban A, et al: Ventilator settings as a risk factor for acute respiratory distress syndrome in mechanically ventilated patients, Intensive Care Med 31:922-926, 2005.
25. Hager DN, Krishman JA et al: Tidal volume reductions in patients with acute lung injury when plateau pressures are not high, Am J Respir Crit Care Med 172:1241-1245, 2005.
26. Ranieri VM, Brienza N, Santostasi S et al: Impairment of lung and chest wall mechanics in patients with acute respiratory distress syndrome: role of abdominal distension, Am J Respir Crit Care Med 156:1082-1091, 1997.
27. Marini JJ, Crooke PS: A general mathematical model for respiratory dynamics relevant to the clinical setting, Am Rev Respir Dis 147:14-24, 1993.
28. Vassilakopoulos T, Petrof BJ: Ventilator-induced diaphragmatic dysfunction, Am J Respir Crit Care Med 169:336-341, 2004.
29. Raps EC, Bird SJ, Hansen-Flashen J: Prolonged muscle weakness after neuromuscular blockade in the ICU, Crit Care Clin 10:799-813, 1994.
30. American Association for Respiratory Care: Positive end expiratory pressure—state of the art after 20 years, Respir Care 33:417-500, 1988.
31. Crotti S, Mascheroni D, Caironi P et al: Recruitment and derecruitment during acute respiratory failure: a clinical study, Am J Respir Crit Care Med 164:131-140, 2001.
32. Suter PM, Fairley HB, Isenberg MD: Optimum end-expiratory pressure in patients with acute pulmonary failure, N Engl J Med 292:284-289, 1975.
33. Lim SC, Adams AB, Simonson DA et al: Intercomparison of recruitment maneuver efficacy in three models of acute lung injury, Crit Care Med 32:2371-2377, 2004.
34. Benito S, Lemaire F: Pulmonary pressure-volume relationship in acute respiratory distress syndrome in adults: role of positive end expiratory pressure, J Crit Care 5:27-34, 1990.
35. Putensen C, Bain M, Hormann C: Selecting ventilator settings according to the variables derived from the quasi static pressure volume relationship in patients with acute lung injury, Anesth Analg 77:436-447, 1993.
36. Servillo G, Svantesson C, Beydon L et al: Pressure-volume curves in acute respiratory failure: automated low flow inflation vs occlusion, Am J Respir Crit Care Med 155:1629-1636, 1997.
37. Brower RG, Lanken PN, MacIntyre N et al: National Heart, Lung, and Blood Institute ARDS Clinical Trials Network. Higher versus lower positive end-expiratory pressures in patients with the acute respiratory distress syndrome, N Engl J Med 351:327-336, 2004.
38. Stewart T, Meade M, LOVS Trial: Presentation at the European Society for Intensive Care Medicine, Barcelona, Spain, Sept 2006.

39. Mercat A: Express Trial. Presentation at the European Society for Intensive Care Medicine, Barcelona, Spain, Sept 2006.
40. Kolobow T, Moretti MP, Fumagalli R et al: Severe impairment in lung function induced by high peak airway pressure during mechanical ventilation, Am Rev Respir Dis 135:312-315, 1987.
41. Habashi NM: Other approaches to open-lung ventilation: airway pressure release ventilation, Crit Care Med 33(3 Suppl):S228-240, 2005.
42. Stock MC, Downs JB, Frolicher DA: Airway pressure release ventilation, Crit Care Med 15:462-466, 1987.
43. Putensen C, Zech S, Wrigge H et al: Long term effects of spontaneous breathing during ventilatory support in patients with ALI, Am J Respir Crit Care Med 164:43-49, 2001.
44. Varpula T, Valta P, Niemi R et al: Airway pressure release ventilation as a primary ventilation mode in ARDS, Acta Anaesth Scand 48:722-731, 2004.
45. Sevransky JE, Levy MM, Marini JJ: Mechanical ventilation in sepsis induced ALI/ARDS—an evidence based review, Crit Care Med 32:S548-553, 2004.
46. Froese AB, Bryan C: High frequency ventilation, Am Rev Respir Dis 135:1363-1374, 1987.
47. Chang HK: Mechanisms of gas transport during high frequency ventilation, J Appl Physiol 56:553-563, 1984.
48. Froese AB, Kinsella JP: High-frequency oscillatory ventilation: lessons from the neonatal/pediatric experience, Crit Care Med 33(3 Suppl):S115-121, 2005.
49. Froese AB: High frequency oscillatory ventilation for ARDS: let's get it right this time, Crit Care Med 25:906-908, 1998.
50. Mehta S, Granton J, MacDonald RJ et al: High-frequency oscillatory ventilation in adults: the Toronto experience, Chest 126:518-527, 2004.
51. Derdak S, Mehta S, Stewart TE et al: Multicenter oscillatory ventilation for acute respiratory distress syndrome trial (MOAT) study investigators. High-frequency oscillatory ventilation for acute respiratory distress syndrome in adults: a randomized, controlled trial, Am J Respir Crit Care Med 166:801-808, 2002.
52. NIH ARDS Network: Comparison of two fluid management strategies in acute lung injury, N Engl J Med 354:2564-2575, 2006.
53. Gillespie DJ, Marsh HMN, Divertie MB et al: Clinical outcome of patients requiring prolonged (>24 hrs) mechanical ventilation, Chest 90:364-382, 1986.
54. Milberg JA, Davis DR, Steinberg KP et al: Improved survival of patients with ARDS: 1983-1993, JAMA 273:306-309, 1995.
55. Ingbar DH, Matthew RA: Lung function in survivors, Crit Care Clin 2:377-380, 1986.
56. Herridge MS, Cheung AM, Tansey CM et al: One-year outcomes in survivors of the acute respiratory distress syndrome, N Engl J Med 348:683-693, 2003.

CHAPTER

16

Management of Obstructive Airway Disease

NEIL R. MACINTYRE

OUTLINE

OBJECTIVES

- Describe the pathophysiology of obstructive airways.
- Discuss approaches to ventilator settings in patients with obstructive lung disease.
- Explain the effects of intrinsic PEEP on mechanical ventilation settings.
- State the outcomes of respiratory failure from obstructive airway diseases.

KEY TERMS

air trapping
ARDS Network
dead space
hypercapnia
hypoventilation
obstructive lung disease
overdistention
permissive hypercapnia

Airflow obstruction is a manifestation of a number of disease processes. Among the most common of these are asthma and chronic obstructive pulmonary disease (COPD). Less common causes include bronchiectasis, cystic fibrosis, bronchiolitis, and other processes involving the small and large airways of the lung. Acute respiratory failure from exacerbation of airflow obstruction is a common occurrence in these diseases. Causes for these acute exacerbations include infection (both bacterial and viral), environmental stresses (e.g., allergens, toxins, and dusts), cardiac abnormalities, and systemic inflammatory processes. In patients with airway disease, respiratory failure is often the end result of a progressive worsening of airflow obstruction over several days.[1] In the asthmatic patient, respiratory failure can occur rapidly, with acute bronchospasm and mucous plugging in *asthma sudden death syndrome*.[1]

PATHOPHYSIOLOGY OF OBSTRUCTIVE AIRWAY DISEASES

Respiratory failure from airflow obstruction is a direct consequence of acute airway narrowing and critical increases in airway resistance. These lead to two important mechanical changes. First, the increased pressures required for airflow may overload respiratory muscles, producing a ventilatory pump failure with spontaneous minute ventilation inadequate for gas exchange.[2] Second, the narrowed airways create regions of the lung that cannot be properly emptied and returned to their normal resting volume. This sometimes is called **air trapping** and produces elevated end-expiratory pressures (intrinsic positive end-expiratory pressure [PEEPi] or auto-PEEP).[3,4] These regions of overinflation put inspiratory muscles at a substantial mechanical disadvantage, which further worsens respiratory muscle function. Overinflated regions also may compress more healthy regions of the lung, impairing ventilation-perfusion ($\dot{V}/\dot{Q}$) matching. The high intrathoracic pressures may also impair cardiac filling. During spontaneous efforts, regions of air trapping and intrinsic PEEP can also function as a threshold load to trigger assisted breaths, which can further overload ventilatory muscles.[4,5]

There are several gas exchange abnormalities that occur with worsening airflow obstruction.[6] First, although there may be a transient hyperventilation due to dyspnea in the asthmatic, worsening respiratory failure in **obstructive lung disease** generally is characterized by **hypoventilation,** producing hypercapnic respiratory failure. Second, overdistended regions of the lung (PEEPi) coupled with underlying emphysematous changes in some patients result in capillary loss and increasing **dead space.** This wasted ventilation further compromises the ability of the respiratory muscles to supply adequate ventilation for alveolar gas exchange. Third, hypoxemia can develop as a consequence of $\dot{V}/\dot{Q}$ mismatch produced from maldistributed ventilation. Alveolar inflammation and flooding, however, are not characteristic features of respiratory failure due to pure airflow obstruction, and thus shunts are less of an issue than in parenchymal lung injury. Fourth, hypoxemia-induced pulmonary vasoconstriction, coupled with chronic pulmonary vascular changes in some airway diseases, overloads the right ventricle, further decreasing blood flow to the lung and making the dead space larger.

All of these issues must be considered in providing mechanical ventilatory support for the patient with respiratory failure from airflow obstruction. Sometimes this support can be accomplished with noninvasive systems as described in Chapter 21. However, the remainder of this chapter will focus on the management of patients requiring endotracheal intubation for ventilatory support.

GOALS OF VENTILATORY SUPPORT

In general, the overall goals of ventilatory support in respiratory failure due to airflow obstruction are similar to overall goals in other forms of respiratory failure—providing adequate gas exchange while minimizing lung injury. There are, however, two other considerations that are particularly important in the patient with airflow obstruction.

First, the development of air trapping and PEEPi creates several challenges in providing mechanical ventilatory support.[4,5] Specifically, PEEPi places ventilatory muscles at a further mechanical disadvantage, imposes significant breath trigger loads on these muscles, reduces right ventricular filling, and raises the baseline (and thus all subsequent inspiratory) pressures. Mechanical ventilatory strategies must focus on minimizing PEEPi and its effects.

Second, narrowed airways produce a high resistance to flow that can result in very high peak airway pressures. Much of this pressure is dissipated in providing gas flow through obstructed airways and therefore does not overdistend distal alveoli. However, the heterogeneous distribution of airflow obstruction seen in most airway diseases means that less obstructed alveolar regions may transiently be exposed to these high peak pressures and thus be at risk for overdistention injury (Figure 16-1). Because of this, clinicians should realize that a high peak pressure, even in the presence of acceptable plateau pressures (i.e., less than 30 cm H_2O), should be avoided.

It is important to realize that managing both of these issues may involve significant reductions in delivered minute ventilation and resulting **hypercapnia.** This is the basis for the concept of **permissive hypercapnia**—accepting the development of a respiratory acidosis to protect the lung and the respiratory muscles.[7,8]

MECHANICAL VENTILATION STRATEGIES

Mode Selection

Generally, severe respiratory failure from airway obstruction is managed during the acute phases with an assist-control (A-C) mode of ventilation. This ensures that all breaths have positive pressure supplied by the ventilator to provide virtually all the work of breathing and unload the acutely overloaded ventilatory muscles.

Choosing flow-volume versus pressure-targeted ventilation for A-C modes depends largely on clinician experience, as the two approaches are far more similar (i.e., both can provide similar frequency-tidal volume [V_T] patterns) than they are different and clinical data showing outcome benefits to one over the other are lacking. Flow-volume targeted A-C ventilation (volume assist-control ventilation [VACV])

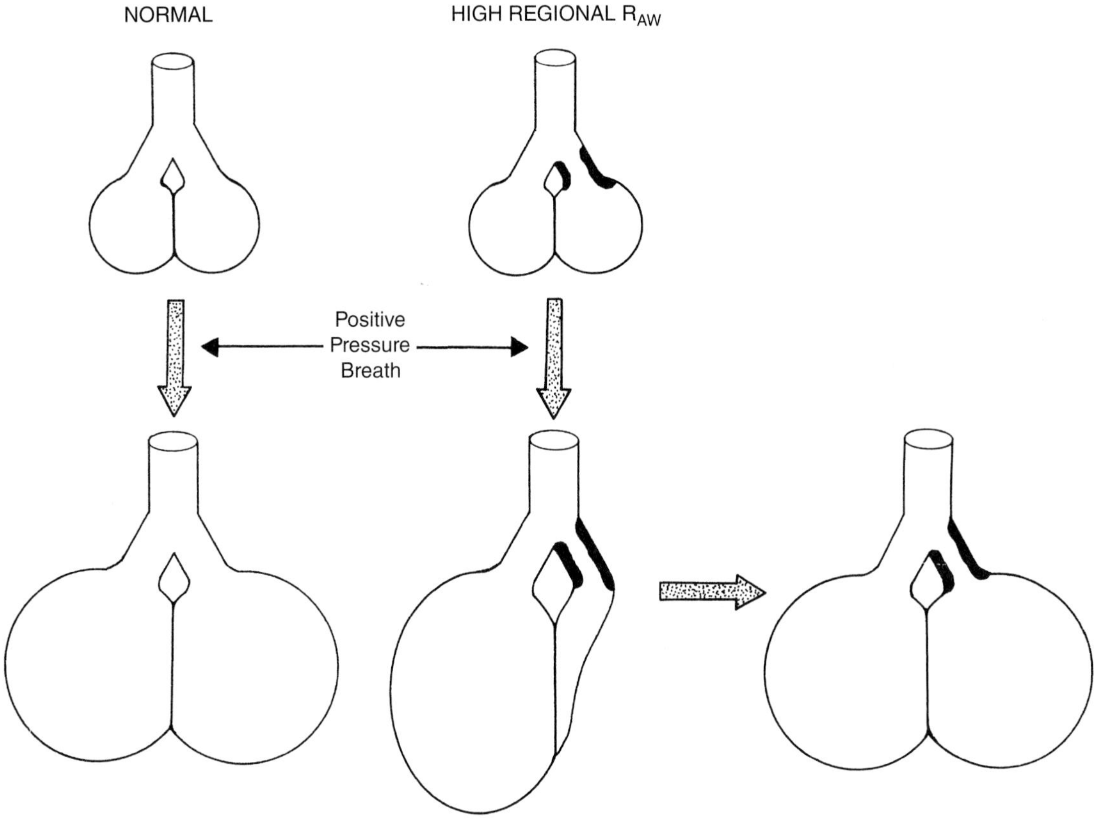

FIGURE 16-1 Regional overdistention and pendelluft effect from heterogeneous distribution of airway properties.

guarantees a certain V_T. This, in turn, gives the clinician substantial control over minute ventilation and CO_2 clearance. Under these conditions, however, airway and alveolar pressures are dependent variables and increase or decrease depending on changes in lung mechanics or patient effort. Thus sudden worsening of airway resistance can cause abrupt increases in airway pressures to preserve minute ventilation. The set flow of VACV during assisted breaths may also produce discomfort in patients with vigorous inspiratory efforts. In contrast, pressure-targeted ventilation (pressure assist-control ventilation [PACV]) does not guarantee a volume but rather controls inspiratory airway pressure. Volume is thus a dependent variable and will change as lung mechanics or patient efforts change. Sudden worsening of airway resistance with pressure-targeted ventilation results in a loss of volume but maximal airway pressures will not rise. Pressure-targeted ventilation also has a variable decelerating flow waveform, which may improve gas mixing[9] and may interact with any patient efforts more synchronously.[10]

On many modern ventilators, a hybrid form of ventilation mode exists that incorporates features of both pressure and flow-volume targeting.[11] Commonly referred to as pressure regulated volume control (PRVC), this mode is basically a pressure-targeted mode with a volume feedback feature. Specifically, with PRVC the clinician selects a V_T and the machine then adjusts the inspiratory pressure to assure this volume. On one hand, this preserves the decelerating variable flow features of pressure targeted breaths while also providing a more constant V_T. On the other hand, the inspiratory pressure limit will vary with PRVC and thus potentially expose healthier lung units to higher volumes and pressures should overall mechanics worsen. Clinical data exist showing that PRVC behaves as designed but outcome benefits have not been demonstrated to date.

In patients with less severe airflow obstruction (e.g., those not in florid respiratory failure or those recovering from an episode of acute respiratory failure), non-A/C modes, such as pressure support (PS) or pressure assist (PACV with a set rate of zero), can be used. The dual control hybrid mode, VS, is functionally pressure support with a feedback control on the inspiratory pressure to assure a target volume.[11] VS attempts to combine some of the synchrony features of pressure targeting with the volume guarantee of flow-volume targeting. These modes, if properly applied, encourage muscle activity to prevent atrophy and allow significant patient control over the ventilatory pattern, which may reduce discomfort. As discussed in more detail below, flow cycling with PS and VS can be unduly delayed in the presence of significant airway obstruction. Care must thus be taken when using these modes to assure that expiratory time is adequate to minimize PEEPi.

Tidal Volume/Frequency/InspiratoryTime

Unlike in parenchymal lung injury, an **ARDS Network** like V_T study has not been done in obstructive diseases. However, because there can be great regional disparity in the degree of airflow obstruction (see Figure 16-1) and because the concept behind lung protective strategies is to protect the more normal and healthier units from ventilator-induced lung injury (VILI),[12-15] it would seem reasonable in patients with respiratory failure from airflow obstruction to start with the ARDS Network V_T target of 6 ml/kg IBW and keep P_{PLAT} below 35 cm H_2O.[16,17] Adjustments can be made as per ARDS Network rules: increases in V_T up to 8 ml/kg IBW for either severe patient-ventilator dys-synchrony or severe respiratory acidosis; decreases in V_T to 5 ml/kg IBW to maintain P_{PLAT} less than 35 cm H_2O. Inspiratory time settings should be of sufficient length for comfort and avoidance of unnecessarily high peak (i.e., flow resistive) pressures (e.g., 0.7 to 1.0 sec).

As noted above, in setting both the minute ventilation and the inspiratory time (and the inspiratory : expiratory [I:E] ratio), minimizing PEEPi must also be an important goal. This can be monitored in several ways.[3-5] First, persistent expiratory flow at the end of the allotted expiratory time suggests incomplete lung emptying and thus the presence of PEEPi (Figure 16-2, breaths A and B). Second, in the presence of PEEPi, a brief prolongation of expiratory time (e.g., decrease in set rate) can allow additional lung emptying such that the subsequent breath would either have a larger V_T (pressure-targeted breath) or lower airway pressures (flow-volume targeted breath). Third, during controlled mechanical ventilation (i.e., no patient efforts), the expiratory hold maneuver can allow PEEPi to equilibrate with circuit pressure and be measured (see Figure 16-2, C). Finally, an esophageal pressure sensor can be used to detect the inspiratory triggering load imposed by PEEPi (see later discussion). The clinical challenge thus is to reduce the total ventilation and I:E ratio as much as possible to minimize this risk while still maintaining an acceptable pH.

It is important to realize that the definition of an acceptable pH has changed dramatically over the last 2 decades. Older approaches attempting to normalize the pH have given way to the idea that hypercapnia and pH values less than 7.20 or even 7.10 are acceptable if the lung can be protected from air trapping, high peak pressures, and **overdistention** injury.[8,14,18] Indeed, there is some emerging evidence (although not universal) that a modest respiratory acidosis may actually may improve cellular injury.[19,20]

In rare cases of severe airway obstruction, heavy sedation (and sometimes neuromuscular blockade) may be required to remove any dys-synchronous patient efforts that may raise peak airway pressures or inappropriately increase minute ventilation.[21] In most patients, however, patient breath triggering (assisted breath) is generally preferred to machine breath triggering (control breath) because it can help improve comfort and forestall ventilatory muscle atrophy (ventilator-induced diaphragmatic dysfunction or VIDD).[22]

In the patient with airflow obstruction, a particularly important problem encountered with patient triggering is the inspiratory threshold load imposed by intrinsic PEEP.[4,5] Simply stated, the intrinsic PEEP must be overcome by the inspiratory muscles before airway pressure and flow change to produce a signal to the ventilator that a patient breath is desired. This is manifested clinically by a patient who appears to be contracting the inspiratory muscles but in whom the ventilator detects no activity. An esophageal balloon often can be helpful in detecting and managing this phenomenon (Figure 16-3). Judicious amounts of extrinsic PEEP in the airway help equilibrate this trapped pressure with pressure throughout the ventilator circuitry.[4,5,23,24] This allows for less effort on the part of the patient to trigger the ventilator. Using an esophageal pressure measurement, proper PEEP application under these circumstances can be shown to be as high as 70% to 80% of the measured intrinsic PEEP.[24] Up to this level, the applied PEEP only affects circuit and airway pressures—not alveolar pressures. Applied PEEP greater than this, however, appears to begin elevating alveolar pressures and thus becomes counterproductive because regional overdistention develops in less

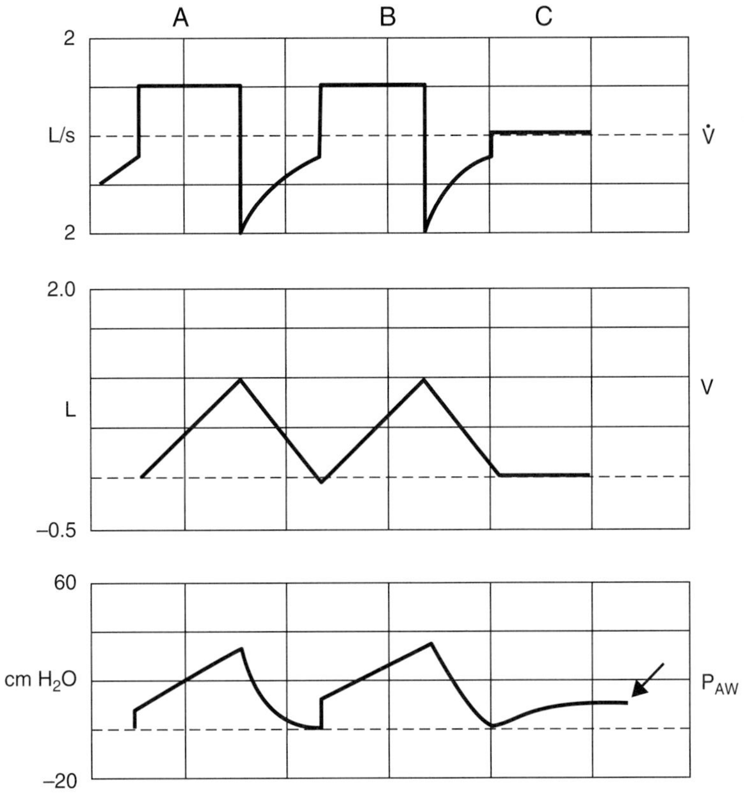

FIGURE 16-2 Effects of air trapping (PEEPi) on controlled mechanical ventilation. Note that in the first two breaths (*A* and *B*), expiratory flow has not returned to baseline before the next breath is given. Note also that an expiratory hold has been applied at the time that the third breath (*C*) should have been given *(arrow)*. Under these conditions, the "trapped" pressure in the lung equilibrates with the ventilator circuit pressure at the end of the expiratory hold.

obstructed regions.[4,5,24] If an esophageal balloon is not available, trial and error can be used to provide applied PEEP to effect this triggering load. Clinically, one would add small increments (e.g., 2 to 5 cm H_2O) and watch the patient's response. If successful, the patient's effort to trigger the breaths should become less as the appropriate level of PEEP is provided. Increasing dyspnea and other signs of increasing intrathoracic pressure (e.g., decreasing blood pressure and worsening of clinical signs of hyperinflation) suggest that excessive PEEP is being provided.

There is a specific cycling problem that can occur with pressure support in patients with airway obstruction. Under these circumstances, the peak flow of the pressure-targeted breath may be diminished and the decelerating flow profile may be quite slow. This may cause a significant prolongation of the pressure support breath because the cycling flow value (often 25% to 35% of the peak flow) may take substantial time to reach. Consequently shortened expiratory times may lead to a buildup of PEEPi.[25] Ways to address this issue are to increase the pressure support flow cycling criteria (e.g., to 50% or more of peak flow) or to switch to pressure assist with a set inspiratory time of an appropriate duration.

Positive End-Expiratory Pressure/ Inspired Oxygen Concentration

As noted previously, because alveolar inflammation, flooding, and collapse are not major features of acute respiratory failure from airflow obstruction, applying PEEP to maintain alveolar recruitment is generally not necessary. Moreover, because applied PEEP can further overdistend obstructed regions, it probably should be avoided unless clear regions of atelectasis or alveolar edema exist. F_{IO_2} adjustments can be used to provide adequate oxygenation (e.g., the ARDS Network goal of 55 to 80 mm Hg or S_{PO_2} of 88 to 95)[16] (see Chapter 15, Table 15-3). As described above, applied PEEP may help patient triggering of assisted breaths in the setting of high levels of intrinsic PEEP.

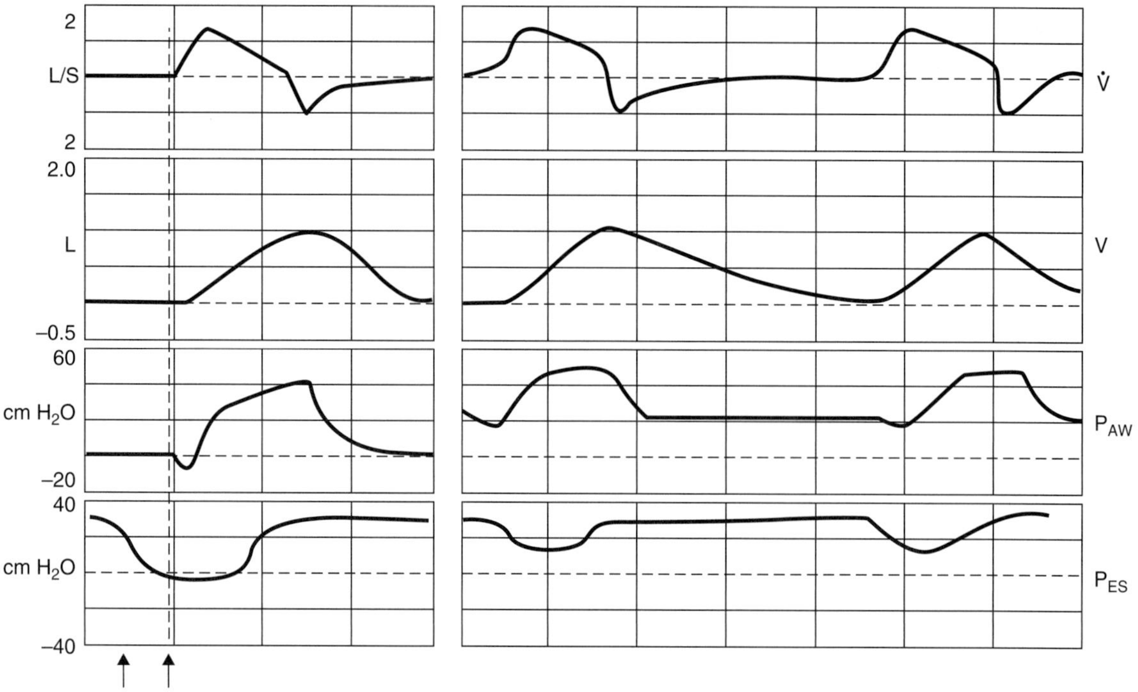

FIGURE 16-3 Effects of air trapping (PEEPi) on triggering assisted breaths. Plotted are volume (V), flow ($\dot{V}$), airway pressure (P_{AW}), and esophageal pressure (P_{ES}) over time. In the left panel, patient effort begins at the first arrow and is reflected by a drop in P_{ES}. Under normal conditions (no PEEPi), there would be a simultaneous drop in P_{AW}, which would trigger the assisted breath. In this case, however, significant PEEPi (i.e., 25 cm H_2O) is present, which must first be overcome by the ventilatory muscles before P_{AW} is changed. Thus P_{ES} changes 25 cm H_2O and 0.7 second elapses before P_{AW} changes and the breath is triggered. This creates a significant triggering work load on the patient. In the right panel, 20 cm H_2O PEEP has been applied in the airway. This does not eliminate the PEEPi but rather equilibrates expiratory pressures in the circuit and the lung. Note that this results in much lower P_{ES} changes being needed to change P_{AW} and trigger breaths.

Other Considerations in Ventilatory Management

In severe airway obstruction, uses of low-density gases (e.g., 80:20, 70:30, or 60:40 helium:O_2 or heliox) can help reduce patient inspiratory work and facilitate lung emptying (recall that driving pressure decreases and/or flow increases through a tube as gas density decreases).[26] If a helium:O_2 gas mixture is used, remember that many flow sensors must be recalibrated to account for the change in gas density. Indeed, some ventilators actually cannot function in the presence of heliox.

In managing patients with airflow obstruction on a ventilator, techniques to deliver bronchodilator aerosols through the ventilator circuitry must be employed. This generally involves in-line circuit nebulizers, although metered dose inhalers with inspiratory circuit-holding chambers are also effective.[27,28] Because endotracheal tubes significantly reduce aerosol delivery, doses usually are increased threefold to fourfold (or even aerosolized continuously) to ensure adequate drug effectiveness.[27,28] Assessment of airway pressures (peak to plateau gradients) or flow-volume patterns can be used to monitor bronchodilator effectiveness. See Chapter 4 for further discussion on aerosol delivery during mechanical ventilation.

In severe refractory asthma, anesthetic gases are sometimes employed to break the bronchospasm.[29] Generally this requires dedicated anesthesia machines rather than intensive care unit ventilators although the support settings should be similar to those described above.

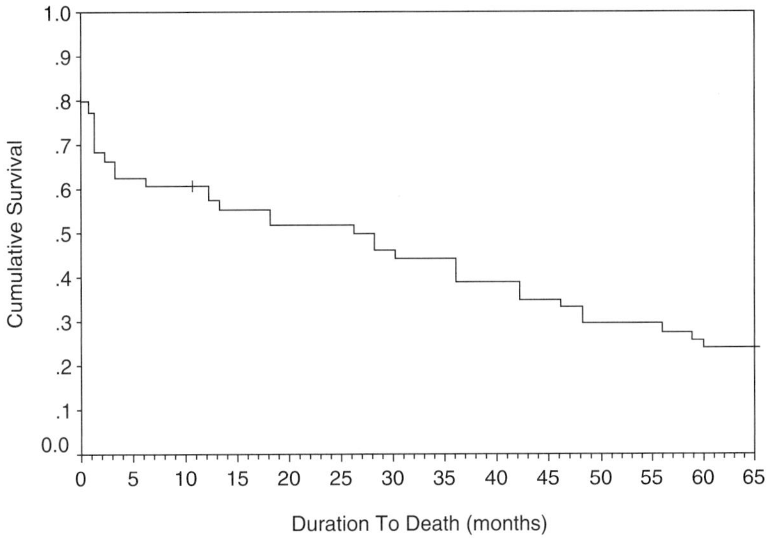

FIGURE 16-4 Mortality in COPD patients requiring mechanical ventilation. Note that in-hospital mortality is 20% to 25%. Note also that a significant mortality risk persists over the ensuing months. (Modified from Ai-Ping C, Lee KH, Lim TK: In-hospital and 5-year mortality of patients treated in the ICU for acute exacerbation of COPD: a retrospective study, Chest 128:518-524, 2005.)

OUTCOMES OF RESPIRATORY FAILURE FROM OBSTRUCTED AIRWAY DISEASE

The outcome of patients with acute airflow obstruction on mechanical ventilators depends on whether the underlying acute airflow obstruction can be reversed. In general, the outcome of patients with asthma is quite good, although there is a certain mortality associated with even the best management of status asthmaticus.[30] This mortality is the result of intractable airflow inflammation and mucous secretion that cannot be overcome by medications and mechanical support. Long-term survivors of mechanical ventilation for asthma, however, generally have respiratory function similar to their baseline.

In contrast to patients with asthma, mortality is substantial in patients with COPD who are receiving mechanical ventilation (although it is still better than in patients with acute lung injury/acute respiratory distress syndrome)[31,32] (Figure 16-4). Unlike asthmatic patients, survivors of respiratory failure from COPD tend to return to baseline lung function very slowly (i.e., weeks to months). Interestingly, in a recent large multicenter study, the need for mechanical ventilation did not influence outcome in patients with COPD admitted to an intensive care unit.[31] However, the risk for rehospitalization and reintubation for patients with COPD is increased greatly after an episode of respiratory failure requiring mechanical ventilation.[31]

KEY POINTS

- Acute respiratory failure can be a consequence of acute airway inflammation in both asthma and COPD.
- Acute respiratory failure from obstructive airway disease is caused by high-resistance workloads on patient muscles, decreased muscle capabilities from hyperinflation, and gas exchange disturbances caused by $\dot{V}/\dot{Q}$ mismatching.
- Goals of mechanical ventilation in obstructive airway disease are generally twofold: prevent overdistention of healthier lung units (keep V_Ts and P low) and reduce air trapping (reduce minute ventilation, lengthen expiratory time).
- Intrinsic PEEP and air trapping can produce an inspiratory triggering load on the patient for assisted/supported breaths; this can be helped by judicious application of circuit PEEP.

ASSESSMENT QUESTIONS

1. True or False. Respiratory failure from airflow obstruction is a consequence of acute airway narrowing and consequent air trapping.
2. True or False. Respiratory failure and obstructive lung disease are often characterized by ventilatory muscle pump failure leading to hypercapnia.
3. True or False. In mechanically ventilated patients with airflow obstruction, the peak to plateau airway pressure gradient is dramatically reduced.
4. True or False. The peak airway pressure is a good indication of lung alveolar stretching pressures in obstructive patients.
5. True or False. To reduce air trapping, a low minute ventilation and resulting hypercapnia may be necessary.
6. True or False. In obstructed patients with significant air trapping, applying PEEP can help reduce the trapped gas volume in the lung.
7. True or False. In obstructed lung disease patients, V_Ts of 10 to 15 ml/kg are recommended.
8. True or False. Heliox mixtures should be used with caution in patients with obstructive lung disease because they may increase air trapping.
9. True or False. In the actively breathing patient (i.e., mechanical breath rate set very low), the expiratory hold maneuver can measure the amount of PEEPi.
10. True or False. In patients with significant air trapping, a triggering load on the ventilatory muscles may develop, which can be somewhat counterbalanced by applying PEEP.

CASE STUDIES

For additional practice, refer to Case Studies 3 and 4 in the appendix at the back of this book.

REFERENCES

1. Fromm RE, Varon J: Acute exacerbations of obstructive lung disease, Postgrad Med 95:101-106, 1994.
2. Tobin MJ: Respiratory muscles in disease, Clin Chest Med 9:263-286, 1988.
3. Marini JJ, Crooke PS: A general mathematical model for respiratory dynamics relevant to the clinical setting, Am Rev Respir Dis 147:14-24, 1993.
4. Smith TC, Marini JJ: Impact of PEEP on lung mechanics and work of breathing in severe airflow obstruction, J Appl Physiol 65:1488-1499, 1988.
5. Gay PC, Rodarte JR, Hubmayr RD: The effects of positive expiratory pressure on isovolume flow and dynamic hyperinflation in patients receiving mechanical ventilation, Am Rev Respir Dis 139:621-626, 1989.
6. Oddo M, Fiehl F, Schaller MD et al: Management of mechanical ventilation in acute severe asthma: practical aspects, Intensive Care Med 32:501-510, 2006.
7. Darioli R, Perret C: Mechanical controlled hypoventilation in status-asthmaticus, Am Rev Respir Dis 129:385-387, 1984.
8. Fiehl F, Perret C: Permissive hypercapnia—how permissive should we be? Am J Respir Crit Care Med 150:1722-1737, 1994.
9. Abraham E, Yoshihara G: Cardiorespiratory effects of pressure controlled ventilation in severe respiratory failure, Chest 98:1445-1449, 1990.
10. MacIntyre NR, McConnell R, Cheng KC et al: Pressure limited breaths improve flow dyssynchrony during assisted ventilation, Crit Care Med 25:1671-1677, 1997.
11. MacIntyre NR, Branson RD: Feedback enhancements on ventilator breaths. In Tobin M, editor: Principles and practice of mechanical ventilation, ed 2, New York, 2006, McGraw-Hill.
12. Plotz FB, Slutsky AS, van Vught AJ et al: Ventilator-induced lung injury and multiple system organ failure: a critical review of facts and hypotheses, Intensive Care Med 30:1865-1872, 2004.
13. Dreyfuss D, Savmon G: Ventilator induced lung injury: lessons from experimental studies, Am J Respir Crit Care Med 157:294-323, 1998.
14. Slutsky AS: ACCP consensus conference: mechanical ventilation, Chest 104:1833-1859, 1993.
15. Gajic O, Frutos-Vivar F, Esteban A et al: Ventilator settings as a risk factor for acute respiratory distress syndrome in mechanically ventilated patients, Intensive Care Med 31:922-926, 2005.
16. NIH ARDS Network: Ventilation with lower tidal volumes as compared with traditional tidal volumes for acute lung injury and the acute respiratory distress syndrome, N Engl J Med 342:1301-1308, 2000.
17. Brower VT, Hager DN, Krishman JA et al: Tidal volume reductions in patients with acute lung injury when plateau pressures are not high, Am J Respir Crit Care Med 172:1241-1245, 2005.
18. Hickling KG, Walsh J, Henderson S et al: Low mortality rate in adult respiratory distress syndrome using low-volume, pressure-limited ventilation with permissive hypercapnia: a prospective study, Crit Care Med 22:1568-1578, 1994.

19. Kavanaugh BP: Therapeutic hypercapnia: careful science, better trials, Am J Respir Crit Care Med 171:96-97, 2005.
20. Kregenow DA, Rubenfeld GA, Hudson LD et al: Hypercapnic acidosis and mortality in acute lung injury, Crit Care Med 34:1-7, 2006.
21. Hansen-Flaschen J, Brazinsky S, Bassles C et al: Use of sedating drugs and neuromuscular blockade in patients requiring mechanical ventilation for respiratory failure, JAMA 266:2870-2875, 1991.
22. Vassilakopoulos T, Petrof BJ: Ventilator-induced diaphragmatic dysfunction, Am J Respir Crit Care Med 169:336-341, 2004.
23. MacIntyre NR, McConnell R, Cheng KC: Applied PEEP reduces the inspiratory load of intrinsic PEEP during pressure support, Chest 111:188-193, 1997.
24. Ranieri VM, Mascia L, Petruzzelli V: Inspiratory effort and measurement of dynamic intrinsic PEEP in COPD patients: effects of ventilator triggering systems, Intensive Care Med 21:896-903, 1995.
25. Jubran A, Van de Graaff WB, Tobin MJ: Variability of patient ventilator interactions with pressure support ventilation in patients with chronic obstructive pulmonary disease, Am J Respir Crit Care Med 152:129-136, 1995.
26. Kass JE, Castriotta RJ: Heliox therapy in acute severe asthma, Chest 107:757-760, 1995.
27. Dhand R: Inhalation therapy with metered-dose inhalers and dry powder inhalers in mechanically ventilated patients, Respir Care 50:1331-1334, 2005.
28. MacIntyre NR: Aerosol delivery through an artificial airway, Respir Care 47:1279-1288. 2002.
29. Rosseel P, Lauwers LF, Baute L: Halothane treatment in life threatening asthma, Intensive Care Med 11:241-246, 1985.
30. Zimmerman JL, Dellinger RP, Shah AN et al: Endotracheal intubation and mechanical ventilation in severe asthma, Crit Care Med 21:1727-1736, 1993.
31. Senoff MG, Wagner DP, Wagner RP et al: Hospital and 1 year survival of patients admitted to ICUs with acute exacerbation of COPD, JAMA 274:1852-1857, 1995.
32. Ai-Ping C, Lee KH, Lim TK: In-hospital and 5-year mortality of patients treated in the ICU for acute exacerbation of COPD: a retrospective study, Chest 128:518-524, 2005.

CHAPTER

17 *Unique Patient Populations*

John H. Sherner*; Lisa K. Moores*

OUTLINE

OBJECTIVES

- Describe mechanical ventilation strategies in neurologically injured patients.
- Explain mechanical ventilation strategies in lung transplantation patients.
- Discuss mechanical ventilation strategies in burn patients.
- State mechanical ventilation strategies in perioperative respiratory failure.

KEY TERMS

bradycardia
cerebral perfusion pressure (CPP)
Glasgow coma scale
Guillain-Barré syndrome (GBS)
high frequency ventilation
hyperkalemia
hyperventilation
hypotension
idiopathic pulmonary fibrosis (IPF)
myasthenia gravis
orthopnea
positive pressure ventilation (PPV)
pulmonary edema
recruitment maneuvers
traumatic brain injury (TBI)

*The opinions contained herein are solely those of the authors and do not represent the opinions or policy of the United States Army or the Department of Defense.

Mechanical ventilation may be indicated for reasons other than parenchymal lung or airway disease. Likewise, restrictive or obstructive lung disease may be present in a variety of specific clinical situations. The objective of this chapter is to highlight the unique features, pathophysiology, and management of specific clinical situations as they relate to mechanical ventilation. In particular, traumatic brain injury, neuromuscular disease, lung transplantation, burn injury, and perioperative patient populations will be addressed. The recognition of the unique issues relevant to each population will allow the provider to optimize the use of mechanical ventilation and adjunctive measures.

BOX 17-1 *Mediators of Secondary Brain Injury in TBI*

Hypoxia
Hypotension
Hypercarbia or hypocarbia
Hyperglycemia or hypoglycemia
Elevated intracranial pressure
Hyperpyrexia

Boldface indicates that it may be directly affected by mechanical ventilation. Cerebral ischemia is the common mechanism.

TRAUMATIC BRAIN INJURY

Traumatic brain injury (TBI) is characterized by primary irreversible injury from the initial insult, and the potential for secondary injury related to physiologic abnormalities and nosocomial complications often seen in critically ill patients. Mechanical ventilation has a direct effect on many key mediators of secondary brain injury, such as hypoxia, hypocarbia or hypercarbia, intracranial pressure (ICP), and cerebral perfusion pressure (CPP) (Box 17-1). In addition to correcting hypoxemia, an effective ventilatory strategy should also allow optimization of cerebral blood flow, usually measured as CPP.

Pathophysiology and Unique Features

Many patients with TBI may have normal pulmonary function and require mechanical ventilation only to maintain an adequate airway. In general, patients with a **Glasgow Coma Scale** score of less than eight are considered unable to protect their airway, and intubation and mechanical ventilation are indicated. However, patients with TBI may have associated respiratory failure in 20% to 50% of cases, from causes such as direct chest trauma, neurogenic pulmonary edema, aspiration, acute respiratory distress syndrome (ARDS), and ventilator associated pneumonia.[1] In such patients, knowledge of the effects of mechanical ventilation on intracerebral pressure is central to management.

Cerebral perfusion pressure (CPP) is defined as the difference between the mean arterial pressure (MAP) and the ICP, with a normal value being 60 to 70 mm Hg. Cerebral blood flow appears to be lowest in the first few hours following injury. **Positive pressure ventilation (PPV)** can therefore have a detrimental effect on CPP if the ventilatory strategy leads to either a rise in the ICP or a drop in the MAP. Deep suctioning, coughing, or other airway manipulation can induce a rise in ICP. Positive intrathoracic pressure may also decrease venous return and lead to a decrease in the MAP. Additionally, hypercarbia induces cerebral vasodilation, which increases ICP. These concerns have prevented widespread implementation of lung protective strategies using positive end-expiratory pressure (PEEP) and low tidal volumes (V_Ts) in patients with TBI, and have led to the previous widespread use of routine **hyperventilation** for head-injured patients. As discussed below, these concerns may not be justified.

TABLE 17-1 *Effect of PEEP on Cranial Pressure and Cardiac Index*

PEEP (cm H_2O)	ICP (mm Hg)	CPP (mm Hg)	CI (L/min/m^2)
0-5	14.7	77.5	3.8
6-10	13.6	80.1	4.0
11-15	13.1	78.9	3.8

From Huynh T, Messer M, Sing RF et al: PEEP alters ICP and CPP in severe traumatic brain injury, *J Trauma* 53(3):488-492, 2002.

Management

As with all ventilated patients, the head of the bed should be kept elevated at 30 degrees not only to minimize aspiration, but also to facilitate venous drainage in this population. Other measures to avoid venous congestion include keeping a midline head position, avoidance of internal jugular catheters if possible, and ensuring that cervical collars, if present, are not constrictive.

PEEP

Traditional teaching has been that high levels of PEEP may lead to elevated ICP, and should be avoided in patients with TBI. This could be particularly problematic in those head-injured patients who develop neurogenic **pulmonary edema** or who have other concomitant lung injury, and may require higher mean airway pressures to maintain adequate oxygenation. While high levels of PEEP may lead to slight increases in ICP in patients with normal ICP, studies suggest that PEEP does not increase ICP in those patients with preexisting elevated ICP.[2,3] Data from a retrospective review show that rising levels of PEEP have no effect on ICP or CPP[4] (Table 17-1). Such data advocate use of PEEP, with appropriate monitoring, in the head-injured population, as the risks of hypoxia outweigh the potential risk of

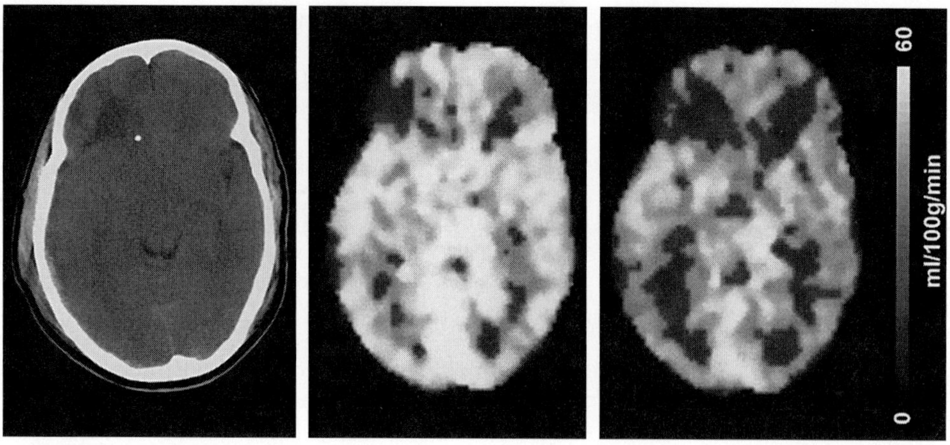

FIGURE 17-1 Effect of hyperventilation on the burden of hypoperfusion. The left panel is the computerized tomographic image. The middle and right panels are perfusion scans. Dark gray areas represent severe hypoperfusion. An increased amount of severe hypoperfusion is noted at P_{CO_2} 26 *(right panel)* compared with P_{CO_2} 35 *(middle panel)*. (From Coles J, Minhas P et al: Effect of hyperventilation on cerebral blood flow in traumatic head injury: Clinical relevance and monitor correlates, Crit Care Med 30(9):1954, 2002.)

decreased CPP from reduced cardiac output or decreased venous return.

Recruitment Maneuvers

The use of **recruitment maneuvers** is also controversial, particularly in patients with TBI, for reasons outlined above. One study actually found a modest decrease in ICP with the use of recruitment maneuvers consisting of inspiratory pressure 40 cm above PEEP for 2 to 3 breath cycles, although an explanation for such a decrease remains unclear.[2] However, other data suggest that the use of a recruitment maneuver employing a peak airway pressure of 60 cm for 30 seconds led to decreased MAP and increased ICP, and therefore decreased CPP and jugular venous oxygen saturation.[5] Given these data, and the limited benefit of recruitment maneuvers in general, they cannot be routinely recommended in patients with TBI. Other components of protective lung ventilation, such as low V_Ts and use of PEEP, have been shown to be feasible in patients with TBI.[2]

Hyperventilation

In the past, hyperventilation was part of the routine management of head-injured patients with increased ICP. However, based on the current data, hyperventilation to P_{CO_2} less than 35 should be limited to cases of refractory ICP, or possibly for acute, short elevations of ICP, as seen with endotracheal suctioning. Prolonged hyperventilation leads to vasoconstriction that will lower ICP but also decreases cerebral blood flow. Recent studies suggest that there is significant heterogeneity in cerebral perfusion, and that hyperventilation leads to an increased amount of severely hypoperfused tissue, even in the setting of normal ICP and CPP values[6] (Figure 17-1). Hyperventilation has not been shown to have a beneficial effect on outcome; in fact patients hyperventilated to a P_{CO_2} of 25 mm Hg for 5 days had a worse outcome than those who were not.[7] In their most recent recommendations, the Brain Trauma Foundation and the American Academy of Neurosurgeons recommend that P_{CO_2} less than 35 mm Hg should be avoided, especially in the first 24 hours after injury, when risk of cerebral ischemia is highest.[8]

Patients who have been chronically hyperventilated should not be rapidly returned to normocapnia. In this situation, the relatively rapid compensatory decrease in cerebrospinal fluid (CSF) bicarbonate that has occurred predisposes to acidemia during normocapnia, which then leads to cerebral hyperemia and increased ICP. The P_{CO_2} of chronically hyperventilated head-injured patients should be slowly returned to normal.[9]

Mode Selection

Most authorities recommend use of traditional modes of ventilation for patients with TBI. No data are available for the use of airway pressure release ventilation (APRV) in this population. There are preliminary data on the use of **high frequency ventilation.** In one retrospective study of 10 patients with severe head injury and ARDS, the authors noted an increase in Pa_{O_2} : F_{IO_2} ratio and decreased ICP when patients

BOX 17-2 *Neuromuscular Disorders That May Result in Respiratory Failure**

Guillain-Barré syndrome
Myasthenia gravis
Quadriplegia
Critical illness polyneuropathy
Botulism
Eaton Lambert syndrome
Polio
Lyme disease
Tick paralysis
Organophosphate toxicity
Polymyositis
Muscular dystrophy
Amyotrophic lateral sclerosis

*Partial list.

were switched from conventional ventilation to high frequency ventilation.[1] Such data warrant further study.

NEUROMUSCULAR DISORDERS

Pathophysiology and Unique Features

Acute respiratory failure can complicate a variety of neuromuscular disorders (Box 17-2), most frequently **Guillain-Barré syndrome (GBS)** and **myasthenia gravis.** Respiratory failure may occur secondary to a combination of weakness of muscles of inspiration, expiration, and the pharyngeal airway.[10] Airway muscle weakness predisposes to aspiration and obstruction, and loss of expiratory muscle strength leads to ineffective cough and poor clearance of secretion. Weak inspiratory muscles are unable to generate large V_Ts, resulting in atelectasis and pulmonary shunt. Complications, such as aspiration, pneumonia, and venous thromboembolic disease, are prevalent and aggravate the respiratory failure associated with neuromuscular weakness.

Assessment

Patients with neuromuscular disease should be assessed for the ability to maintain a patent airway. A number of clinical findings are suggestive of respiratory compromise and are summarized in Box 17-3.[11,12] Inability to speak clearly or a nasal quality to the voice may indicate impending airway failure. Immobility of the soft palate or a decreased or absent gag reflex on examination is also an indicator of inadequate airway protective mechanisms. Additionally, the patient should be assessed for ventilatory muscle strength. **Orthopnea,** inability to speak in full sentences, or paradoxical inward abdominal motion on inspiration all indicate respiratory muscle weakness and fatigue. An exaggerated drop in forced vital capacity (FVC) when supine (decreased 8% to 19% in normals) also suggests respiratory weakness. In general, an FVC of less than 15 ml/kg or maximum inspiratory force of less than 25 cm H_2O is considered to be an indication for prophylactic intubation and mechanical ventilation.[13] Of note, hypercarbia is a late finding. A decreasing FVC on serial monitoring is also a reliable indicator of respiratory failure and need for mechanical ventilation.[14]

BOX 17-3 *Factors Associated With Respiratory Failure in GBS*

Time from onset to admission less than 7 days
Inability to stand
Inability to lift elbows or head
FVC less than 60% predicted
Absence of cough
Rapid decrease in FVC
Peripheral and axial muscle involvement
Bulbar muscle involvement

Data from references 11 and 12.
FVC, Forced vital capacity.

Management

Approximately 15% to 30% of patients with GBS will require mechanical ventilation.[10] Patients with inability to maintain an airway or inadequate respiratory muscle function, as assessed by the above techniques, should be intubated and mechanically ventilated. Care should be taken during intubation because these patients are prone to autonomic dysfunction, which can result in exaggerated **hypotension** or **bradycardia** with induction anesthetic agents. Furthermore, the use of succinylcholine or other depolarizing muscular blockers should be avoided due to the risk of **hyperkalemia**.

Mode Selection

Patients with some degree of preservation of function in their respiratory muscles (FVC 5 to 10 ml/kg) may do well with pressure support ventilation (PSV), which may allow better synchronization with the ventilator. Many patients, however, will not maintain even this degree of strength and will therefore require a mode of full support, such as assist-control or synchronized intermittent mandatory ventilation (SIMV). SIMV was the preferred mode in many reports in the older literature.[15] Larger V_Ts (10 to 15 ml/kg) have traditionally been used to maintain patient comfort, and may be acceptable as long as plateau airway pressures remain less than 30 cm H_2O. Our experience suggests that APRV is effective in providing patient comfort and preventing atelectasis and pneumonia in this population. Most patients with neuromuscular disorders will require aggressive pulmonary toilet, including frequent suctioning and chest percussion. Again it should be noted that such patients may be prone to episodes of bradycardia or hypotension during airway manipulation as a result of autonomic instability.

Outcome

Patients requiring mechanical ventilation have increased mortality, usually secondary to complications. In one series, 21 of 79 patients with GBS had significant respiratory compromise. Thirteen patients required mechanical ventilation and tracheostomy, and had significantly increased duration of hospital stay.[16] Roughly one third of patients requiring mechanical ventilation can be weaned in the first 2 weeks, although even lower rates of successful early weaning have been reported.[13,17] Early tracheostomy should be considered, particularly in the elderly and in those with preexisting lung disease, dysautonomias, or involvement of axial muscle groups. Most authorities recommend proceeding to tracheostomy after 2 weeks of mechanical ventilation unless the clinical course is rapidly improving.[10]

LUNG TRANSPLANTATION

Lung transplantation is increasingly used as a therapy for end-stage lung disease. The number of potential recipients, however, far exceeds the number of available donors. This is in part due to a low rate of lung procurement from potential donors. In one series, lungs were harvested from only 13% of potential donors.[18] Appropriate use of mechanical ventilation of potential donors may help increase the supply of available donor lungs. Additionally, mechanical ventilation is obviously central to the early management of lung transplant recipients.

Donor Care

Pathophysiology

The process of brain death leads to a cascade of physiologic events that may be harmful to potential donor organs, including the lungs. Initially, brain death causes excessive sympathetic stimulation that may lead to increased pulmonary capillary permeability. Combined with aggressive volume resuscitation, this predisposes the donor lungs to pulmonary edema.[19] Additionally, brain death is accompanied by a cytokine-mediated proinflammatory response, which further contributes to pulmonary edema and acute lung injury. Finally, potential donors frequently have associated pulmonary complications, including aspiration, neurogenic pulmonary edema, pneumonia, or pulmonary trauma.

All of these factors can lead to a low PaO_2/FIO_2 ratio, which may make the lungs less acceptable for donation. Based on traditional criteria, a PaO_2/FIO_2 ratio greater than 300 has been required for lung donation[20] (Box 17-4). One study demonstrated that 45% of potential donors had a ratio less than 300, but had normal chest x-rays and low plateau pressures.[21] Recent studies of such patients suggest that optimization of ventilatory management may allow for enough improvement in oxygenation to render such traditionally unacceptable lungs suitable for donation. Studies have confirmed equivalent outcomes in recipients of donor lungs managed in such a fashion

BOX 17-4 *Standard Criteria for Lung Donation*

- PO_2/FIO_2 ratio greater than 300, $FIO_2 = 1.0$
- PEEP = 5 cm H_2O
- Clear chest x-ray
- Age less than 55 years*
- Absence of chest trauma
- Absent aspiration, sepsis, or purulent secretions
- Smoking history of less than 20 pack years
- Absent history of malignancy

*The Lung Work Group proposed new criteria to include virtually any donor age up to 65 years and an absence of lung injury from smoking.
From Rosengard B, Feng S, Alfrey E et al: Report of the Crystal City meeting to maximize the use of organs recovered from the cadaveric donor, *Am J Transplant* 2(8):701-709, 2002.

compared with donor lungs meeting more stringent criteria.[18]

Management

Aggressive management of brain-dead patients to optimize lung procurement typically includes monitoring of central venous pressure, diuresis, steroids, and judicious use of fluids to maintain adequate arterial pressure, with vasopressor use as needed. An intravenous bolus of Solu-Medrol 15 mg/kg once a patient has been declared brain dead has been demonstrated to improve oxygenation and lung procurement, most likely by mediating the proinflammatory response that follows brain death.[22] Patients require frequent endotracheal suctioning and often bronchoscopy to evaluate and clear secretions.

The optimum ventilatory strategy for potential multiorgan donors remains undefined. There is general agreement that the lowest FIO_2 necessary to maintain a PaO_2 of at least 80 mm Hg should be employed. The use of serial (every 2 hours) recruitment maneuvers to prevent atelectasis has been advocated. A recent survey indicates that historically most patients were ventilated with V_Ts of approximately 10 ml/kg with relatively low levels of PEEP.[21] The Lung Work Group, a meeting of several transplant-related organizations, recommends the use of V_Ts of 10 to 12 ml/kg and low levels of PEEP (5 cm H_2O)[23] (Box 17-5). Similarly, another study of aggressive donor management advocates the use of relatively high V_Ts.[24] Such recommendations are contrary to the low V_T approach advocated by the ARDS Network study group, however. It is important to note that what might be best for gas exchange may be detrimental to lung tissue and other potential donor organs, perhaps by worsening the overall inflammatory state. Because of this, others have advocated a low V_T approach for mechanical ventilation of donor lungs.[19] A randomized, controlled trial evaluating a lung protective ventilatory strategy in potential organ donors is underway and should help define the best approach to these patients.

BOX 17-5 *Recommendations for Donor Management*

The airway:
- Bronchoscopy
- Frequent suctioning and aspiration precautions
- Albuterol therapy for wheezing (may improve lung fluid clearance)

Mechanical ventilation:

Adequate oxygenation:
- PO_2 greater than 100 mm Hg, $FIO_2 = 0.40$, or O_2 saturation greater than 95%

Adequate ventilation:
- Maintain pH 7.35-7.45 and PCO_2 30-35 mm Hg
- PEEP + 5 cm H_2O
- Tidal volume 10-12 ml/kg
- Peak airway pressures less than 30 mm Hg

Fluid management and monitoring:
- CVP at a minimum; PA catheter desirable
- Arterial line and pulse oximetry

Judicious fluid resuscitation to ensure end-organ perfusion:
- CVP 6-8 mm Hg, PCWP 8-12 mm Hg
- Urine output 1 ml/kg/hr
- Colloid as the fluid of choice for volume resuscitation
- Albumin with normal PT, PTT; FFP with coagulopathy
- Hemoglobin greater than 10 g/dl

From Rosengard B, Feng S, Alfrey E et al: Report of the Crystal City meeting to maximize the use of organs recovered from the cadaveric donor, *Am J Transplant* 2(8):701-711, 2002.
FFP, Fresh frozen plasma; *PT,* prothrombin time; *PTT,* partial thromboplastin time.

Perioperative Care of Transplant Recipients

Pathophysiology

Lung allografts are denervated below the anastomosis, which results in loss of cough reflex and the normal mucociliary transport system. These deficits predispose the donor lung to retention of secretions, atelectasis, and pneumonia. Donor lungs are also prone to pulmonary edema. In particular, ischemia reperfusion injury is a form of noncardiogenic pulmonary edema manifested by worsening oxygenation, radiographic infiltrates, and worsening pulmonary compliance. The development of ischemia-reperfusion injury may be related to abnormalities of the donor lungs, or to prolonged ischemia or other poor preservation techniques (Figure 17-2).

Single lung transplantation may lead to significant alterations in ventilation-perfusion ($\dot{V}/\dot{Q}$) matching, which are dependent upon the underlying disease process of the recipient. Such $\dot{V}/\dot{Q}$ mismatch can complicate ventilatory management, particularly with the occurrence of ischemia-reperfusion injury or another insult requiring higher level support. In recipients with pulmonary hypertension, ventilation

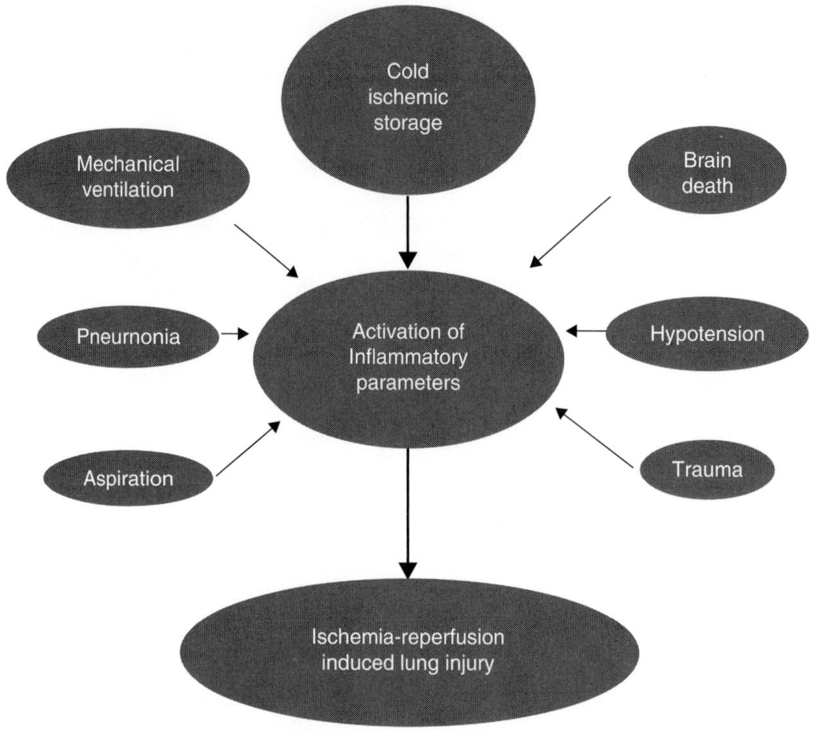

FIGURE 17-2 Events in donor lungs that may aggravate ischemia-reperfusion injury. (Modified from de Perrot M, Liu M, Waddell T et al: Ischemia-reperfusion-induced lung injury, Am J Respir Crit Care Med 167:491, 2003.)

will be evenly distributed but the allograft will receive the majority of perfusion secondary to the increased pulmonary pressure in the native lung. In **idiopathic pulmonary fibrosis (IPF)** or other fibrotic conditions, the majority of both ventilation and perfusion go to the allograft. In emphysema, the compliant native lung receives the majority of ventilation, while the allograft receives the majority of blood flow. If ischemia-reperfusion injury occurs, oxygenation will worsen. Attempts at correction by increasing PEEP may further worsen oxygenation, as most of the PEEP will be preferentially directed to the native lung, leading to hyperexpansion. Continued expansion of the native lung leads to diaphragmatic alterations that may worsen atelectasis of the allograft.[25] Furthermore, hyperexpansion will lead to increased pulmonary vascular resistance of the native lung, further shunting blood to the dysfunctioning allograft. Additionally, hyperinflation can cause barotrauma and hemodynamic consequences by reducing venous return.

Phrenic nerve injury is a usually transient complication of lung transplantation, occurring more often in bilateral lung recipients. This complication usually manifests as difficulty weaning from ventilatory support, and may require tracheostomy and prolonged mechanical ventilation. There are reports of successful use of noninvasive ventilation to treat cases of posttransplant phrenic nerve palsy.[26]

Management

Peak airway pressures should be maintained under 30 cm H_2O, and perhaps under 25 cm H_2O.[27] The use of either volume or pressure controlled modes of ventilation has been advocated by various groups. As recently transplanted lungs are prone to pulmonary edema, close attention to fluid balance is required, with a negative balance the typical goal. Aggressive pulmonary toilet, including frequent suctioning within the endotracheal tube and chest physiotherapy, is required due to loss of cough and normal mucociliary clearance mechanisms.

Although the majority of recipients can be weaned and extubated in the first 48 hours following transplantation, a portion will have increasing needs for ventilatory support because of ischemia-reperfusion injury. Data suggest that the incidence can be reduced by the use of low potassium preservation fluids, avoidance of donor lung hyperinflation, and controlled flow reperfusion with leukocyte depletion. Diuresis and supportive care are the cornerstones of management. Experimental data suggest that there may also be a role for inhaled nitric oxide and/or prostacyclin in this patient population.[28]

Reperfusion-ischemia injury in the single lung transplant recipient with emphysema may respond to conservative measures. Chest physiotherapy should be used. The patient should be positioned with the better functioning lung down, which in the case of significant reperfusion injury means the allograft side up, to increase perfusion to the more functioning lung. Acceptance of a respiratory acidosis may be preferable to interventions, which may lead to worsening hyperexpansion. In refractory cases, effective use of independent lung ventilation has been described.[27] With the use of a dual lumen endotracheal tube and separate ventilators, the native lung can be ventilated with low PEEP and low tidal volumes to decrease hyperexpansion. Simultaneously, the dysfunctioning allograft can receive increasing levels of PEEP to facilitate recruitment. However, the narrow lumen of dual lumen tubes is prone to obstruction, and frequent suctioning is required. Additionally, the tube must be precisely positioned and the placement closely monitored to prevent displacement and occlusion of lobar bronchial orifices.

BURN INJURIES

Pathophysiology and Unique Features

Patients with burn injuries are susceptible to lung injury by a variety of mechanisms. Direct toxic effects of smoke inhalation can lead to airway inflammation, with resultant small airway obstruction and atelectasis. Secondary lung injury from the systemic inflammatory response, pneumonia, and sepsis may also cause or contribute to respiratory insufficiency. The prevalence of ARDS in burn patients requiring mechanical ventilation has been estimated at 54%.[29] Coexistent inhalational injury or development of pulmonary complications both increase the mortality of patients suffering burns.[30]

Assessment

Signs of inhalational injury may be absent until several days after the injury. The presence of carbonaceous sputum strongly suggests inhalational injury. Fiberoptic bronchoscopy to look for airway edema, erythema, or ulceration is indicated. Proximal airways may also be normal in the case of inhalation of small particles that deposit in the distal airways and alveoli. Xenon 133 $\dot{V}/\dot{Q}$ scanning should be performed to confirm inhalational injury when suspected clinically.[31]

Management

In general, lung protective ventilation with avoidance of excessive airway pressures should be employed. However, a growing body of evidence supports the use of high frequency ventilation in the burn population.[32] Initially used as "rescue" therapy for patients with a requirement for high F_{IO_2} or high airway pressures, there appears to be a trend toward earlier use. High frequency percussive ventilation may have benefits over oscillatory ventilation, perhaps due to enhanced mucokinesis.[33] See Chapter 25 on high frequency ventilation for further discussion regarding the use of these modalities. There are data that aerosolized heparin and acetylcysteine may reduce pulmonary complications in burn patients with inhalational injury.[34]

PERIOPERATIVE RESPIRATORY FAILURE

Pathophysiology and Unique Features

The most frequent indication for mechanical ventilation in the perioperative patient is apnea from unreversed anesthetic agents. General anesthesia results in atelectasis and a 20% reduction in functional residual capacity (FRC) in all patients. Additionally, several medications commonly used in the perioperative period may have specific effects on the respiratory system. As examples, high dose fentanyl may lead to chest wall rigidity and result in increased airway pressures, and nitroprusside may overcome pulmonary hypoxic vasoconstriction and lead to $\dot{V}/\dot{Q}$ mismatching and hypoxemia. Patients undergoing cardiothoracic surgery may be prone to a number of complications, ranging from atelectasis to phrenic nerve injury and diaphragmatic dysfunction that can contribute to respiratory failure.[35]

Management

Patients with lung disease may require prolonged perioperative mechanical ventilation, with management dictated by their underlying respiratory disorder. Most modes of ventilation are acceptable in the perioperative patient population. Evidence continues to mount that a low V_T strategy is beneficial, even in patients without preexistent lung disease or acute lung injury. In a study of patients without lung injury that included a largely perioperative population, the odds ratio for developing acute lung injury was 1.3 for every 1 ml/kg of V_T greater than 6 ml/kg.[36]

CONCLUSIONS

Unique patient populations may develop respiratory failure and require mechanical ventilation due to a variety of pathophysiologic mechanisms. In general, ventilatory strategies employing low V_Ts (6 to 10 ml/kg) and the use of PEEP with avoidance of airway pressures higher than 30 cm H_2O are safe and prudent. Knowledge of the unique pathophysiology present in each of these patient populations will allow appropriate use of mechanical ventilation and avoidance of iatrogenic complications.

KEY POINTS

- Unique patient populations develop respiratory failure by specific pathophysiologic mechanisms. Knowledge of these mechanisms can guide ventilatory management, and preventive and adjunctive therapy.
- The main goal of ventilatory management in TBI is avoidance of hypoxemia, hypotension, and other mediators of secondary brain injury.
- Available data suggest that use of PEEP has little effect on ICP, particularly in patients with already elevated ICP. Patients with TBI should not be excluded from lung protective ventilatory strategies. High frequency ventilation may be an emerging therapy for this population.
- Hyperventilation with PCO_2 less than 35 mm Hg should be avoided in patients with TBI except in the situation of acute herniation.
- Patient comfort and avoidance of complications are the goals of ventilatory management for patients with neuromuscular respiratory failure. Higher V_Ts (10 to 12 ml/kg) with avoidance of plateau airway pressures greater than 30 cm H_2O are acceptable.
- The process of brain death is characterized by sympathetic stimulation and cytokine-mediated inflammation, which may make the lungs less suitable for donation. Aggressive management, including appropriate mechanical ventilation, may increase organ procurement; however, the optimal ventilatory strategy remains undefined.
- Avoidance of peak airway pressures greater than 25 to 30 mm Hg is essential for lung transplant recipients.
- Ischemia-reperfusion injury may complicate the early course of lung transplant recipients. Recipients with chronic obstructive pulmonary disease may have significant $\dot{V}/\dot{Q}$ mismatch, and mechanical ventilation may lead to hyperexpansion of the native lung. Patient positioning with the better functioning lung down and independent lung ventilation are management options.
- High frequency ventilation appears to reduce respiratory complications in patients with burn injury.
- The use of lung protective ventilation (V_T 6 to 10 ml/kg) in perioperative patients may decrease the rate of development of acute lung injury.

ASSESSMENT QUESTIONS

1. True or False. In brain-injured patients, in addition to supporting gas exchange, mechanical ventilation settings must also take into account ICP and CPP.
2. True or False. Permissive hypercapnia is appropriate for all patients with TBI.
3. True or False. TBI can produce a neurogenic form of ARDS.
4. True or False. Intrathoracic pressures have no relationship to ICP.
5. True or False. While PEEP may have some effect on ICP, correcting the hypoxia with judicious application of PEEP outweighs this risk in most patients with brain injury.
6. True or False. Hyperventilation and hypocapnia will reliably reduce ICP for days.
7. True or False. In patients with neuromuscular respiratory failure, PEEP and/or sigh breaths can be helpful in minimizing atelectasis.

ASSESSMENT QUESTIONS—cont'd

8. True or False. A cause of respiratory failure in a recently lung-transplanted patient is the development of ischemia-reperfusion injury.

9. True or False. In the brain-dead patient who will be a lung transplant donor, it is critical to maintain lung protective ventilatory support to optimize the viability of the donated lung.

10. True or False. One cause of respiratory failure in a lung transplant patient is phrenic nerve injury during the transplantation process.

REFERENCES

1. Salim A, Miller K, Dangleben D et al: High-frequency percussive ventilation: an alternative mode of ventilation for head-injured patients with ARDS, J Trauma 57:542, 2004.
2. Wolf S, Schurer L, Trost HA et al: The safety of the open lung approach in neurosurgical patients, Acta Neurochir (Supp) 81:99, 2002.
3. McGuire G, Crossley D, Richards J et al: Effects of varying levels of PEEP on ICP and CPP, Crit Care Med 25:1059, 1997.
4. Huynh T, Messer M, Sing RF et al: PEEP alters ICP and CPP in severe traumatic brain injury, J Trauma 53:488, 2002.
5. Bein T, Kuhr LP, Bela S et al: Lung recruitment maneuver in patients with cerebral injury: effects on ICP and cerebral metabolism, Intensive Care Med 28:554, 2002.
6. Coles J, Minhas P, Fryer TD et al: Effect of hyperventilation on cerebral blood flow in traumatic head injury: Clinical relevance and monitor correlates, Crit Care Med 9:1950, 2002.
7. Muizelaar J, Marmarou A, Ward JR et al: Adverse effects of prolonged hyperventilation in patients with severe head injury: a randomized clinical trial, J Neurosurg 75:731, 1991.
8. Bullock R, Chestnut R, Clifton G: Guidelines for the management of severe head injury: brain trauma foundation, Eur J Emerg Med 3(2):109, 1996.
9. Yundt K, Diringer M: The use of hyperventilation and its impact on cerebral ischemia in the treatment of traumatic brain injury, Crit Care Clin 13(1):163, 1997.
10. Hund E, Borel C, Cornblath DR et al: Intensive management and treatment of severe Guillain-Barre syndrome, Crit Care Med 21(3):433, 1993.
11. Orlikowski D, Prigent H, Sharshar T et al: Respiratory dysfunction in Guillain-Barre syndrome, Neurocrit Care 1(4):415, 2004.
12. Sharshar T, Chevret S: Early predictors of mechanical ventilation in Guillain-Barre syndrome, Crit Care Med 31(1):278, 2003.
13. Borel C, Guy J: Ventilatory management in critical neurologic illness, Neurol Clin 13(3):627, 1995.
14. Chevrolet J, Deleamont P: Repeated vital capacity measurements as predictive parameters for mechanical ventilation need and weaning success in the Guillain-Barre syndrome, Am Rev Respir Dis 144(4):814, 1991.
15. Ropper A, Kehne S: Guillain-Barre syndrome: management of respiratory failure, Neurology 35(11):1662, 1985.
16. Gracey D, McMichan J, Divertie MB et al: Respiratory failure in Guillain-Barre syndrome: a 6-year experience, Mayo Clin Proc 52(12):742, 1982.
17. Lawn N, Wijdicks E: Tracheostomy in Guillain-Barre syndrome, Muscle Nerve 22(8):1058, 1999.
18. Straznicka M, Follette D, Eisner MD et al: Aggressive management of lung donors classified as unacceptable: excellent recipient survival one year after transplantation, J Thoracic Cardiovasc Surg 124(2):250, 2002.
19. Smith M: Physiologic changes during brain stem death—lessons for management of the organ donor, J Heart Lung Transplant 23(9S):S217, 2004.
20. de Perrot M, Snell G, Babcock WD et al: Strategies to optimize the use of currently available lung donors, J Heart Lung Transplant 23(10):1127, 2004.
21. Mascia L, Bosma K, Pasero D et al: Ventilatory and hemodynamic management of potential organ donors: An observational survey, Crit Care Med 34(2):321, 2006.
22. Follette D, Rudich S, Babcock WD et al: Improved oxygenation and increased lung donor recovery with high-dose steroid administration after brain death, J Heart Lung Transplant 17:423, 1998.
23. Rosengard B, Feng S, Alfrey E et al: Report of the Crystal City meeting to maximize the use of organs recovered from the cadaver donor, Am J Transplant 2:701, 2002.
24. Gabbay E, Williams T, Griffiths A et al: Maximizing the utilization of donor organs offered for lung transplantation, Am J Respir Crit Care Med 160:265, 1999.
25. Simpson K, Garrity E: Perioperative management in lung transplantation, Clin Chest Med 18(2):277, 1997.
26. Callegari G, Fracchia C: Modalities of ventilation in lung transplantation, Monaldi Arch Chest Dis 53(5):543, 1998.
27. de Perrot M, Liu M, Waddell T et al: Ischemia-reperfusion-induced lung injury, Am J Respir Crit Care Med 167:490, 2003.
28. Lau C, Patterson G, Palmer S: Critical care aspects of lung transplantation, J Intensive Care Med 19(2):83, 2004.
29. Dancey D, Hayes J, Gomez M et al: ARDS in patients with thermal injury, Intensive Care Med 25(11):1231, 1999.

30. Rue L, Cioffi W, Mason A et al: Improved survival of burned patients with inhalation injury, Arch Surg 128(7):772, 1993.
31. Pruitt B: Critical care management of the severely burned patient. In: Parillo J, Dellinger R, editors: Critical care medicine: Principles of diagnosis and management in the adult, St. Louis, 2005, Mosby.
32. Cartotto R, Ellis S, Smith T: Use of high-frequency oscillatory ventilation in burn patients, Crit Care Med 33(3S):S175, 2005.
33. Cioffi W, Graves T, McManus W: High-frequency percussive ventilation in patients with inhalation injury, J Trauma 29(3):350, 1989.
34. Desai M, Mlcak R, Richardson J et al: Reduction in mortality in pediatric patients with inhalation injury with aerosolized heparin/N-acetylcysteine therapy, J Birm Care Rehabil 32:344, 1998.
35. Weiman D, Ferdinand F, Bolton J et al: Perioperative respiratory management in cardiac surgery, Clin Chest Med 14(2):283, 1993.
36. Gajic O, Dara A, Mendez J et al: Ventilator-associated lung injury in patients without acute lung injury at the onset of mechanical ventilation, Crit Care Med 32(9):1817, 2004.

CHAPTER

18 Discontinuing Mechanical Ventilation

Neil R. MacIntyre

OUTLINE

OBJECTIVES

- Explain the determinants of ventilated dependence.
- List techniques to assess the potential for ventilatory discontinuation.
- Discuss the criteria for removing an artificial airway.
- Describe the management of patients not yet ready for ventilatory discontinuation.

KEY TERMS

muscle fatigue
muscle overload
partial support
spontaneous breathing trial (SBT)
ventilator dependence
ventilator discontinuation
weaning
weaning techniques
wean screen

As respiratory failure stabilizes and begins to reverse, clinical attention shifts to the ventilator withdrawal process. In these patients, continued ventilator dependency is caused by two fundamental problems: (1) disease-imposed factors—mechanical/gas exchange issues that continue to require positive pressure ventilation; and (2) clinician-imposed factors—either clinician delay in recognizing the ability of a patient to have the ventilator discontinued or inappropriate ventilator settings that overload respiratory muscles, preventing recovery (Figure 18-1). With respect to this latter point, several large clinical trials have clearly demonstrated that many current assessment/management strategies cause considerable undue delay in ventilator withdrawal.[1] For example, the two large randomized trials of **weaning** conducted in the 1990s both showed that commonly used assessments and ventilator **weaning techniques** were often associated with several days of delayed **ventilator discontinuation.**[2,3] Moreover, recent trials of protocol-driven ventilator discontinuation procedures have clearly demonstrated that traditional standard care is often associated with significant delays in ventilator withdrawal.[4,5] Estimates are that these traditional standard care approaches result in the ventilator discontinuation process constituting up to 40% of the time a patient is on a ventilator.[6,7]

Clearly, ventilator management should be aimed at getting the patient off ventilator support as rapidly as possible. Delayed discontinuation from mechanical ventilatory support exposes patients to unnecessary

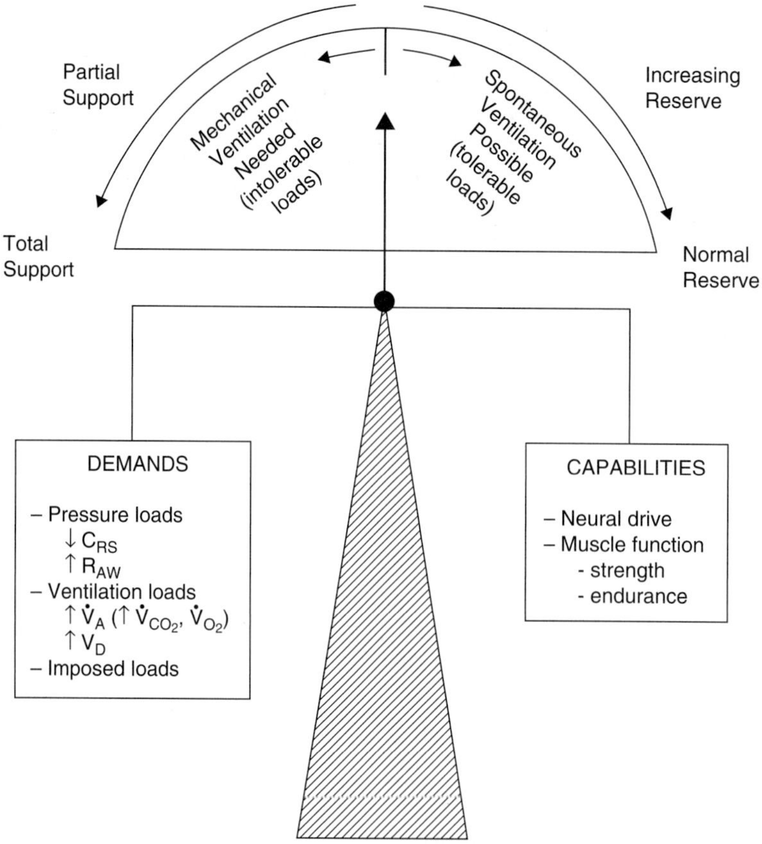

FIGURE 18-1 Causes of ventilator dependency. Depicted is a balance with capabilities on the right and demands on the left. When demands outstrip capabilities, ventilatory dependency exists. C_{RS}, Respiratory system compliance; R_{AW}, airway restrictions; $\dot{V}_A$, alveolar ventilation; V_{CO_2}, CO_2 production; V_{O_2}, oxygen consumption; V_D, dead space.

risks of infection, stretch injury, sedation needs, airway trauma, and costs. The discontinuation process must be done with proper caution and monitoring, however, because premature withdrawal has its own problems. These include loss of airway protection, cardiovascular stress, suboptimal gas exchange, and muscle overload and fatigue. **Muscle overload** and **fatigue** are of particular concern because it may take 24 hours or more of muscle rest (i.e., reintubation and high levels of mechanical support) to recover fatigued ventilatory muscles.[8]

CONSIDERING VENTILATION DISCONTINUATION

In general, when a patient's underlying respiratory disease begins to stabilize and reverse, consideration for ventilator discontinuation should begin. A recent multisociety-sponsored evidence-based task force (hereafter referred to as the Task Force)[1] has recommended that a patient should be considered a candidate for withdrawal *if:*

1. The lung injury is stable/resolving.
2. The gas exchange is adequate with low positive end-expiratory pressure (PEEP)/F_{IO_2} requirements (e.g., PEEP less than 5 to 8 cm H_2O, F_{IO_2} less than 0.4 to 0.5)
3. Hemodynamics are stable without a need for pressors.
4. There is the capability to initiate spontaneous breaths.

This information is usually readily available and the Task Force recommends that these issues be assessed daily (i.e., the daily **wean screen**).[1] An extrapolation of this concept could be taken to the postsurgical arena where respiratory recovery is often rapid and the wean screen could be done on a more frequent basis (e.g., every hour).

ASSESSING THE POTENTIAL FOR DISCONTINUATION

A number of parameters have been found to be associated with ventilator discontinuation success

TABLE 18-1 *Commonly Reported Criteria to Predict Discontinuation Success*

Mechanical Factors	MV < 15 L/min
	MIF < −25 cm H_2O
	VC > 10 ml/kg
	$f/V_T < 105$
	Work <5 joules/min (exclusive of endotracheal tube work)
	PTI < 0.15
Integrated Factors	CROP index >13[7]
	Weaning score based on compliance, resistance, V_D/V_T, $PaCO_2$, and $f/V_T < 3$[8]
	Weaning index (PTI × MV for $PaCO_2$ of $40/V_T$) < 4[33]
	Neural network[13]
Patient Assessment	Lack of: Dyspnea
	Accessory muscle use
	Abdominal paradox
	Agitation/anxiety/tachycardia

f, Frequency; *MV*, minute ventilation; *$PaCO_2$*, partial pressure of carbon dioxide; *PTI*, pressure–time index; *VC*, vital capacity; *V_D*, dead-space volume; *V_T*, tidal volume.

or failure.[9-12] A summary of the better studied parameters is given in Table 18-1. Some of these are readily obtained (e.g., vital capacity [VC], minute ventilation [MV], frequency/tidal volume [f/V_T] ratio, muscle force generated during 20 seconds of effort against a closed airway maximum inspiratory force [MIF], and patient observations). Other parameters, however, require more sophisticated measurements. For instance, an esophageal balloon to measure esophageal pressure (P_{ES}, an estimate of pleural pressure) is necessary to assess patient muscle loads. Muscle loads can be expressed as either work or pressure-time products (PTPs) per breath (work = $\int P_{ES} \cdot V_T$, PTP = $\int P_{ES} \cdot T_i$).[13-16] These indices of muscle load can be expressed with respect to time (i.e., work/min), to ventilation (i.e., work/liter) or to maximum muscle strength (i.e., PTP/MIF). Multiplying the PTP/MIF by the inspiratory time fraction (T_i/T_{tot}) results in the pressure-time index (PTI), which can be a useful predictor of fatigue.[14]

Integrated factors also have been employed.[9] The CROP index multiplies dynamic compliance by PaO_2/PAO_2 (arterial O_2 pressure/alveolar O_2) by MIF and divides this product by respiratory rate to determine a single integrated value reflecting the important ventilator dependence determinants. Other integrated scores incorporate P_{ES} load calculations[8] and may use neural networks.[17] Important clinical assessment criteria include subjective dyspnea, accessory muscle use, diaphoresis, tachycardia, abdominal paradox, and subjective comfort.

Analyses of receiver-operator characteristics (ROC curves) have shown none of these indices alone to be sufficiently sensitive and specific to be used in clinically predicting discontinuation success.[1,9] Moreover, the likelihood ratios for all of these parameters (i.e., the percentage increase is predicting success using the parameter), although always statistically significant, are not large enough to be of use in making a decision on an individual patient. Because of these limitations the Task Force does not recommend routinely using these parameters in clinical practice.[1] Instead, because the direct assessment of spontaneous breathing capabilities for up to 2 hours has been shown in several randomized trials to be the most effective way to shorten the ventilator discontinuation process,[2,4] the Task Force has recommended that those passing the daily wean screen be assessed with a formal **spontaneous breathing trial (SBT).**

The SBT involves an integrated patient assessment during spontaneous breathing with little or no ventilator assistance (e.g., T-piece trial or using either 1 to 5 cm H_2O continuous positive airway pressure [CPAP] or 5 to 7 cm H_2O of pressure support from the ventilator).[1,2,12] The Task Force further recommends that no single parameter be used to judge SBT success or failure. Rather, an integrated assessment of the respiratory pattern (especially the development of tachypnea), hemodynamic status (especially tachycardias, bradycardias, or blood pressure swings), gas exchange (especially SpO_2 decreases), and patient comfort (especially the development of anxiety or diaphoresis). The Task Force emphasizes that the trial must last at least 30 minutes but no longer than 120 minutes.[1] If it is not clear that the patient is an SBT success at the 120-minute mark, then the patient should be considered an SBT failure.

NEXT STEPS FOR PATIENTS WITH SUCCESSFUL SPONTANEOUS BREATHING TRIAL

A patient who successfully completes an SBT has been shown in multiple studies to have a high likelihood of tolerating ventilator discontinuation permanently.[9] Discontinuation, however, should be considered a two-step process. In successfully performing an SBT, the first step, removing positive pressure ventilation, is accomplished. The second step is removing the artificial airway.

The decision to remove the artificial airway depends on a different set of assessments than those used to determine ventilator removal.[1,9] First, artificial airway removal must be done only in patients with the ability to protect the airway. Thus patients must demonstrate good coughing strength and minimal need for suctioning (e.g., no more than every 2 hours). Second, alertness and the ability to follow commands can greatly improve the success rate of artificial airway removal. This is the rationale behind protocols to reassess and minimize sedation needs on a regular basis.[18,19] Third, in borderline cases, the decision to remove the artificial airway may need to take into account the difficulty anticipated in replacing the airway if needed.

Because ventilator discontinuation and artificial airway removal are not exact sciences, a certain reintubation rate is to be expected for even the most skilled of clinicians. Large surveys suggest that 10% to 15% reintubation rates are typical for most well-run ICUs.[20] Rates significantly above or below this range should prompt reassessment of potentially either overaggressive (high reintubation rates) or underaggressive (low reintubation rates) practices.

Several small studies have suggested that noninvasive ventilation (NIV) can be used to avert reintubations in recently extubated patients with chronic obstructive pulmonary disease (COPD) who are failing.[21,22] This concept may also extend to COPD patients who have failed an SBT, but are judged capable of protecting their airway. In these patients the artificial airway is removed and ventilatory support is supplied with NIV. Importantly, these uses of NIV appear to be restricted to the COPD population because larger studies of these practices in non-COPD patients have shown no benefit to NIV.[23]

MANAGING THE NOT-YET-READY-TO-BE-DISCONTINUED PATIENT

Patients who fail an SBT pose an important management challenge. A first step in addressing this challenge is to determine the reasons for failure. Common causes for failed discontinuation and continued **ventilator dependence** are:

1. Respiratory drive failure involving inability of the patient to generate a reliable respiratory drive because of central nervous system (CNS) injury or drugs.[24]
2. Oxygenation failure involving rapid hemoglobin desaturation from loss of expiratory pressure and/or inspired O_2 concentration (FIO_2)
3. Cardiovascular failure involving dysrhythmias and/or hypotension from catechol release, edema formation, or coronary hypoxemia caused by the loss of ventilatory support.[25]
4. Muscle failure involving muscle overload from abnormal respiratory system impedances in the setting of weakened, fatigued, or metabolically disturbed muscles.[13,26-31]

Depending upon the clinical venue, certain forms of failure may be more common. For example, coronary care units may see more cardiac problems; neurologic units may see more respiratory drive failures.

Once a cause of ventilator dependence has been established, a management plan can be developed. This plan first must focus on the cause of the ventilator dependency identified above (e.g., improving respiratory drive, improving cardiac function, improving gas exchange etc.). The plan must also focus on managing the ventilator and the patient's respiratory muscle loading because these can be equally as important in optimizing outcome.

Ventilator management of these patients should focus on preventing ventilator-induced lung injury (VILI)[32] and properly loading the respiratory muscles. Strategies to prevent VILI are covered in Chapters 10 and 15 and involve minimizing tidal and maximal stretch and avoiding collapse/reopening stresses in atelectatic units. Proper muscle loading should prevent both fatigue and atrophy. Fatigue results from inadequate or dys-synchronous ventilatory support and can damage sarcomeres.[26,27] Atrophy (sometimes referred to as ventilator-induced diaphragmatic dysfunction or VIDD) results from lack of neural stimulation and muscle activity.[33]

The ideal mode should thus be an assisted form of ventilation that provides nonfatiguing synchronous respiratory muscle loading. Volume-assisted (VA) breaths (volume assist-control ventilation [VACV] with low backup rate) permits patient effort to trigger most breaths but generally is designed to do the bulk of the ventilation work after triggering. To allow more patient work to be done, the VACV backup rate can be reduced to allow low-level pressure support (PS) or unassisted spontaneous breaths to occur (synchronized intermittent mandatory ventilation or SIMV). In contrast, pressure-assisted (PA) breaths (pressure assist-control ventilation [PACV] with low backup rate), and stand-alone pressure support ventilation (PSV) not only permit patient triggering but are also designed to do significant sharing of the ventilation work with each patient breath.[34] Patient work is thus determined by the inspiratory pressure setting; intermittent unassisted or low-level assisted spontaneous breaths are not necessary. Studies comparing these different modes in this patient-recovery clinical setting are few. In general, consistent loading with variable flow pressure-targeted breaths appears easier to synchronize with patient efforts and is less complicated to adjust than alternating VA and spontaneous breath types using SIMV.[35] It must be pointed out, however, that SIMV was the first **partial support** mode invented, has been used successfully for decades, and is still commonly used today.

If VA breaths are used, the tidal volume should be set according to the National Institutes of Health (NIH) ARDS Network rules (4 to 8 ml/kg; see Chapter 15).[36] Synchrony of VA breaths with patient effort can often be achieved with proper flow and timing adjustments. If PA or PS breaths are used, the pressure level should focus on comfort and assuring that the tidal volume is also within the NIH ARDS Network rules. Generally this involves pressure settings between 10 and 25 cm H_2O. The rise time adjustments and inspiratory timing (set inspiratory time with PA and flow cycling criteria with PS) can be used to maximize synchrony and comfort.[37]

An important consideration is whether the level of support should be decreased over time (i.e., decrease PA or PS pressure or decrease the VACV backup rate, thereby allowing increasing spontaneous or PS breaths with SIMV). This is the traditional concept of ventilator weaning and is based upon the notion that progressive loading (exercising) of the respiratory muscles would hasten the transition to unassisted spontaneous ventilation. However, there is no good evidence that loading recovering respiratory muscle above that required for breath triggering and comfortable breathing provides any physiologic benefit.[9] Moreover, the Task Force found no good evidence that gradual support reduction improved outcome and only added to ventilator management complexity.[1] The recommendation thus was to set a comfortable level of assisted ventilation (mode not important) and then not adjust it unless the patient worsened. It is important to re-emphasize that a critical additional part of this Task Force recommendation is that it must always be coupled with the daily wean screen and subsequent SBT in those passing the screen.

THE IMPACT OF NEWER FEEDBACK CONTROLLERS ON DISCONTINUATION

The earliest approaches to feedback controllers involved adjusting the machine breath rate with SIMV according to the delivered minute ventilation. This was commonly referred to as minimum minute ventilation (MMV).[38] As noted above, because SIMV modes are less comfortable and more complex and because weaning mandatory breaths have not been shown to improve outcomes when compared with stable support and daily wean screens/SBTs, MMV is less commonly used today.

On many modern ventilators, pressure-targeted modes can have a feedback controller of the inspiratory pressure to assure a minimal V_T.[38] With pressure assist-control, this is termed pressure regulated volume control (PRVC); with pressure support this is termed volume support (VS). With these modes, a reduced effort or worsening mechanics would result in the ventilator automatically increasing the inspiratory pressure target; with increased effort or improving mechanics the ventilator would automatically reduce the inspiratory pressure target. A more sophisticated approach is to also add an end tidal CO_2 monitor to guide the inspiratory pressure setting.

Some have speculated that these techniques could be used to automatically decrease support to wean patients as their clinical status improved. A problem with this concept, however, is that if the minimal V_T is set too low, resulting dyspnea may increase effort and thereby further reduce support inappropriately. Conversely, an inappropriately high V_T may never stimulate patient efforts and thus no pressure reduction will ever occur. Perhaps more importantly, however, is the fact that the Task Force, as noted above, found no evidence that gradual support reduction accelerated the ventilator discontinuation process. Thus until good outcome data are obtained that support these approaches, automated weaning procedures cannot be routinely recommended at the present time. One conceptual application for PRVC and VS in the discontinuation process might be in the patient with a fluctuating respiratory drive, for example, during sleep or with sedation. Under these conditions these modes might provide an appropriate safety net for patients receiving pressure-targeted support.

More complex approaches to "automated weaning" exist. One, adaptive support ventilation (ASV), uses respiratory system mechanics to set the ventilator to deliver the frequency-V_T combination resulting in the lowest ventilator work (and thus lowest mechanical stress applied to the lung).[39,40] The ventilator contribution to the total work of breathing can also be automatically titrated downward. In small trials, often of relatively straightforward postsurgical patients, ASV effectively reduces ventilatory support. Randomized trials of ASV versus aggressive protocol-driven SBT-focused discontinuation strategies, however, do not exist. Other novel approaches to automated discontinuation provide an automated pressure support reduction based upon such things as the respiratory pattern or the respiratory drive as reflected in the P0.1 (the airway pressure generated by a patient against a closed shutter after 100 msec of effort).[41] Another pressure support reduction approach culminating in an SBT is based upon the respiratory pattern and the end tidal CO_2.[42] This latter approach has recently been studied in a randomized controlled trial but, unfortunately, the control group was not an aggressive SBT-based approach. Thus any benefits ascribed to this new approach must be viewed with caution. Finally, in the future, the potential to drive the level of ventilatory support based upon diaphragm electromyogram or patient work exists.[43] The idea behind these approaches would be to titrate the level of ventilatory support based upon patient respiratory drive and/or mechanical loading. While conceptually attractive, these approaches are not commercially available and clearly need to be tested in outcome studies versus aggressive SBT-based discontinuation approaches.

APPROACHES FOR THE DIFFICULT-TO-WEAN PATIENT

Patients consistently failing SBTs despite apparent stabilization or even reversal of their underlying disease comprise one of the most challenging management problems in the ICU. On occasion, an extubation attempt might be warranted in such patients if only to convince the care team that the irritant and loading effects of the artificial airway are not the cause of the SBT failure. Similarly, a tracheostomy might be done to eliminate the effects of the endotracheal tube as a cause of discontinuation failure.[44,45]

In those patients, however, who are truly ventilator dependent after 14 to 21 days despite disease stabilization or reversal, different management approaches might be indicated.[46] These are discussed in more detail in Chapter 19. In general, these approaches involve comprehensive multidisciplinary rehabilitation interventions in addition to ventilatory support. These interventions are aimed at optimizing all of the other factors that are contributing to the patient's reliance on life support (e.g., nutrition, physical therapy, psychosocial support, etc). From the ventilatory support perspective, a gradual support reduction strategy (weaning) might be appropriate in this population because this is the approach used by most experts in the field.

A consistent recommendation from numerous observational trials is to wean patients to about 50% of their maximal support levels (i.e., 50% of their initial PA or PS inspiratory pressure settings) without using daily SBTs. When that has been achieved, daily SBTs are re-instituted.[46] Subsequent decisions on ventilator withdrawal are then based on the assessments described above. Unfortunately, ventilator discontinuation success in this population remains near 50% to 60% (see Chapter 19).

KEY POINTS

- The ventilator discontinuation process is a critical component of ICU care.
- Ventilator dependency is caused by both disease factors and clinician management factors.
- The daily wean screen and subsequent SBT in those passing the screen is now the gold standard for ventilator withdrawal assessment and should be done in virtually all patients recovering from respiratory failure.
- The decision to remove the artificial airway in those successfully passing an SBT requires further assessments of the patient's ability to protect the airway.
- Managing the patient who fails the SBT is one of the biggest challenges facing ICU clinicians.
- In general, simple, stable forms of partial support that provide comfortable ventilatory support are what is required between the daily wean screen/SBT.

ASSESSMENT QUESTIONS

1. True or False. The failure to recognize the patient's ability to be discontinued from the ventilator is a major cause of iatrogenic delays in ventilatory discontinuation.
2. True or False. Patients should be screened daily for stability/reversibility of the disease process, gas exchange, hemodynamics, and capabilities for spontaneous breathing.

ASSESSMENT QUESTIONS—cont'd

3. True or False. Measurements of VC and MIF are critical in determining a patient's ability to tolerate ventilator discontinuation.
4. True or False. Measurements of patient's workload have been shown to be very effective in guiding clinical decision making for ventilator discontinuation.
5. True or False. The SBT is the most effective way of determining a patient's ability to tolerate ventilator discontinuation.
6. True or False. The SBT should only be done with the ventilator removed and the patient breathing spontaneously.
7. True or False. A gag reflex must be present for an extubation to be successful.
8. True or False. Reintubation rates should be less than 1 percent in a well-run respiratory care unit.
9. True or False. If a patient fails a spontaneous breathing trial, it is wise to delay another 3 to 4 days before trying it again.
10. True or False. In between failed SBTs, the literature advocates repeated attempts to reduce the level of support (e.g., pressure support reductions or IMV rate reductions).

CASE STUDIES

For additional practice, refer to Case Study 5 in the appendix at the back of this book.

REFERENCES

1. ACCP/SCCM/AARC Task Force: Evidence based guidelines for weaning and discontinuing mechanical ventilation, Chest 120 (6 Suppl):375S-395S, 2001.
2. Esteban A, Frutos F, Tobin MJ et al: A comparison of four methods of weaning from mechanical ventilation, N Engl J Med 332:345-350, 1995.
3. Brochard L, Ramos A, Benito S et al: Comparison of these methods of gradual withdrawal from ventilatory support during weaning from mechanical ventilation, Am J Respir Crit Care Med 50:896-903, 1994.
4. Ely EW, Baker AM, Dunagan DP et al: Effect on the duration of mechanical ventilation of identifying patients capable of breathing spontaneously, N Engl J Med 335:1864-1869, 1996.
5. Kollef MH, Shapiro SD, Silver P et al: A randomized controlled trial of protocol directed vs physician directed weaning from mechanical ventilation, Crit Care Med 25:567-574, 1997.
6. Esteban A, Alia I, Ibanez J et al: Modes of mechanical ventilation and weaning. A national survey of Spanish hospitals. The Spanish Lung Failure Collaborative Group, Chest 106:1188-1193, 1994.
7. Esteban A, Anzueto A, Alia I et al: How is mechanical ventilation employed in the intensive care unit? An international utilization review, Am J Respir Crit Care Med 161:1450-1458, 2000.
8. Laghi F, D'Alfonso N, Tobin MJ: Pattern of recovery from diaphragmatic fatigue over 24 hours, J Appl Physiol 79:539-546, 1995.
9. MacIntyre NR, Cook DJ, Guyatt G, editors: Weaning mechanical ventilation: the evidence base, Chest 120 (Suppl 6):375-473, 2001.
10. Sahn SA, Lakschminarayan MB: Bedside criteria for the discontinuation of mechanical ventilation, Chest 63:1002-1005, 1973.
11. Morganroth ML, Morganroth JL, Nett LM et al: Criteria for weaning from prolonged mechanical ventilation, Arch Intern Med 144:1012-1016, 1984.
12. Yang K, Tobin MJ: A prospective study of indexes predicting outcome of trials of weaning from mechanical ventilation, N Engl J Med 324:1445-1450, 1991.
13. Tobin MJ: Respiratory muscles in disease, Clin Chest Med 9:263-286, 1988.
14. Collett PW, Perry C, Engel LA: Pressure time product, flow, and oxygen cost of resistive breathing in humans, J Appl Physiol 58:1263-1272, 1985.
15. Bellemare F, Grassino A: Effect of pressure and timing or contraction on human diaphragm fatigue, J Appl Physiol 53:1190-1195, 1982.
16. MacIntyre NR, Leatherman NE: Mechanical loads on the ventilatory muscles: a theoretical analysis, Am Rev Respir Dis 139:968-973, 1989.
17. Ashutosh K, Hyukjoon L, Mohan CK et al: Prediction criteria for successful weaning from respiratory support, Crit Care Med 20:1295-1301, 1992.
18. Park G, Coursin D, Ely EW et al: Balancing sedation and analgesia in the critically ill, Crit Care Clin 17:1015-1027, 2001.
19. Schweickert WD, Gehlbach BK, Pohlman AS et al: Daily interruption of sedative infusions and complications of critical illness in mechanically ventilated patients, Crit Care Med 32:1272-1276, 2004.
20. Rothaar RC, Epstein SK: Extubation failure: magnitude of the problem, impact on outcomes, and prevention, Curr Opin Crit Care 9:59-66, 2003.
21. Nava S, Ambrosini N, Clini E et al: Non invasive ventilation in the weaning of patients with respiratory failure due to COPD, Ann Intern Med 128:721-728, 1998.
22. Girault C, Daudenthun I, Chevron V et al: Non invasive ventilation as a systematic extubation and weaning technique in acute chronic respiratory failure, Am J Respir Crit Care Med 160:86-92, 1999.

23. Esteban A, Frutos-Vivar F, Ferguson ND et al: Noninvasive positive-pressure ventilation for respiratory failure after extubation, N Engl J Med 350:2452-2460, 2004.
24. Argov Z, Mastaglia FL: Disorders of neuromuscular transmission caused by drugs, N Engl J Med 301:409-413, 1979.
25. Lemaire F, Teboul JL, Cinotti L et al: Acute left ventricular dysfunction during unsuccessful weaning from mechanical ventilation, Anesthesiology 69:171-179, 1988.
26. Hussain SNA, Simkus T, Roussos C: Respiratory muscle fatigue: a cause of ventilatory failure in septic shock, J Appl Physiol 58:2033-2040, 1985.
27. Roussos CS, Macklem PT: Diaphragmatic fatigue in man, J Appl Physiol 43:189-197. 1977.
28. Agusti AGN, Torres A, Estopa R et al: Hypophosphatemia as a cause of failed weaning: the importance of metabolic factors, Crit Care Med 12:142-143, 1984.
29. Molloy DW, Dhingra S, Solven F et al: Hypomagnesemia and respiratory muscle power, Am Rev Respir Dis 129:497-498, 1984.
30. Bark H, Heimer D, Chaimowitz C et al: Effect of chronic renal failure on respiratory muscle strength, Respiration 54:151-163, 1988.
31. Pingleton SK, Harmon GS: Nutritional management in acute respiratory failure, JAMA 257:2094-2099, 1987.
32. Plotz FB, Slutsky AS, van Vught AJ et al: Ventilator-induced lung injury and multiple system organ failure: a critical review of facts and hypotheses, Intensive Care Med 30:1865-1872, 2004.
33. Vassilakopoulos T, Petrof BJ: Ventilator-induced diaphragmatic dysfunction, Am J Respir Crit Care Med 169:336-341, 2004.
34. Banner MJ, Kirby RR, MacIntyre NR: Patient and ventilator work of breathing and ventilatory muscle loads at different levels of pressure support ventilation, Chest 100:531-533, 1991.
35. MacIntyre NR, McConnell R, Cheng KC et al: Pressure limited breaths improve flow dys-synchrony during assisted ventilation, Crit Care Med 25:1671-1677, 1997.
36. NIH ARDS Network: Ventilation with lower tidal volumes as compared to traditional tidal volumes in acute lung injury and acute respiratory distress syndrome, N Engl J Med 342:1301-1308, 2000.
37. MacIntyre NR, Ho LI: Effects of initial flow rate and breath termination criteria on pressure support ventilation, Chest 99:134-138, 1991.
38. MacIntyre NR, Branson RD: Feedback enhancements on ventilator breaths. In Tobin M, editor: Principles and practice of mechanical ventilation, ed 2, New York, 2006, McGraw-Hill.
39. Cassina T, Chiolero R, Mauri R et al: Clinical experience with adaptive support ventilation for fast-track cardiac surgery, J Cardiothor Vasc Anesth 17:571-575, 2003.
40. Petter AH, Chiolero RL, Cassina T et al: Automatic "respirator/weaning" with adaptive support ventilation: the effect on duration of endotracheal intubation and patient management, Anesth Analg 97:1743-1750, 2003.
41. Iotti GA, Braschi A: Closed loop support of ventilatory workload: the P0.1 controller, Resp Care Clin North Am 7:441-451, 2001.
42. Lellouche F, Mancebo J, Jolliet P et al: A multicenter randomized trial of computer-driven protocolized weaning from mechanical ventilation, Am J Respir Crit Care Med 174:894-900, 2006.
43. Sinderby C, Navalesi P, Beck J et al: Neural control of mechanical ventilation in respiratory failure, Nat Med 5:1433-1436, 1999.
44. Rumback MJ, Newton M, Truncale T et al: A prospective randomized study comparing early percutaneous dilatational tracheotomy to prolonged translaryngeal intubation (delayed tracheotomy) in critically ill medical patients, Crit Care Med 32:1689-1694, 2004.
45. Griffiths J, Barber VS, Morgan L et al: Systematic review and meta analysis of studies of the timing of tracheostomy in adult patients undergoing artificial ventilation, BMJ 330:1243-1257, 2005.
46. MacIntyre NR, Epstein SK, Carson S et al: Management of patients requiring prolonged mechanical ventilation, Chest 128:3937-3954, 2005.

CHAPTER

19 *Prolonged Mechanical Ventilation*

CHRISTOPHER E. COX; SHANNON S. CARSON

OUTLINE

OBJECTIVES

- Explain the epidemiology and outcomes of prolonged mechanical ventilation.
- Review issues related to the role and timing of tracheostomy for prolonged mechanical ventilation.
- List effective ways to wean patients requiring prolonged mechanical ventilation.
- Describe multidisciplinary approaches to improving patient outcome.

KEY TERMS

acute lung injury (ALI)
acute physiology and chronic health evaluation (APACHE)
disease management programs
endotracheal tube
percutaneous dilatational tracheostomy (PDT)
polyneuropathy
pressure-regulated volume control (PRVC)
tracheostomy
ventilator dependence
weaning

Patients requiring prolonged mechanical ventilation (PMV) represent a growing number of critical care outliers. This population is estimated to make up 5% to 10% of all patients in U.S. intensive care units (ICUs), yet they use almost a third of ICU resources. The long-term outcomes of this primarily elderly patient group are relatively poor, and the demands on family members and health care providers are significant. These patients may also create patient access limitations in ICUs because of their prolonged lengths of stay. Patients, their families, clinicians, and policymakers all struggle with the challenges of PMV.

PROLONGED MECHANICAL VENTILATION

A starting point for PMV discussion begins with clarification about how this group is defined. In some ways, the many (and varied) definitions of PMV in the medical literature have led to more confusion than clarity. Some clinicians and investigators have described PMV as receiving more than 2 days of ventilation, others by receiving as many as 29 days. Considering that worldwide, the median duration of ventilation is 3 days and that 75% of persons are ventilated for less than or equal to 7 days, it would be reasonable to consider a week or more somewhat prolonged.[1] Still, few clinicians would likely consider a person with septic shock and acute respiratory distress syndrome (ARDS) to have an especially prolonged course if they were liberated from mechanical ventilation after 10 days.

In an attempt to unify the literature, a recent consensus group has recommended the following definition to describe PMV: ventilation for at least 21 days (for 6 or more hours a day), with or without a **tracheostomy.**[2] The choice of 21 days of mechanical ventilation is consistent with Center for Medicare and Medicaid Services (CMS) designations for PMV. This definition captures the true outliers of critical care, for whom the disproportionate use of ICU and health care resources is most pronounced. Patients requiring 21 days of mechanical ventilation consistently reflect the condition of persistent single or multiple organ failure, muscle atrophy, frequent delirium, and recurrent infection that are often referred to as chronic critical illness.

A frequently encountered definition for PMV or chronic critical illness is the requirement of tracheostomy for prolonged mechanical ventilation. Reflected in Diagnosis Related Code (DRG) 483 (now DRG 541: ventilation for ≥ 96 hours plus placement of tracheostomy for non-ENT reasons *with* a major surgical procedure, and DRG 542: ventilation for ≥ 96 hours plus placement of tracheostomy for non-ENT reasons *without* a major surgical procedure), this definition has allowed for population-based studies of PMV using administrative databases. Studies using this definition must be interpreted in the context of changing physician practice toward earlier placement of tracheostomies.[3] It is likely that between 75% and 90% of persons ventilated for at least 21 days will have had a tracheostomy placed during the acute hospitalization and qualify for DRG 541 or 542, so there is considerable overlap between these definitions in terms of group composition.

The specific definition for PMV is more relevant to interpretation of medical literature than it is to the daily practice in a given ICU. From a physician or patient's point of view, any day of mechanical ventilation beyond the initial period of stabilization or beyond the immediate postoperative period is too long, and attention is immediately directed toward liberation from mechanical ventilation.

EPIDEMIOLOGY OF PMV

Although PMV patients are a minority population in ICUs, their numbers are growing annually.[3] It has been estimated that between 5% and 10% of persons admitted to ICUs annually receive PMV.[4,5] However, both large cohort and international epidemiologic studies have shown that up to 24% of all ventilated patients and as many as 33% of persons ventilated for more than 2 days may receive tracheostomies.[6,7] Considering that approximately 30% to 50% of all persons admitted to ICUs require mechanical ventilation, there are more PMV patients than people might expect. These numbers are supported by a recent review of the National Inpatient Survey Sample that demonstrated that there were 88,000 discharges during 1997 under DRG 483, 52% of whom were 65 years of age or older.[8] This also is similar to the roughly 45,000 Medicare-eligible patients who received DRG 541 or 542 codes in 2005.[9]

In one state population–based study, the incidence of tracheostomy placement for prolonged mechanical ventilation increased from 8.3/100,000 population in 1993 to 24.2/100,000 population in 2002 (Figure 19-1). This increase is out of proportion to that of the increase in incidence of mechanical ventilation itself.[3] Given that the incidence of respiratory failure increases significantly after age 65 and that the population is aging remarkably as the baby boom generation approaches age 65, it is likely that the burden of chronic critical illness will only increase further in the coming decade.[10]

Economics of PMV

Discussion of economics is difficult to separate from the process of PMV care. Despite numbering only sixtieth in total discharges among Medicare recipients by diagnostic group, PMV patients rank third in summative Medicare inpatient charges (more than $8 billion in 2005) and first in inpatient charges per individual patient.[9] The posthospital costs per patient have been estimated at close to $150,000 (adjusted to inflation for 2005) during the first year after discharge, as well.[11] Since the institution of the prospective payment system in 1997, hospitals have been paid more or less a set amount by patient diagnosis with

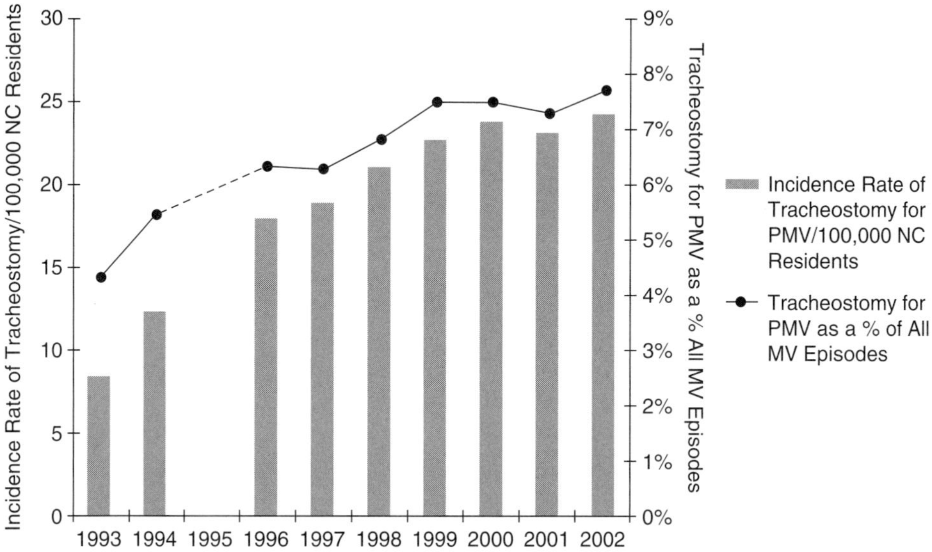

FIGURE 19-1 The bars represent the annual incidence rate of tracheostomy placement for prolonged mechanical ventilation (*PMV*) per 100,000 North Carolina (*NC*) state residents (values on the left *y*-axis). The line represents annual tracheostomy placement for PMV as a percentage of all patients who required mechanical ventilation (*MV*) for acute respiratory failure (values on right *y*-axis). The dashed line represents interpolated data points for the year 1995. (Modified from Cox CE: Increase in tracheostomy for prolonged mechanical ventilation in North Carolina, 1993-2002, Crit Care Med 32(11):2219-2226, 2004.)

minor adjustments for geographic area and other factors. DRG 541 and 542 have a high Medicare reimbursement rate because of their prolonged hospital stays and high costs of care. Therefore, hospitals have an incentive to limit PMV patients' length of stay so that they may minimize costs and maximize reimbursement. However, many patients' hospital stays become prolonged enough that the hospitals lose money on their care, even with the addition of "outlier" payment adjustments.[12]

Hospitals have found that costs for PMV patients can be limited by reducing the length of ICU care and by reducing overall length of stay. One can view the process of PMV care over the course of a year like a compartment of constant area that is subdivided within various partitions: acute hospital care, post-acute care, and home (Figure 19-2). Before the proliferation of long-term acute care (LTAC) facilities and other institutions providing care to PMV patients, hospitals were relegated to keeping PMV patients in-house until they were stable enough to transfer home or to a nursing facility. To achieve cost savings, some groups established in-hospital, non–ICU-based **weaning** and respiratory care units.[13] Over time, many more hospitals established referral patterns to LTAC facilities and highly skilled nursing facilities with ventilator capabilities. This allowed earlier transfer of PMV patients from the acute hospital ICU setting. Now, as shown in Figure 19-2, the typical PMV patient's process of care will likely include a number of institutions before eventual home discharge.

PMV Patients

PMV patients represent all age groups (Figure 19-3). Nonetheless, the median age of PMV patients in many series is around 65 years. There is no strong gender difference among these persons, and patients tend to be evenly divided between surgical and medical ICUs. Frequently, patients are survivors of sepsis, trauma, or other causes of multiorgan failure and **acute lung injury (ALI)** or ARDS. Nontrauma patients generally have more than one comorbid condition, especially underlying renal disease, chronic obstructive pulmonary disease (COPD), congestive heart failure (CHF), or diabetes. Underlying vascular disease is also common.

Ventilator-Dependent Patients

As with acute ventilatory failure, the list of factors associated with the development of **ventilator dependence** is long (Box 19-1). These factors are mostly clinical in nature, but process of care issues can be involved as well. PMV patients have survived

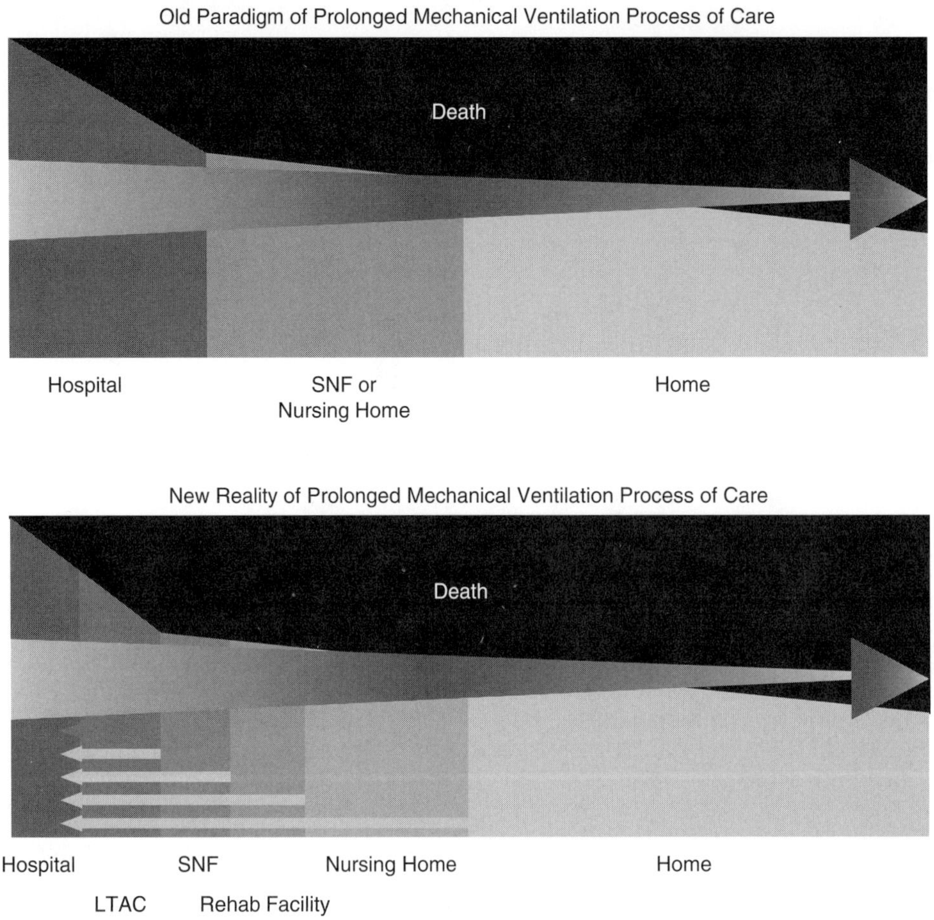

FIGURE 19-2 These diagrams represent the overall change in PMV process of care that has evolved over the past few decades. Previously, patients were managed for extended periods in acute care hospitals until they were weaned and ready for transfer to a facility or home. Now, hospitals are discharging PMV patients sooner to a variety of post–acute care facilities. As patients navigate these facilities, they remain at high risk for hospital readmission.

the acute phase of their illness, but the sequelae of the acute insults leave them unable to sustain spontaneous ventilation. These sequelae can be directly related to their acute illness (e.g., fibrotic phase of ARDS, critical illness polyneuropathy), or related to interventions prompted by the acute illness (e.g., upper airway obstruction due to tracheostomy). Critical illness **polyneuropathy** is a particularly important causal factor in PMV. In one study, up to 95% of patients requiring more than 28 days of ICU care had neurophysiologic evidence of chronic partial denervation of muscle, consistent with previous critical illness polyneuropathy.[14] These findings were evident up to 5 years after ICU discharge.

Predicting the Need for PMV

Clinical research has identified a few predictors of the need for prolonged ventilation measured during the index hospitalization. These include a witnessed aspiration event, failed extubation, nosocomial pneumonia, high **acute physiology and chronic health evaluation (APACHE)** III score, advanced age, poor prior functional status, and primary disease.[4,15] However, a satisfactory model for reliably predicting ventilator days on an individual patient level has not yet been published.

REDUCING THE LIKELIHOOD OF PMV

There are many factors associated with the duration of ventilation that are not amenable to intervention, such as illness severity, age, comorbidities, and primary diagnosis. However, there are certain process-of-care characteristics that may help lower the risk of PMV. These include tight glycemic control in

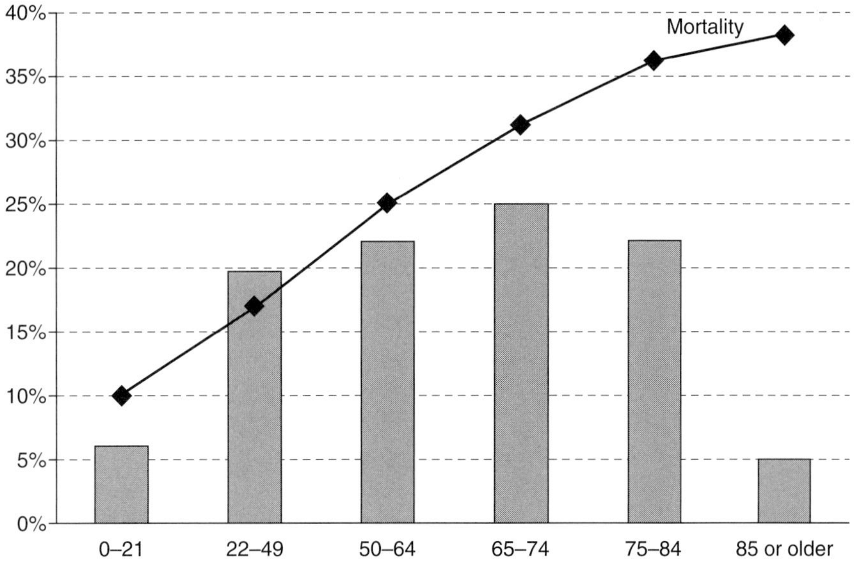

FIGURE 19-3 This figure shows the total percent of the estimated 88,000 PMV patients managed in the United States annually by age group (columns) and each age group's hospital mortality rate. (Data from the Nationwide Inpatient Sample, 1997. Modified from Carson SS: The epidemiology and costs of chronic critical illness, Crit Care Clin 18(3):461-476, 2002.)

surgical patients, screening for and performance of spontaneous breathing trials, and the use of low tidal volumes among ALI patients. The importance of strict glucose control has been shown to decrease the duration of mechanical ventilation and incidence of PMV in both medical and surgical populations.[15a,15b] Prevention of ICU-associated complications is known to decrease duration of mechanical ventilation, especially prevention of ventilator-associated pneumonia and catheter-associated bloodstream infection. Handwashing, barrier protocols, head of bed elevation, line insertion protocols and checklists, and sterile maintenance of ventilator components and tubing are simple measures that can have a significant impact on ventilator days in an ICU.

As described above, an important factor in the development of PMV is critical illness polyneuropathy. Use of neuromuscular blockers and high-dose steroids, two risk factors for polyneuropathy, should be limited to conditions in which they are absolutely indicated. In fact, the availability of intravenous infusions of sedatives, especially in combination with adequate doses of narcotics, has eliminated the use of neuromuscular blocking agents almost entirely in many ICUs. With regard to steroids, the largest randomized trial of high-dose steroids for persistent ARDS indicates that steroid use does not decrease mortality.[16] High-dose steroids initiated more than 14 days into the course of ARDS were associated with higher mortality compared with patients who received placebo. Steroid use was associated with more ventilator-free days in 28 days; however, the risk of neuromyopathy was higher.

When continuous infusions of sedatives are required, daily interruption of sedative infusions to allow awakening of patients should be a standard part of the sedation protocol.[17] Recent data indicate that use of continuous infusions of short-acting sedatives such as propofol (with daily interruption) results in fewer ventilator days when compared with intermittent dosing of lorazepam, a longer-acting sedative.[18] Oversedation interferes with performance during spontaneous breathing trials and complicates assessments of readiness for extubation. Implementation of evidence-based sedation protocols that include regular assessments of responsiveness using validated scales is the most effective way to prevent this complication.

TIMING FOR TRACHEOSTOMY PLACEMENT

Prolonged intubation via an **endotracheal tube** may be uncomfortable for patients and lead to the development of psychological distress. Endotracheal intubation also typically requires sedation and analgesia—a

BOX 19-1 *Mechanisms Associated With Ventilator Dependence*

Systemic factors
Chronic comorbid conditions (e.g., malignancy, COPD, immunosuppression)
Overall severity of illness
Nonpulmonary organ failure
Hyperglycemia
Poor nutritional status

Mechanical factors
Increased work of breathing
Reduced respiratory muscle capacity
Critical illness polyneuropathy
Steroid myopathy
Disuse myopathy
Isolated phrenic nerve/diaphragmatic injury (e.g., after surgery)
Imbalance between increased work of breathing and respiratory muscle capacity
Upper airway obstruction (e.g., tracheal stenosis) preventing decannulation

Iatrogenic factors
Failure to recognize withdrawal potential
Inappropriate ventilator settings leading to excessive loads/discomfort
Imposed work of breathing from tracheotomy tubes
Medical errors

Complications of long-term hospital care
Recurrent aspiration
Infection (e.g., pneumonia, sepsis)
Stress ulcers
Deep venous thrombosis
Other medical problems developing in the PMV care venue

Psychological factors
Sedation
Delirium
Depression
Anxiety
Sleep deprivation

Process-of-care factors
Absence of weaning (and sedation) protocols
Inadequate nursing staffing
Insufficient physician experience

From MacIntyre NR, Epstein SK, Carson S et al: Management of patients requiring prolonged mechanical ventilation: report of a NAMDRC consensus conference, Chest 128:3937-3954, 2005.

factor that may contribute to a prolonged need for ventilatory support (see above). For selected patients who require (or are expected to require) ventilatory support for longer than average, placement of a tracheostomy has the attraction of allowing for reductions in sedation, easier patient communication, decreased work of breathing because of lower airway resistance, and enhanced airway clearance with suctioning.[19]

There is wide variation in physician practice regarding the timing of tracheostomy placement, likely because of the lack of data to guide this decision making. Previous consensus recommendations have suggested waiting until 21 days or more of ventilation before placing tracheostomies.[20] However, physicians have clearly begun to place tracheostomies earlier over time.[3] A recent analysis of the Project Impact database, including more than 43,000 patients, showed that the median duration of ventilation before tracheostomy placement was 9 days, while 75% of tracheostomies were placed by the fourteenth day of ventilation.[21] A survey of European ICUs reported that the tracheostomies were placed at a median of 12 days of ventilation in a total of 11% of ventilated patients.[22]

One systematic review found that there is no appreciable difference in the duration of ventilation or the incidence of airway injury based on early versus late placement of a tracheostomy.[23] The difficulty of comparing studies that use different definitions of early and late placement of tracheostomies is worth noting, however. A more recent meta-analysis of five studies and 400 patients found that although early (range 0 to 7 days) versus late (8 or more days) tracheostomy placement was not associated with either a reduction in mortality or the development of pneumonia, it did result in 9 fewer ventilator days and 15 fewer ICU days.[24] Although it remains debatable as to whether tracheostomy timing affects patient outcome, early placement of tracheostomies does allow for quicker transfer to specialized inpatient wards and to postacute care institutions that focus on weaning.

The impact of tracheostomy placement on patients' quality of life versus a longer course of ventilation via an endotracheal tube is unclear. Would patients consider the possible benefits of early tracheostomy (a chance to communicate and possibly earlier liberation from the ventilator) to be worth the risk of complications and a visible neck scar if the procedure could be avoided? There is no easy answer for questions like these based on the current medical literature. Larger randomized clinical trials are still necessary to determine if mortality is impacted by early tracheostomy. These randomized trials will depend on some method to predict who will require prolonged ventilation. However, as stated above, reliable methods of predicting who will require PMV from the perspective of the first few days of ventilation have not been validated.

Placing a Tracheostomy

Tracheostomies may be placed in the operating room or at the bedside. The popularity of bedside tracheostomies placed by the percutaneous dilatational technique has resulted in the rapid growth of this procedure over time. Also, **percutaneous dilatational tracheostomy (PDT)** has allowed persons not formally trained in surgery to perform this intervention because of the relative simplicity of the tracheostomy kits. For selected patients, PDT may be a good option because of lower costs, lack of need for patient transport, and slightly fewer postoperative complications.[25] Patients who have deviant anatomy or are obese are better suited for conventional surgical tracheostomies.

OUTCOME OF PMV PATIENTS

Outcomes of PMV can be considered from the perspective of patients, their families, providers, and society using measures of weaning success, survival, quality of life, functional status, emotional health, caregiver burden, and cost-effectiveness.

Disposition

Because of residual physical and cognitive limitations and unresolved medical issues (including continued ventilator dependence in some cases), fewer than 20% of PMV patients are discharged directly home from the acute care hospital. Most are transferred to another hospital or a postacute care venue, such as a skilled nursing facility, an LTAC hospital, or an inpatient rehabilitation facility. Frequently, PMV survivors require further graduated facility-based care after the initial transfer. Unfortunately, up to 60% may require readmission to an acute care hospital within the first year after discharge.

Weaning Success

The success of long-term weaning in the acute hospital setting ranges from 57% to 80% of hospital survivors, depending on access to weaning facilities. Weaning success in LTAC hospitals ranges from 70% to 90% of survivors, and time to weaning averages 40 days in most series. This may depend somewhat on selection criteria for each LTAC hospital, but process-of-care differences may be a factor as well.[26-28] One study found significant differences in weaning success and time to weaning for patients managed by two different physician groups in the same hospital.[29] The physician group that was more aggressive with spontaneous breathing trials and that were present in the hospital for longer periods of each day achieved better outcomes for their patients.

Survival

Hospital mortality for PMV ranges from 19% to 61% in published series, but hospital mortality is informative only in the context of the type of hospital reporting outcomes and their access to alternative weaning sites.[22,30] For example, one hospital reporting a low mortality rate (19%) also reports a low weaning rate (57%), suggesting that a large proportion of patients are transferred to weaning facilities.[30] Actual hospital mortality for PMV, therefore, depends in part on outcomes from the next institution. Population-based studies that include data from a multitude of acute hospital types report hospital mortality rates of 25% to 39%.[3,31] These mortality rates do not differ significantly from those reported for overall populations of patients requiring mechanical ventilation.

The risk of death after hospital discharge for PMV patients remains as high as 25% to 50%. Therefore long-term survival of PMV patients is a more useful outcome than hospital mortality from the patient's perspective. In most studies, between 50% and 77% of PMV patients will have died by 1 year after ICU admission. Long-term survival for recipients of critical care in general is best predicted by severity of acute illness, comorbidities, previous functional status, and to some extent, age. These same variables may be predictive of long-term outcome in PMV patients; however, reliable survival prediction models have not yet been validated.[26]

Quality of Life and Functional Status

PMV survivors on average report significant functional status limitations in basic activities of daily living, even 1 year after the index hospitalization. Most have at least one to two limitations in simple functioning, such as walking, ability to feed oneself, toileting, and taking medications without assistance. It is easy to assume that PMV survivors would report poor quality of life given their newly acquired functional limitations and critical illness–associated symptoms. Interestingly, studies have shown that in general PMV survivors' perceived quality of life is similar to

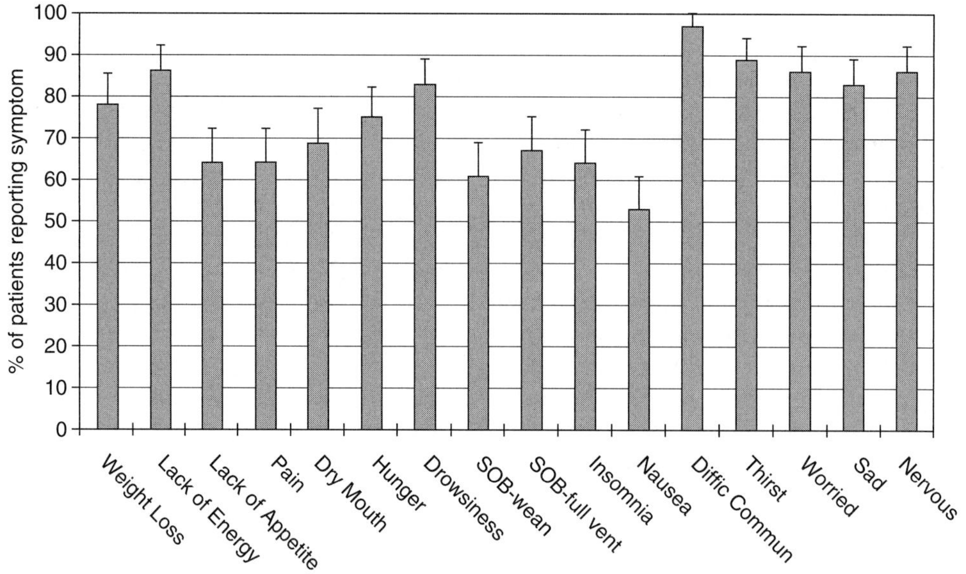

FIGURE 19-4 Prevalence of physical and psychological symptoms among chronically critically ill patients providing self-reports. The figure shows the percentage of patients providing symptom self-reports (n = 36) who responded that the symptom was present. Error bars represent sem. *SOB-wean,* Shortness of breath during weaning; *SOB-full vent,* shortness of breath during full ventilator support; *Diffic commun,* difficulty communicating. (Modified from Nelson JE: The symptom burden of chronic critical illness, Crit Care Med 32(7):1527-1534, 2004.)

that reported by other survivors of critical care. Patients evidently adapt to their altered physical capacities fairly well.

It is worth noting that a significant percentage of PMV patients are not captured in studies of health-related quality of life because they are either unable to complete telephone interviews or have died before the point of study follow-up. It is likely that physical and cognitive dysfunction that is advanced enough to prohibit telephone access would be associated with lower perceived quality of life, but this is yet to be confirmed. It is known that during hospitalization, chronically critically ill patients experience a high degree of symptoms ranging from pain, dyspnea, hunger and thirst, to frustration with limitations of communication (Figure 19-4).[32] Clinicians must remain sensitive to this symptom burden in all patients, regardless of prognosis.

Cost-Effectiveness

An emotionally charged issue relevant to society is whether PMV provision is cost-effective. Given the extremely high costs of these patients coupled with their poor survival and functional status, this is an important question to consider. Only one formal study of PMV cost-effectiveness exists, though.[32a] In this study, the authors reported that the value of PMV provision exceeds standard societal benchmarks of cost-effectiveness when patient age exceeded age 68 and when the likelihood of in-hospital survival was less than 50%. However, in first world nations, the suggestion of withholding PMV from patients based on economic factors is unrealistic at the current time. In second and third world nations, these concerns may be more of a reality because of limited technologies and resources. Given both the expansion of the elderly population in Western Europe and North America and the increasing limitations of national health care outlays in the coming decade, the unlimited provision of PMV to patients regardless of prognosis certainly will become more widely discussed and debated.

MOST EFFECTIVE WAYS TO WEAN PMV PATIENTS

Few data exist to support specific weaning protocols for PMV patients in the acute hospital setting. The experience in the LTAC setting has not been widely published either. However, weaning in the post–acute care setting is often protocol-driven and performed by non-physician providers. In one LTAC setting, Scheinhorn et al compared a therapist-implemented weaning protocol to a historical control of physician-directed, non–protocol-based weaning from 2 prior years.[33] They found that although the therapist-implemented protocol did not improve overall weaning success, it did reduce the time to wean and overall length of stay by 12 and 7 days, respectively.

There is yet no consensus about the best weaning strategy or protocol for PMV patients. In general, most providers agree that alternating periods of ventilator support with advancing periods of spontaneous breathing is the best current strategy of weaning PMV patients.[2] There is evidence, however, that gradual reduction in the level of pressure support alone may result in weaning rates similar to those of advancing duration of spontaneous breathing trials.[34] Given hemodynamic stability and resolution of acute medical and surgical issues, many clinicians wean the level of ventilator support to the equivalent of 10 to 15 cm H_2O of pressure support before beginning periods of unsupported spontaneous breathing through the tracheostomy tube. On the other hand, some have found that introducing spontaneous breathing trials can safely be done early, even from relatively high levels of initial support, if the respiratory rate to tidal volume (f/V_T ratio) is less than 80 and possibly 100 breaths/min/L.[33]

The ratio of spontaneous breathing exercise to rest may be increased based on the patient's success with initial trials of spontaneous breathing. It may be difficult to standardize the rate at which periods of spontaneous breathing should be advanced since patients' illness severity, muscle strength, and other physical and mental factors can vary widely by individual. The risks of overly quick advancement include fatiguing patients, whereas advancing too slowly increases length of stay and cumulative rate of ventilator-associated complications. Still, many short-term and long-term care institutions have successfully maintained weaning protocols for PMV patients that emphasize early recognition of readiness and rapid advancement of spontaneous breathing trials as tolerated.

It is not clear that any specific ventilation mode is superior to another with regard to the speed and overall success with which liberation from full support can be achieved. However, most clinicians prefer to use pressure support (PS) when possible because of its similarity to the characteristics of spontaneous breathing, including variable flow rates and tidal volumes. Volume modes are acceptable also. The combination of synchronized intermittent mandatory ventilation (SIMV) and PS is not recommended because of the unnatural combination of resultant tidal volumes and flow patterns for patients who are presumably not significantly sedated. This mode has previously been discredited as beneficial to the weaning process in large clinical trials. If the delivery of a set minute ventilation is imperative, either volume or pressure assist-control or possibly **pressure-regulated volume control (PRVC)** modes may be helpful. Because a mandatory minimum minute ventilation can be delivered within specific pressure limits, PRVC may be particularly useful if a lack of staffing limits in-house after-hours coverage of PMV patients.

Predicting Weaning Success

Weaning success is relatively easy to define in the acute ICU setting because it is marked by the successful removal of an endotracheal tube. However, among PMV patients who are ventilated via a tracheostomy, weaning success is less clear because the PMV weaning process can require short periods of ventilation after 2- to 3-day periods of spontaneous breathing before a patient is completely liberated from mechanical ventilation. At the present time, the recommended definition for PMV weaning success is complete removal from ventilation for 7 consecutive days.[2] A requirement for nocturnal noninvasive ventilation does not exclude patients from classification as being liberated from ventilation.

Predictors of successful weaning among 334 DRG 483 patients who survived acute hospitalization, 57% of whom were successfully weaned, included younger aged, nonmedical admissions, who after having an operation, were able to walk in the hall, and were able to eat without the need for either enteral or parenteral feeding.[30]

INTERVENTIONS TO IMPROVE PMV OUTCOMES

PMV patients have numerous physical, emotional, and social needs. Therefore, we believe that a multidisciplinary team approach to care may be the best way to hasten weaning, rehabilitation, and recovery of functional independence. Further, protocolization of care when possible helps to streamline the overall process for team members. This team approach should be considered in both the acute and post–acute care settings (Box 19-2).

Physicians should be skilled in ventilator management because even chronic PMV patients may have complicated ventilator issues. Physical, occupational,

BOX 19-2 *Components of Rehabilitative Model of Post-ICU Weaning*

Physician service
- Physician experienced in ventilator care/ weaning
- Hospitalist vs. practitioner model
- Leader of multidisciplinary team that meets weekly
- Assess patient daily
- Order plan of treatment (best practice model, standard order sets)
- Approve, order, and monitor nonphysician-care protocols

Clinical case manager
- Nurse experienced in PMV setting
- Lead multidisciplinary conferences
- Ensure communication between team members and resolve disputes
- Ensure that care plan is carried out
- Ensure policy and procedure uniformity
- Monitor protocol compliance

Nutrition support
- Registered dietitian
- Initial and follow-up evaluation
- Goal setting (e.g., transition from parenteral to enteral nutrition), enteral and oral feeding, optimize energy and protein delivery, tailored to volume sensitivity and organ dysfunction (e.g., congestive heart failure, renal disease, hepatic disease, diabetes mellitus, fluid and electrolyte balance)
- Prompt laboratory testing as appropriate

Bedside nursing
- Registered nurse, licensed practical nurse, assistants with experience with ventilator patients
- Cross-training with respiratory care practitioners (e.g., suctioning techniques, mechanical ventilator awareness)
- Training in patient and family education
- Adherence to policies and procedures
- Meticulous nursing care with focus on protocols involving tracheostomy care, indwelling lines, feeding tubes, and bladder catheters
- Good communication with other team members

Respiratory therapy
- Certified and registered therapists
- Competence in use of all equipment/ procedures (e.g., suctioning, aerosol therapy, invasive and noninvasive mechanical ventilation, airway care)
- Patient assessment: judgment of dyspnea, comfort, anxiety
- Management of weaning per protocol as indicated
- Communication to patient and care team

Pharmacy support
- Registered pharmacists with experience in geriatric dosing
- Review of medication profiles and minimization of overuse
- Focus on minimizing sedatives
- Involvement in patient, family, staff education

Rehabilitation service
- Physical therapist
- Extremity training
- Ambulation, all muscle groups training
- Respiratory muscle training
- Occupational therapist
- Activities of daily living
- Speech therapist
- Swallowing evaluation and therapy
- Early teaching using communication tools

Psychological services
- Professionals (psychologists/psychiatrists)
- Patient and family evaluation
- Anxiety vs. delirium
- Counseling
- Aspects of geriatric and palliative care

Social services
- Experienced social workers with access to pastoral care
- Patient and family education and counseling in hospital
- Problem solving
- Palliative care aspects of treatment
- Discharge planning (include all above disciplines and participate early)
- Liaison with:
  - Durable medical equipment vendors
  - Home health care services (Visiting Nurse Association)
  - Local community hospital
  - Ambulance companies
  - Power company

From MacIntyre NR, Epstein SK, Carson S et al: Management of patients requiring prolonged mechanical ventilation: report of a NAMDRC consensus conference, Chest 128:3937-3954, 2005.

and speech therapy providers are essential in speeding patients' rehabilitation and ability to communicate. Nutritional specialists are needed to address issues of malnutrition after a course of prolonged critical care. A nursing staff that has experience with this population is helpful as well. PMV patients have unique medical and emotional needs and common issues affecting their families. Nurses with a specialized skill set are best able to recognize and address these issues. Respiratory therapists are critical in the supportive care and weaning of these patients. Finally, psychiatrists and psychologists can be important team members since the courses of many PMV patients are complicated by depression, anxiety, and delirium.

PMV patients come from an ICU atmosphere that emphasizes central venous access, placement of bladder catheters, widespread use of broad-spectrum antibiotics, polypharmacy, and frequent use of blood gas and laboratory testing. Removal of patients from the acute ICU environment when they are hemodynamically stable lessens the invasive approach to care and reduces complications. Patients who are free of indwelling vascular and bladder catheters are much less prone to infectious complications. Mobilization of awake patients at the bedside or with ambulation while being bag ventilated is also of likely benefit in improving overall strength and advancing rehabilitation while the weaning process is ongoing.

The high readmission and mortality rates for PMV patients after hospital discharge are concerning. These complex patients obviously warrant careful discharge planning after weaning. Inpatient or outpatient rehabilitation services are often necessary for patients who demonstrate sufficient cognitive abilities. Family education regarding tracheostomy care, O_2 therapy, medications and side effects, expected complications, and available resources should begin well before the anticipated discharge to home. The emotional and financial burden of PMV upon caregivers during hospitalization is high, and physical burdens increase when patients are eventually discharged home. Research is ongoing with regard to **disease management programs** that may help improve outcomes for patients after discharge and decrease caregiver burden.[35,36]

Post–Acute Care Facilities and Respiratory Care Units in PMV Care

Clinicians should be aware that there are many complementary facilities that specialize in PMV care, though they have a geographic concentration in the Northeast and Southeast. LTAC hospitals, some specialized skilled nursing and inpatient rehabilitation facilities, and dedicated ventilator weaning facilities may all be present to assist in the subacute and chronic care of PMV patients. Some acute care hospitals also have dedicated in-house units to offload PMV patients from busy ICUs.

Although there is no clear evidence that care in these facilities improves survival compared with an acute care setting, these institutions appear to reduce the overall costs of patient care. Many post–acute care facilities also have the benefit of multidisciplinary care teams, including respiratory therapy, physical and occupational therapy, speech therapy, and nutritionists with special expertise in PMV patients' unique needs.

It is important to stress that there is no uniform level of care across any type of post–acute care facility. Many judiciously select patients with a high likelihood of weaning success and early discharge because their reimbursement from some providers is driven by length of stay in a way similar to that of acute care hospitals. Others have limited staffing that precludes care provision for patients with more than a moderate amount of medical complexity. It is helpful for clinicians to familiarize themselves with the post–acute care facilities in their area of practice so that they can make referrals that are appropriate for their patients' level of need.

Palliative Care in the PMV Population

Although many persons who survive prolonged mechanical ventilation report good or excellent quality of life in long-term follow-up, the fact remains that most PMV patients will have died within 1 year after initial critical care provision—perhaps after cycling through multiple care facilities. As described in the section on quality of life, PMV patients report a sobering array of symptoms that providers often underappreciate[32] (see Figure 19-4). Effective symptom palliation, therefore, is an essential component in the care of PMV patients. This entails awareness of common symptoms such as thirst, dyspnea, pain, and anxiety. It is a special challenge to provide adequate palliation using sedatives, analgesics, and other pharmacologic interventions without compromising wakefulness, airway clearance, and strength. On the other hand, skillful management of symptoms will facilitate the weaning and rehabilitation process by reducing physiologic stress and improving patient cooperation and motivation. Palliative care interventions should not be reserved only for patients considered to be terminal or unweanable. Active management of symptoms should proceed in parallel with weaning and rehabilitation in a concurrent model of palliative care. Many hospitals now have palliative care specialists, and their expertise should be called upon frequently for the PMV patient.

SUMMARY

Providing care to persons who receive PMV is challenging and expensive. A team approach to the unique medical, emotional, and rehabilitation needs of this population seems to work best. The natural history of recovery from PMV is best measured in months, not weeks. Clinicians who practice in acute care hospitals should investigate post–acute care facilities that can help facilitate the process of care for PMV patients. Patients who do not have access to such facilities will benefit from the multidisciplinary rehabilitation-based care model that characterizes most post–acute care facilities.

KEY POINTS

- PMV is defined by consensus statement as ventilation for at least 21 days (for 6 or more hours a day), with or without tracheostomy.
- Between 5% and 10% of persons admitted to ICUs receive PMV. The incidence of PMV has been increasing as more patients survive the acute phases of multiorgan failure.
- PMV patients are predominantly elderly and have multiple comorbidities. Unresolved multiorgan failure, including ARDS and critical illness polyneuropathy, are common risk factors.
- Prevention of ICU-related complications, such as nosocomial infections, hyperglycemia, and oversedation, can decrease the likelihood of PMV.
- Between 50% and 77% of PMV patients die within 1 year of ICU admission. Survivors have significant functional limitations. Those who are able to respond report satisfactory health-related quality of life.
- Weaning patients from PMV usually entails alternating periods of spontaneous breathing with periods of rest on full ventilator support.
- A multidisciplinary approach to care to optimize nutrition, mobility, symptom control, and emotional support is the standard of care to achieve optimal outcomes.

ASSESSMENT QUESTIONS

1. What is the overall trend in PMV incidence?
2. What are risk factors for long-term mortality from PMV?
3. What clinical factors may predict the need for prolonged ventilation?
4. What process-of-care interventions can help prevent PMV?
5. Does the timing of tracheostomy placement affect survival or weaning success?
6. How do approaches to ventilator weaning of the PMV patient differ from weaning for the typical ventilated patient?
7. What is the role of post–acute care facilities in the care of PMV patients?
8. How do post–acute care facilities that specialize in the management of PMV patients affect long-term outcome?
9. What are common causes of discomfort for the PMV patient?
10. Does palliation of symptoms for PMV patients interfere with weaning?

REFERENCES

1. Esteban A, Anzueto A, Frutos F et al: Characteristics and outcomes in adult patients receiving mechanical ventilation: a 28-day international study, JAMA 287:345-355, 2002.
2. MacIntyre NR, Epstein SK, Carson S et al: Management of patients requiring prolonged mechanical ventilation: report of a NAMDRC consensus conference, Chest 128:3937-3954, 2005.
3. Cox CE, Carson SS, Holmes GM et al: Increase in tracheostomy for prolonged mechanical ventilation in

North Carolina, 1993-2002, Crit Care Med 32:2219-2226, 2004.
4. Seneff MG, Zimmerman JE, Knaus WA et al: Predicting the duration of mechanical ventilation. The importance of disease and patient characteristics, Chest 110:469-479, 1996.
5. Wagner DP: Economics of prolonged mechanical ventilation, Am Rev Respir Dis 140:S14-S18, 1989.
6. Quality of Life After Mechanical Ventilation Among the Aged Investigators: 2-month mortality and functional status of critically ill adult patients receiving prolonged mechanical ventilation, Chest 121:549-558, 2002.
7. Esteban A, Anzueto A, Alia I et al: How is mechanical ventilation employed in the intensive care unit? An international utilization review, Am J Respir Crit Care Med 161:1450-1458, 2000.
8. Carson SS, Bach PB: The epidemiology and costs of chronic critical illness, Crit Care Clin 18:461-476, 2002.
9. Services CfMaM. www.cms.hhs.gov. Accessed August 8, 2005.
10. Behrendt CE: Acute respiratory failure in the United States: incidence and 31-day survival, Chest 118:1100-1105, 2000.
11. Douglas SL, Daly BJ, Gordon N et al: Survival and quality of life: short-term versus long-term ventilator patients, Crit Care Med 30:2655-2662, 2002.
12. Seneff MG, Wagner D, Thompson D et al: The impact of long-term acute-care facilities on the outcome and cost of care for patients undergoing prolonged mechanical ventilation, Crit Care Med 28:342-350, 2000.
13. Gracey DR, Hardy DC, Koenig GE: The chronic ventilator-dependent unit: a lower-cost alternative to intensive care, Mayo Clin Proc 75:445-449, 2000.
14. Fletcher SN, Kennedy DD, Ghosh IR et al: Persistent neuromuscular and neurophysiologic abnormalities in long-term survivors of prolonged critical illness, Crit Care Med 31:1012-1016, 2003.
15. Kollef MH, Ahrens TS, Shannon W: Clinical predictors and outcomes for patients requiring tracheostomy in the intensive care unit, Crit Care Med 27:1714-1720, 1999.
15a. van den Berghe G, Wouters P, Weekers F et al: Intensive insulin therapy in the critically ill patients, N Engl J Med 345(19):1359-1367, 2001.
15b. Hermans G, Wilmer A, Meersseman W et al: Impact of intensive insulin therapy on neuromuscular complications and ventilator dependency in the medical intensive care unit, Am J Respir Crit Care Med 175(5):480-489, 2007.
16. Steinberg KP, Hudson LD, Goodman RB et al: Efficacy and safety of corticosteroids for persistent acute respiratory distress syndrome, N Engl J Med 354:1671-1684, 2006.
17. Kress JP, Pohlman AS, O'Connor MF et al: Daily interruption of sedative infusions in critically ill patients undergoing mechanical ventilation, N Engl J Med 342:1471-1477, 2000.
18. Carson SS, Kress JP, Rodgers JE et al: A randomized trial of intermittent lorazepam versus propofol with daily interruption in mechanically ventilated patients, Crit Care Med 34:1326-1332, 2006.
19. Heffner JE: The role of tracheotomy in weaning, Chest 120:477S-481S, 2001.
20. Plummer AL, Gracey DR: Consensus conference on artificial airways in patients receiving mechanical ventilation, Chest 96:178-180, 1989.
21. Freeman BD, Borecki IB, Coopersmith CM et al: Relationship between tracheostomy timing and duration of mechanical ventilation in critically ill patients, Crit Care Med 33:2513-2520, 2005.
22. Frutos-Vivar F, Esteban A, Apezteguia C et al: Outcome of mechanically ventilated patients who require a tracheostomy, Crit Care Med 33:290-298, 2005.
23. Maziak DE, Meade MO, Todd TR: The timing of tracheotomy: a systematic review, Chest 114:605-609, 1998.
24. Griffiths J, Barber VS, Morgan L et al: Systematic review and meta-analysis of studies of the timing of tracheostomy in adult patients undergoing artificial ventilation, BMJ 330:1243-1246, 2005.
25. Freeman BD, Isabella K, Lin N et al: A meta-analysis of prospective trials comparing percutaneous and surgical tracheostomy in critically ill patients, Chest 118:1412-1418, 2000.
26. Carson SS, Bach PB, Brzozowski L et al: Outcomes after long-term acute care. An analysis of 133 mechanically ventilated patients, Am J Respir Crit Care Med 159:1568-1573, 1999.
27. Pilcher DV, Bailey MJ, Treacher DF et al: Outcomes, cost and long term survival of patients referred to a regional weaning centre, Thorax 60:187-192, 2005.
28. Scheinhorn DJ, Chao DC, Hassenpflug MS et al: Post-ICU weaning from mechanical ventilation: the role of long-term facilities, Chest 120:482S-484S, 2001.
29. Bach PB, Carson SS, Leff A: Outcomes and resource utilization for patients with prolonged critical illness managed by university-based or community-based subspecialists, Am J Respir Crit Care Med 158:1410-1415, 1998.
30. Engoren M, Arslanian-Engoren C, Fenn-Buderer N: Hospital and long-term outcome after tracheostomy for respiratory failure, Chest 125:220-227, 2004.
31. Dewar DM, Kurek CJ, Lambrinos J et al: Patterns in costs and outcomes for patients with prolonged mechanical ventilation undergoing tracheostomy: an analysis of discharges under diagnosis-related group 483 in New York State from 1992 to 1996, Crit Care Med 27:2640-2647, 1999.
32. Nelson JE, Meier DE, Litke A et al: The symptom burden of chronic critical illness, Crit Care Med 32:1527-1534, 2004.
32a. Cox CE, Carson SS, Govert JA et al: Economic evaluation of prolonged mechanical ventilation, Crit Care Med 35:1918-1927, 2007.
33. Scheinhorn DJ, Chao DC, Stearn-Hassenpflug M et al: Outcomes in post-ICU mechanical ventilation: a therapist-implemented weaning protocol, Chest 119:236-242, 2001.

34. Vitacca M, Vianello A, Colombo D et al: Comparison of two methods for weaning patients with chronic obstructive pulmonary disease requiring mechanical ventilation for more than 15 days, Am J Respir Crit Care Med 164:225-230, 2001.
35. Daly BJ, Douglas SL, Kelley CG et al: Trial of a disease management program to reduce hospital readmissions of the chronically critically ill, Chest 128:507-517, 2005.
36. Douglas SL, Daly BJ, Kelley CG et al: Impact of a disease management program upon caregivers of chronically critically ill patients, Chest 128:3925-3936, 2005.

CHAPTER

20 Mechanical Ventilation During Transport and Cardiopulmonary Resuscitation

Richard D. Branson; Jay A. Johannigman

OUTLINE

OBJECTIVES

- List the techniques for providing ventilation during cardiopulmonary resuscitation and compare and contrast the safety and efficacy of each.
- List the standards for ventilation during cardiopulmonary resuscitation (CPR) using both expired air resuscitation and ventilation devices.
- Describe the problem of "death by hyperventilation" and explain techniques to avoid this problem.
- Describe the components of an impedance threshold device and the effects of the device on ventilation and circulation during CPR.
- Describe the process of transporting the mechanically ventilated patient.
- Compare and contrast the use of manual ventilation and a transport ventilator during transport.
- List the risks and benefits of transporting the mechanically ventilated patient.

KEY TERMS

American Heart Association (AHA) device classification system
bag-valve resuscitators
barrier device
cricoid pressure
expired air resuscitation (EAR)
gas consumption
gastric insufflation
impedance threshold device (ITD)
O_2-powered breathing devices (OPDs)
Sellick maneuver

Ventilation in emergency care and transport represents a significant challenge to the health care team. The need for rapidly available, rugged, light-weight ventilation devices is crucial to success in both cases. Training and preparation are also important to ensure appropriate application of devices and retention of skills. In this chapter, ventilatory support during cardiopulmonary resuscitation (CPR) and mechanical ventilation during transport are discussed.

VENTILATION DURING CARDIOPULMONARY RESUSCITATION

Ventilatory support during CPR can be accomplished using an array of methods and devices. These include **expired air resuscitation (EAR),** including mouth-to-mouth (MO-MO) and mouth-to-mask (MO-MA) resuscitation, and the use of mechanical ventilators. Appropriate application of these techniques depends on the clinical situation, rescuer training, and availability of equipment.

Standards for Ventilation and Devices

Several agencies have published recommendations for the use and evaluation of emergency ventilation devices. These include the American Heart Association (AHA), the Emergency Care Research Institute (ECRI), the American Society of Testing and Materials (ASTM), and the International Standards Organization (ISO).[1-9] Of these, the AHA provides standards for the depth and timing of ventilation and device characteristics.[1] The remaining agencies suggest standards for rate and volume but are more focused on the testing of devices.

In 2005, AHA recommendations underwent one of the most comprehensive changes regarding ventilation standards. Perhaps most important is the suggestion that early in spontaneous cardiac arrest, cardiac compressions are more important than ventilation. This means that in the out of hospital setting, it is more important to continue cardiac compression than to worry about timing for ventilation. For adults, ventilation standards include a frequency (f) of 8 to 10 breaths per minute with a tidal volume (V_T) of 0.5 to 0.6 L (6 to 7 ml/kg) and an inspiratory time of 1.0 to 2.0 seconds. This corresponds with an inspiratory flow of 30 to 40 L/min.[1] The use of longer inspiratory times and slower flows is recommended to prevent **gastric insufflation.**[10,11] It is important to note that this slow inspiratory flow is only advantageous in the patient without an instrumented airway. ISO and ASTM standards suggest a V_T of 0.6 L and an f of 12 breaths per minute.

According to AHA guidelines,[1] all devices used for ventilation can be classified according to a scale. The **American Heart Association (AHA) device classification system** follows and is referred to during device descriptions.

Class I—A therapeutic option that is usually indicated, always is acceptable, and is considered useful and effective.

Class II—A therapeutic option that is acceptable, is of uncertain efficacy, and may be controversial.

Class IIa—A therapeutic option for which the weight of evidence is in favor of its usefulness and efficacy.

Class IIb—A therapeutic option that is not well established by evidence but may be helpful and probably is not harmful.

Class III—A therapeutic option that is inappropriate, is without scientific supporting data, and may be harmful.

Lung Compliance After Cardiac Arrest

Changes in compliance and resistance after cardiopulmonary arrest have been attributed to pulmonary aspiration, pulmonary venous congestion, effects of chest compressions, and pulmonary embolism.[12-14] Fillmore and colleagues made comparisons of arterial blood gases (ABGs) to postmortem lung weights and found that the lightest lungs were associated with the best ABGs.[12]

Ornato and associates measured ventilation during CPR and estimated pulmonary compliance during cardiac arrest to be 0.022 L/cm H_2O, or about one quarter of normal lung compliance.[15] Davis and colleagues evaluated lung compliance in the emergency department after cardiac arrest.[16] Twenty-five patients requiring CPR because of cardiac arrest were studied immediately after discontinuation of CPR. A super-syringe technique was used to construct compliance curves. Data from the study are shown in Figure 20-1. The mean compliance was 0.051 L/cm H_2O, a value more than twice that reported by Ornato and associates. These findings have implications for future emergency ventilation research and interpretation of previous studies. The use of longer inspiratory times and slower flows during CPR is, in part, related to the suspected low lung compliance (0.02 L/cm H_2O). Based on findings that lung compliance is twice that previously reported, ventilation strategies might be modified.

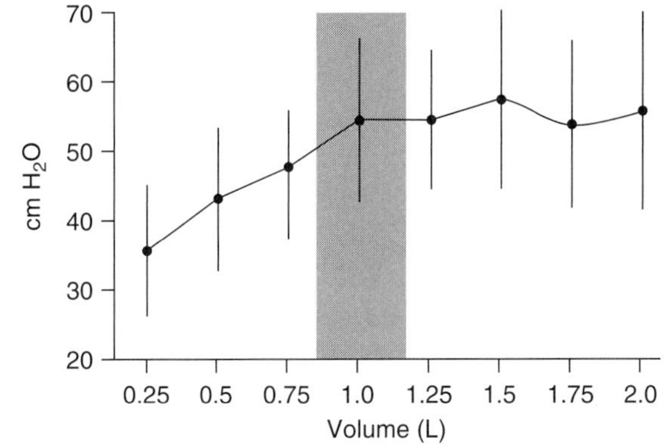

FIGURE 20-1 Mean pulmonary compliance of 25 patients after cardiac arrest.

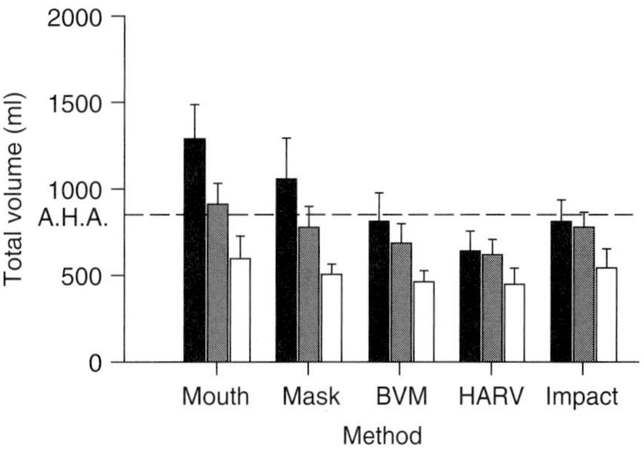

FIGURE 20-2 Delivered V_T of five methods of ventilation. (From Johannigman JA, Branson RD, Davis K et al: Techniques of emergency ventilation: a model to evaluate tidal volume, airway pressure, and gastric insufflation, J Trauma 31:93-98, 1991.)

Another variable affecting delivered V_T is esophageal opening pressure. Because airway pressure is increased to deliver volume in the face of increased pulmonary impedance, gastric insufflation results. Based on work by Ruben and associates, esophageal opening pressure is approximately 20 cm H_2O.[10]

TECHNIQUES OF EMERGENCY VENTILATION

Expired Air Resuscitation

Description

EAR includes MO-MO, MO-MA, and mouth-to-nose ventilation. MO-MO ventilation is the oldest method of EAR, with origins in biblical times.[17] MO-MO ventilation is accomplished by the rescuer placing his or her mouth over the victim's mouth while maintaining an open airway. While observing the victim's chest, the rescuer should watch the chest rise and fall, listen for air escaping during exhalation, and feel the exhaled air flow. During EAR, a V_T of 0.5 to 0.6 L should be delivered over a period of 1.0 second, 8 to 10 times per minute. During EAR it is impractical to measure the V_T delivered. The general guideline is to continue inspiration until there is a visible chest rise. This results in a minute ventilation ($\dot{V}_E$) of 4.0 to 6.0 L/min and an inspiratory : expiratory (I:E) ratio of 1:4 or 1:5. The most recent AHA guidelines suggest that there is no need to synchronize breaths and cardiac compressions.[18]

Assessment

MO-MO ventilation has been recommended for basic life support (BLS) since 1974. The major advantages of MO-MO are availability, ease of use, universal application, large reservoir volume (the delivered volume is limited only by the rescuer's vital capacity, which is 3 to 4 times the necessary V_T), and the fact that no equipment is necessary.

Numerous publications have shown that MO-MO is effective in providing AHA-recommended V_Ts, regardless of lung compliance.[19-24] Johannigman and colleagues[24] found that MO-MO was superior to MO-MA, bag-valve mask (BVM), and ventilator-to-mask ventilation with respect to delivered V_T (Figure 20-2). However, it was also associated with the greatest amount of gastric insufflation.[24] The increase in gastric insufflation is related to the ability of the rescuer to deliver a larger, more forceful volume when pulmonary impedance is increased.

Other data provided by Johannigman and colleagues[24] demonstrate that at normal lung compliance, gastric insufflation during MO-MO ventilation is low (Figure 20-3). This is in agreement with work by Melker and Banner.[25]

Disadvantages of MO-MO ventilation include low delivered O_2 concentration (F_{DO_2}), gastric insufflation, unpleasantness of the task, fear of the possibility of disease transmission, and actual disease transmission.

During EAR, F_{DO_2} is approximately 16% to 18%, allowing for an alveolar O_2 tension of 52 to 76 mm Hg, assuming a barometric pressure of 747 mm Hg and partial arterial pressure of carbon dioxide (Pa_{CO_2}) of 40 mm Hg. This range of arterial O_2 pressure (Pa_{O_2}) is associated with an O_2 saturation of approximately 90. During MO-MO, F_{DO_2} can be increased by increasing inspired O_2 concentration

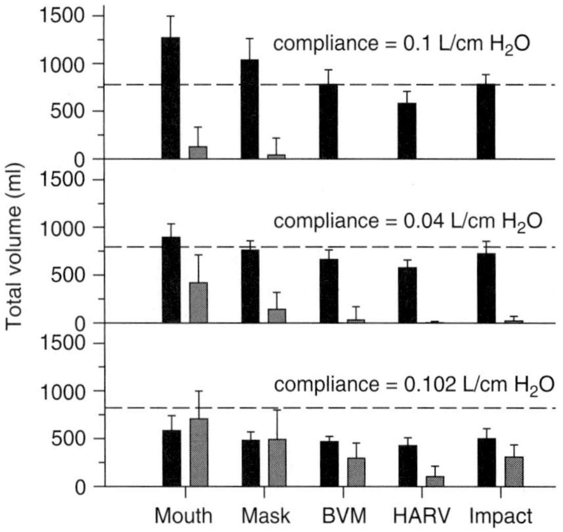

FIGURE 20-3 **Comparison of delivered V_T versus gastric insufflation. Dashed line represents AHA minimum volume of 800 ml.** (From Johannigman JA, Branson RD, Davis K et al: Techniques of emergency ventilation: a model to evaluate tidal volume, airway pressure, and gastric insufflation, J Trauma 31:93-98, 1991.)

(FIO_2) of the rescuer. Hess and colleagues evaluated the change in FDO_2 when the rescuer was wearing a nasal cannula with O_2 flows of 6 L/min and 10 L/min.[26] They found an FDO_2 of 16% during EAR, 27% at an O_2 flow of 6 L/min, and 31% at an O_2 flow of 10 L/min. Hess and colleagues suggested that in the absence of other devices, O_2 breathing by the rescuer is a viable method of delivering adequate V_T and elevated FDO_2.

In a lung model study, Rottenberg and associates found an FDO_2 of 18% during EAR and an FDO_2 of 32% when the rescuer was breathing O_2 via a nasal cannula at 10 L/min.[27] They also evaluated the role of oral inspiration of O_2 via the supply tubing at 15 L/min. With this technique, the rescuer places the connecting tubing between his or her lips and inspires just before ventilating the mannequin. Lastly, rescuers breathed air from a manually triggered demand valve. The demand valve is placed between the rescuer's lips and the manual trigger activated. In this instance, the rescuers were essentially ventilating themselves with 100% O_2 via the demand valve before ventilating the mannequin. Breathing O_2 from the supply tubing allowed an FDO_2 of 37%, and inspiring from the demand valve provided an FDO_2 of 78%. The authors concluded that patients at risk for cardiac arrest could have O_2 "on hand" in the home to allow family members to use supplemental O_2 during resuscitative efforts. They likewise suggested having O_2 available in high-risk areas, such as swimming pools.

Both of these studies make reasonable comments about the potential usefulness of increasing rescuer FIO_2 to increase FDO_2. However, it is more than likely that wherever O_2 is available, other methods of ventilation—for example, MO-MA or BVM—probably will be available. In the study by Rottenberg and associates, it is unclear why, if the rescuer has a demand valve, he or she does not use it to ventilate the patient. These data do prove, however, that FDO_2 can be increased by increasing rescuer FIO_2.

Cricoid Pressure

Gastric insufflation with the potential sequelae of pulmonary aspiration is a problem whenever ventilation via an unprotected airway is attempted. Using less forceful inspirations, longer inspiratory times, and smaller V_Ts are effective strategies in limiting gastric insufflation.[25]

Another technique to prevent gastric insufflation is the use of **cricoid pressure,** often referred to as the **Sellick maneuver.**[28] Sellick described this method in 1961 as a method to prevent regurgitation during induction of anesthesia and endotracheal intubation. By pushing down on the cricoid membrane, the esophagus is collapsed against the cervical vertebrae. In children, cricoid pressure has been shown to prevent gastric insufflation during mask ventilation up to a peak inspiratory pressure of 40 cm H_2O.[29] Vanner and associates found that a cricoid force of 40 newtons increased esophageal opening pressure to a mean of 38 mm Hg in anesthetized adults.[30]

Cricoid pressure is a fairly simple technique, but it is not without complications. If excessive pressure is applied, the trachea can also be collapsed, causing complete airway obstruction. An important clinical point surrounds the release of cricoid pressure. Since the esophagus is collapsed, cricoid pressure can stimulate regurgitation. Once cricoid pressure is begun, it should not be released until intubation of the trachea is accomplished. There are also reports of gastric rupture occurring when the patient regurgitates during application of cricoid pressure.[31,32]

Disease Transmission

Concern about disease transmission has become a major issue regarding MO-MO resuscitation.[33-38] Ornato and colleagues found that 40% of basic cardiac life support (BCLS) instructors, including health care workers, public service workers, and lay persons, would hesitate to perform MO-MO for fear of contracting a disease.[33]

Additional surveys have found that although many BCLS providers say that they would perform MO-MO on a stranger (97%), only half (44%) would do CPR on a patient known to or suspected to have acquired immunodeficiency syndrome (AIDS).[34] Link and associates found that 48% of medical residents employed in New York City hospitals reported a moderate to major concern about contracting AIDS from a patient.[35]

The AHA has addressed the issue of infection risk during CPR.[1,36] When a patient is known to be "high risk," recommendations regarding ventilation techniques include the following:

1. Rescuers who have an infection that may be transmitted by blood or saliva or believe that they have been exposed to such an infection should not perform MO-MO if other methods are available (e.g., MO-MA or BVM).
2. Individuals have a duty to respond to the CPR needs of high-risk patients using MO-MA ventilation of adequate design to BVM device and should be trained in their use.
3. Early intubation should be encouraged when equipment and trained professionals are available.[36]

The effect of these suggestions on bystander CPR has been debated.[37,38] Bystander CPR is primarily performed by family members and public health service personnel.[1] In the latter case, equipment designed to obviate the need for MO-MO contact is available. In the former, the caregiver is knowledgeable of the patient's health history and is quite frequently a relative. The issue then may be more academic than practical.

There remains, however, a reluctance on the part of many people to perform MO-MO resuscitation. Although the risk of infection is small, there are reports of possible cases of infection after CPR. These include infection with *Mycobacterium tuberculosis,*[39] meningococcus,[40] herpes simplex virus,[41-43] shigella,[44] and salmonella.[45]

In essence, health care policy has added to the confusion on this issue. Although the risk of infection is reported to be very low, and the risk of human immunodeficiency virus (HIV) transmission even smaller, recommendations are made that devices to prevent MO-MO contact be available in high-risk areas.[36,46] The city of New York has even made the availability of infection control equipment for CPR in public places mandatory.[47]

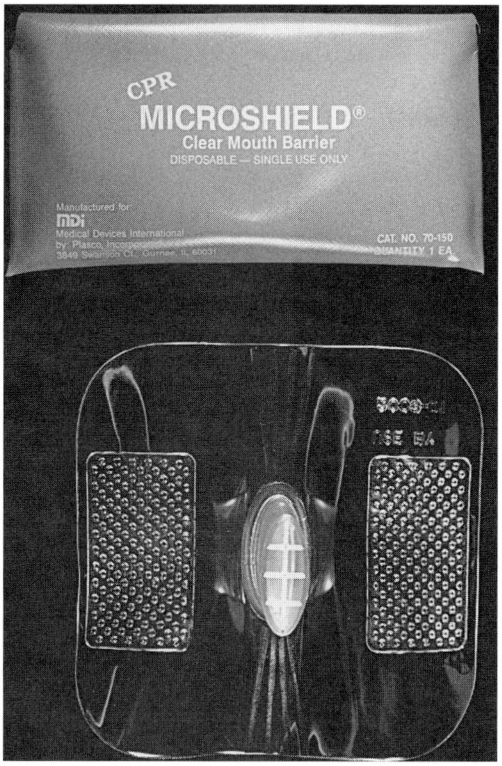

FIGURE 20-4 Barrier device used for CPR.

Debate about the true risk of infection from performing CPR may be futile. The unpleasantness of the task of MO-MO breathing (contact with vomitus, blood, and the like) and even the minute possibility of infection mandate that we develop cost-effective, readily available, safe, and efficacious alternatives to MO-MO breathing.

Barrier Devices

Description

A **barrier device** is a flexible sheet that typically contains a valve or filter that separates the rescuer from the patient (Figure 20-4). Barrier devices are, quite frankly, a disposable version of the "handkerchief" recommended by Waters as a protective device some 50 years ago.[48] Barrier devices are sometimes called face shields, but should not be confused with face masks. An effective barrier device should have the following characteristics:

- Have universal application—conform to the anatomy of patients of all sizes and shapes.
- Be small, lightweight, and easy to carry.
- Have minimal airflow resistance.

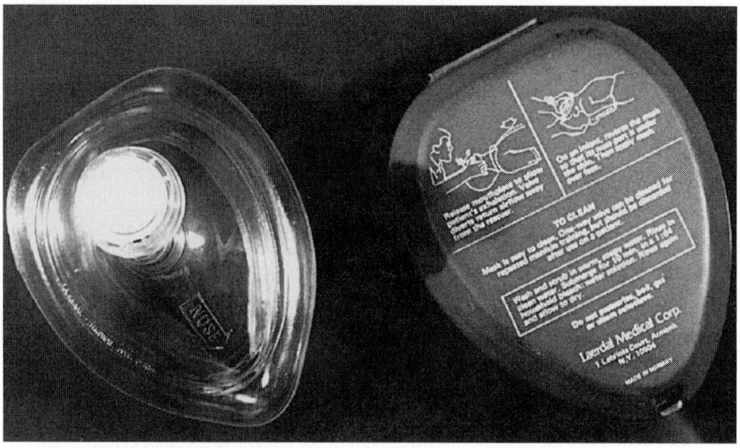

FIGURE 20-5 Mouth-to-Mask (MO-MA) resuscitation device.

- Prevent cross-infection (victim to rescuer and vice versa).
- Resist tearing.

Assessment

Few evaluations have been made on the safety and efficacy of barrier devices. Anecdotal reports of the ability of barrier devices to prevent movement of HIV-infected broth[49,50] have been published. A mannequin study found that use of a barrier device allowed similar ventilation as MO-MO ventilation without a barrier device.[51] In a 1985 health devices report, barrier devices were believed to be inferior to face masks with respect to creating an effective seal on the face.[8] There is also some concern that barrier devices may slip if the patient's face is wet and that during prolonged resuscitation efforts, the plastic sheet may tear away from the central valve.[52,53]

Rossi and colleagues compared MO-MA, mouth-to-tube, and mouth-to-barrier device methods of ventilation in the laboratory.[54] Using a motorized calibration syringe, they delivered a V_T of 1.0 L to a mannequin and test lung. Inspiratory and expiratory pressures and valve leakage were measured. Rossi and colleagues concluded that resistance to airflow was excessive in several of the devices tested. This has been confirmed by Simmons, who found that the MICROSHIELD device created 17 cm H_2O back pressure at a flow of 50 L/min.[55]

Simmons and coworkers also compared volume delivered to a mannequin using MO-MO with three barrier devices.[56] They reported a volume of 1.0 L using MO-MO, 0.25 L using the Kiss of Life, 0.75 L using the MICROSHIELD, and 0.64 L using the Res-Cue Key. The reasons for these disparities are unclear.

If anything can be said definitely about barrier devices, it is that more research is necessary to determine their safety and efficacy. The AHA considers barrier devices as class IIb (acceptable, possibly helpful).

Mouth-to-Mask

Description

MO-MA ventilation devices can be as simple as a face mask or include a face mask, O_2 inlet, nonrebreathing valve (NRV) extension tube, filter, and mouth piece (Figure 20-5). Both devices can be used effectively, but the latter incorporates components that help protect the rescuer and patient from cross-contamination.

Desirable characteristics of an MO-MA device include a clear, soft mask capable of making an effective seal with the patient's face; an O_2 inlet nipple; an NRV that diverts expired flow away from the rescuer; low-flow resistance; no back leak; and a filter with low-flow resistance that is not adversely affected by humidity or vomitus. Dead space should be considered in pediatric applications. In adults, a dead space of less than 200 ml is acceptable.

Assessment

MO-MA ventilation was shown to be an effective method of ventilation as early as 1954 by Elam and colleagues.[57] Safar and McMahon described the first MO-MA device (Laerdal pocket mask) in 1958,[58] and Safar described the role of O_2 supplementation in 1974.[59] The technique of MO-MA ventilation has been recommended for more than a decade by the AHA as the method of choice before endotracheal intubation unless a rescuer with experience with BVM is present. Despite the use of the mask, proximity of the rescuer to the victim continues to be the major deterrent to widespread use of MO-MA ventilation.

MO-MA ventilation has been shown to be superior to BVM ventilation in a number of studies.[18-23,60-63] Hess and Baran found that higher volumes were provided with MO-MA compared with BVM by one rescuer using a mannequin and a test lung.[19] In this study, mean delivered volume with MO-MO was 0.73 L, with MO-MA was 0.6 L, and with BVM was 0.3 L. When two people used the BVM device, one to hold the mask seal and one to squeeze the bag, delivered volumes increased to 0.58 L. Interestingly, the authors found no difference in performance of any of these techniques related to operator experience. This is contrary to the AHA statement concerning the use of BVM if an experienced user is present. Hess and Baran's work suggests that even with experience, BVM by a single rescuer is inadequate.[19] Seidelin and colleagues agreed, recommending that ventilation should be provided by MO-MA until a third rescuer arrives to allow two-person BVM.[22]

Johannigman and colleagues[24] found that MO-MA ventilation consistently provided higher V_Ts than BVM or ventilator-to-mask ventilation. At normal compliance, 0.1 L/cm H_2O, Johannigman and colleagues found that MO-MO, MO-MA, BVM, and ventilator-to-mask techniques provided adequate V_Ts with little to no gastric insufflation (see Figure 20-3). At a compliance of 0.04 L/cm H_2O, which is near the value measured clinically, they found that MO-MO ventilation provided the largest V_Ts but also produced gastric insufflation equivalent to 50% of the V_T. MO-MA ventilation produced similar V_Ts but with approximately half the gastric insufflation of MO-MO. Johannigman and colleagues made a further plea for early use of MO-MA during single-rescuer CPR.[24]

Studies by Sainsbury and associates[19] and Lawrence and Sivaneswaran[21] also have demonstrated the superiority of MO-MA compared with BVM. More recently, Thomas and colleagues evaluated MO-MA ventilation using a mannequin[60] and in anesthetized patients.[61,63] The authors had anesthesia residents provide MO-MA or BVM ventilation, both with an O_2 flow of 15 L/min, to 30 subjects (American Society of Anesthesiologists [ASA] class I or II) requiring general anesthesia. Residents were given "brief tuition" by the investigators and used a Laerdal pocket mask or Laerdal silicone resuscitator for ventilation. During a 4-minute period, airway pressure, CO_2, and O_2 concentrations were measured. The authors found that BVM provided a mean F_{DO_2} of 0.95 and mean delivered carbon dioxide (F_{DCO_2}) of 0.05. MO-MA yielded a mean F_{DO_2} of 0.54 and mean F_{DCO_2} of 0.14. Despite the higher F_{DCO_2}, mean expired CO_2 was equivalent between the groups, suggesting no adverse effect on CO_2 removal. Arterial O_2 saturation as measured by pulse oximetry was also equal between the two ventilation methods.

Thomas and Weber also suggested using MO-MA during two-rescuer CPR but with an alternative strategy.[60] Rather than having one rescuer provide ventilation while the other performs compressions, they suggested that one rescuer hold the mask and provide airway control (head-tilt, chin-lift) while the second rescuer provides both ventilation and compressions. During conventional two-rescuer CPR, V_T was lower and respiratory rate was higher than during modified CPR. Although the compression rate was slowed during modified CPR, the delivered V_T was significantly improved. The authors postulated that reducing the ventilation : compression ratio from 1:5 to 2:15 would increase the number of compressions while maintaining gas exchange by virtue of the larger V_T.

One of the disadvantages related to use of MO-MA is the inability to increase F_{DO_2}. Safar demonstrated an FDO_2 of 0.54 using MO-MA at a V_T of 1.0 L, frequency of 12 beats/min, and O_2 flow of 15 L/min.[59] In an effort to increase F_{DO_2}, Johannigman and Branson[64] recommended placing the O_2 inlet valve of the MO-MA device above the NRV and allowing the rescuer to inspire from the continuous O_2 flow during patient expiration. This so-called "inhalation technique" was compared with conventional MO-MA ventilation in a mannequin and lung model to determine the effect on F_{DO_2}. O_2 flows of 5 L/min, 10 L/min, and 15 L/min were used. Figure 20-6 demonstrates the increase in F_{DO_2} seen with the inhalation technique. Interestingly, at a flow of 15 L/min, mean F_{DO_2} was 0.43, not far from that originally reported by Safar.[59] Using the inhalation technique, F_{DO_2} was increased to a mean of 0.71. Johannigman and Branson also noted that increasing O_2 flow was associated with increased delivered V_T.[64] This is particularly evident at high O_2 flows, in which rescuer expiratory effort is supplemented by the O_2 flow. At an O_2 flow of 15 L/min and inspiratory time of 1.5 seconds, an additional 375 ml of O_2 (250 ml/sec) is added to the rescuer's effort. The authors cited previous work demonstrating the superiority of MO-MA ventilation and suggested

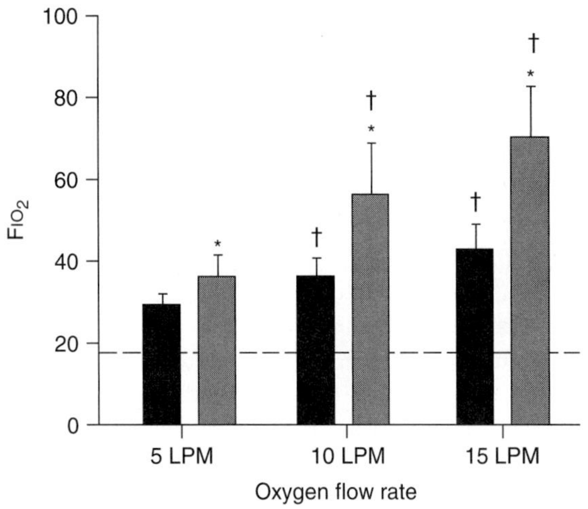

FIGURE 20-6 FDO_2 **at different** O_2 **flows using standard and inhalation technique.** (From Johannigman JA, Branson RD: Oxygen enrichment of expired gas for mouth to mask resuscitation, Respir Care 36:99-103, 1991.)

that O_2 supplementation using the inhalation technique might represent the ventilatory method of choice in early CPR before endotracheal intubation.

Stahl and associates studied five MO-MA devices and evaluated the FDO_2 delivered to a test lung at two combinations of frequency and V_T (500 ml × 20 breaths/min and 90 ml × 12 breaths/min).[65] A ventilator was used to keep rate and volume constant while O_2 flow to the MO-MA device was varied from 2 L/min to 14 L/min in 2-L increments. The devices performed similarly, with the limiting factor being dead-space volume of the mask. As dead-space volume increased, so did FDO_2. The authors recommended that during MO-MA ventilation, (1) high O_2 flows be used (14 L/min) and (2) slow inspirations be used.

Thomas and colleagues studied the effects of increasing O_2 flow to the Laerdal pocket mask.[66] Using a recording mannequin, the authors had 24 volunteers provide MO-MA ventilation for 90 seconds with O_2 flows of 5 L/min, 10 L/min, 15 L/min, and 20 L/min. Similar to previous work, Thomas and colleagues found that as O_2 flow increased, inspired CO_2 decreased and V_T was enhanced. The authors recommended that if MO-MA is used, a flow of 20 L/min is preferable.

Palmisano and colleagues evaluated the effect of supplementary O_2 flow on MO-MA ventilation in a pediatric model.[67] They demonstrated an FDO_2 of 0.50 with an O_2 flow of 5 L/min when V_T was 100 ml and frequency was 20 beats/min. Increasing O_2 flow to 15 L/min served to increase FDO_2 to 0.60, but also increased delivered volume to 221 ml, a 121% increase. The authors also pointed out the adverse effects of the ill-advised attempt of introducing O_2 flow below the nonrebreathing valve. In this case, high flows interfere with function of the NRV.

Hess and colleagues have compared MO-MA devices and found considerable variability in device performance.[68] Hess and colleagues attributed differences in device performance to design characteristics. Specifically, they suggest that differences are the result of:

1. Ability of the mask to fit the face and achieve a seal
2. Resistance to flow through the NRV
3. Size and shape of the mask, which either aids or hinders the rescuer's grip

MO-MA ventilation, when combined with supplemental O_2, is arguably the safest, most effective method of ventilatory support in the unintubated patient when one rescuer is present. Resistance to use of MO-MA devices may be related to rescuer proximity to the patient with the attendant fears of disease transmission and the unpleasantness of the task. MO-MA also may appear unsophisticated when compared with BVM. Another issue may be related to a hindering of communication of the rescuer performing MO-MA ventilation.

BAG-VALVE DEVICES

Description

Bag-valve resuscitators consist of a self-inflating bag, an O_2 reservoir, and an NRV (Figure 20-7). The operator ventilates the patient by squeezing the self-inflating bag, which forces air into the NRV and to the patient. The self-inflating bag typically is made of a resilient material, such as rubber, silicone, or polyvinylchloride. Most self-inflating bags have a volume of approximately 2.0 L for adults. When the operator releases the bag, it returns to its resting inflated position. During re-expansion, the bag fills with room air via a one-way valve on the rear of the bag or with O_2 from an O_2 reservoir. O_2 reservoirs usually are classified as "tube" or "bag" reservoirs based on their construction and appearance. During the exhalation phase, the patient's expired air is directed away from the self-inflating bag to ambient space by the NRV. NRVs have numerous designs, including duck-bill

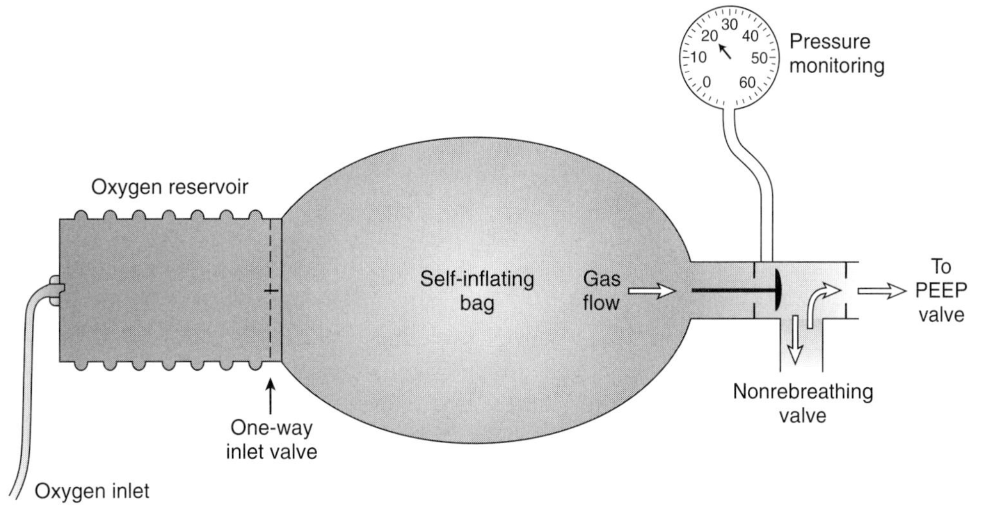

FIGURE 20-7 Schematic of a manual resuscitator.

valves, spring-disk valves, spring-ball valves, diaphragm valves, and leaf valves.

An ideal self-inflating resuscitator would have the following characteristics:[69]

1. Volume delivery—Bag volume should be capable of delivering the desired V_T when squeezed with one hand.
2. F_{DO_2}—An F_{DO_2} of 0.85 to 1.0 should be available for CPR. The reservoir should be lightweight and unobtrusive.
3. Self-inflating bag characteristics—The construction of the bag should allow rapid refill so that faster respiratory rates can be provided as required. The bag should not require gas flow to inflate, and the material used for construction should allow the operator a "feel" for patient impedance characteristics.
4. Nonrebreathing valve—The NRV should prevent any back leak of patient expired gases into the self-inflating bag, have a low resistance to inspiratory and expiratory flow (less than 5 cm H_2O pressure decrease at 50 L/min), and possess a minimum dead space (less than 30 ml for adults). The NRV should be transparent to allow detection of vomitus or other obstructions and perform effectively at high-O_2 flows.
5. Pressure relief valve—Adult resuscitators should not have a pressure relief valve. Pediatric devices should use a 35- to 40-cm H_2O pressure relief valve, which may be overridden if required.
6. Options—For selected situations, the bag-valve device should allow attachment of a spirometer to measure expired volumes, a positive end-expiratory pressure (PEEP) valve, and a tap for monitoring airway pressure with an aneroid manometer.
7. Construction—The resuscitator bag should be lightweight, easily held in one hand, easy to disassemble, easy to clean, and impossible to reassemble improperly. The device should be rugged and able to perform in adverse conditions of temperature.

Bag-Valve Device Performance

The performance of bag-valve devices has been the subject of significant interest.[70] Controversy regarding BVM use is presented below.

Ventilation Efficacy

Numerous studies have evaluated the ability of rescuers to provide ventilation to models using BVM. Uniformly, results have shown that one-rescuer BVM is ineffective.[19,22-25,61,71,72] These reports suggest diminished volume delivery resulting from the inability of a single rescuer to use one hand to hold the mask securely while maintaining airway patency (head-tilt, chin-lift) and squeezing the bag with the other hand. Results from these studies vary widely, with a minimum value reported by Hess and Baran[19] of 300 ml up to 700 ml reported by Seidelin and colleagues.[23] Even with the wide variability in results, it can easily be concluded that BVM by one rescuer is typically ineffective.

Several suggestions have been made to improve ventilation provided by BVM. Cummins and associates and Barnes and Adams have evaluated the face and thigh squeeze, or so-called FATS, technique.[73,74] This method is used in prehospital care to increase delivered volume. The rescuer kneels and places the victim's head between his or her knees. One hand holds the mask and provides the head-tilt/chin-lift by pulling up on the mandible. The remaining hand squeezes the bag against the rescuer's thigh in an attempt to maximize bag deflation.

Increasing volume delivery during BVM also can be accomplished by using two rescuers.[75] Similarly, when two hands are used to squeeze the bag, V_T is enhanced. Hess and Baran[20] found that delivered volume almost doubled when using two-person BVM and two-hand compression of the bag (from 300 to 580 ml). Practically speaking, in the prehospital setting, it is unlikely to have the luxury of two rescuers to perform ventilation.

Other factors affecting BVM performance include mask design,[76] respiratory impedance,[77] hand size,[78,79] and volumetric feedback.[80] In general, a soft, pliable, inflatable sealing mask improves the face-to-mask seal and increases V_T. As pulmonary compliance decreases or resistance increases, delivered volume decreases, and larger hands are associated with larger V_Ts. Volumetric feedback improves volume delivery by allowing the rescuer to get a feel for adequate volume delivery.

Branson and colleagues recorded breath-by-breath volumes during bag-valve-endotracheal tube ventilation during CPR in the emergency department.[81] These results showed mean V_Ts during CPR were 571 ml at a frequency of 24 breaths/min. Mean peak airway pressures were 41 cm H_2O, and the average inspiratory time was 1.1 second. These values are considerably different from AHA guidelines and suggest that some type of volume or frequency monitor might improve the efficiency of bag-valve ventilation.

Most of the work related to BVM has surrounded the issue of V_T delivery. In recent years the performance related to respiratory frequency has received more scrutiny. The work by Branson et al demonstrated a respiratory frequency of 24 breaths per minute while the AHA guideline stipulated 10 to 12 breaths/min.[81] The current AHA standard of 8 to 10 breaths would mean that this finding represents a threefold increase in observed versus desired breaths. Aufderheide et al have shown that at these respiratory frequencies there is an increase in intrathoracic pressure, a decrease in coronary perfusion pressure, and reduced survival from cardiac arrest. Increased ventilation rates and increased ventilation duration impede venous blood return to the heart, decreasing hemodynamics and coronary perfusion pressure during cardiopulmonary resuscitation. It has also been shown that there is a direct and immediate transfer of the increase in intrathoracic pressure to the cranial cavity with each positive pressure ventilation, also reducing cerebral perfusion pressure. The reduced amount of blood flowing through the pulmonary bed during cardiopulmonary resuscitation tends to be overventilated, compromising hemodynamics to both the heart and brain and resulting in ventilation-perfusion mismatch.[82-86]

This problem has been termed "death by hyperventilation" and suggests that both education of caregivers and tools to monitor appropriate ventilation are necessary to achieve appropriate ventilation.

Delivered Oxygen Concentration

Numerous reports have evaluated the ability of resuscitators to deliver a desired F_{DO_2}.[87-96] According to the ASTM[8] and ISO,[9] F_{DO_2} should be 0.85, with an O_2 reservoir in use and an O_2 flow of 15 L/min. The AHA recommends an F_{DO_2} of 1.0 or "the highest possible O_2 concentration should be administered as soon as possible to all patients with cardiac or respiratory arrest."[1] This recommendation seems to be prudent, but no studies have proved that an F_{DO_2} of 1.0 is superior to an F_{DO_2} of 0.5. In fact, it could be speculated that an F_{DO_2} of 1.0 might accentuate reperfusion injury. The required, safe F_{IO_2} during CPR is a matter of some controversy and requires some sound scientific investigation for clarification.

Cases with an F_{DO_2} of less than 0.85 have been reported with bag-valve devices and are related to high minute ventilation, insufficient reservoir volume, and ambient temperatures less than 0° C.[87-96] Most current resuscitator designs are capable of delivering a minimum F_{DO_2} of 0.85 during CPR.

Nonrebreathing Valve Performance

The NRV is the heart of the resuscitation bag. According to the ASTM, the NRV should resist breakage, function in the presence of vomitus, allow flows of up to 30 L/min without sticking, and continue to function at extremes of temperature (−18° C to +50° C).[8]

Studies of NRV competence in the presence of vomitus have shown adequate performance in most cases.[87-96] Several devices have failed at low temperatures when condensation freezes the valve's components.[96] Reports have also shown that many devices fail the "drop test" of falling 1 m to a concrete floor.[93-96]

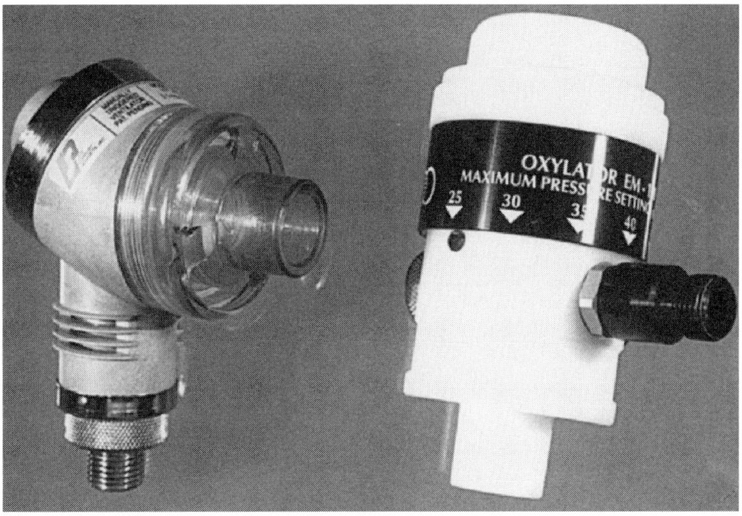

FIGURE 20-8 Two manually triggered O_2-powered breathing devices.

Back leak through an NRV should be minimal to prevent rebreathing, and most devices produce few problems with valve incompetence. Several cases of NRV failure caused by misassembly have been reported, which underscores the need for operator vigilance.[96]

Hess and Simmons found that resistance to flow of NRV in adult resuscitators was variable.[97] They found three devices that exceeded the 5-cm H_2O back pressure standard at a flow of 50 L/min specified by the ASTM.[8] Hess and Simmons suggested that the increased flow resistance of some NRVs could prolong expiration and cause air-trapping, which might lead to barotrauma or further impediment to ventilation. They also suggested that NRVs with high flow resistance might contribute to fatigue of the rescuer squeezing the bag.

Spontaneous breathing through the NRV of resuscitators has been an area of some controversy.[98,99] Hess and colleagues evaluated the imposed work of breathing created during simulated spontaneous breathing via the NRV of 11 disposable resuscitators.[95] They found that both inspiratory and expiratory work of breathing was elevated. Imposed work of breathing increased with the application of PEEP and with increased patient flow demand. Measurements of work in this study were quite high (up to 2.0 J/L) and represent a 10- to 100-fold increase compared with the imposed work of common intensive care ventilators.[100] Hess et al recommended that the practice of allowing spontaneous breathing via disposable resuscitator bags be abandoned.

Bag-valve mask ventilation remains the most popular method of ventilatory support by BLS providers in the field.[101] One way to limit V_T and prevent gastric distention in adults is to use a bag designed for pediatric use. This limits the maximum V_T that can be delivered. Many factors previously discussed allow BVM to be used extensively despite the plethora of evidence suggesting its inefficiency. Effort in the area of provider education may be the answer to problems with BVM, rather than introduction of new ventilatory techniques.

OXYGEN-POWERED BREATHING DEVICES

Description

O_2-powered breathing devices (OPDs) are frequently called demand valves. Both the ASTM and the ISO have created standards for OPDs.[8,9] A typical OPD consists of a demand valve that can be manually triggered or patient triggered (Figure 20-8). The OPD is connected to a 50-psig source of gas and connects to the patient via a standard 15/22-mm connector. During manual activation of the demand valve, the operator depresses the actuator, allowing flow to travel to the patient. According to the ASTM standard, this flow should be restricted to 40 L/min to prevent excessive ventilation and gastric distention. Modern OPDs also limit the available airway pressure via a pressure-limiting valve and limit the length of inspiratory time. In the latter case, inspiration is terminated after 3 seconds, even if the operator continues to depress the actuator. During spontaneous breathing, the demand valve is pressure-triggered and allows a flow of up to 100 L/min for patient demand.

Assessment

The history of OPDs indicates problems with the devices. A number of studies have shown failure of the pressure-limiting devices within the OPD and subsequent high airway pressure (greater than 100 cm H_2O).[102-105] Pradis and Caldwell have reported a case of pneumocephalus resulting from OPD-to-mask ventilation caused by excessive airway pressures.[104] Much of this work was done before limiting flow during manual ventilation to 40 L/min.

More recently, Menegazzi and colleagues evaluated the use of the OPD in a model, providing ventilation via OPD to mask and OPD to endotracheal tube.[106] Using a mannequin system similar to that developed by Johannigman and colleagues,[24] Menegazzi and colleagues found no difference in delivered V_Ts between BVM and OPD-to-mask. They did, however, report significantly increased gastric insufflation with BVM. This difference was attributed to the high inflation pressures and flows that can be developed during BVM compared with the fixed steady flow of 40 L/min provided by the OPD. Menegazzi and Winslow[106] suggested that OPD-to-mask ventilation was superior to BVM in preventing gastric insufflation in this model. They did, however, suggest that clinical studies be performed before widespread use of the OPD.

Mesezzo and associates compared the OPD with a bag-valve device for ventilation of a model via an endotracheal tube. They found similar delivered V_Ts at all levels of compliance tested. Additionally, they reported a higher airway pressure with the bag-valve device compared with the OPD (31 cm H_2O versus 13 cm H_2O at normal lung compliance). These authors suggested that the lower airway pressures were caused by the fixed 40-L/min inspiratory flow and that demand valve ventilation through an endotracheal tube may be preferable.[107] One limitation of the OPD is the inability of the rescuer to detect patient compliance.

The history of the OPD is a major limitation to its adoption. However, devices that meet the ASTM standard can probably be used safely and effectively. Clinical studies of the OPD in the field are necessary before widespread use can be recommended. The AHA rates the OPD as class II.

Ventilator-to-Mask Ventilation

Description

Transport ventilators for prehospital care and CPR are typically machine-triggered, volume-limited, time-cycled devices.[107-110] They are typically simple, having one or two controls, providing only one mode, no PEEP, and strictly a 1.0 F_{IO_2}. The AHA has suggested that automatic transport ventilators meeting the following criteria are class I devices:

- Have a lightweight connector with a standard 15/22-mm connector
- Have a lightweight (2-5 kg), compact, rugged design
- Operate in all environmental conditions and extremes of temperature
- Have a peak pressure limit of 60 cm H_2O with an option of 80 cm H_2O
- Have an audible alarm when the peak pressure limit is exceeded
- Have minimal **gas consumption**
- Have minimum gas compression volume in the circuit
- Deliver an F_{IO_2} of 1.0
- Have an inspiratory time of 2.0 seconds for adults and 1.0 second for children with corresponding peak inspiratory flow rates of 30 L/min and 15 L/min, respectively
- Have at least two respiratory frequency settings[1]

Additionally, the AHA lists desirable features, which include a pressure manometer, separate rate and volume controls, and a low-pressure alarm.

Descriptions of prehospital ventilators and desirable characteristics have been published.[108,110] These are similar to those listed by the AHA, and descriptions follow.

Operational Characteristics

All ventilators used in prehospital care should be time or volume cycled. Modified pressure-cycled devices have been used by skilled clinicians, although their general use is discouraged. Constant flow rate ventilators are preferred, but nonconstant flow ventilators can be used successfully. Inspiratory flow rate and V_T should be affected minimally by changes in airway resistance and lung-thorax compliance (less than 10% change). Ideally, gas consumption to power the ventilator's system components should be zero. Low-level gas consumption (less than 5 L/min) is acceptable but decreases the ventilator's operating time.

Portability

Size and weight are the chief concerns. Orientation of controls and handles for carrying the device are also important. Generally, a weight less than 4 kg is considered desirable.

Power Source

Ventilators that require pneumatic and electronic power sources require compressed O_2 and a direct current power source (battery); thus *two* perishable power sources are necessary. There are tradeoffs, however, with these two types of ventilators. Electronically powered ventilators provide more precise control of variables and do not consume gas during operation. Either type of ventilator is thus adequate.

Ease of Operation

Operation of the ventilator should be as simple as possible with the minimum number of controls. Each control should be labeled as to function, effects, and possible hazards. When possible, a diagram of the circuit and its proper connection to the patient should be printed on the side or back panel of the ventilator. Ventilators used in prehospital care *do not* need a variable F_{IO_2}, continuous positive airway pressure (CPAP), or a variety of ventilatory modes. In our study of prehospital ventilatory support, 95% of patients remained apneic during transport. Addition of a demand-flow valve adds size and weight to the ventilator and can also increase gas consumption. Some transport ventilators position the demand-flow valve on the endotracheal tube. This can result in inadvertent extubation or kinking of the tube because of the weight of the demand-flow valve. As stated previously, independent control knobs for V_T and ventilator rate should be available. An important, and often overlooked, feature is the "manual inhalation" control push button. This allows the operator to control ventilator rate and V_T manually, independent of the ventilator's settings, in special situations. This control is also helpful during auscultation of breath sounds to confirm proper endotracheal tube placement.

Assembly and Disassembly

The ventilator breathing circuit and exhalation valve should be simple, and incorrect assembly should be impossible. Likewise, high-pressure hoses from the gas source to the ventilator and from ventilator to patient should not be interchangeable such that misassembly can occur. If a valve is used to control the flow of inspiratory and expiratory gases (such as an NRV), it should be easily cleaned of vomitus, blood, and secretions.

Safety

The number of safety devices is limited by the small size of transport ventilators. A high-pressure relief valve, which vents gas to the atmosphere at a preselected peak inflation pressure (PIP) (typically 60 to 80 cm H_2O for adults and 30 to 40 cm H_2O for children), should be required on transport ventilators. Activation of the high-pressure limit should be signaled by a visual or audible alarm to alert the operator. The ventilator also should have an antiasphyxia valve. If gas or electric power supplies are exhausted, the patient should be able to breathe ambient air without excessive resistance. Battery-powered ventilators should be equipped with a "low battery" signal that indicates when 1 hour of power remains. Loss of O_2 power supply to a transport ventilator should activate audible or visual alarms, or both.

Durability

Extremes of temperature and humidity should not adversely affect the operation of transport ventilators. These ventilators should be capable of operating at a moment's notice, even after prolonged periods of storage, and should be able to withstand rough treatment and still operate properly. Occasionally, transport ventilators are used in hazardous environments and should, therefore, have protective cases that can withstand erosion by chemicals or other foreign substances.

Maintenance

Preventive maintenance should be performed periodically by the manufacturer or a trained technician. Routine maintenance should be minimal.

Breathing Valve

One distinct feature incorporated in ventilators used in prehospital care is a breathing or inhalation/exhalation valve mechanism. This valve is connected to the ventilator by corrugated or high-pressure tubing and directs inspiratory and expiratory gases to and from the patient. The valve may be simple, such as an NRV, or it can be complicated. Some of these valves may house an NRV, a pressure-limiting valve, a demand-flow valve, and an antiasphyxia valve. As a result, several connecting ports on these breathing valves are required to accommodate additional valves. The connecting ports should have different inside and outside diameters such that improper connection cannot occur. Resistance to inhalation and exhalation should be low (less than 3 cm H_2O/L/sec). The weight of the breathing valve should be minimal (less than 0.3 kg) because heavy or awkward valves can cause kinking of the endotracheal tube or accidental extubation. Also, this valve should be easy to clean.

Assessment

Evaluations of the ability of transport ventilators to deliver adequate V_Ts have been published.[110-115] These studies, however, typically deal with a model of an intubated patient. We have presented data regarding use of transport ventilators in the prehospital environment, but also only in intubated patients.[101]

Johannigman and colleagues[24] found that a transport ventilator with an adjustable flow control delivered more consistent V_Ts than BVM. The ventilator provided smaller V_Ts than MO-MO or MO-MA ventilation but had significantly less gastric insufflation than either of those techniques.[20] A ventilator with a fixed flow provided smaller V_Ts.

Greenslade compared volumes delivered to a mannequin with MO-MO, MO-MA, BVM, and ventilator-to-mask ventilation during one-rescuer CPR.[113] This fascinating study had rescuers perform CPR in the back of a moving ambulance with each ventilation technique. Greenslade found that MO-MO allowed the largest $\dot{V}_E$ and most successful number of compressions per minute. Use of the ventilator and manual resuscitator resulted in the smallest $\dot{V}_E$ and lowest number of compressions. He recommended that MO-MA be used in unintubated patients and that ventilators be reserved for intubated patients. Greenslade further suggested that "keeping ambulance speed below 30 mph and using O_2 supplemented mouth to mask ventilation . . . appear to offer the best chance of success in unintubated patients receiving one-operator CPR."[113]

Greenslade would recommend that BLS squads perform O_2-supplemented MO-MA until endotracheal intubation is performed, after which time the bag-valve, OPD, or ventilator works effectively. One advantage of the ventilator is that it frees up a rescuer to perform other tasks. A disadvantage is the loss of "feel" for pulmonary compliance.

AHA recommendation for a ventilator with a fixed flow of 30 L/min may be confusing. Because the ventilator most often is used in intubated patients, there is no advantage to a slow inspiratory flow. In fact, the slow inspiratory flow creates two distinct disadvantages:

1. It makes it impossible to make up for leaks around a mask if used in an unintubated patient.
2. If a higher frequency is desired (e.g., for head injury), air-trapping may result because of insufficient expiratory time.

Although a fixed flow setting may be useful, the ventilator should have a provision for increasing flow.

IMPEDENCE THRESHOLD DEVICE

The **impedance threshold device (ITD)** is a spring-loaded valve that limits air entry into the lungs during recoil of the chest wall following cardiac compressions. The effect it has is that, on the downstroke of the compression, air is forced out of the lung. When the chest is released, air normally returns to the lungs as a consequence of the negative pressure. The ITD prevents this return of gas into the lungs and results in a negative intrathoracic pressure. The negative intrathoracic pressure enhances venous return and improves cardiac output.

Early reports of the ITD demonstrate improved hemodynamic performance, but outcome studies have shown mixed results. Because the ITD improves hemodynamic performance, AHA rates it a class IIa device.[116-121]

TRANSPORT OF THE MECHANICALLY VENTILATED PATIENT

Rationale for Transport

Critically ill patients in the intensive care unit (ICU) frequently require diagnostic testing or therapeutic procedures that cannot be performed at bedside. These include computed tomography (CT) scans, angiography, and magnetic resonance (MR) imaging. When transportation is deemed necessary, every effort should be made to "take the ICU with the patient." This includes taking the appropriate personnel and providing for ventilation, care, and monitoring similar to those provided in the ICU.

Preparation

Ensuring a safe and uneventful transport begins long before any movement actually occurs. In elective situations, patience is the operative word. Time taken before transport to stabilize hemodynamics, oxygenation, and ventilation is well spent. Electrolyte abnormalities should be corrected and the necessary invasive monitoring devices (arterial line, pulmonary artery catheter, intracranial pressure monitor) placed and secured.

Although a special transport team is deemed necessary for interhospital transport, intrahospital transport can best be accomplished by personnel familiar

TABLE 20-1 *Staff Who Must Accompany and Remain With Patients Who Must Leave the ICU**

Purpose: In recognizing the need to observe closely ICU patients during periods of time when the patient must be outside the ICU for studies or procedures, the following guidelines are established.

TYPE OF PATIENT	ACCOMPANYING STAFF
Stable patient with only an IV line	Staff to be determined by head nurse and ICU director
Stable patient with arterial line only	RN
Patient on ventilator	RN and RT
Patient with pulmonary artery catheter or any vasoactive drips	RN and resident†
Patient with arterial line, ventilator, and pulmonary artery catheter	RN, resident,† and RT
Any unstable patient	RN, resident,† and RT

From Smith J, Flemming S, Cernaianu A: Mishaps during transport from the intensive care unit, Crit Care Med 18:278-281, 1990.

ICU, Intensive care unit; *IV*, intravenous; *RN*, registered nurse; *RT*, respiratory therapist.

*If appropriate staff cannot be assembled to accompany the patient, the patient's attending physician should be contacted. The attending physician will decide whether the patient can be transported safely without the specified staff or whether the study should be cancelled. The attending physician will indicate his or her decision in the form of an order.

†For patients managed by the medical residents, one of the unit residents must accompany the patient. For patients managed by the surgical resident, a resident from the primary surgical service must accompany the patient. A medical student may not substitute for the RN or a resident.

with the patient. The type and number of personnel should be commensurate with the degree of support required and the severity of patient illness.[122] Our ICU guidelines require that a respiratory therapist (RT) and a nurse attend the transport of any mechanically ventilated patient. We also find it useful in many cases to enlist orientees and students to assist in physically moving the patient and equipment to and from the destination. Smith and colleagues[123] have published guidelines (Table 20-1) for accompanying staff based loosely on the therapeutic intervention scoring system (TISS).[124] This system allows for as few as two attendants (one nurse and one transporter) for transporting stable patients, and up to three attendants (one physician, one RT, and one nurse) for critically ill patients. These guidelines were developed at a teaching hospital and therefore may not apply to community hospitals, where physicians are not as readily available.

Once personnel are assembled, delineation of roles and responsibilities should be established. The nurse or physician should be in a position to observe the electrocardiographic (ECG) monitor and reach intravenous (IV) pumps to manipulate pharmacologic agents. The RT should be positioned at the head of the bed to ensure adequate control of the airway and provide ventilatory support. As always, the "team approach" is essential for a safe, successful transport.

Equipment

Equipment for transport must be similar to that used in the ICU in terms of performance, yet be portable, small, lightweight, and rugged. Of course compromises must be made, and complexity often gives way to simplicity for the sake of size and reliability. The following items are essential for in-hospital transport of the mechanically ventilated patient (Table 20-2).

Portable Monitor

A portable ECG monitor capable of monitoring two pressure channels should accompany all patients. This allows continuous monitoring of heart rate, rhythm, and arterial blood pressure. The second pressure channel may be used for patients with a pulmonary artery catheter or those who need intracranial pressure monitoring. The monitor should be small and lightweight, but provide a display large enough and bright enough to be seen from 8 to 10 feet away. This is particularly important when the patient is isolated from the caregivers, as occurs during a CT scan. The monitor should have its own rechargeable power supply that continuously charges while connected to AC power. A typical transport takes approximately 80 minutes,[122-124] 10 to 20 minutes of which are spent in transit to the respective destinations. Based on these figures, a portable monitor

TABLE 20-2 *Essential Equipment for Transport of the Mechanically Ventilated Patient*

EQUIPMENT	CAPABILITY
Portable monitor	ECG; two pressure channels for monitoring arterial blood pressure and pulmonary artery pressures or intracranial pressure
Portable ventilator or self-inflating bag	IMV and/or AMV; PEEP; PEEP compensation of the demand valve; disconnect alarm; manual breath control; separate frequency and V_T controls; low gas consumption
Airway maintenance	Laryngoscope; endotracheal tubes 6-9 mm; ID curved and straight laryngoscope blades; oral and nasal airways; stylet; Magill forceps; batteries; tape
Drug box	Epinephrine; sodium bicarbonate; atropine; calcium chloride; IV fluids—D_5W and lactated Ringer's solution; IV tubing; other drugs currently being delivered in the ICU—sedatives, paralytic agents, vasoactive agents, and antiarrhythmics
Infusion pumps	Must operate reliably from an internal battery
Stethoscope	Auscultation of breath and heart sounds; measurement of blood pressure

AMV, Assisted mechanical ventilation; *D_5W*, 5% dextrose (in water); *ECG*, electrocardiogram; *ICU*, intensive care unit; *ID*, internal diameter; *IMV*, intermittent mechanical ventilation; *IV*, intravenous; *PEEP*, positive end-expiratory pressure; *V_T*, tidal volume.

should be capable of operating at least 2 hours without recharging. When possible, the monitor should be powered by a permanent AC power supply while the patient is stationary.

Monitoring blood pressure noninvasively during transport is essential when the patient lacks arterial access. However, recent work by Runcie and associates demonstrates that noninvasive blood pressure (NIBP) underestimates systolic blood pressure by 13% to 21% and overestimates diastolic pressure by 5% to 27% during transport when compared with direct measurement.[125,126] These inaccuracies have been ascribed to movement of the patient or simply the difference between the two techniques in a heterogeneous group of critically ill patients.[126,127] In any event, trends are to be followed. Whenever direct measurement of arterial blood pressure is precluded, intermittent manual oscillometric values should be ascertained.[128,129]

Ventilator

Ventilatory support during transport has been the subject of several investigations.[130-137] Hurst and associates,[130] Gervais and colleagues,[131] and Braman and co-workers[132] all have demonstrated that manual ventilation with a self-inflating bag during transport can lead to unintentional respiratory alkalosis. In each of these studies, episodic hypotension and cardiac dysrhythmias were associated with this rapid change in acid-base status. Gervais and colleagues demonstrated that hyperventilation could be avoided if V_T and $\dot{V}_E$ were monitored with a portable spirometer.[131] All three studies suggest that use of a transport ventilator avoids unintentional hyperventilation and is superior to manual ventilation during transport.

Weg and Haas recently reported that manual ventilation of critically ill patients during transport can be accomplished without detriment.[133] They compared blood gases and pH values obtained while patients were being manually ventilated to values obtained while patients were mechanically ventilated in the ICU. In their group of 20 patients, only one was found to have acute respiratory alkalosis (pH increased 0.13 unit and $Pa{CO_2}$ decreased 9 mm Hg). However, in their report, there was a tendency for pH to increase and $Pa{CO_2}$ to decrease during periods of manual ventilation. They also had one patient who had an increase in $Pa{CO_2}$ of 13 mm Hg. Weg and Haas concluded that use of a transport ventilator is unnecessary and expensive. However, the reality of transport cannot guarantee this, and interoperator variability is inevitable.[134] Therefore, we consider that use of a transport ventilator or a system allowing delivered V_T to be measured is the preferred method of ventilatory support during transport. A typical transport ventilator is shown in Figure 20-9.

Characteristics of a Ventilator for Intrahospital Transport

Operational Characteristics

Ideally, the transport ventilator should be capable of operating in both the intermittent mandatory

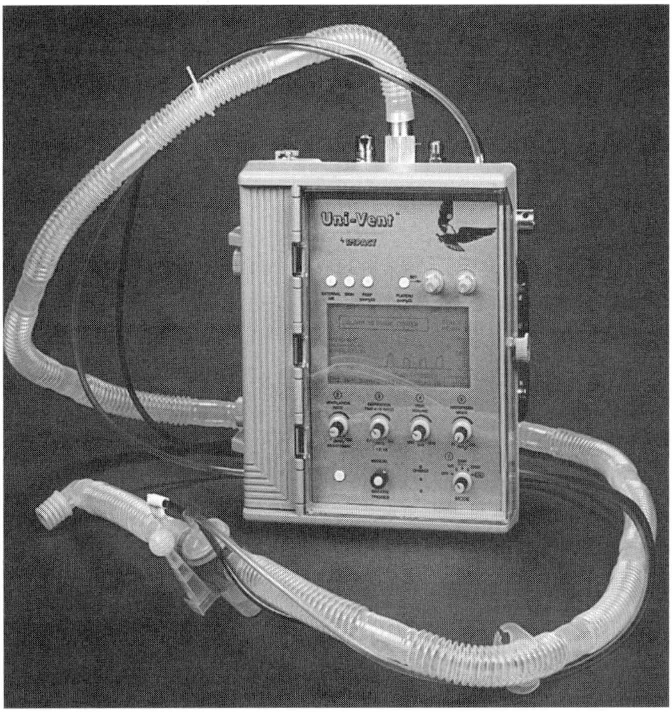

FIGURE 20-9 A typical transport ventilator (Impact 754, Impact Medical, West Caldwell, N.J.).

ventilation (IMV) and assisted mechanical ventilation (AMV) modes. However, a single mode may be acceptable if most patients are managed in the ICU with that technique. There should be separate controls for respiratory frequency (*f*) and V_T, and the delivered V_T should be within 10% of set V_T regardless of PIP. A continuously adjustable F_{IO_2} is generally unnecessary in adults in whom 100% O_2 is acceptable. Infants at risk for developing retrolental fibroplasia (RLF) should be ventilated with the appropriate F_{IO_2}. It should be remembered that delivery of a precise F_{IO_2} requires an air tank and air-O_2 blender, thus increasing the cost, complexity, weight, and size of the transport system. Alternatively, some transport ventilators use Venturi systems that entrain room air to decrease F_{IO_2} and increase O_2 source life.[122,123] The application of PEEP/CPAP should be possible, and a demand valve, able to compensate for elevated baseline pressures, should be available if IMV is used. A basic alarm system, consisting of a low-pressure/disconnect and high-pressure alarm, also must be included.

Portability

Size and weight are chief concerns for transport ventilators. A weight less than 5 kg is desirable, and the ventilator's dimensions should make it easy to mount it or lay it on the bed. Orientation of controls should be in a single plane and inadvertent movement of dials difficult.

Power Source

Pneumatically powered and operated ventilators have been considered preferable to those requiring electronic control.[109] The reasoning has suggested that if two power sources are required, the likelihood of failure is doubled with a device requiring both gas and electric (battery) supplies. As usual, there are tradeoffs with each type of ventilator. Although pneumatic ventilators require only one power source, they often consume gas for operation, depleting the gas source more quickly. Conversely, although an electronically controlled device has the possibility of battery failure, these ventilators generally provide more precise control of settings, are less likely to be affected by fluctuations in source gas pressure, and do not consume as much gas during operation. Both types have been used successfully.[130-138]

Gas Consumption

Under ideal circumstances, all gas leaving the O_2 cylinder is delivered to the patient. However, pneumatic and fluidic logic circuits often consume gas to control inspiration and expiration. In some cases, gas is also consumed by pneumatic components of electronically controlled ventilators.[136] Gas consumption is defined as gas used by the ventilator for operating circuits or valves, which is exhausted into the atmosphere and not delivered to the patient. Campbell et al have shown that gas consumption can be affected by the set $\dot{V}_E$, lung compliance, PEEP, and F_{IO_2}. These factors affect ventilators differently based on the principle of operation.[137] Acceptable levels of gas consumption are less than 5 L/min.

Safety

The number and complexity of safety devices are limited by the small size of transport ventilators. A high-pressure relief valve that vents gas into the atmosphere at a preselected PIP is essential. Activation of the high-pressure limit should be signaled by a visual or audible alarm to alert the operator. An antiasphyxia valve that allows the patient to breathe from ambient air in the event of gas source failure is also desirable. Battery-powered ventilators should be equipped with a "low-battery" signal that indicates when 1 hour of power remains. Loss of O_2 power to the ventilator also should result in an audible or visual alarm.

Durability

Transport ventilators should be built to withstand the harsh treatment given them during movement. Control knobs should be protected to keep them from being broken off or cracked. If the ventilator is accidentally dropped from the bed, it should withstand the shock and continue operating. If it fails after impact, it should fail closed (no gas delivery) or open to ambient air (no pressure rise).

Ease of Operation

A delicate balance between operational flexibility and simplicity must be maintained. Most transport ventilators have controls for V_T and *f*. Additional controls should include mode selection, inspiratory time or I:E, alarm settings, PEEP (if applicable), and a manual breath control. Sensitivity should be preset at a minimum level or should be adjustable by the clinician.

Ancillary Equipment for Ventilators

All ventilators require a self-contained O_2 supply source. Both compressed gas cylinders and liquid systems can fulfill this need. Intrahospital transport usually is accomplished with an E cylinder or two E cylinders yoked together. This provides 630 L and 1260 L of gas, respectively. We routinely use two E cylinders and whenever possible operate the ventilator from stationary sources at the destination. For longer transports, an H cylinder containing 6900 L may be required. Although the H cylinder provides a substantially larger supply of gas, it is 152 cm in height and weighs 68 kg, and an additional member of the transport team is required just to move it. Movement of a cylinder of this size must be accomplished carefully because of potential dangers should it fall from an upright position.

Liquid O_2 systems can provide 860 cubic feet of gaseous O_2 for every cubic foot in the liquid stage. However, most liquid systems cannot operate at 50 psig, which is necessary for proper ventilator operation. Additionally, should liquid O_2 be spilled, its extremely low temperature may result in thermal injury.

Humidification is frequently overlooked during transport of ventilated patients.[139] This is in part the result of the impracticality of transporting the patient with the humidifier used in the ICU. The logistics and dangers of transporting an electrically powered, position-dependent, water-filled device are exasperating. However, some humidification should be used because delivery of anhydrous medical gases to the tracheobronchial tree can cause tissue damage in less than 30 minutes.[140] A passive humidification device, or "artificial nose," may be used. These devices collect the patient's own respired heat and moisture and return them during the following inspiration. Artificial noses are not as efficient as heated humidifiers but are particularly suited for use during transport.[141] Use of an artificial nose may result in a progressive increase in breathing-circuit resistance, and the patient should be monitored for signs of respiratory distress.[142] Also, premoistening an artificial nose is inadvisable. It does not improve efficiency and serves only to further increase the flow resistance of the device.

Airway Maintenance Equipment

Airway management is a primary concern during transport and frequently is the responsibility of the RT. During movement of the patient, the possibility of disconnecting or pulling out tubes (e.g., endotracheal or IV) is increased. Therefore movement of the patient should be done slowly, with one member of the team solely responsible for maintaining the airway in place. This member should also lead the team in deciding when movement should take place so that movement is coordinated and efficient. This is usually accomplished by counting down from five and coordinating movement on the count of one. While away from the ICU, the transport team should carry all the necessary supplies for airway management (see Table 20-2). The patient's endotracheal tube should be secured. Our practice is to use adhesive tape to hold endotracheal tubes in place. We have not found it necessary to carry a cricothyrotomy tray with the team because in extreme emergencies it can be brought quickly to the patient by surgeons capable of performing the procedure.

Infusion Pumps

Continuous delivery of fluids and pharmacologic agents should not be interrupted during transport. Infusion pumps can be easily attached to IV poles and are usually capable of operating for several hours on internal batteries. These devices should have alarms to warn of infusion problems and should be as small and lightweight as possible. When the patient is receiving enteral nutrition, we usually elect to discontinue feeding during transport.

Drug Box

A drug box with all pharmacologic agents necessary to manage emergency situations should accompany the team. Additionally, extra IV fluids, IV tubing, and other drugs currently being delivered should be available.

Stethoscope

The stethoscope is essential equipment for all members of the team. Without fancy electronics, it can detect the quality or presence of breath sounds and heart sounds and can assist in the manual measurement of blood pressure. Frequent use of the stethoscope is recommended to ensure patient safety.

Additional Equipment

In selected cases, it may be advantageous for the transport team to carry a pulse oximeter and a defibrillator. Pulse oximetry can detect inadequate O_2 saturation before overt clinical signs.[143] However, if an FIO_2 of 1.0 is used, the incidence of hypoxemia during transport is low. If an oximeter is used, it should have its own battery, be relatively insensitive to motion, and like all other equipment be as small and lightweight as possible.

A defibrillator may be necessary when transferring patients with known cardiac disease. In some cases, the defibrillator may be part of the ECG monitor, in which case additional equipment is unnecessary. The defibrillator should have its own power supply and meet size and weight requirements.

Physiologic Effects and Risks of Transport

The detrimental physiologic effects and risks of intrahospital transport have been described by several authors. However, there is difficulty in comparing results because some reports consider ECG lead disconnection a complication of transport, whereas others consider only physiologic changes.

Taylor and colleagues described their experience transporting 50 patients with acute cardiac disease.[144] All patients had continuous ECG monitoring, and a defibrillator accompanied every trip. Forty-two of 50 patients were noted to have arrhythmias during transport, and of these, 22 were considered life-threatening, requiring immediate treatment. The average length of transport in this survey was 57 minutes. The authors noted that transportation also resulted in an increase in heart rate but no consistent change in blood pressure. No patient died during transport. Taylor and colleagues concluded that ECG monitoring of these patients was essential, and they speculated that patient movement in and of itself may predispose the patient to arrhythmias.

Waddell published results of a prospective trial of patient transport in 1975.[145] He studied 55 patients transported to and from the ICU during a 5-month period and reported that "one patient a month suffered major cardiorespiratory collapse or death as a direct result of movement." In one instance, movement resulted in renewed bleeding from a pelvic fracture and death. In two cases, movement was associated with cardiac arrhythmia and hypotension, and in one case, airway obstruction occurred. In the second part of his study, Waddell demonstrated that 70 postoperative patients could be moved without incident. Waddell recommended that critically ill patients should be moved only when absolutely necessary and that preparation and stabilization of the patient were essential to limit adverse effects.

Ehrenwerth and associates retrospectively studied 204 critically ill patients transported to the ICU and identified only three instances in which the transport process resulted in morbidity.[146] They concluded that critically ill adults could be transported safely.

Insel and colleagues described the cardiovascular changes during transport of patients after major surgery from the operating room to the ICU.[147] They recorded heart rate and blood pressure preoperatively, at 30 minutes, at 15 minutes, and immediately before transport; in the elevator; on arrival; and 30 minutes after arrival at their destination. They demonstrated that cardiovascular instability was common during transport and attributed most of the changes to the emergence from anesthesia. Additionally, they reported cases of hypotension, hypertension, and ventricular fibrillation before or just after arrival at the ICU. Insel and colleagues stated that "transport itself has little hemodynamic impact."

Rutherford and Fisher studied 49 patients during transport from a medical ICU.[148] They classified patients into three groups according to level of support required:

1. ECG monitoring only
2. Invasive hemodynamic monitoring plus ECG
3. Mechanical ventilation or pharmacologic cardiovascular support plus ECG and invasive monitoring

They observed a 45% incidence of life-threatening complications during transport, including five episodes of systolic blood pressure less than 80 mm Hg, four episodes of respiratory distress, three disconnections of central venous lines, and two dysrhythmias requiring pharmacologic intervention and cardioversion. Rutherford and Fisher concluded that "transport should be kept to an absolute minimum."[148]

In 1987, separate studies by Braman and associates[132] and Gervais and colleagues[131] demonstrated the adverse effects of unintentional hyperventilation during transport, as previously discussed. However, Braman and associates also reported other complications during transport. In two instances, ventilator malfunction was associated with a deterioration in patient condition. This was caused by battery failure and disconnection of the O_2 source. Five patients demonstrated significant hypotension, one had bradycardia, and one had premature ventricular contractions (16/min). In this study, an LP-6 ventilator was used for ventilation during transport. It is unclear whether any adverse effects were related to the increased work of breathing seen with this ventilator in the IMV mode.[149-151] Braman and associates also suggested that "tests be kept to a minimum" and that improvements in ventilatory support "may substantially reduce the risk for serious complications."[132]

Indeck and colleagues prospectively evaluated the risk, cost, and benefits of 103 transports to and from the ICU.[125] They defined complications as a change in O_2 saturation greater than 5%, a change in blood pressure of 20 mm Hg for longer than 5 minutes, a change in heart rate of 20 beats/min for longer than 5 minutes, and a change in respiratory frequency greater than 5 breaths/min for more than 5 minutes. During these transports, they recorded 113 significant physiologic changes. Most changes occurred in blood pressure (46/113), followed by heart rate (24/113), respiratory rate (23/113), and O_2 saturation (20/113). Indeck and colleagues also documented whether the test being performed outside the ICU altered patient management. They concluded that in their series, 76% of tests resulted in no change in patient treatment. Although no patient died or had significant morbidity, Indeck and colleagues suggest that "the decision to transport must be weighed carefully in the face of a greater than 76% chance that the result will not alter management."[125]

Smith and colleagues prospectively studied 125 patients requiring intrahospital transport for "mishaps" related to transport.[123] Although most of these mishaps seem inconsequential (ECG lead disconnect), the 14% incidence of monitor power failure is disturbingly high. This study demonstrated that one third of all transports are associated with mishaps in various degrees. However, no patient died during transport.

The diverse opinions and findings by the previous authors leave questions regarding the safety and efficacy of transport. We recently completed a prospective cohort study of 100 transports.[126] Using the method of Indeck and colleagues,[125] we monitored the patient during transport, and a control patient remaining in the ICU with a similar APACHE (Acute Physiology and Chronic Health Evaluation) II score. We found the incidence of physiologic complications and equipment failures to be similar in the two groups (71 versus 64 and 5 versus 4, respectively). We also monitored ABGs and found no differences during transport compared with ICU blood gases. Our study demonstrates that the "mishaps" and "complications" often attributed to transport are experienced by critically ill patients in the ICU as well. This suggests that the nature of the patient's illness is more important than the act of transport. Commonly reported complications of transport are shown in Box 20-1.

BOX 20-1 *Common Complications During Transport of the Mechanically Ventilated Patient*

Cardiovascular
Arrhythmia
Hypotension
Hypertension
Tachycardia
Bradycardia
Myocardial ischemia
Worsening heart failure
Cardiac arrest

Respiratory
Hypoventilation
Hyperventilation
Hypoxemia
Barotrauma

Neurologic
Elevated intracranial pressure
Increased anxiety

Other
Increased risk of ventilator-associated pneumonia
Bleeding or hemorrhage
Hypothermia
Effects of altitude on physiology*

Equipment failure/Mishaps
Airway obstruction
Extubation
Intubation of right mainstem bronchus
Gastric aspiration around endotracheal tube cuff
Loss of battery power to monitoring equipment or ventilator
Damage to equipment due to mishandling or falls
Loss of oxygen supply
Failure to reproduce ICU ventilation parameters with a portable ventilator or manual ventilator (loss of PEEP, failure to trigger, inappropriate V_T or frequency)
Effects of altitude on equipment performance*
Loss of venous access/indwelling vascular catheters
Interruption of medications—continuous and intermittent
Inadequate chest tube drainage

ICU, Intensive care unit; *PEEP,* positive end expiratory pressure; V_T, tidal volume.
*Unique to air transport.

KEY POINTS

- During CPR, a slow inspiratory time should be used to prevent gastric insufflation.
- During expired air resuscitation, the delivered O_2 concentration is approximately 16% to 18%.
- Death by hyperventilation refers to negative hemodynamic effects caused by too rapid a respiratory rate during CPR.
- The inspiratory threshold device improves venous return by creating a negative intrathoracic pressure.
- A barrier device is intended to protect the caregiver during expired air resuscitation.
- The use of a ventilator during CPR can reduce gastric insufflation and prevent hyperventilation.
- During CPR volume constant ventilators should be used.
- Transportation of the critically ill mechanically ventilated patient can result in significant complications.
- Manual ventilation during transport has been associated with hyperventilation, respiratory alkalosis, and cardiac compromise.
- Portable ventilators should be rugged and light weight, and provide ventilation similar to ICU ventilators.
- Important characteristics of portable ventilators include work of breathing, battery life, and gas consumption.
- The key to successful in-hospital transport is preparation and planning.

ASSESSMENT QUESTIONS

1. What is the approximate delivered O_2 concentration during expired air resuscitation?
   - A. 20% to 21%
   - B. 16% to 18%
   - C. 15% to 16%
   - D. 19% to 20%
2. During CPR, hyperventilation is associated with:
   - I. Improved oxygenation
   - II. Decreased venous return
   - III. Increased intrathoracic pressure
   - IV. Reduced cardiac output
     - A. I, II, and III
     - B. II, III, and IV
     - C. I, III, and IV
     - D. All of the above
3. True or False. A slow inspiratory flow and long inspiratory time during ventilation with a face mask helps reduce gastric insufflation.
4. The inspiratory threshold device creates which of the following effects during CPR?
   - I. Negative intrathoracic pressure
   - II. Improved venous return
   - III. Positive intrathoracic pressure
   - IV. Decreased venous return
     - A. I and II
     - B. I and IV
     - C. II and IV
     - D. II and III
5. What does death by hyperventilation refer to?
   - A. Excessive ventilation causing hypoxemia
   - B. Excessive ventilation causing hyperoxia
   - C. Excessive ventilation causing hypocarbia
   - D. Excessive ventilation causing decreased venous return and cardiac output
6. Current AHA standards call for what combination of rate and V_T during adult CPR?
   - A. 10 to 12 breaths/min and 600 to 800 ml
   - B. 8 to 10 breaths/min and 500 to 600 ml
   - C. 10 to 15 breaths/min and 1000 ml
   - D. 8 to 10 breaths/min and 800 to 1000 ml
7. The Sellick maneuver refers to pressure applied to:
   - A. the costochondral cartilage.
   - B. the Sellick cartilage.
   - C. the cricoid membrane.
   - D. the hyoid membrane.
8. Which of the following are disadvantages of MO-MO resuscitation?
   - I. Possible disease transmission
   - II. Low delivered O_2
   - III. Possibility of gastric insufflation
   - IV. Unpleasantness of the task
     - A. I, II, and III
     - B. I, II, and IV
     - C. I and II only
     - D. All of the above
9. Breathing through the NRV of a BVM is associated with:
   - A. a decreased work of breathing.
   - B. an increased work of breathing.
   - C. hypoxemia.
   - D. hypocarbia.
10. Manual ventilation during transport is associated with which of the following?
    - I. Hypercarbia
    - II. Hypocarbia
    - III. Alkalosis
    - IV. Cardiac arrhythmias
      - A. I, II, and III
      - B. II, III, and IV
      - C. II and III
      - D. All of the above
11. Which of the following are commonly reported complications of in-hospital transport?
    - I. Hypotension
    - II. Cardiac arrhythmias
    - III. Hypoxemia
    - IV. Equipment failure
    - V. Hypothermia
    - VI. Respiratory alkalosis
      - A. I, II, III, and VI
      - B. I, II, III, V, and VI
      - C. I, II, III, IV, and VI
      - D. All of the above

ASSESSMENT QUESTIONS—cont'd

12. The safety of manual ventilation can be improved by monitoring what parameters?
A. Blood pressure and heart rate
B. V_T and respiratory rate
C. Intracranial pressure and blood pressure
D. V_T and PaO_2

13. Important characteristics of portable ventilators for in-hospital transport include:
I. battery life.
II. gas consumption.
III. work of breathing.
IV. size and weight.
A. I, II, and III
B. I and III
C. I, III, and IV
D. All of the above

14. Battery life of a portable ventilator can be affected by
I. PEEP.
II. FIO_2.
III. $\dot{V}_E$.
IV. altitude.
A. I and II
B. I and III
C. I, II, and III
D. All of the above

15. True or False. Manual ventilation and use of a portable ventilator provide similar consistency of ventilation.

REFERENCES

1. International Liaison Committee on Resuscitation. 2005 international consensus on cardiopulmonary resuscitation and emergency cardiovascular care science with treatment recommendations, Circulation 112:III-1-III-136, 2005.
2. Emergency Care Research Institute: Manually operated resuscitators, Health Devices 1:13-17, 1971.
3. Emergency Care Research Institute: Manual resuscitators, Health Devices 8:133-146, 1979.
4. Emergency Care Research Institute: Gas-powered resuscitators, Health Devices 8:24-38, 1978.
5. Emergency Care Research Institute: Gas-powered pulmonary resuscitators, Health Devices 18:362-363, 1989.
6. Emergency Care Research Institute: Pulmonary resuscitators, Health Devices 17:348-354, 1988.
7. Emergency Care Research Institute: Exhaled air pulmonary resuscitators (EAPR's) and disposable manual pulmonary resuscitators (DMPR's), Health Devices 18:333-352, 1989.
8. American Society of Testing Materials: Standard specifications for minimum performance and safety requirements for resuscitators intended for use with humans, Designation F 920-985, Philadelphia, 1985, ASTM.
9. International Standards Organization: International Standard ISO 8382:1988(E): resuscitators intended for use with humans, New York, 1988, American National Standards Institute.
10. Ruben H, Knudsen EJ, Carugti G: Gastric insufflation in relation to airway pressure, Acta Anaesth Scand 5:107-114, 1961.
11. Melker RJ: Recommendations for ventilation during cardiopulmonary resuscitation: time for a change? Crit Care Med 13:882-883, 1985.
12. Fillmore SJ, Shapiro M, Killip J: Serial blood gas studies during cardiopulmonary resuscitation, Ann Intern Med 72:465-470, 1970.
13. Gilston A: Clinical and biochemical aspects of cardiac resuscitation, Lancet 2:1039-1043, 1965.
14. Himmelhoch SR, Dekker A, Gazzaniga AB et al: Closed-chest cardiac resuscitation: a prospective clinical and pathological study, N Engl J Med 270:118-122, 1964.
15. Ornato JP, Bryson BL, Donovan PJ et al: Measurement of ventilation during cardiopulmonary resuscitation, Crit Care Med 11:79-82, 1983.
16. Davis K, Johannigman JA, Johnson RC et al: Lung compliance following cardiac arrest, Acad Emerg Med 2:874-878, 1995.
17. 11 Kings 4:31-35 The Bible, King James Version.
18. Ristagno G, Gullo A, Tang W et al: New cardiopulmonary resuscitation guidelines 2005: importance of uninterrupted chest compression, Crit Care Clin 22(3):531-538, 2006.
19. Sainsbury DA, Davis R, Walker MC: Artificial ventilation for cardiopulmonary resuscitation, Med J Aust 141:509-511, 1984.
20. Hess D, Baran C: Ventilatory volumes using mouth-to-mouth, mouth-to-mask, and bag-valve-mask techniques, Am J Emerg Med 3:292-296, 1985.
21. Lawrence PJ, Sivaneswaran N: Ventilation during cardiopulmonary resuscitation: which method? Med J Aust 143:443-446, 1985.
22. Harrison RR, Maull KI, Keenan RL et al: Mouth-to-mask ventilation: a superior method of rescue breathing, Ann Emerg Med 11:74-76, 1982.
23. Seidelin PH, Stolarek IH, Littlewood DG: Comparison of six methods of emergency ventilation, Lancet 2:1274-1275, 1986.
24. Johannigman JA, Branson RD, Davis K et al: Techniques of emergency ventilation: a model to evaluate

tidal volume, airway pressure, and gastric insufflation, J Trauma 31:93-98, 1991.
25. Melker RJ, Banner MJ: Ventilation during CPR: two-rescuer standards reappraised, Ann Emerg Med 14:397-402, 1985.
26. Hess D, Kapp A, Kurtek W: The effect of delivered oxygen concentration of the rescuer's breathing supplemental oxygen during exhaled gas ventilation, Respir Care 30:691-694, 1985.
27. Rottenberg EM, Dzwonczyk R, Reilley TE et al: Use of supplemental oxygen during bystander-initiated CPR, Ann Emerg Med 23:1027-1030, 1994.
28. Sellick BA: Cricoid pressure to control regurgitation of stomach contents during induction of anesthesia, Lancet 2:404-406, 1961.
29. Moynihan RJ, Brock-Utne JG, Archer JH et al: The effect of cricoid pressure on preventing gastric insufflation in infants and children, Anesthesiology 78:652-656, 1993.
30. Vanner RG, O'Dwyer JP, Pryle BJ et al: Upper oesophageal sphincter pressure and the effect of cricoid pressure, Anaesthesia 47:95-100, 1992.
31. Ralph SJ, Wareham CA: Rupture of the oesophagus during cricoid pressure, Anaesthesia 46:40-41, 1991.
32. Barker SJ, Karagianes T: Gastric barotrauma: a case report and theoretical considerations, Anesth Analg 64:1026-1028, 1985.
33. Ornato JP, Hallagan LF, McMahon SB et al: Attitudes of BCLS instructors about mouth to mouth resuscitation during the AIDS epidemic, Ann Emerg Med 19:151-156, 1990.
34. Pane GA, Salness KA: A survey of participants in a mass CPR training course, Ann Emerg Med 16:1112-1116, 1987.
35. Link RN, Feingold AR, Charap MH et al: Concerns of medical and pediatric house officers about acquiring AIDS from their patients, Am J Public Health 78:455-459, 1988.
36. American Heart Association: Supplemental guidelines: Risk of infection during CPR training and rescue, JAMA 262:2714-2715, 1989.
37. Fluck RR, Sorbello JG: Mouth to mouth resuscitation by lay rescuers—should they or shouldn't they? Respir Care 35:831-832, 1990.
38. Durbin CG: Mouth to mask resuscitation by lay rescuers—will they or won't they? Respir Care 35:832-834, 1990.
39. Heilman KM, Muscheheim C: Primary cutaneous tuberculosis resulting from mouth to mouth respiration, N Engl J Med 273:1035-1036, 1965.
40. Feldman HA: Some recollections of the meningococcal disease, JAMA 220:1107-1112, 1972.
41. Hendricks AA, Shapiro EP: Primary herpes simplex infection following mouth to mouth resuscitation, JAMA 243:257-258, 1980.
42. Finkelhorn RS, Lampman JH: Herpes simplex infection following cardiopulmonary resuscitation, JAMA 243:650, 1980.
43. Harris MJ, Wendel RT: Transmission of herpes simplex during cardiopulmonary resuscitation, Compr Ther 10:15-17, 1984.
44. Todd MA, Bell JS: Shigellosis from cardiopulmonary resuscitation, JAMA 243:331, 1980.
45. Ahmad F, Senadhira DC, Charters J et al: Transmission of salmonella via mouth-to-mouth resuscitation, Lancet 335:787-788, 1990.
46. Mamby SA: A plea for CPR equipment in public places, N Engl J Med 322:1161, 1990.
47. Hodgin L: New law in the Big Apple mandates CPR infection control equipment, Occup Health Safety 61:56-58, 1992.
48. Waters RM: Simple methods for performing artificial respiration, JAMA 123:559-561, 1943.
49. Don Michael A, Forrester JS: Mouth to mouth ventilation: the dying art, Am J Emerg Med 10:156-161, 1992.
50. Lightsey DM, Shah PK, Forrester JS et al: A human immunodeficiency virus resistant airway for cardiopulmonary resuscitation, Ann J Emerg Med 10:73-77, 1992.
51. Rossi R, Ahnefeld FW: Expired air resuscitation in emergency situations with Ambu-Life key, Notfallmedizin 16:3-7, 1990.
52. Baskett PJF: Advances in cardiopulmonary resuscitation, Br J Anaesth 69:182-193, 1992.
53. Westfall MD: Kiss of life mask: evaluation or opinion? (Letter) Am J Emerg Med 10:616, 1992.
54. Rossi R, Lindner KH, Ahnefeld FW: Devices for expired air resuscitation, Prehospital Disaster Med 8:123-126, 1993.
55. Simmons M: Resistance to flow through the valves of three face shield CPR barrier devices, Respir Care 39:1068, 1994.
56. Simmons M, Deao D, Moon L: Bench evaluation: three face shield barrier devices, Respir Care 40:618-623, 1995.
57. Elam JO, Brown ES, Elder JD Jr: Artificial respiration by mouth-to-mask method, N Engl J Med 250:749-754, 1954.
58. Safar P, McMahon M: Mouth to airway emergency artificial respiration, JAMA 166:1459-1461, 1958.
59. Safar P: Pocket mask for emergency artificial ventilation and oxygen inhalation, Crit Care Med 2:273-276, 1974.
60. Thomas AN, Weber EC: A new method of two-resuscitator CPR, Resuscitation 26:173-176, 1993.
61. Thomas AN, O'Sullivan K, Hyatt J et al: A comparison of bag mask and mouth mask ventilation in anaesthetized patients, Resuscitation 26:13-21, 1993.
62. Tolley PM, Watts J, Hickman JA: Comparison of the use of the laryngeal mask and face mask by inexperienced personnel, Br J Anaesth 69:320-321, 1992.
63. Thomas AN, Bergesio R, Hyatt J et al: Mouth mask ventilation: use of a Pall Ultipor breathing system and effect of mask design (abstract), Br J Anaesth 69:527P-528P, 1992.
64. Johannigman JA, Branson RD: Oxygen enrichment of expired gas for mouth to mask resuscitation, Respir Care 36:99-103, 1991.
65. Stahl JM, Cutfield GR, Harrison GA: Alveolar oxygenation and mouth to mask ventilation: effects of oxygen insufflation, Anaesth Intensive Care 20:177-186, 1992.
66. Thomas AN, Hyatt J, Chen JL et al: The Laerdal pocket mask: effects of increasing supplementary oxygen flow, Anaesthesia 47:967-971, 1992.

67. Palmisano JM, Moler FW, Galura C et al: Influence of tidal volume, respiratory rate, and supplemental oxygen flow on delivered oxygen fraction using a mouth to mask ventilation device, J Emerg Med 11:685-689, 1993.
68. Hess D, Ness C, Oppel A et al: Evaluation of mouth to mask ventilation devices, Respir Care 34:191-195, 1989.
69. Hess DR: Manual and gas powered resuscitators. In: Branson RD, Hess DR, Chatburn RL, editors: Respiratory care equipment, Philadelphia, 1999, Lippincott Williams and Wilkins, pp 187-202.
70. Barnes TA: Emergency ventilation techniques and related equipment, Respir Care 37:673-694, 1992.
71. Elling R, Politis J: An evaluation of emergency medical technicians ability to use manual ventilation devices, Ann Emerg Med 12:765-768, 1983.
72. Giffen PR, Hope CE: Preliminary evaluation of a prototype tube-valve-mask ventilator for emergency artificial ventilation, Ann Emerg Med 20:262-266, 1991.
73. Cummins RO, Austin D, Graves JR et al: Ventilation skills of emergency medical technicians: a teaching challenge for emergency medicine, Ann Emerg Med 15:1187-1192, 1986.
74. Barnes TA, Adams G: Ventilatory volumes using mouth to mouth, bag-valve-mask, and pocket face mask (abstract), Respir Care 36:1292, 1991.
75. Jesudian MC, Harrison RR, Keenan RL et al: Bag-valve-mask ventilation: two rescuers are better than one: preliminary report, Crit Care Med 13:122-123, 1985.
76. Stewart RD, Kaplan R, Penrock B et al: Influence of mask design on bag-mask ventilation, Ann Emerg Med 14:403-406, 1985.
77. Hess D, Goff G: The effects of two-hand versus one-hand ventilation on volumes delivered during bag-valve ventilation at various resistances and compliances, Respir Care 32:1025-1028, 1987.
78. Augustine JA, Seidel DR, McCabe JB: Ventilation performance using a self-inflating anesthesia bag: effect of operator characteristics, Am J Emerg Med 5:267-270, 1987.
79. Hess D, Goff G, Johnson K: The effect of hand size, resuscitator brand, and use of two hands on volumes delivered during adult bag-valve ventilation, Respir Care 34:805-810, 1989.
80. Powers WE: Evaluation of a training method that uses volumetric feedback with bag-valve-mask ventilation techniques (abstract), Respir Care 33:942-943, 1988.
81. Branson RD, Davis K, Johnson RC et al: Manual ventilation during cardiopulmonary resuscitation (abstract), Respir Care 39:1068, 1994.
82. Aufderheide TP, Sigurdsson G, Pirrallo RG et al: Hyperventilation-induced hypotension during cardiopulmonary resuscitation, Circulation 27;109(16): 1960-1965, 2004.
83. Aufderheide TP, Lurie KG: Death by hyperventilation: A common and life-threatening problem during cardiopulmonary resuscitation, Crit Care Med 32(9 Suppl):S345-S351, 2004.
84. Yannopoulos D, Tang W, Roussos C et al: Reducing ventilation frequency during cardiopulmonary resuscitation in a porcine model of cardiac arrest, Respir Care 50(5):628-635, 2005.
85. Aufderheide TP: The problem with and benefit of ventilations: should our approach be the same in cardiac and respiratory arrest? Curr Opin Crit Care 12(3):207-212, 2006.
86. Yannopoulos D, Aufderheide TP, Gabrielli A et al: Clinical and hemodynamic comparison of 15:2 and 30:2 compression-to-ventilation ratios for cardiopulmonary resuscitation, Crit Care Med 34(5):1444-1449, 2006.
87. Priano L, Ham J: A simple method to increase FDO_2 of resuscitator bags, Crit Care Med 6:48-49, 1978.
88. Fitzmaurice MW, Barnes TA: Oxygen delivery performance of three adult resuscitation bags, Respir Care 25:928-933, 1980.
89. LeBovet L: 1980 assessment of eight adult manual resuscitators, Respir Care 25:1136-1142, 1980.
90. Barnes TA, Watson MW: Oxygen delivery performance of four adult resuscitation bags, Respir Care 27:139-146, 1982.
91. Barnes T, Watson M: Oxygen delivery performance of old and new designs of the Laerdal, Vitalograph, and AMBU adult manual resuscitators, Respir Care 28:1121-1128, 1983.
92. Phillips GD, Showronski GA: Manual resuscitators and portable ventilators, Anaesth Intensive Care 14:306-313, 1986.
93. Campbell TP, Stewart RD, Kaplan RM et al: Oxygen enrichment of bag-valve-mask units during positive-pressure ventilation: a comparison of various techniques, Ann Emerg Med 17:232-235, 1988.
94. Barnes TA, Potash R: Evaluation of five disposable operator powered adult resuscitators, Respir Care 34:254-261, 1989.
95. Barnes TA, McGarry W: Evaluation of ten disposable manual resuscitators, Respir Care 35:960-968, 1990.
96. Barnes TA, Stockwell DL: Evaluation of ten manual resuscitators across an operational temperature range of −18EC to 50EC, Respir Care 36:161-172, 1991.
97. Munford BJ, Wishaw KJ: Critical incidents with nonrebreathing valves, Anaesth Intensive Care 18:560-563, 1990.
98. Hess D, Simmons M: An evaluation of the resistance to flow through the patent valves of twelve adult manual resuscitators, Respir Care 37:432-438, 1992.
99. Mills PJ, Baptiste J, Preston J et al: Manual resuscitators and spontaneous ventilation: an evaluation, Crit Care Med 19:1425-1431, 1991.
100. Stemp LI: Manual resuscitators and spontaneous ventilation—an evaluation (letter), Crit Care Med 20:1496, 1992.
101. Hess D, Hirsch C, Marquis-D'Amico C et al: Imposed work and oxygen delivery during spontaneous breathing with adult disposable manual ventilators, Anaesthesia 81:1256-1263, 1994.
102. Johannigman JA, Branson RD, Johnson DJ et al: Out-of-hospital ventilation: bag-valve device versus

transport ventilator, Acad Emerg Med 2:719-724, 1995.
103. Osborn HH, Kayen D, Horne H et al: Excess ventilation with oxygen powered resuscitators, Am J Emerg Med 2:408-413, 1984.
104. Pradis IL, Caldwell EJ: Traumatic pneumocephalus: a hazard of resuscitators, J Trauma 19:61-63, 1979.
105. Fasi TH, Lucas BG: An evaluation of some mechanical resuscitators for use in the ambulance service, Ann R Coll Surg Engl 62:291-293, 1980.
106. Menegazzi JJ, Winslow HJ: In-vitro comparison of bag-valve-mask and the manually triggered oxygen powered breathing device, Acad Emerg Med 1:29-33, 1994.
107. Mesezzo VN, Lukitsch K, Menegazzi J et al: Comparison of delivered volumes and airway pressures when ventilating through an endotracheal tube with bag valve versus demand valve, Prehosp Disaster Med 9:24-28, 1994.
108. Branson RD: Intrahospital transport of critically ill mechanically ventilated patients, Respir Care 37:775-795, 1992.
109. Branson RD, McGough EK: Transport ventilators. In: Banner MJ, editor: Problems in critical care: positive pressure ventilation, Philadelphia, 1990, JB Lippincott, pp 254-274.
110. Austin PA, Campbell RS, Johannigman JA et al: Transport ventilators in 2001, Respir Care Clin North Am 8:1-32, 2002.
111. Nolan JP, Baskett JF: Gas-powered and portable ventilators: an evaluation of six models, Prehosp Disaster Med 7:25-34, 1972.
112. McGough EK, Banner MJ, Melker RJ: Variations in tidal volume with portable transport ventilators, Respir Care 37:233-239, 1992.
113. Campbell RS, Davis K, Johnson DJ et al: Laboratory and clinical evaluation of the Impact 750 portable ventilator, Respir Care 37:29-36, 1992.
114. Johannigman JA, Branson RD, Campbell RS et al: Laboratory and clinical evaluation of the MAX transport ventilator, Respir Care 35:952-959, 1990.
115. Greenslade GL: Single operator cardiopulmonary resuscitation in ambulances, Anaesthesia 46:391-394, 1991.
116. Lurie KG, Coffeen P, Shultz J et al: Improving active compression-decompression cardiopulmonary resuscitation with an inspiratory impedance valve, Circulation 91:1629-1632, 1995.
117. Plaisance P, Lurie KG, Payen D: Inspiratory impedance during active compression-decompression cardiopulmonary resuscitation: A randomized evaluation in patients in cardiac arrest, Circulation 101:989-994, 2000.
118. Plaisance P, Lurie KG, Vicaut E et al: Evaluation of an impedance threshold device in patients receiving active compression-decompression cardiopulmonary resuscitation for treatment of out of hospital cardiac arrest, Resuscitation 61:265-271, 2004.
119. Wolcke BB, Mauer DK, Schoefmann MF et al: Comparison of standard cardiopulmonary resuscitation versus the combination of active compression-decompression cardiopulmonary resuscitation and an inspiratory impedance threshold device for out-of-hospital cardiac arrest, Circulation 108:2201-2205, 2003.
120. Aufderheide TP, Pirrallo RG, Provo TA et al: Clinical evaluation of an inspiratory impedance threshold device during standard cardiopulmonary resuscitation in patients with out-of-hospital cardiac arrest, Crit Care Med 33:734-740, 2005.
121. Lurie KG, Mulligan KA, McKnite S et al: Optimizing standard cardiopulmonary resuscitation with an inspiratory impedance threshold valve, Chest 113:1084-1090, 1998.
122. Smith IV, Flemming S, Bekes CE: Written policy and patient transport from the intensive care unit (letter), Crit Care Med 15:1162, 1987.
123. Smith I, Flemming S, Cernaianu A: Mishaps during transport from the intensive care unit, Crit Care Med 18:278-281, 1990.
124. Keene AR, Cullen DJ: Therapeutic intervention scoring system: update 1983, Crit Care Med 11:1-8, 1983.
125. Indeck M, Peterson S, Smith J et al: Risk, cost and benefit of transporting ICU patient for special studies, J Trauma 28:1020-1025, 1988.
126. Hurst JM, Davis K Jr, Johnson DJ et al: Cost and complications during in-hospital transport of critically ill patients: a prospective study (abstract), J Trauma 31:1717, 1991.
127. Runcie CJ, Reeve W, Reidy J et al: A comparison of measurements of blood pressure, heart rate and oxygenation during inter-hospital transport of the critically ill, Intensive Care Med 16:317-322, 1990.
128. Runcie CJ, Reeve WG, Reidy J et al: Blood pressure measurement during transport, Anaesthesia 45:659-665, 1990.
129. Gallagher TJ, Melker RJ: Transport of the critically ill/injured patient. In: Civetta JM, Taylor RW, Kirby RR, editors: Critical care, Philadelphia, 1988, JB Lippincott, pp 1579-1588.
130. Hurst JM, Davis K, Branson RD et al: Comparison of blood gases during transport using two methods of ventilatory support, J Trauma 29:1637-1640, 1989.
131. Gervais HW, Eberle B, Konietzke D et al: Comparison of blood gases of ventilated patients during transport, Crit Care Med 15:761-764, 1987.
132. Braman SS, Dunn SM, Amico C et al: Complications of inter-hospital transport in critically ill patients, Ann Intern Med 107:469-473, 1987.
133. Weg JG, Haas CF: Safe intra-hospital transport of critically ill ventilator dependent patients, Chest 96:631-635, 1989.
134. Adams KS, Branson RD, Hurst JM: Variabilities in delivered tidal volume and respiratory rate during manual ventilation (abstract), Respir Care 31:986, 1986.
135. Park GR, Manara AR, Bodenham AR et al: The pneuPAC ventilator with new patient valve and air compressors, Anaesthesia 44:419-424, 1989.
136. Johannigman JA, Branson RD, Campbell RS et al: Laboratory and clinical evaluation of the MAX transport ventilator, Respir Care 35:952-959, 1990.
137. Campbell RS, Austin PA, Matacia GM et al: Battery life of eight portable ventilators: Effect of control

variable, PEEP, and FIO_2, Respir Care 47:1173-1183, 2002.

138. Campbell RS, Davis K Jr, Johnson DJ et al: Laboratory and clinical evaluation of the Uni-Vent 750 portable ventilator, Respir Care 37:29-36, 1992.
139. Shelly MP, Park GR, Warren RE: Portable lung ventilators: the potential risk from bacterial colonisation, Intensive Care Med 12:328-331, 1986.
140. Chalon J, Loew DAY, Malebranche J: Effect of dry anesthetic gases on the tracheobronchial epithelium, Anesthesiology 37:338-343, 1972.
141. Branson RD, Hurst JM: Laboratory evaluation of moisture output of seven airway heat and moisture exchangers, Respir Care 32:741-747, 1987.
142. Ploysonsang Y, Branson RD, Rashkin MC et al: Pressure flow characteristics of commonly used heat-moisture exchangers, Am Rev Respir Dis 138:675-678, 1988.
143. Adams KS, Branson RD, Hurst JM: Monitoring oxygenation with oximetry during transport, Respir Manage Nov/Dec:63-69, 1987.
144. Taylor JO, Landers CF, Chulay JD et al: Monitoring high-risk cardiac patients during transportation in hospital, Lancet 2:1205-1208, 1970.
145. Waddell G: Movement of critically ill patients within hospital, Br Med J 2:417-419, 1975.
146. Ehrenwerth J, Sorbo S, Hacker A: Transport of critically ill adults, Crit Care Med 14:543-547, 1986.
147. Insel J, Weissman C, Kemper M et al: Cardiovascular changes during transport of critically ill and post-operative patients, Crit Care Med 14:539-542, 1986.
148. Rutherford WF, Fisher CJ: Risks associated with in-house transportation of the critically ill (abstract), Clin Res 34:414, 1986.
149. Kacmarek RM, Stanek KS, McMahon KM et al: Imposed work of breathing during synchronized intermittent mandatory ventilation provided by five home care ventilators, Respir Care 35:405-414, 1990.
150. Branson RD, Davis K Jr: Work of breathing imposed by five ventilators used for long-term support: The effects of PEEP and simulated patient demand, Respir Care 40:1270-1278, 1995.
151. Austin PA, Campbell RS, Johannigman JA et al: Work of breathing characteristics of seven portable ventilators, Resuscitation 49:163-172, 2001.

CHAPTER

21

Noninvasive Mechanical Ventilation

NICHOLAS S. HILL

OUTLINE

OBJECTIVES

- Explain the role of noninvasive ventilation in the treatment of acute respiratory failure.
- List the types of respiratory failure that are most successfully treated with noninvasive ventilation.
- Describe the signs of success and failure of noninvasive ventilation.
- Compare and contrast noninvasive ventilators with invasive ventilators.
- Understand when each type of ventilator is most successful in the application of noninvasive ventilation.
- Compare and contrast interfaces (masks, helmet, etc.) for the delivery of noninvasive ventilation.

KEY TERMS

asynchrony
critical care ventilators
diaphragm pacers
glossopharyngeal (frog) breathing
mask bag
nasal pillows
noninvasive positive-pressure ventilation (NPPV)
noninvasive ventilation (NIV)
obesity hypoventilation syndrome (OHS)
standard nasal masks

Noninvasive ventilation (NIV) is mechanical ventilation administered without an invasive artificial airway. Many types of noninvasive ventilators have been developed since the first description of a prototype negative-pressure "tank" ventilator 150 years ago. "Tank" ventilators such as the iron lung were the mainstay of mechanical ventilatory assistance during the polio epidemics that occurred from the 1920s through the 1950s[1] and still see limited use in some respiratory care units in Italy and Spain.[2] For practical purposes, however, NIV now refers to positive-pressure ventilation administered via a mask or "interface" that directs pressurized gas into the upper airway. Since the late 1980s, NIV has assumed an increasingly important role in the management of patients with both acute and chronic forms of respiratory failure.[3] This chapter takes a practical approach to the administration of NIV to patients with respiratory failure, focusing on indications for use in different diagnostic categories, selection of appropriate patients, and techniques of administration.

RATIONALE FOR THE USE OF NONINVASIVE VENTILATION

Invasive mechanical ventilation has proven to be effective and reliable, but an endotracheal airway, whether an acute translaryngeal or chronic tracheostomy, predisposes to complications as follows[4]:

- Traumatic complications, such as hemorrhage or tracheal laceration
- Infectious complications related to bypassing the airway defense system
- Discomfort and interference with communication and swallowing

Airway intubation interferes with normal airway clearance mechanisms, such as cough and ciliary function, and serves as a continual irritant, increasing mucus production and necessitating intermittent suctioning. It also necessitates the use of sufficient sedation and analgesia to maintain a desired level of calmness and comfort, which can retard the weaning process from mechanical ventilation. By avoiding these complications, NIV has the potential of improving patient outcomes, enhancing patient comfort and satisfaction, shortening lengths of ICU and hospital stays, and reducing the cost of care. However, it must be emphasized that the patients who are to receive NIV must be selected carefully.

INDICATIONS FOR NONINVASIVE VENTILATION: ACUTE APPLICATIONS

Best Established Indications

Chronic Obstructive Pulmonary Disease

Exacerbations of Chronic Obstructive Pulmonary Disease. In the setting of an exacerbation of chronic obstructive pulmonary disease (COPD), NIV consisting of pressure support and positive end-expiratory pressure (PEEP) or so-called "bilevel" positive airway pressure (PAP) is well-suited to avert respiratory failure. The lower expiratory pressure counterbalances auto-PEEP, reducing the inspiratory threshold load, whereas the inspiratory pressure "boost" actively assists inhalation. The combination of a higher inspiratory pressure and lower expiratory pressure is more effective than either pressure alone in reducing diaphragmatic work of breathing in COPD patients[5] and can serve as a "crutch" to support COPD patients during exacerbations while medical therapy is given time to work.

Multiple randomized controlled trials and meta-analyses have established that NIV, compared with standard therapy, more rapidly reduces respiratory rate, improves dyspnea and gas exchange, reduces intubations from an average rate of 50% to 20%, and lowers mortality compared with standard therapy.[6-10] In European studies, NIV also reduces hospital lengths of stay as well, but this has not been confirmed in North America, where lengths of stay overall tend to be much shorter than in Europe. The strength of the evidence justifies use of NIV for COPD exacerbations as a standard of care unless there are contraindications. Randomized controlled or prospective studies have also shown that COPD exacerbations respond well to NIV when complicated by pneumonia[11] or that occur in the setting of a do-not-intubate (DNI) status,[12] or postoperative[13] or postextubation respiratory failure[14] (Box 21-1).

Facilitation of Weaning in COPD Patients. When patients with COPD exacerbations are intubated because they are not candidates for NIV initially or fail a trial of NIV, multiple controlled trials have demonstrated that NIV can be used to permit earlier extubation, even if these patients have failed multiple "T" piece weaning trials.[15,16] Early extubation to NIV increases eventual weaning rates, shortens the duration of ventilator use and hospital length of stay, reduces the occurrence of nosocomial pneumonia, and reduces mortality. This approach should

BOX 21-1 *Diagnoses and Categories of Acute Respiratory Failure Treated With Noninvasive Ventilation: Levels of Evidence*

Obstructive diseases
COPD (A)
Asthma (B)
Cystic fibrosis (C)
Upper airway obstruction (C)

Restrictive diseases (Mainly long-term setting)
Kyphoscoliosis (C)
Neuromuscular disease (C)
Obesity hypoventilation syndrome (C)

Hypoxemic respiratory failure
Acute pulmonary edema (A*)
Pneumonia (B†)
ARDS (C)
Trauma (C)

Categories of acute respiratory failure
Facilitation of weaning (A)
Immunocompromised patients (A)
Postoperative respiratory failure (B)
Extubation failure (B‡)
Do-not-intubate patients (C‡)

Letters in parentheses indicate level of evidence: *A*, multiple controlled trials; *B*, a single supportive controlled trial; *C*, uncontrolled trials, case reports.
CPAP, Continuous positive airway pressure; *COPD*, chronic obstructive pulmonary disease; *CHF*, congestive heart failure.
*Strongest evidence for CPAP (continuous positive airway pressure) of 10-12 cm H_2O.
†Mainly for COPD patients.
‡Mainly in COPD or CHF patients.

be considered whenever intubated COPD patients are failing "T" piece or spontaneous breathing trials, but it should be used with caution—only in patients who are otherwise excellent candidates for NIV, can breathe without any assistance for at least 5 minutes, can tolerate levels of pressure support deliverable by mask (i.e., inspiratory pressure < 20 cm H_2O), and are not a "difficult intubation."

Acute Cardiogenic Pulmonary Edema

The beneficial effects of positive airway pressure have long been known in patients with acute pulmonary edema. The increased functional residual capacity (FRC) opens collapsed alveoli and rapidly improves compliance and oxygenation. The increased intrathoracic pressure reduces transmyocardial pressure and has preload and afterload reducing effects, enhancing cardiac function in patients with left ventricular dysfunction who are afterload dependent.

A number of randomized controlled trials have demonstrated that noninvasive continuous positive airway pressure (CPAP 10 to 12.5 cm H_2O) alone dramatically improves dyspnea and oxygenation and lowers intubation rates in patients with acute pulmonary edema compared with standard O_2 therapy.[17-19] Subsequent studies evaluating the efficacy of NIV (i.e., pressure support plus PEEP) compared with either O_2 therapy or CPAP alone[20-22] have shown benefits similar to those previously demonstrated for CPAP, but one study raised the possibility that myocardial infarction rate may be higher with NIV.[20]

More recently, a number of meta-analyses evaluating these studies have confirmed the benefits of CPAP, even showing a significant reduction in mortality compared with O_2 therapy.[23,24] They found equal efficacy of NIV and CPAP with regard to reducing intubation, lengths of stay, and mortality, and no increase in the myocardial infarction rate was attributable to NIV use. However, some studies have found that NIV reduces dyspnea and improves gas exchange better than CPAP alone.[20,21] Therefore, by virtue of its greater simplicity and potentially lower cost, CPAP alone is generally regarded as the initial noninvasive modality of choice for cardiogenic edema patients, but NIV is substituted if patients treated initially with CPAP remain dyspneic or hypercapnic. Considering the demonstrable benefits of noninvasive positive airway pressure in patients having acute cardiogenic pulmonary edema, it should be considered a standard of care to treat such patients in emergency settings. More early responders are incorporating it into their emergency protocols to reduce the need for emergency intubations in the field.[25]

Immunocompromised Patients

Immunocompromised patients (i.e., those with human immunodeficiency virus (HIV) and *Pneumocystis* pneumonia or following solid organ or bone marrow transplantation) have poor outcomes when treated with invasive mechanical ventilation. Nosocomial infections and fatal bouts of septicemia are common complications, and those with hematologic malignancies may encounter fatal airway hemorrhages caused by thrombocytopenia and platelet dysfunction. NIV offers a way to prevent such complications and improve outcomes.

Randomized trials on patients with acute respiratory failure related to solid organ transplantation or hematologic malignancy have demonstrated reduced intubation and mortality rates compared with controls.[26,27] NIV was begun in these patients before respiratory failure became severe, and even then, the mortality rate in the NIV group was 50% compared with 80% in the conventionally treated group.[27] Thus NIV should be considered early during the development of respiratory failure in immunocompromised patients as a way to avoid intubation and its attendant mortality.

INDICATIONS SUPPORTED BY WEAKER EVIDENCE

Box 21-1 lists other causes of acute respiratory failure supported by single randomized trials, multiple historically controlled or cohort series, or sometimes conflicting evidence. Nonetheless, NIV offers potential benefit for these applications and may be tried in appropriately selected patents.

Other Obstructive Diseases

Asthma Exacerbations

Based on retrospective series, NIV probably improves gas exchange and avoids intubation in patients with respiratory failure caused by asthma exacerbations; remarkably, however, there is only one randomized trial supporting its use for this application—in patients who were not hypercapnic. In this trial,[28] NIV improved FEV_1 more rapidly and reduced the hospitalization rate compared with sham controls. One study also demonstrated that peak flow improved more rapidly when bronchodilator aerosol was administered via a "bilevel" device than via a standard nebulizer. Thus it is conceivable that NIV would benefit patients with severe asthma exacerbations as an initial therapy to reverse airway obstruction more rapidly, but presently, most clinicians use it if patients are not responding adequately and remain dyspneic after initial bronchodilator therapy.

Cystic Fibrosis

NIV has been used mainly as a bridge to transplantation for patients with cystic fibrosis who deteriorate.[30] These patients may remain severely hypercapnic and require aggressive management of secretion retention, but NIV permits avoidance of intubation.

Hypoxemic Respiratory Failure

Hypoxemic respiratory failure is characterized by severe hypoxemia ($Pao_2/Fio_2 < 200$), respiratory distress, tachypnea (>30/min) and a non-COPD cause such as acute respiratory distress syndrome (ARDS), acute pneumonia, trauma, and acute pulmonary edema. With the exception of acute cardiogenic pulmonary edema and pneumonia in COPD or immunocompromised patients, however, the evidence to support the use of NIV in these patients is weak, and the modality should be used selectively and with caution. Some randomized studies on hypoxemic respiratory failure have observed reductions in the need for intubation, shortened ICU lengths of stay, and even mortality in the NIV group as opposed to controls,[31,32] but it is difficult to draw firm conclusions about individual diagnostic groups within this very broad category. NIV should be started only in carefully selected patients within this group, and intubation should be contemplated if there is not a substantial improvement in oxygenation within the first hour ($Pao_2/Fio_2 > 150$ or so).

Extubation Failure

Patients who develop respiratory failure after extubation according to standard criteria are at high risk for morbidity and have mortality rates up to 40%.[33] NIV has been suggested as a way to avoid reintubation and improve outcomes. Earlier randomized studies[34,35] comparing NIV to standard O_2 therapy found no reduction in reintubation attributable to NIV and one even found a significantly increased ICU mortality in the NIV group. Only approximately 10% of patients in these trials had COPD, however, and the increased mortality was thought to be related to a 10-hour delay in reintubations in the NIV group compared with controls.[35] Two subsequent randomized trials[14,15] on patients deemed to be at "high risk" for extubation failure found that NIV reduced the need for reintubation and ICU mortality. Forty to fifty percent of patients in these trials had COPD or congestive heart failure (CHF), and in one of the trials[14] most of the benefit was attributable to the COPD subgroup. These data support the use of NIV in patients at "high risk" of extubation failure, particularly if they have COPD, CHF, and/or hypercapnia. However, early indiscriminate use of NIV in patients who have risk factors for extubation failure but do not meet standard criteria for NIV initiation is discouraged. Patients with extubation failure treated with NIV should be monitored closely and delays in needed intubation avoided.

Postoperative Respiratory Failure/Insufficiency

Both CPAP and NIV have been used in two ways for postoperative patients: to prevent postoperative complications after high-risk surgeries and to treat frank postoperative respiratory failure. When used prophylactically after major abdominal surgery[36] or thoracoabdominal aneurysm repair,[37] CPAP (10 cm H_2O) reduces the incidence of hypoxemia, pneumonia, atelectasis, and intubations compared with standard treatment. Prophylactic use of NIV reduces the occurrence of restrictive lung syndrome in obese patients after bariatric surgery[38] and improves oxygenation following coronary artery bypass surgery.[39] In the only randomized study of NIV in patients with postoperative respiratory failure, post–lung resection patients had reduced intubation and mortality rates if treated with NIV compared with standard management.[13] Although these studies strongly support the idea that NIV is useful in the postoperative setting to prevent and treat respiratory complications and failure, it is difficult to make specific recommendations because of the different surgeries and positive-pressure techniques evaluated.

Do Not Intubate Status

NIV to treat DNI and palliative care patients has been controversial because some argue that there is little to lose by trying NIV in a dying patient and others counter that this is apt to add to patient discomfort and prolong suffering in a patient's final hours. Prospective cohort series[40,41] demonstrate that many DNI patients treated with NIV actually survive the hospitalization, depending on the diagnosis. In one series, 43% of 114 such patients survived to hospital discharge, 75% for CHF patients and 53% for COPD patients, whereas hospital survivals for patients with pneumonia or an underlying malignancy were in the range of 25%. The presence of a cough and an awake mental status also imparted a favorable prognosis (25%). Thus it is possible to identify, on the basis of diagnosis and some simple clinical observations, patients with a favorable chance of surviving the hospitalization, and NIV could be used in these as a form of life support with the hope of "bridging" them through their acute illness. There might also be reasons to use NIV in patients with poor prognoses for survival if the goal is to palliate—to alleviate dyspnea or prolong the dying process slightly so that the patient has time to settle affairs or say goodbye to loved ones. As recommended by a recent consensus statement by a Society of Critical Care Medicine task force on NIV, it is necessary for patient, family, and caregivers to be clear on these goals and to cease promptly if the goals aren't being accomplished.[42]

Other Acute Applications of Noninvasive Ventilation

Fiberoptic Bronchoscopy

In separate randomized trials, CPAP alone (up to 7.5 cm H_2O) and NIV improved oxygenation and reduced postprocedure respiratory failure in patients with severe hypoxemia undergoing bronchoscopy compared with those receiving conventional O_2 supplementation.[43,44] Successful bronchoscopy using NIV has also been reported in hypercapnic COPD patients with pneumonia.[45] The evidence supports the idea that NIV improves gas exchange and reduces potential complications during fiberoptic bronchoscopy, especially when risks of intubation are deemed high such as in immunocompromised patients or in those with bleeding diatheses. However, patients must be monitored closely and the caregiver team must be prepared for the possible need for emergent intubation.

Preoxygenation Before Intubation

A recent randomized trial of NIV in critically ill patients with hypoxic respiratory failure showed that preoxygenation with NIV before intubation improved O_2 saturation during and after intubation and decreased the incidence of O_2 desaturations below 80% during intubation.[46] This approach is promising but should be further studied before routine use can be recommended. This also begs the question whether, if NIV improves oxygenation substantially, intubation was really necessary in all of the patients.

SELECTION GUIDELINES FOR NONINVASIVE VENTILATION IN ACUTE RESPIRATORY FAILURE

Determinants of Success/Failure

Selection of appropriate patients for NIV is critical for optimizing success rates and deriving benefit. Knowledge of factors that predict success or failure is helpful in selecting good candidates for NIV. Such factors compiled from previous studies are shown in Box 21-2. In effect, the predictors indicate that patients who are most likely to succeed with NIV have incipient, but not far advanced, respiratory failure. They suggest that there is a "window of opportunity" for implementation of NIV when success is most likely. NIV should be started when

BOX 21-2 *Predictors of Success of Noninvasive Ventilation in Acute Respiratory Failure*

Cooperative patient
Intact neurologic function
Good synchrony with ventilator
APACHE II score not too high (<29)
pH > 7.25
Intact dentition
Air leaking well-controlled
Able to control secretions
Within first 2 hours of NIV use*:
- Reduced respiratory rate (<30/min)
- Reduced accessory muscle use
- Improved gas exchange ($Pa{O_2}/FI{O_2}$ > 150)

*Strongest predictors of success.

patients have evidence of acute respiratory distress and increased Acute Physiology and Chronic Health Evaluation II (APACHE II) scores, but not too late, when patients are approaching respiratory arrest, have very advanced CO_2 retention and acidemia, have high APACHE II scores, and are unable to cooperate.

Predictors of success differ slightly between patients with hypercapnic and hypoxemic forms of respiratory failure. A chart to predict failure of COPD patients on NIV identified pH < 7.25, respiratory rate = 35, APACHE II score > 29, and Glasgow Coma Scale score = 11 as independent predictors,[47] whereas a recent prospective multicenter study on NIV to treat patients with ARDS identified a simplified acute physiology score (SAPS) II score of = 34 and a $Pa{O_2}/FI{O_2}$ ratio = 175 after the first hour as independent predictors.[48] In both analyses, the response to NIV after the first hour or two had more predictive value than baseline values.

In hypercapnic respiratory failure, a rise in pH and improving mental status (presumably reflecting a drop in $Pa{CO_2}$) predicts success, whereas, not surprisingly, a substantial early improvement in oxygenation bodes well in patients with hypoxemic respiratory failure. These observations highlight the importance of a "2-hour checkpoint" after which, if the patient is not improving sufficiently, prompt intubation should be contemplated rather than risk further deterioration and the need for a riskier emergent intubation.

Selection Process

The selection process for **noninvasive positive-pressure ventilation (NPPV)** in acute respiratory failure is based on criteria used in randomized controlled trials and these are listed in Box 21-3. This is

BOX 21-3 *Selection Guidelines for Use of Noninvasive Ventilation to Treat Acute Respiratory Failure*

1. Appropriate diagnosis with potential reversibility over hours to days*
2. Ascertain need for ventilatory assistance
   a. Moderate to severe respiratory distress
   b. Tachypnea (>24/min for COPD, >30/min for hypoxemia)
   c. Accessory muscle use or abdominal paradox
   d. Blood gas abnormality
   e. pH < 7.35, $Pa{CO_2}$ > 45, or
   f. $Pa{O_2}/FI{O_2}$ < 200
3. Exclude patients with contraindications to NPPV
   a. Respiratory arrest/apnea
   b. Medically unstable (hemodynamic instability, transmural myocardial ischemia, unstable angina or arrhythmia, massive upper gastrointestinal bleed)
   c. Unable to protect airway
   d. Excessive secretions
   e. Uncooperative or agitated
   f. Unable to fit mask
   g. Recent upper airway or gastrointestinal surgery

COPD, Chronic obstructive pulmonary disease; *$Pa{CO_2}$,* arterial carbon dioxide; *$Pa{O_2}/FI{O_2}$,* arterial oxygen/inspired oxygen ratio; *NPPV,* noninvasive positive-pressure ventilation.

a simple two-step process, the first of which is to identify patients who need ventilatory assistance on the basis of clinical and blood gas indicators. Patients with milder derangements are likely do well without ventilatory assistance.

The second step excludes patients needing ventilatory assistance but who would be better managed invasively. Box 21-3 also lists contraindications to NIV, most of which are relative. Judgment must be exercised when deciding whether patients have excessive secretions or medical instability or uncooperativeness. Sedation may help to enhance cooperativeness. Hypercapnic coma and severe obtundation are no longer considered contraindications. Patients with hypercapnic coma (Glasgow Coma Scale score < 8) have success and mortality rates with NPPV that are equivalent to those of similar noncomatose patients.[49]

The underlying cause and potential reversibility of the acute respiratory failure are also important considerations in patient selection. In this regard, NPPV may be viewed as a "crutch" that assists the patient through a critical interval of hours or days, allowing time for other therapies, such as diuretics, bronchodilators, or corticosteroids to act. Severe, less reversible forms of respiratory failure that will require prolonged periods of ventilatory support, such as ARDS with multiorgan dysfunction, should be managed invasively.

LONG-TERM APPLICATIONS OF NONINVASIVE VENTILATION

Restrictive Thoracic Disease

Patients with chronic hypoventilation syndromes due to neuromuscular disease, chest wall or spinal deformity, and obesity hypoventilation syndrome (OHS) respond gradually over a few weeks to initiation of nocturnal NIV. The benefits consist of improved symptoms and gas exchange, better sleep, and resolution of cor pulmonale (if initially present). Although no studies have yet directly compared nasal and mouthpiece NPPV, mouthpiece NPPV may be used for long-term ventilatory support in patients with severe neuromuscular diseases who have virtually no measurable vital capacity.[50]

Temporary withdrawal of nocturnal nasal ventilation from patients with chronic respiratory failure caused by restrictive thoracic diseases results in worsening nocturnal gas exchange, daytime symptoms, and sleep quality, offering strong evidence that NPPV is effective in reversing nocturnal hypoventilation and improving symptoms in these patients.[51,52] More recently a randomized, controlled trial of NPPV for patients with amyotrophic lateral sclerosis (ALS) showed a 205-day survival advantage compared with controls in those with intact bulbar function. These patients also had improvements in quality of life and sleep-related symptoms. Patients with impaired bulbar function experienced no survival advantage but did improve symptomatically.[53] Predictors of a favorable response to NIV for ALS patients were orthopnea and hypercapnia.[54]

Long-term follow-up studies on several hundred patients using NIV for 3 to 5 years have observed very favorable rates for NIV continuation (and hence survival) among patients with postpolio syndrome, most myopathies, and kyphoscoliosis.[55,56] Survivals for ALS were less favorable because the underlying disease progresses more rapidly. Thus the evidence clearly shows multiple benefits for NPPV in patients with restrictive thoracic disease, establishing it as the ventilatory modality of first choice for these patients if there are no contraindications.

Chronic Obstructive Pulmonary Disease

The most controversial long-term application of NIV has been for severe "stable" COPD. This application was first proposed as a way to rest the mechanically disadvantaged respiratory muscles in patients with severe COPD that were thought to be chronically fatigued. Early trials found that intermittent daytime sessions using negative-pressure wrap ventilators improved daytime gas exchange and inspiratory and expiratory muscle strength in patients with severe COPD.[57] Longer-term controlled studies failed to demonstrate the same favorable effects of intermittent negative-pressure ventilation in patients with severe COPD.[58] In addition, COPD patients tolerated the wrap ventilators poorly, using them for less time daily than recommended, and having trouble sleeping during use.[59]

These disappointing results stimulated interest in the use of positive-pressure NIV for severe COPD. Two 3-month crossover trials using the BiPAP device (Respironics, Inc., Murrysville, Pa.) yielded conflicting results. In one,[60] only 7 of 19 patients completed the trial, and improvement was detected only in tests of neuropsychological function and not in nocturnal or daytime gas exchange, sleep quality, pulmonary functions, exercise tolerance, or symptoms. In the other study, 14 of 18 patients completed the study, and NIV improved nocturnal and daytime gas exchange, total sleep time, and quality of life scores.[61] The substantial differences in baseline characteristics of patients entering these trials may explain the conflicting results. Patients entering the favorable study had greater hypercarbia ($Pa\text{CO}_2$ 56 mm Hg versus 46 mm Hg) and more nocturnal O_2 desaturations despite having less severe airway obstruction (FEV_1 0.81 L versus 0.54 L) than patients in the unfavorable trial. This supports the hypothesis that the subgroup of patients most likely to benefit from NIV is that with substantial daytime CO_2 retention ($Pa\text{CO}_2 > 50$ to 55 mm Hg) and nocturnal O_2 desaturations. A recent controlled trial of COPD patients with chronic retention ($Pa\text{CO}_2 > 50$ mm Hg) demonstrated less increase in $Pa\text{CO}_2$, less deterioration of quality of life, and a trend toward fewer hospital days after 2 years of nocturnal NIV compared with O_2-treated controls.[62] Only 47 patients completed the trial out of 90 enrolled.

Thus compared with O_2 therapy alone, NIV maintains gas exchange and quality of life and probably reduces the need for hospitalization in patients with severe stable COPD who have substantial CO_2 retention. However, the evidence is not highly conclusive and patient adherence with the therapy remains a major challenge.

Obesity Hypoventilation

Obesity hypoventilation syndrome (OHS) is the combination of hypercapnia and obesity (BMI > 30) in the absence of other causes for hypoventilation, such as hypothyroidism or neuromuscular disease. Obesity has reached epidemic proportions in many Western countries and OHS has become a very common reason for initiating NIV.[63] Predisposing factors for OHS include upper airway resistance due to anatomic narrowing, impairment of respiratory system mechanics related to the obesity, blunted central ventilatory drive, and deficiency of or resistance to the respiratory stimulant leptin.[64] Approximately 90% of OHS patients have underlying obstructive sleep apnea (OSA) and may respond to CPAP treatment alone.[65] Some of these patients have persisting hypoventilation despite CPAP therapy and are candidates for noninvasive positive-pressure ventilation (NPPV), which enhances nocturnal alveolar, resets the respiratory center sensitivity for CO_2, and lowers daytime $Paco_2$.

NIV also relieves clinical symptoms such as morning headache, daytime hypersomnolence, and edema; improves quality of life; and reduces the need for hospitalization in OHS patients.[66] The high inspiratory impedance encountered in some very obese individuals may necessitate high inflation pressures to adequately treat OHS. The mean inspiratory and expiratory pressures in one study on patients with an average body mass index (BMI) of 42 were 18 and 7 cm H_2O, respectively.[63] Evidence and guidelines to assist with the decision between CPAP and NIV are lacking, but most clinicians start with CPAP alone if OSA is present and NIV if OSA is lacking (and central sleep apnea/hypoventilation is presumably contributing) or hypoventilation is severe ($Paco_2$ > 50 to 55 mm Hg). Patients begun on CPAP are switched to NIV if hypoventilation fails to improve within the first few weeks to months. One small series described initiation of deteriorating OHS patients on NIV, then switching to CPAP once they were stabilized.[67]

Selection Guidelines

When to Start Noninvasive Ventilation

A number of characteristics permit selection of appropriate candidates with chronic respiratory failure for NIV (Box 21-4). Most clinicians recommend starting NIV for patients with neuromuscular disease when they have symptoms attributable to nocturnal hypoventilation (morning headaches) and associated poor sleep quality (daytime hypersomnolence), but before the occurrence of daytime hypoventilation and well before the onset of a respiratory crisis. Ward et al[68] found that most patients with nocturnal hypoventilation developed daytime hypoventilation and required initiation of NIV within the next 2 years. Thus the authors recommended initiation of NIV at the onset of nocturnal hypoventilation and not to await the onset of diurnal hypoventilation. Medicare guidelines permit initiation even when patients are asymptomatic if they have severe respiratory muscle weakness or restriction (see Box 21-4), but adherence may be difficult in such patients if they are not motivated by the desire for symptom relief. Secondary considerations for initiation of NIV include a history of repeated hospitalizations for bouts of respiratory failure.

Indications for Noninvasive Ventilation in Obesity Hyperventilation Syndrome and Severe, Stable Chronic Obstructive Pulmonary Disease

Patients with OHS should have a polysomnogram and should be placed on CPAP if they are found to have OSA. If they have substantial CO_2 retention, arterial blood gases should be monitored, and if there is no improvement, positive inspiratory pressure (i.e., NIV) should be added to enhance ventilatory assistance. For reimbursement, improvement on NIV should be documented using a repeat sleep study or arterial blood gas, according to Medicare guidelines.

For COPD patients, the threshold value for CO_2 retention is higher than for restrictive thoracic diseases ($Paco_2 \geq 52$ mm Hg). This is because of several studies that failed to show benefit of NIV among normocapnic or mildly hypercapnic COPD patients. Evidence of nocturnal hypoventilation should be shown, as evidenced by sustained nocturnal O_2 desaturation on the usual level of O_2 supplementation, and OSA should be excluded on clinical grounds (see Box 21-4).

CONTRAINDICATIONS TO LONG-TERM NONINVASIVE VENTILATION

Patients should be excluded from consideration for NIV if they are unable to protect their airway

BOX 21-4 *Guidelines for Initiating Noninvasive Ventilation in Patients With Chronic Respiratory Failure* Restrictive Thoracic Disorders*

1. Symptomatic despite optimal medical therapy† and
2. Severe pulmonary dysfunction:
   a. FVC < 50% predicted or
   b. Maximal inspiratory pressure > –60 cm H_2O or
3. Gas exchange disturbance:
   a. Chronic CO_2 retention ($PaCO_2$ > 45 mm Hg) or
   b. Nocturnal hypoventilation (as evidenced by O_2 sat <88% for >5 consecutive min while breathing room air) or
4. Other considerations:
   a. Repeated hospitalizations for hypercapnic respiratory failure

Chronic obstructive pulmonary disease

1. Symptomatic despite optimal medical therapy and
2. Gas exchanges disturbance:
   a. Chronic CO_2 retention ($PaCO_2$ ≥ 52 mm Hg) and
   b. Nocturnal hypoventilation (as evidenced by O_2 sat < 89% for ≥5 consecutive min while breathing usual FIO_2) and
3. Obstructive sleep apnea excluded (on clinical grounds; sleep study needed only if clinically indicated; if OSA present, CPAP indicated initially)
4. Other considerations:
   a. Repeated hospitalizations for hypercapnic respiratory failure

Obesity hypoventilation/central sleep apnea

1. Sleep polysomnogram showing OSA or central sleep apnea
2. If OSA, failure to improve on CPAP alone
3. If central sleep apnea, sustained desaturations (O_2 sat < 89% for >5 consecutive min)
4. Evidence of improvement in nocturnal hypoventilation (by oximetry or polysomnogram)

Adapted from Hill NS: Noninvasive mechanical ventilation. In Albert RK, Spiro SG, Jett J, editors: Clinical respiratory medicine, ed 2, St. Louis, 2005, Mosby.

*Based on Medicare guidelines for reimbursement of noninvasive ventilation. Medicare guidelines do not recognize repeated hospitalizations as a reason for reimbursement and appeal may be necessary if that is justification.

†O_2 therapy alone may exacerbate CO_2 retention and should be avoided in hypercapnic patients with restrictive thoracic disorders.

BOX 21-5 *Contraindications to Long-Term Noninvasive Ventilation*

- Uncooperative, unmotivated patient
- Inadequate financial or caregiver resources
- Rapidly progressive neuromuscular disease with bulbar dysfunction
- Unable to protect airway
- Uncontrollable secretions
- Unable to fit mask

adequately because of swallowing impairment or excessive secretions, particularly if combined with a weakened cough mechanism (Box 21-5). If such patients desire aggressive support, they should undergo tracheostomy placement. The patient's diagnosis is also an important consideration. Those with stable or slowly progressive neuromuscular diseases or chest wall deformities are the best candidates. Others, such as those with hypoventilation due to central or obstructive sleep apnea who have failed a trial of nasal CPAP, are also good candidates. On the other hand, patients with rapidly progressive neuromuscular processes such as Guillain-Barré syndrome, particularly if there is upper airway involvement, are poor candidates.

TECHNIQUES AND EQUIPMENT FOR NONINVASIVE VENTILATION

Noninvasive Positive-Pressure Ventilation

NPPV consists of a positive-pressure ventilator connected by way of tubing to a mask or "interface" that applies positive air pressure to the nose or mouth, or both. Relative advantages and disadvantages of different masks are shown in Table 21-1.

TABLE 21-1 *Advantages and Disadvantages of Different Interfaces*

	NASAL	ORONASAL	HELMET	MOUTHPIECE
Comfort	+++	++	+++	++
Claustrophobia	+	++	++	+
Rebreathing	+	++	+++	+
Lowers CO_2	+	++	+	++
Permits expectoration	++	+	+	++
Permits speech*	++	+	+	+
Permits eating*	++	+	+	+
Noisy	+	+	+++	+

+, Less likely; ++, more likely; +++, very likely.
*During use.

Interfaces

Nasal Masks

Nasal masks are the most commonly used interface for chronic respiratory failure because they are relatively comfortable and permit normal speech, swallowing, and expectoration. In a study on naïve subjects with chronic restrictive or obstructive conditions, Navalesi et al[69] found that traditional nasal masks were sensed as more comfortable than nasal prongs or full face masks, but were less efficient than full face masks at eliminating CO_2. Manufacturers now offer numerous modifications of the nasal mask that fit into several basic categories.

Standard Nasal Masks. Standard nasal masks were initially developed to provide CPAP for OSA and consist of triangular clear plastic domes that fit over the nose (Figure 21-1). A soft cuff makes contact with the skin around the perimeter of the nose to form an air seal. These masks must be properly fitted to minimize pressure over the bridge of the nose, which may cause redness, skin irritation, and occasionally ulceration. Thin silicone flaps are used to create an effective air seal with minimal strap tension, and forehead "spacers" are often used to minimize pressure on the bridge of the nose. Strap systems that hold the masks in place are important for patient comfort. Various approaches have been used to enhance patient comfort, including an additional thin plastic flap or a baffle system (Figure 21-2) to further reduce the strap tension necessary to maintain an air seal and gel-containing seals, some that have heat molding capabilities and have also been introduced to enhance patient comfort.

Nasal Pillows. Nasal pillows or "seals" consist of small rubber cones that are inserted directly into the nostrils (Figure 21-3). By moving the air sealing surfaces away from the eyes, these reduce claustrophobic reactions and permit use of eyeglasses during use. They are helpful for patients with nasal bridge irritation or ulceration caused by standard nasal masks because they eliminate contact with the bridge of the nose. However, they can cause irritation in the nostrils, so some patients alternate between different types of masks as a way of minimizing discomfort.

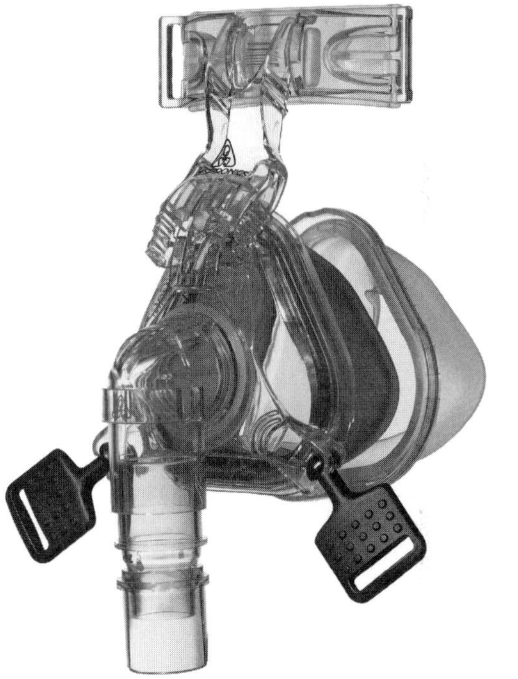

FIGURE 21-1 Example of standard nasal mask. Gel cushion enhances comfort on forehead. Comfort Gel Nasal Mask. (Courtesy Respironics, Inc.)

Nasal Minimasks. These were developed for patients unhappy with the size of nasal masks and pressure of nasal "pillows" on the nostrils (Figure 21-4). They are designed to cover the nostrils with a minimal amount of material, but they may be less secure than the other masks, dislodging when patients move because they are often held in place using only strap connections.

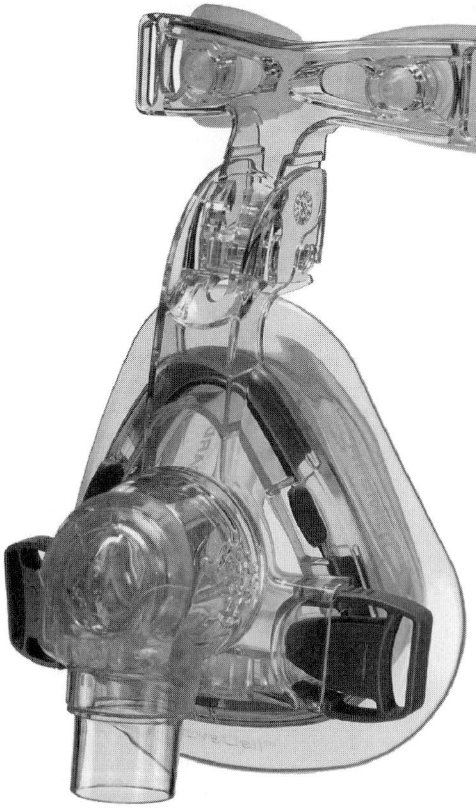

FIGURE 21-2 Nasal mask with baffle on silicon seal to minimize leaking under mask seal. (Courtesy ResMed, Inc.)

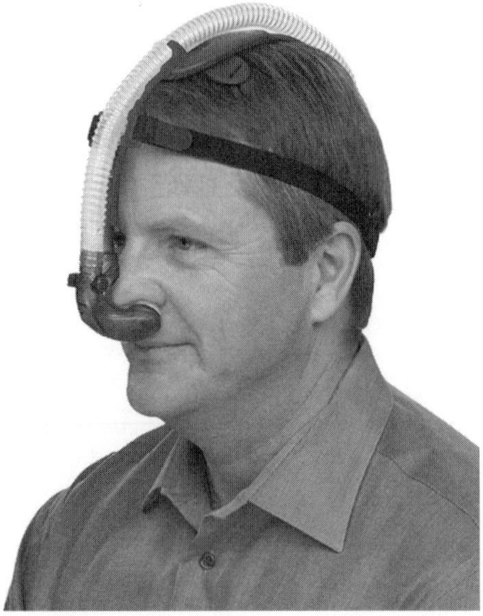

FIGURE 21-3 Nasal "pillows" or "prongs" fit into nostrils. (Courtesy Puritan Bennett, Pleasanton, Calif.)

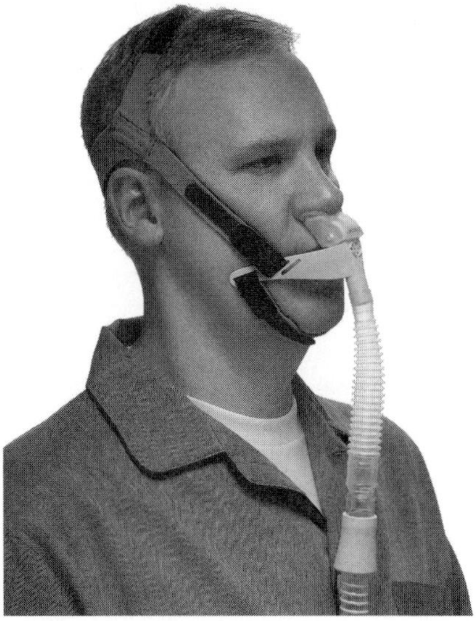

FIGURE 21-4 Minimask fits snugly on the nose and eliminates seal over nasal bridge. (Courtesy Respironics, Inc.)

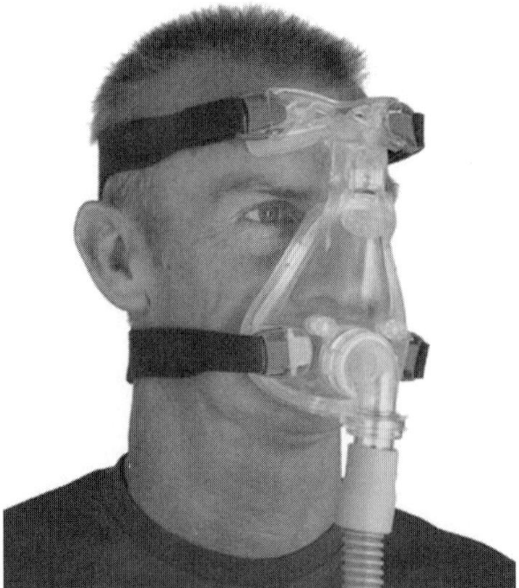

FIGURE 21-5 Oronasal mask. (Courtesy ResMed, Inc.)

Custom Kits. Although kits for custom molding have been available commercially, they are expensive and require time and skill for successful application. They were used more often in the past when fewer mask choices were available but are rarely used now because a suitable commercially available mask can almost always be found.

Oronasal or Full Face Masks. These masks cover both the nose and mouth (Figure 21-5). Their main advantage over nasal masks is that they reduce air leaking through the mouth most, an advantage particularly in the acute setting. The air seals are

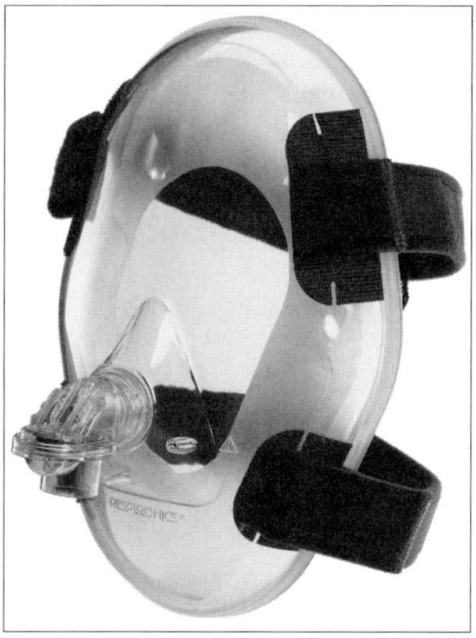

FIGURE 21-6 **Total Face Mask seals around perimeter of face, away from nose and mouth.** (Courtesy Respironics, Inc.)

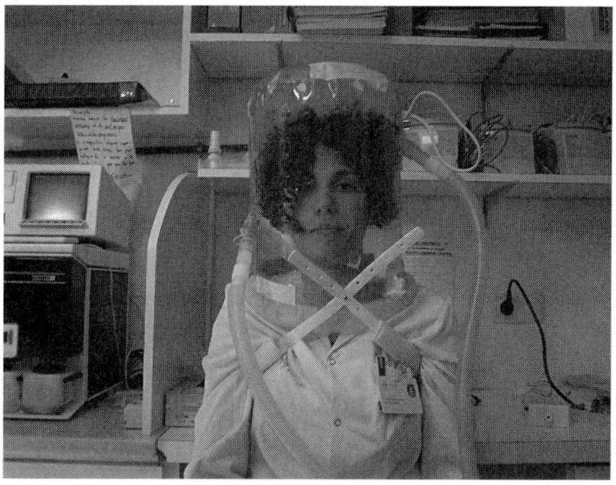

FIGURE 21-7 **Helmet interface.** (From Albert RK, Slutsky A, Ranieri VM et al: Clinical critical care medicine, Philadelphia, 2006, Mosby.)

similar to those of nasal masks, attempting to maximize comfort and minimize air leaks. They have built-in valves to prevent rebreathing and asphyxiation in the event of ventilator malfunction. Because of concerns that vomiting into a full face mask could cause aspiration, full face masks have straps that allow rapid removal. Some have incorporated designs that attempt to stabilize the chin to minimize air leaking under the air seal. Compared with the nasal mask, full face masks interfere more with speech and eating, have more dead space, and are less comfortable. However, they are more efficient at removing CO_2 and for this reason are usually preferred over nasal masks to treat acute respiratory failure.

The Total Face Mask (Respironics, Inc.) (Figure 21-6) is a larger version of an oronasal mask that seals around the perimeter of the face.[70] It removes the sealing gasket from the nose and mouth to the perimeter of the face. It easily accommodates most facial shapes and sizes and can be rapidly applied by fastening just two Velcro straps behind the head. Although some patients find it frightening and refuse to try it, most find it comfortable and no more claustrophobic than standard oronasal masks because it has optical grade plastic at eye level.

Helmet. The helmet (Figure 21-7) has been used primarily in Italy and has not yet been approved for use with NIV by the FDA in the United States. It consists of an inflatable plastic cylinder that fits over the head and seals around the neck and shoulders with straps under the axillae. Studies evaluating its use in COPD patients[71] show that it is more comfortable and reduces facial ulcerations compared with a full face mask. However, it is less efficient at CO_2 removal than a full face mask and because it can cause problems with triggering and cycling during pressure support ventilation, it appears to be best suited for applying CPAP in patients with acute cardiogenic edema. To prevent rebreathing, high air flow rates are necessary, which render the helmet much noisier than the full face mask (100 dB versus 70 dB, respectively).[72] Thus although the helmet has some advantages over the full face mask, it is limited by less efficient CO_2 removal, excessive noisiness, and higher cost, even in countries where it is available.

Oral Interfaces

Commercially available oral interfaces use a mouthpiece inserted into a lip seal that is strapped tautly around the head to minimize air leakage around the air seal (Figure 21-8). A strapless version that seals using flanges that fit inside and outside of the lips is custom-made at certain centers. It can be easily expectorated if necessary and has been shown to be quite useful for long-term, full-time ventilatory assistance in patients with severe neuromuscular disease, some of whom have little or no measurable vital capacity.[73] For daytime use, mouthpieces can be mounted on a goose-neck device on a wheelchair, permitting patients to remain mobile while receiving ventilatory assistance.

Headgear

The straps used to hold the interface in place are important for comfort. The number of connections

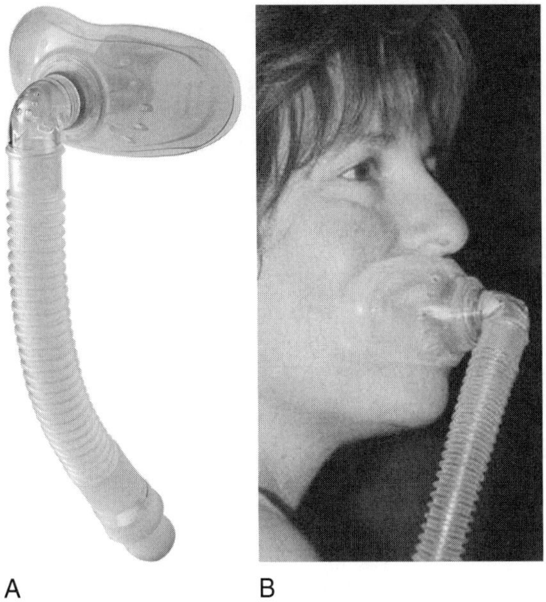

FIGURE 21-8 A, Oral mouth seal. **B,** Oral mouth seal in position on a patient. (Courtesy Fisher & Paykell Healthcare, Laguna Hills, Calif.)

BOX 21-6 *Important Parameters to Monitor During Noninvasive Ventilation*

Subjective responses
- Patient comfort
- Discomfort related to the mask
- Respiratory distress

Vital signs and physical findings
- Respiratory and heart rate
- Blood pressure
- Ability to cough and raise secretions
- Accessory muscle use

Ventilator function
- Patient-ventilator synchrony
- Tidal volume ≥6 ml/kg
- Air leaking
- Waveforms (if available)

Gas exchange
- Continuous oximetry
- Change in $PaCO_2$ if hypercapnic
- Change in pH

varies from two for some "minimasks" to five for some oronasal masks. The more connections, the more stable the interface, but claustrophobia becomes a concern. Most strap systems use soft, stretchable material fastened with Velcro, but abrasions can occur if the edges are too rough. For long-term applications, head caps may help to hold straps in place. Minimizing strap tension just to the point of controlling air leaks can enhance comfort.

Ventilators for Positive-Pressure Noninvasive Ventilation

NPPV may be administered using **critical care ventilators** (designed mainly for invasive ventilation in the acute setting), ventilators designed especially for acute applications of NIV, or portable positive-pressure ventilators designed mainly for use in the home. The choice of ventilator depends largely on practitioner preference and patient needs. For example, some practitioners prefer the enhanced alarm and monitoring capabilities of critical care ventilators for acute applications of NIV. For chronic use in the home, simplicity and portability are important features, where most practitioners prefer portable pressure-limited devices.

Critical Care Ventilators

Many of the microprocessor-controlled ventilators currently used in critical care units can be adapted for NIV. These offer an array of volume-limited or pressure-limited modes and sophisticated monitoring and alarm capabilities. Advantages over so-called "bilevel" positive-pressure devices include the presence of O_2 blenders, accurate tracking of tidal and minute volumes, and a dual limb circuit with an active exhalation valve that minimizes rebreathing (Box 21-6). Most practitioners use the pressure support mode with these ventilators because of enhanced comfort,[74] combining it with PEEP. These ventilators are not tolerant of air leaks that inevitably occur with NIV, causing difficulty with triggering and cycling, and triggering annoying alarms. Many newer critical care ventilators incorporate "NIV" modes that automatically improve leak tolerance and compensating abilities, disable nuisance alarms, and permit adjustments to limit inspiratory time. Masks and circuitry for the application of NIV via critical care ventilators should not have built-in exhalation valves that will interfere with proper function. Some mask manufacturers have dyed plastic parts of masks meant for use with critical ventilators blue so that they can be easily identified.

Portable Volume-Limited and Hybrid Ventilators

Portable volume-limited ventilators (Figure 21-9) are used to administer NIV mainly to patients with

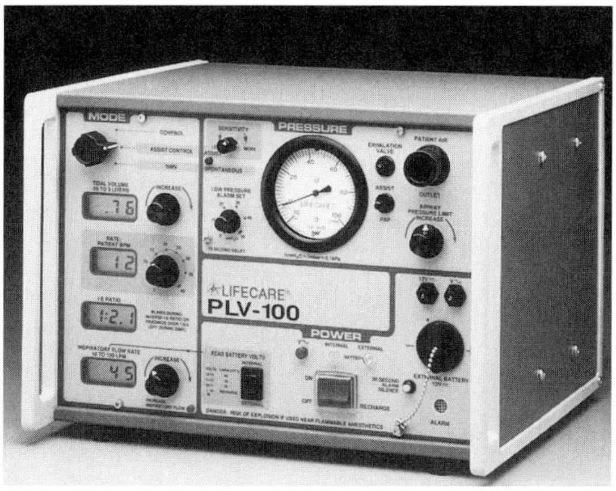

FIGURE 21-9 Portable volume-limited ventilator. (PLV-100, Courtesy Respironics, Inc.)

chronic respiratory failure. These are more commonly used to administer ventilation via a tracheostomy for patients in a chronic care facility or at home, but when used to deliver NIV, are usually set in the assist-control mode to allow for spontaneous patient triggering, and the backup rate is usually set at slightly below spontaneous patient breathing rate. Currently available volume-limited ventilators have more alarm- and pressure-generating capabilities than most portable pressure-limited ventilators, and they may be better suited to patients in need of full-time ventilation or those with severe chest wall deformity or obesity who need high inflation pressures. They also permit "stacking" of breaths—the administration of multiple breaths to a patient who closes the glottis in-between ventilator breaths to achieve a large tidal volume that can be used to achieve higher air flows to enhance cough.[75] This technique is of greatest use to neuromuscular disease patients with weakened expiratory muscles but intact bulbar function.

"Hybrid" ventilators (Figure 21-10) offer both pressure- and volume-limited modes and are suitable for use in both the acute and long-term settings. Examples of such ventilators include the LTV series (Pulmonetics, Inc., Minneapolis, Minn.), Achieva (Puritan Bennett, Inc., Pleasanton, Calif.), and HT50 (Newport, Inc., Newport Beach, Calif.). Because some of these devices are no larger than a laptop computer, they are popular among patients who wish to receive ventilatory assistance while sitting in a wheelchair. They have the sophisticated alarm and monitoring capabilities of critical care ventilators and can be built with optional O_2 blenders, but are more portable and usually cost considerably less. However, they cost considerably more than "bilevel" positive-pressure devices and have not been used as often to deliver NIV.

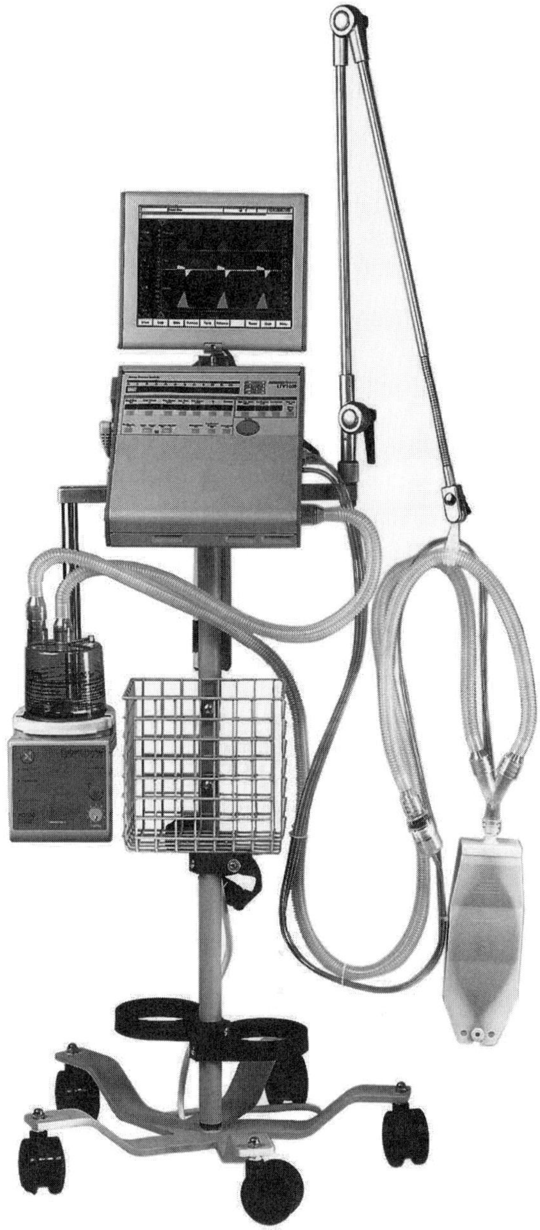

FIGURE 21-10 "Hybrid" ventilator. (LTV 1000, Courtesy Pulmonetics, Inc.)

Bilevel Pressure-Limited Ventilators

Portable ventilators that deliver pressure assist or pressure support ventilation (often referred to as "bilevel" devices) have seen increasing use in recent years. The prototype "bilevel" device was the "BiPAP" (Respironics, Inc., Murrysville, Pa.), introduced during the

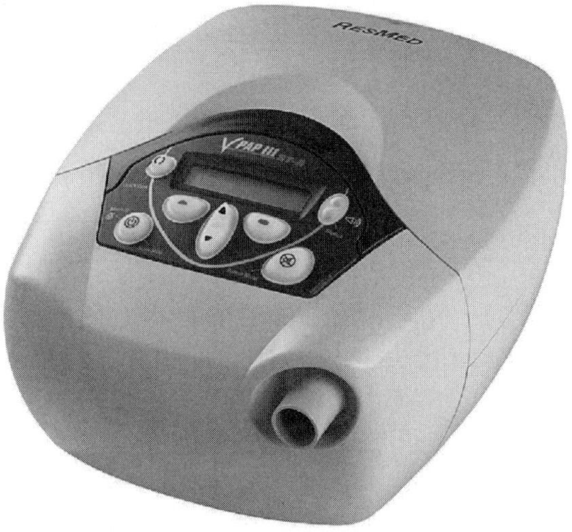

FIGURE 21-11 **Portable "bilevel" ventilator, suitable for home or hospital use.** (VPAP ST-A, Courtesy ResMed, Inc.)

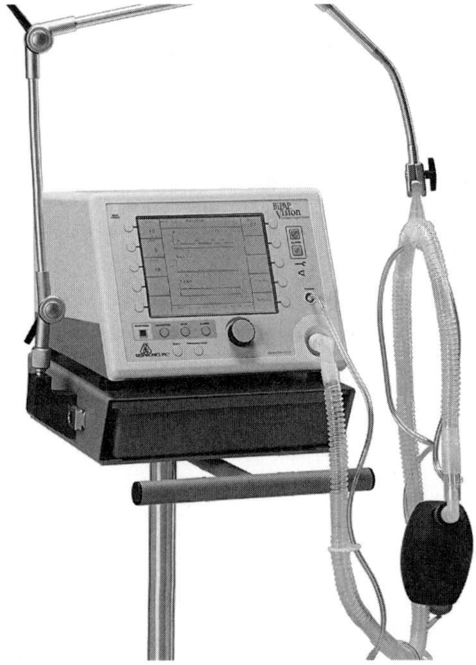

FIGURE 21-12 **"Bilevel" ventilator designed for acute applications of NIV. Has graphic screen and O_2 blender.** (BiPAP Vision, Courtesy Respironics, Inc.)

late 1980s,[78] but numerous versions of this approach are now available from many manufacturers (Figure 21-11).

"Bilevel" devices deliver a preset inspiratory positive airway pressure (IPAP) that is combined with positive end-expiratory pressure (PEEP or EPAP). The difference between the IPAP and EPAP is the level of inspiratory assistance, or pressure support. Pressure support modes provide sensitive inspiratory triggering and expiratory cycling mechanisms (usually by sensing changes in flow), potentially allowing excellent patient-ventilator synchrony, reducing diaphragmatic work, and improving patient comfort.[77] Because these devices are lighter (5 to 10 kg), more compact (<0.025 m^3), and have fewer alarms than critical care or portable volume-limited ventilators, they are preferred for patients requiring only nocturnal use in the home. Most have limited IPAP (up to 20 to 35 cm H_2O, depending on the ventilator) and oxygenation capabilities and lack alarms or battery backup systems. Also, unlike volume-limited ventilators, "bilevel" pressure-limited devices are able to increase inspiratory airflow to compensate for air leaks, thereby potentially providing better support of gas exchange during leakage. O_2 supplementation is via a T-connector in the ventilator tubing or connector directly in the mask, the latter providing a slightly higher FIO_2. Even at flow rates of 15 L/min, the maximum recommended by manufacturers, the FIO_2 is only 45% to 50%,[78] insufficient for many patients with hypoxemic respiratory failure.

The BiPAP Vision (Respironics, Inc.) (Figure 21-12) was designed for both invasive and noninvasive acute care applications, although it is used mainly for noninvasive FIO_2. Equipped with an O_2 blender, it provides high FIO_2s and has more sophisticated alarm and monitoring systems than the traditional "bilevels" (including a graphic screen). It also features an adjustable rise time (the time taken to reach target inspiratory pressure) and inspiratory time limits that can help with comfort and synchrony during NIV. Because of these features, the Vision has been well received as a device for the administration of NIV in acute care hospitals.

Because they have a single ventilator tube, rebreathing may occur during use of "bilevel" ventilators that could interfere with the ability to augment alveolar ventilation.[79] The rebreathing can be minimized by using masks with in-mask exhalation ports, which are associated with less rebreathing than in-circuit valves,[80] use of nonrebreathing valves, or EPAP pressures of 4 cm H_2O or greater, which ensure higher bias flows during exhalation.[79] In one study of patients receiving long-term nasal ventilation, a valve designed to minimize rebreathing (Plateau Valve, Respironics, Inc.) did not lower nocturnal transcutaneous PCO_2 or daytime $PaCO_2$

compared with a standard in-tubing exhalation valve, probably because of frequent air leaking through the mouth.[81]

Body Ventilators

In the past, NIV was provided by so-called "body" ventilators that achieved popularity during the polio epidemics of the 1920s through 1950s. These include negative-pressure ventilators and ventilators that worked via the effect of gravity on diaphragm motion (abdominal displacement ventilators).[82] Negative-pressure ventilators include tank ventilators (such as the iron lung) and the smaller, more portable wrap (or jacket) and cuirass (or shell) ventilators. The wrap ventilator consists of an impermeable nylon jacket suspended by a rigid chest piece that fits over the chest and abdomen. The cuirass ventilator is a rigid plastic or metal dome fitted over the chest and abdomen. Negative-pressure ventilators expand the lungs by intermittently applying a subatmospheric pressure to the chest wall and abdomen, and expiration occurs passively by elastic recoil of the lung and chest wall. The tank is the most efficient and the cuirass the least efficient of these ventilators.

Abdominal displacement ventilators include the rocking bed, which rocks up and down through an arc of 40 degrees with the fulcrum at hip level. With the patient lying supine on the mattress, it uses gravity to slide the abdominal contents and hence the diaphragm cephalad and caudad. The intermittent pressure abdominal respirator, or pneumobelt, is worn by a sitting patient and consists of a corset that holds an inflatable bladder firmly against the anterior abdomen. Inflation of the bladder compresses the abdominal contents, forcing the diaphragm upward, and bladder deflation permits gravity to pull the diaphragm back down. Both of these devices work best in patients with diaphragm paralysis who have a relatively normal body habitus. Because of their bulkiness and inconvenience relative to positive-pressure NIV, these devices and the negative-pressure ventilators are used rarely today, although some centers in Italy and Spain still use them mainly for patients with acute exacerbations of COPD.[83]

Other Types of Ventilatory Assistance

Although not technically forms of "mechanical" ventilation, diaphragm pacing and glossopharyngeal breathing are ventilatory methods used in selected patients to enhance independence from mechanical ventilation. **Diaphragm pacers** consist of a radiofrequency transmitter and antenna that signal a surgically implanted receiver and electrode to stimulate the phrenic nerve. An intact phrenic nerve and diaphragm are usually required for successful application, but intercostal nerve implantation can be used when the phrenic nerves are damaged. Patients with high spinal cord quadriplegia and chronic hypoventilation, especially children, are the main users of pacers, to gain freedom from invasive positive-pressure ventilation.[84]

Glossopharyngeal or "frog" breathing uses intermittent gulping motions of the tongue and pharyngeal muscles to force air into the trachea and saw wide use by patients during the polio epidemics.[85] The technique can be used to provide freedom from mechanical ventilation for periods of up to several hours, even in severely compromised patients. Use is limited to patients who have intact upper airway musculature, more or less normal lungs and chest walls, and the ability to learn the technique. Good candidates include those with high spinal cord injuries, postpolio syndrome, and appropriate patients with other neuromuscular diseases.

APPLICATION OF NONINVASIVE POSITIVE-PRESSURE VENTILATION

Initiation

Interface and Ventilator Selection

Techniques for initiation of NPPV are similar in the acute and long-term settings except that the level of urgency differs. In both settings, initiation must be tailored for each individual patient. In the acute setting, the interface and ventilator must be selected rapidly, so it is advisable to attach a **mask bag** containing a variety of types and sizes of masks and straps to a noninvasive ventilation cart or to use masks that fit most individuals and can be rapidly applied. In the chronic setting, it is also useful to have a variety of interfaces readily available, but mask interchanges can be made over periods of days to weeks rather than minutes. In both settings, implementation by experienced practitioners who can impart a sense of confidence and reassurance is helpful.

The oronasal mask is usually the preferred initial choice for acute applications of NIV. A randomized trial observed that the nasal mask was associated with a greater initial intolerance rate related to mouth leaks.[86] On the other hand, the nasal mask, if tolerated, was as effective as the oronasal mask in avoiding intubation and may be preferable in patients with claustrophobia or the need to expectorate frequently.

For long-term applications, the nasal mask is rated as more comfortable by patients.[69] Thus transitioning from an oronasal to a nasal mask should be contemplated after the first few days if NPPV use is to continue.

Proper mask fit is key for the successful application of NIV. Selection of a mask that is too large necessitates excessive tightening of the straps to minimize air leakage. Thus a properly fitting oronasal mask should be just large enough to accommodate the nose and mouth.

With regard to ventilator selection, both pressure-limited and volume-limited ventilators have been used with similar success rates. In the acute setting, portable "bilevel" ventilators are the most commonly used to deliver NIV, at least in certain regions of the United States,[87] although "bilevel" devices especially designed for acute applications of NIV such as the Vision have been gaining popularity. Critical care ventilators are used less often, but are suitable choices.

In the long-term setting, portable "bilevel" devices are the most commonly used because of their low cost, ease of use, and portability. Portable volume-limited ventilators are used mainly for patients with continuous need for mechanical ventilation because of their enhanced alarming capabilities and the option to stack breaths to enhance coughing.

Ventilator Settings

To begin NPPV, the technique should be explained to the patient and motivation reinforced. The mask should be placed gently on the patient's face and ventilation started. Cooperative patients may feel more comfortable if they hold the mask themselves. Initial ventilator pressures should be relatively low to enhance patient comfort and acceptance. Typical initial settings on pressure-limited ventilators are 8 to 12 cm H_2O for inspiratory and 4 to 5 cm H_2O for expiratory pressures (pressure support of 5 to 10 cm H_2O and PEEP of 4 to 5 cm H_2O). Inspiratory pressure or tidal volume should be adjusted upward as tolerated to provide adequate ventilatory assistance and alleviate respiratory distress. The aim should be to provide as much ventilatory assistance as needed without rendering the patient intolerant with excessive inspiratory pressure.

Expiratory pressure is usually kept in the 4 to 5 cm H_2O range, but may be increased to counterbalance autoPEEP in COPD patients who are struggling to trigger the ventilator, treat hypoxemia, or eliminate obstructive apneas. The difference between inspiratory and expiratory pressure is the pressure support, and it is important to remember that inspiratory pressure must be increased along with expiratory pressure to maintain the same level of pressure support. For volume-limited ventilation, initial tidal volumes range from 10 to 15 ml/kg to compensate for air leaks.

Patients with ARDS may need higher pressures to alleviate respiratory distress and achieve adequate oxygenation than hypercapnic patients. One study[88] found that pressure support levels of 10 to 15 cm H_2O with a PEEP of 5 cm H_2O were most effective at reducing dyspnea, but a higher PEEP (10 cm H_2O) was more effective at optimizing oxygenation despite worsening dyspnea. Thus optimization of pressures requires the balancing of sometimes conflicting aims: higher levels of oxygenation versus enhanced comfort and minimization of dyspnea.

The ventilator is usually set to allow patient triggering (assist-control mode). The ventilator backup rate is usually set below the spontaneous breathing rate to permit the patient to determine the breathing rate while the backup rate prevents apneas. If the aim is to entrain the patient's breathing and minimize respiratory muscle work, as may be the case during sleep in neuromuscular disease patients, the backup rate can be set higher (15 to 20/min).

In the acute setting, once the patient is synchronizing with the ventilator and appears to be tolerant, the head straps can be tightened. These should be adjusted to minimize air leakage, particularly into the eyes, but two fingers should still fit easily under the strap. Most manufacturers have developed ways to minimize facial trauma, such as forehead cushions and soft silicon seals, and these should be used as recommended.

General Considerations

With the exception of patients with acute pulmonary edema who have well humidified airways and usually require NIV for no more than a few hours, humidification is recommended to enhance comfort and moisten secretions.[89] For "bilevel" devices, humidification should be delivered using heated passover devices. Heat and moisture exchangers should be avoided because they interfere with triggering and cycling. O_2 supplementation is administered via the blender on critical care ventilators and some "bilevel" ventilators, or directly via a cannula connected to the mask or T-connector in the ventilator tubing when using other "bilevel" ventilators. It is adjusted to maintain the desired O_2 saturation, usually >90%. Nasogastric tubes are not used routinely, even with full face masks.

Adaptation and Monitoring

Acute Applications

For acute applications, the first hour or two are critical in achieving successful adaptation, and close monitoring is very important during this period. This should be undertaken in an ICU or step-down unit with monitoring of multiple parameters (Box 21-6). Coaching and encouragement are usually required to help the patient achieve tolerance and keep the mouth shut if a nasal mask has been selected. Synchronization with the ventilator is important to achieve reduction in breathing effort. Instructions such as "try to take slow deep breaths and let the machine breathe for you" may be helpful.

The patient's subjective response to NIV is more important than with invasive ventilation. Discomfort and agitation lead to intolerance and failure unless addressed promptly. Verbal reassurances and judicious sedation may be very helpful, but sedation should be used cautiously, titrating carefully using low doses. A recent survey of pulmonary specialists and intensivists in North America and Europe revealed that most avoided the use of sedation for NIV, citing lack of experience and fear of excessive sedation that might suppress spontaneous breathing as the major reasons.[90] Most physicians who use sedation favor either benzodiazepines or opioids singly. Studies are lacking to demonstrate the efficacy of sedation in NIV, which probably explains some of the reluctance to use it as well.

Vital signs and indices of respiratory muscle effort should improve within the first 2 hours if NIV is likely to be successful.[49,91] Respiratory and heart rates should drop promptly if adequate inspiratory support is being administered, and in patients with COPD, accessory muscle activity should abate. If these improvements fail to occur, adjustments in pressure and measures to enhance synchrony should be tried, but if unsuccessful, prompt intubation should be contemplated to avoid unnecessary delays that could precipitate a respiratory crisis.

Gas exchange should also improve promptly, another indicator of success.[49] Oxygenation is monitored continuously using pulse oximetry, with F_{IO_2} adjusted to maintain the desired O_2 saturation. Arterial blood gases should be obtained at baseline, after 1 to 2 hours, and then as clinically indicated. Initiation in dyspneic patients should not be delayed pending blood gas results, but having baseline measures is helpful in interpreting the response to therapy. In hypercapnic patients, Pa_{CO_2} need not drop rapidly as long as other indicators of response are favorable, but a persistently low pH or a substantial rise in Pa_{CO_2} despite NIV therapy should raise concerns.

The traditional "bilevel" devices lack sophisticated monitoring and alarm capabilities but even newer "bilevel" devices and critical care ventilators may provide misleading feedback in the presence of air leaks. If a reliable measure can be obtained, though, a tidal volume of 6 to 7 ml/kg should be targeted while adjusting inspiratory pressure.

Close bedside monitoring is essential until the patient's respiratory status stabilizes. Although NIV can be easily administered on general medical wards, the acuity of the patient's illness and need for close monitoring should dictate the location of administration. If a patient is alert, capable of calling for help, and stable off ventilatory assistance for at least 30 minutes, transfer to a regular medical floor can be considered. Some patients treated with NIV for acute respiratory failure should be considered for long-term home NIV, if they meet Medicare guidelines for reimbursement. Ideally, this should be nocturnal use only, but some patients with notable weakness due to neuromuscular disease may require more ventilatory assistance to maintain stability.

Long-Term Applications

In the chronic setting, adaptation requires a much longer period of time than in the acute setting, mainly because the patient must become sufficiently comfortable to sleep using the ventilator. The patient is instructed to initiate NIV at home for 1- or 2-hour trial periods during the daytime, and then to try to fall asleep after attaching the device at bedtime. The patient is encouraged to leave the equipment on as long as tolerated, but is allowed to remove it if desired. During this period, frequent contact with an experienced home respiratory therapist helps to assure proper use and adjustment. Some patients successfully sleep through the night within days of initiation, but others require several months. Occasional patients are unable to adapt successfully to NPPV, usually because of mask intolerance. In these patients, trials with alternative noninvasive ventilators, such as negative pressure or abdominal ventilators, may still be successful. Considering that a negative-pressure device may exacerbate or even induce sleep apnea,[92] sleep apnea should be excluded in such patients first.

For follow-up of long-term NIV, patients should be seen every few weeks by a physician during the initial adaptation period. At the time of office follow-up, symptoms and physical signs are assessed for evidence of nocturnal hypoventilation or cor pulmonale. Spirometry is indicated, particularly in patients with

TABLE 21-2 *Complications and Adverse Effects of Noninvasive Ventilation and Possible Remedies*

COMPLICATION/ADVERSE EFFECT	REMEDY
MASK-RELATED PROBLEMS	
Discomfort	Minimize strap tension
Nasal redness, ulceration	Check mask fit
Poor fit	Try new mask
AIR PRESSURE– AND FLOW-RELATED PROBLEMS	
Sinus and ear pain	Lower mask pressure
Nasal dryness	Humidification
Nasal congestion	Decongestants, nasal steroids
Gastrointestinal insufflation	Lower pressures, simethicone
AIR LEAKING	
Under mask	Reseat mask, tighten straps
Through mouth	Close mouth, chin straps
Into eyes/conjunctivitis	Tighten straps, new mask
ASYNCHRONY	
Failure to trigger	New ventilator
Failure to cycle	Shorten inspiratory time
Failure to ventilate	Ventilator that compensates
MAJOR COMPLICATIONS (INFREQUENT)	
Aspiration	Position head at 45 degrees
Pneumothorax	Chest tube, lower pressure
Respiratory/cardiac arrest	No delay of needed intubation

progressive neuromuscular syndromes. Daytime arterial blood gases or pulse oximetry and end-tidal or transcutaneous P_{CO_2} levels should be obtained at the time of visits or when symptoms worsen. Although there is no consensus on the ideal target level, values for daytime Pa_{CO_2} ranging from 40 mm Hg to 60 mm Hg are usually associated with good control of symptoms, as long as nocturnal hypoventilation is controlled and sleep quality is improved.

Nocturnal monitoring using pulse oximetry, multichannel recorders, or, if there are problems with adaptation, full polysomnography is also useful after adaptation to NIV to assure adequacy of oxygenation and ventilation. These follow-up studies should await the achievement of at least 4 hours of sleep nightly to be revealing. Once a patient has been stabilized, blood gases need to be obtained only infrequently, perhaps once or twice yearly.

Common Problems and Possible Remedies

Interface-Related Problems

When used on properly selected patients, NIV is usually safe and well tolerated. Either in acute or chronic settings, the most commonly encountered problems are related to the interface (Table 21-2). Patients often complain of mask discomfort, which can be alleviated by minimizing strap tension, or trying different mask sizes or types. The most common error is to select a mask that is too large, necessitating excessive strap tension to minimize leaks. Claustrophobic reactions are also commonly encountered and lead to mask intolerance. Allowing patients to hold the mask in place initially, switching to masks that don't impede the field of vision, or judicious use of sedation can help.

Other commonly encountered mask-related problems include erythema, pain, or ulceration on the bridge of the nose related to pressure from the mask seal. Minimizing strap tension, using artificial skin, or switching to alternative masks such as nasal "pillows" can alleviate this problem. Newer masks that have softer silicone seals than earlier versions plus the routine use of artificial skin have rendered this problem infrequent in many units.

Air Pressure– and Flow-Related Problems

Excessive air pressure leading to sinus or ear pain is a common complaint, alleviated by lowering pressure temporarily, and then gradually raising it again as tolerance improves. Patients may also complain of dryness or congestion of the nose or mouth. Large air leaks through the nose cause mucosal desiccation and increase nasal resistance.[93] For dryness, nasal saline or gels or efforts to reduce air leaking may help. Heated passover humidifiers may also be helpful. During long-term applications, dryness may be particularly problematic in dry climates or during winter. For nasal congestion, inhaled corticosteroids or decongestants or oral antihistamine-decongestant combinations may be used. Air insufflation into the gastrointestinal tract is also common, but it usually doesn't interfere with tolerance or efficacy, probably because inflation pressures are low compared with those used with invasive ventilation.

Air Leaking

Air leaking is ubiquitous with NIV because it is difficult to maintain a tight mask seal and, during nasal mask ventilation, air commonly leaks through the mouth. Large air leaks interfere with efficacy because the ability of the ventilator to compensate may be exceeded and mask pressure falls. With smaller leaks, patient-ventilator synchrony is disrupted because of difficulty sensing onset of patient inspiration (triggering) or expiration (cycling). Ventilators differ considerably in their ability to compensate for leaks, although as a class the "bilevels" tend to compensate better than traditional critical care ventilators.[94]

Strategies to control leaking include using a well-fitting mask with properly tightened straps. If air leaking occurs under the mask seal, the first response should be to pull the mask outward and reseat it rather than to merely tighten the straps, which increases the likelihood of nasal bridge ulcers. Air leaking through the mouth can be controlled by asking the patient to keep their mouth shut or adding chinstraps, neither of which is highly effective. Switching to an oronasal mask may be more effective. It is important to recall that "bilevel" ventilators have intentional fixed leaks to permit removal of CO_2, and these ports should not be occluded. During long-term applications, air leaking occurs during the majority of sleep in many patients, but fortunately, gas exchange is usually well maintained.[95] Leaks may still contribute to arousals and poor sleep quality, however, and ventilatory assistance may occasionally be compromised.

Asynchrony

Asynchrony renders NIV ineffective because the breath is not timed properly to reduce work of breathing. Agitation commonly contributes to asynchrony, related to many factors including anxiety or claustrophobia, delirium, and mask discomfort among others. Possible remedies include verbal reassurance, efforts at enhancing comfort either by readjusting or changing the interface, adjusting ventilator settings to enhance comfort, or once again judicious sedation. In patients with severe COPD who have PEEPi, increases in applied PEEP may facilitate triggering.

Other causes of asynchrony include air leaking as discussed above, which contributes to failure to trigger or cycle. Some newer ventilators are able to subtract out leak flow to sense triggering. To avoid "hangup" or expiratory asynchrony—the persistence of inspiratory flow and pressure despite the onset of patient expiratory efforts—some ventilators incorporate controls that allow limitations of inspiratory time or the operator can switch to controlled modes of ventilation that cycle based on a timer. Proprietary mechanisms such as Autotrak (Respironics, Inc.) that use a combination of factors such as breathing pattern learned from previous breaths and a moving signal that renders the cycling mechanism more sensitive as inspiration continues offer another approach.

Rebreathing

As discussed above, rebreathing is a concern during "bilevel" ventilation because of the single ventilator circuits, but dual circuits as found on critical care ventilators eliminate the problem. Rebreathing has been reported to interfere with the efficacy of NIV in COPD patients under special circumstances, but using expiratory pressures of 4 cm H_2O or greater and exhalation valves situated in the mask directly over the nose tends to minimize the problem. Although rebreathing has never been shown to contribute to failure of NIV in an actual clinical setting, measures to minimize the problem make sense as long as they don't add too much to the discomfort or complexity of administering NIV.

Major Complications

Fortunately, major complications of NIV are rare if patients are carefully selected. Concerns have been raised that NIV might predispose to problems with aspiration, especially if oronasal masks are used. In fact, the opposite appears to be the case. Studies consistently show a substantial drop in health care–acquired pneumonias when NIV is used compared with patients ventilated invasively.[96] Of course, patients at risk for aspiration—those with swallowing problems or difficulty clearing secretions—should be managed invasively. Pneumothoraces can occur during NIV although they are unusual compared with invasive ventilation presumably because relatively low inflation pressure is used. More serious complications such as respiratory or cardiac arrests can occur during NIV, just as they can during invasive ventilation. For this reason, acutely ill patients must be monitored closely and, if possible, intubated when there is evidence of lack of improvement, before a respiratory or cardiac crisis occurs.

SUMMARY AND CONCLUSIONS

NIV, mainly in the form of NPPV, has established itself as an important ventilator modality. In the acute setting, NIV is preferred to invasive positive-pressure ventilation for selected patients with COPD exacerbations because of reduced morbidity and mortality, the possibility of reduced costs, and enhanced patient comfort. NIV is also suitable for initial mechanical ventilatory assistance in patients with a variety of other forms of acute respiratory failure, including those with acute pulmonary edema or an immunocompromised status, as long as selection guidelines are observed. These are designed to identify patients at risk of needing mechanical ventilatory assistance, while excluding those who are too ill to be safely managed noninvasively. Also the patient should have a reversible cause of respiratory failure that is unlikely to require prolonged continuous ventilatory support.

NIV is also considered the ventilatory modality of first choice for many forms of chronic respiratory failure, including neuromuscular diseases, chest wall restrictive processes, and central and obesity hypoventilation. Here, NIV offers comfort, convenience, safety, and cost advantages over invasive positive-pressure ventilation. Ideal candidates should require only intermittent ventilatory assistance and have intact upper airway function, but NIV has been successfully applied even in patients requiring continuous assistance and those with bulbar dysfunction. Although relatively few randomized controlled trials have been performed to evaluate the efficacy of NIV in the various forms of chronic respiratory failure, the approach is well accepted in patients with neuromuscular disease, and either CPAP or NIV appear to be effective in most patients with obesity hypoventilation. NIV has not been firmly established in patients with chronic respiratory failure due to COPD, but those with substantial hypercarbia and sleep-disordered breathing appear to be the ones most likely to benefit.

KEY POINTS

- NIV is most successful in the treatment of acute exacerbations of chronic respiratory failure and in the treatment of hypoxemia resulting from cardiogenic pulmonary edema.
- Success of NIV is best judged clinically by reduced respiratory muscle effort, slowing respiratory frequency, and improved O_2 saturation in the first 1 to 2 hours of support.
- Failure of the clinical staff to recognize the failure of NIV can result in a worse outcome for the patient.
- Traditional ICU ventilators may offer advantages in providing NIV in acute illness.
- Noninvasive ventilators work with a fixed leak and allow improved leak compensation and reduced triggering effort compared with traditional ventilators.
- PEEP during NIV reduces work to trigger caused by auto-PEEP and helps prevent CO_2 rebreathing.
- Long-term use of NIV is most successful in patients with postpolio syndrome, most myopathies, and kyphoscoliosis.
- A full face mask is ideal for acute care by virtue of reduced leaking and improved elimination of CO_2.
- A nasal mask is ideal for long-term care owing to improved patient comfort and tolerance.
- Critical to the success of NIV is the cooperation of the patient. Gaining the patient's trust and slowly introducing NIV over the first hour greatly enhances success.
- NIV should be initiated at a PEEP of 4 to 5 cm H_2O and a minimum inspiratory pressure until the patient becomes comfortable with the technique.
- Common factors confounding successful use of NIV include air leaks, dry gas, mask discomfort, and asynchrony.

ASSESSMENT QUESTIONS

1. Complications of translaryngeal intubation include
   A. traumatic complications (bleeding).
   B. infectious complications (pneumonia).
   C. discomfort and interference with communication and swallowing.
   D. impaired cough.
   E. requirement for excess sedation.
   F. all of the above.
2. Evidence-based indications for the use of NIV, that demonstrate improved outcomes include
   I. COPD exacerbations.
   II. asthma.
   III. acute cardiogenic pulmonary edema.
   IV. cystic fibrosis.
   V. immunocompromised patients.
      A. I, II, III, and V
      B. I, III, and IV
      C. I, III, and V
      D. All of the above
3. True or False. The use of NIV in hypoxemic respiratory failure should be used cautiously.
4. During the use of NIV for hypoxemic respiratory failure, intubation should be considered if
   A. $Pa{O_2}$ does not double in the first 24 hrs.
   B. $Pa{CO_2}$ does not decrease by at least 50%.
   C. pH falls below 7.35.
   D. $Pa{O_2}/F{IO_2}$ does not increase above 150 in the first hour.
   E. None of the above
5. NIV is most likely to be successful when these factors are present:
   I. Disease process reversible in hours to days
   II. Moderate severity of respiratory failure
   III. Accessory muscle use
   IV. Severe hypoxemia
   V. Abdominal paradox
      A. I, III, and V
      B. I, II, III, and IV
      C. I, II, III, and V
      D. All of the above
6. NIV is most likely to fail when these factors are present:
   I. Excessive secretions
   II. Hemodynamic instability
   III. Uncooperative patient
   IV. Poor mask fit
   V. Unstable respiratory drive
      A. I, II, and III
      B. I, II, and IV
      C. II, III, and IV
      D. All of the above
7. Benefits of long-term use of NIV in patients with restrictive thoracic diseases include
   A. improved sleep.
   B. resolution of right heart failure.
   C. improved gas exchange.
   D. all of the above.
8. Initiation of NIV in the patient with chronic respiratory failure may be considered when the following symptoms are present:
   I. Morning headaches
   II. Daytime hypersomnolence
   III. Hypocarbia
   IV. Respiratory muscle weakness
      A. I, II, and III
      B. I, II, and IV
      C. I, III, and IV
      D. All of the above
9. Contraindications to NIV include
   I. inability to protect the airway.
   II. slowly developing respiratory failure.
   III. rapidly developing respiratory failure.
   IV. hypercarbia.
      A. I and II
      B. I and III
      C. I and IV
      D. All of the above
10. True or False. Nasal masks are preferred to full face masks in the acute care of the patient with an exacerbation of COPD.
11. The major advantage of the full face mask (oronasal mask) compared with the nasal mask is
    A. comfort.
    B. reduced skin breakdown.
    C. reduced CO_2 rebreathing.
    D. elimination of leaks.

Continued

ASSESSMENT QUESTIONS—cont'd

12. Major limitations of the helmet interface include
- **I.** hypoxemia.
- **II.** high noise levels.
- **III.** CO_2 rebreathing.
- **IV.** cost.
- **V.** leaks.
  - **A.** II, III, and IV
  - **B.** II, IV, and V
  - **C.** III, IV, and V
  - **D.** All of the above

13. The major advantage of the noninvasive ventilators or bilevel devices over a critical care ventilator is
- **I.** leak compensation.
- **II.** reduced rebreathing.
- **III.** fewer alarms.
- **IV.** improved monitoring.
  - **A.** II and III
  - **B.** I and II
  - **C.** I and III
  - **D.** II and IV
  - **E.** All of the above

14. The major advantage of critical care ventilators over the noninvasive ventilators or bilevel devices is
- **I.** leak compensation.
- **II.** reduced rebreathing.
- **III.** fewer alarms.
- **IV.** improved monitoring.
  - **A.** I and II
  - **B.** I and III
  - **C.** II and III
  - **D.** II and IV
  - **E.** All of the above

15. The nasal mask is associated with greater discomfort during NIV in the acutely ill patient due to
- **A.** air leaks through the mouth.
- **B.** rebreathing.
- **C.** claustrophobia.
- **D.** hypoxemia.

16. True or False. The success of NIV is highly dependent on the clinician gaining the patient's confidence.

17. Commonly encountered problems with NIV include
- **I.** mask discomfort.
- **II.** claustrophobia.
- **III.** air leaks.
- **IV.** rebreathing.
- **V.** asynchrony.
  - **A.** I, III, and V
  - **B.** I, II, III, and IV
  - **C.** I, III, IV, and V
  - **D.** II, III, and IV
  - **E.** All of the above

18. Major complications of NIV are rare but include
- **I.** pneumonia.
- **II.** aspiration of gastric contents.
- **III.** pneumothorax.
- **IV.** pulmonary embolism.
  - **A.** I and II
  - **B.** II and III
  - **C.** II and IV
  - **D.** III and IV
  - **E.** All of the above

REFERENCES

1. Wilson JL: Acute anterior poliomyelitis, N Engl J Med 206:887-893, 1932.
2. Corrado A, Gorini M, Villella G et al: Negative pressure ventilation in the treatment of acute respiratory failure: an old noninvasive technique reconsidered, Eur Resir J 9:1531-1544, 1996.
3. Mehta S, Hill NS: Noninvasive ventilation. State of the art, Am J Respir Crit Care Med 163:540-577, 2001.
4. Pingleton SK: Complications of acute respiratory failure, Am Rev Respir Dis 137:1463-1469, 1988.
5. Appendini L, Palessio A, Zanaboni S et al: Physiologic effects of positive end-expiratory pressure and mask pressure support during exacerbations of chronic obstructive pulmonary disease, Am J Respir Crit Care Med 149:1069-1076, 1994.
6. Kramer N, Meyer TJ, Meharg J et al: Randomized, prospective trial of noninvasive positive pressure ventilation in acute respiratory failure, Am J Respir Crit Care Med 151:1799-1806, 1995.
7. Brochard L, Mancebo J, Wysocki M et al: Noninvasive ventilation for acute exacerbations of chronic obstructive pulmonary disease, N Engl J Med 333:817-822, 1995.
8. Celikel T, Sungur M, Ceyhan B et al: Comparison of noninvasive positive pressure ventilation with standard medical therapy in hypercapnic acute respiratory failure, Chest 114:1636-1642, 1998.

9. Lightowler J, Wedjicha JA, Elliott MW et al: Noninvasive positive pressure ventilation for the treatment of respiratory failure due to exacerbations of chronic obstructive pulmonary disease (Cochrane Review), BMJ 326:185-189, 2003.
10. Keenan SP, Kernerman PD, Cook DJ et al: Effect of noninvasive positive pressure ventilation on mortality in patients admitted with acute respiratory failure: a meta-analysis, Crit Care Med 25:1685-1692, 1997.
11. Confalonieri M, Potena A, Carbone G et al: Acute respiratory failure in patients with severe community-acquired pneumonia, Am J Respir Crit Care Med 160:1585-1591, 1999.
12. Levy M, Tanios MA, Nelson D et al: Outcomes of patients with do-not-intubate orders treated with non-invasive ventilation, Crit Care Med 32:2002-2007, 2004.
13. Auriant I, Jallot A, Herve P et al: Noninvasive ventilation reduces mortality in acute respiratory failure following lung resection, Am J Respir Crit Care Med 164:1231-1235, 2001.
14. Ferrer M, Valencia M, Nicolas JM et al: Early noninvasive ventilation averts extubation failure in patients at risk: a randomized trial, Am J Respir Crit Care Med 173:164-170, 2006.
15. Nava S, Gregoretti C, Fanfulla F et al: Noninvasive ventilation to prevent respiratory failure after extubation in high-risk patients, Crit Care Med 33:2465-2470, 2005.
16. Ferrer M, Esquinas A, Arancibia F et al: Noninvasive ventilation during persistent weaning failure. A randomized controlled trial, Am J Respir Crit Care Med 168:70-76, 2003.
17. Vaisanen IT, Rasanen J: Continuous positive airway pressure and supplemental oxygen in the treatment of cardiogenic pulmonary edema, Chest 92:481-485, 1987.
18. Bersten AD, Holt AW, Vedig AE et al: Treatment of severe cardiogenic pulmonary edema with continuous positive airway pressure delivered by face mask, N Engl J Med 325:1825-1830, 1991.
19. Lin M, Yang YF, Chiang HT et al: Reappraisal of continuous positive airway pressure therapy in acute cardiogenic pulmonary edema. Short-term results and long-term follow-up, Chest 107:1379-1386, 1995.
20. Mehta S, Jay GD, Woolard RH et al: Randomized, prospective trial of bilevel versus continuous positive airway pressure in acute pulmonary edema, Crit Care Med 25:620-628, 1997.
21. Crane SD, Elliott MW, Gilligan P et al: Randomised controlled comparison of continuous positive airways pressure, bilevel non-invasive ventilation, and standard treatment in emergency department patients with acute cardiogenic pulmonary oedema, Emerg Med J 21:155-161, 2004.
22. Nava S, Carbone G, DiBattista N et al: Noninvasive ventilation in cardiogenic pulmonary edema: A multicenter randomized trial, Am J Respir Crit Care Med 168(12):1432-1437, 2003.
23. Masip J, Betbese AJ, Paez J et al: Non-invasive pressure support ventilation versus conventional oxygen therapy in acute cardiogenic pulmonary oedema: a randomised trial, Lancet 356:2126-2132, 2000.
24. Winck JC, Azevedo LF, Costa-Pereira A et al: Efficacy and safety of non-invasive ventilation in the treatment of acute cardiogenic pulmonary edema—a systematic review and meta-analysis, Crit Care 10:R69, 2006.
25. Hubble MW, Richards ME, Jarvis R et al: Effectiveness of prehospital continuous positive airway pressure in the management of acute pulmonary edema, Prehosp Emerg Care 10(4):430-439, 2006.
26. Hilbert G, Gruson D, Vargas F et al: Noninvasive ventilation in immunosuppressed patients with pulmonary infiltrates, fever, and acute respiratory failure, N Engl J Med 344:481-487, 2001.
27. Antonelli M, Conti G, Bufi M et al: Noninvasive ventilation for treatment of acute respiratory failure in patients undergoing solid organ transplantation: a randomized trial, JAMA 283:235-241, 2000.
28. Soroksky A, Stav D, Shpirer I: A pilot prospective, randomized, placebo-controlled trial of bi-level positive airway pressure in acute asthmatic attack, Chest 123:1018-1025, 2003.
29. Pollack CV Jr, Fleisch KB, Dowsey K: Treatment of acute bronchospasm with beta-adrenergic agonist aerosols delivered by a nasal bilevel positive airway pressure circuit, Ann Emerg Med 26:552-557, 1995.
30. Hodson ME, Madden BP, Steven MH et al: Noninvasive mechanical ventilation for cystic fibrosis patients—a potential bridge to transplantation, Eur Respir J 4:524-527, 1991.
31. Antonelli M, Conti G, Rocco M et al: A comparison of noninvasive positive-pressure ventilation and conventional mechanical ventilation in patients with acute respiratory failure, N Engl J Med 339:429-435, 1998.
32. Ferrer M, Esquinas A, Leon M et al: Noninvasive ventilation in severe hypoxemic respiratory failure. A randomized clinical trial, Am J Respir Crit Care Med 168:1438-1444, 2003.
33. Epstein SK, Ciubotaru RL, Wong JB: Effect of failed extubation on the outcome of mechanical ventilation, Chest 112:186-192, 1997.
34. Keenan SP, Powers C, McCormack DG et al: Noninvasive positive-pressure ventilation for postextubation respiratory distress: a randomized controlled trial, JAMA 287:3238-3244, 2002.
35. Esteban A, Frutos-Vivar F, Ferguson ND et al: Noninvasive positive-pressure ventilation for respiratory failure after extubation, N Engl J Med 350(24):2452-2460, 2004.
36. Squadrone V, Coha M, Cerutti E et al: Continuous positive airway pressure for treatment of postoperative hypoxemia: a randomized controlled trial, JAMA 293: 589-595, 2005.
37. Kindgen-Milles D, Muller E et al: Nasal continuous positive airway pressure reduces pulmonary morbidity and length of stay following thoracoabdominal aortic surgery, Chest 128:821-828, 2005.
38. Joris JL, Sottiaux TM, Chiche JD et al: Effect of bi-level positive airway pressure (BiPAP) nasal ventilation on the postoperative pulmonary restrictive syndrome in obese patients undergoing gastroplasty, Chest 111:665-670, 1997.
39. Gust R, Gottschalk A, Schmidt H et al: Effects of continuous (CPAP) and bi-level positive airway pressure (BiPAP) on extravascular lung water after extuba-

tion of the trachea in patients following coronary artery bypass grafting, Intensive Care Med 22:1345-1350, 1996.
40. Levy M, Tanios MA, Nelson D et al: Outcomes of patients with do-not-intubate orders treated with noninvasive ventilation, Crit Care Med 32:2002-2007, 2004.
41. Schettino G, Altobelli N, Kacmarek RM: Noninvasive positive-pressure ventilation reverses acute respiratory failure in select "do-not-intubate" patients, Crit Care Med 34:5317-5323, 2006.
42. Curtis RJ, Cook DJ, Sinuff T et al: Noninvasive positive pressure ventilation in critical and palliative care settings: understanding the goals of therapy, Crit Care Med (in press).
43. Maitre B, Jaber S, Maggiore SM et al: Continuous positive airway pressure during fiberoptic bronchoscopy in hypoxemic patients. A randomized double-blind study using a new device, Am J Respir Crit Care Med 162:1063-1067, 2000.
44. Antonelli M, Conti G, Rocco M et al: Noninvasive positive-pressure ventilation vs. conventional oxygen supplementation in hypoxemic patients undergoing diagnostic bronchoscopy, Chest 121(4):1149-1154, 2002.
45. Da Conceicao M, Genco G, Favier JC et al: Fiberoptic bronchoscopy during noninvasive positive-pressure ventilation in patients with chronic obstructive lung disease with hypoxemia and hypercapnea, Ann Fr Anesth Reanim 19:231-236, 2000.
46. Baillard C, Fosse JP, Sebbane M et al: Noninvasive ventilation improves preoxygenation before intubation in hypoxic patients, Am J Respir Crit Care Med 174: 171-177, 2006.
47. Confalonieri M, Garuti G, Cattaruzza MS et al: Italian noninvasive positive pressure ventilation (NPPV) study group. A chart of failure risk for noninvasive ventilation in patients with COPD exacerbation, Eur Respir J 25:348-355, 2005.
48. Antonelli M, Conti G, Moro ML et al: Predictors of failures of noninvasive positive pressure ventilation in patients with acute hypoxemic respiratory failure: a multi-center study, Intensive Care Med 27:1718-1728, 2001.
49. Gonzalez Diaz G, Alcaraz AC, Talavera JCP et al: Noninvasive positive-pressure ventilation to treat hypercapnic coma secondary to respiratory failure, Chest 127:952-960, 2005.
50. Bach JR, Alba AS, Saporito LR: Intermittent positive pressure ventilation via the mouth as an alternative to tracheostomy for 257 ventilator users, Chest 103:174-182, 1993.
51. Hill NS, Eveloff SE, Carlisle CC et al: Efficacy of nocturnal nasal ventilation in patients with restrictive thoracic disease, Am Rev Respir Dis 101:516-521, 1992.
52. Masa Jimenez JF, de Cos Escuin JS, Vicente CD et al: Nasal intermittent positive pressure ventilation. Analysis of its withdrawal, Chest 107:382-388, 1995.
53. Bourke SC, Tomlinson M, Williams TL et al: Effects of non-invasive ventilation on survival and quality of life in patients with amyotrophic lateral sclerosis: a randomized controlled trial, Lancet Neurol 5:140-147, 2006.
54. Bourke SC, Bullock RE, Williams TL et al: Noninvasive ventilation in ALS: Indications and effect on quality of life, Neurology 61:171-177, 2003.
55. Leger P, Bedicam JM, Cornette A et al: Nasal intermittent positive pressure. Long-term follow-up in patients with severe chronic respiratory insufficiency, Chest 105:100-105, 1994.
56. Simonds AK, Elliott MW: Outcome of domiciliary nasal intermittent positive pressure ventilation in restrictive and obstructive disorders, Thorax 50:604-609, 1995.
57. Braun NM, Marino WD: Effect of daily intermittent rest of respiratory muscles in patients with severe chronic airflow limitation (CAL), Chest 85:59S-60S, 1984.
58. Hill NS: Noninvasive ventilation in chronic obstructive pulmonary disease, Resp Care 49:72-89, 2004.
59. Zibrak JD, Hill NS, Federman ED et al: Evaluation of intermittent long-term negative pressure ventilation in patients with severe chronic obstructive pulmonary disease, Am Rev Respir Dis 138:1515-1523, 1988.
60. Strumpf DA, Millman RP, Carlisle CC et al: Nocturnal positive pressure ventilation via nasal mask in patients with severe chronic obstructive pulmonary disease, Am Rev Respir Dis 144:1234-1239, 1991.
61. Meecham Jones DJ, Paul EA, Jones PW: Nasal pressure support ventilation plus oxygen compared with oxygen therapy alone in hypercapnic COPD, Am J Respir Crit Care Med 152:538-544, 1995.
62. Clini E, Sturani C, Rossi A et al: Rehabilitation and Chronic Care Study Group, Italian Association of Hospital Pulmonologists (AIPO). The Italian multicentre study on noninvasive ventilation in chronic obstructive pulmonary disease patients, Eur Respir J 20:529-538, 2002.
63. Janssens JP, Derivaz S, Breitenstein E et al: Changing patterns in long-term noninvasive ventilation: A 7-year prospective study in the Geneva Lake area, Chest 123:67-79, 2003.
64. Olson AL, Zwillich C: The obesity hypoventilation syndrome, Am J Med 118:948-956, 2005.
65. Berger KI, Ayappa I, Chatramontri B et al: Obesity hypoventilation syndrome as a spectrum of respiratory disturbances during sleep, Chest 120:1231-1238, 2001.
66. Masa JF, Celli BR, Riesco JA et al: The obesity hypoventilation syndrome can be treated with noninvasive mechanical ventilation, Chest 119:1102-1107, 2001.
67. Piper AJ, Sullivan CE: Effect of short-term NIPPV in the treatment of patients with severe obstructive sleep apnea and hypercapnia, Chest 105:434-440, 1994.
68. Ward S, Chatwin M, Heather S et al: Randomized controlled trial of non-invasive ventilation (NIV) for nocturnal hypoventilation in neuromuscular and chest wall disease patients with daytime normocapnia, Thorax 60:1019-1024, 2005.
69. Navalesi P, Fanfulla F, Frigerio P et al: Physiologic evaluation of noninvasive mechanical ventilation delivered by three types of masks in patients with

chronic hypercapnic respiratory failure, Crit Care Med 28:1785-1790, 2000.
70. Criner GJ, Travaline JM, Brennan KJ et al: Efficacy of a new full face mask for noninvasive positive pressure ventilation, Chest 106:1109-1115, 1994.
71. Antonelli M, Pennisi MA, Pelosi P et al: Noninvasive positive pressure ventilation using a helmet in patients with acute exacerbation of chronic obstructive pulmonary disease, Anesthesiology 100:16-24, 2004.
72. Cavaliere F, Conti G, Costa R et al: Noise exposure during noninvasive ventilation with a helmet, a nasal mask, and a facial mask, Intensive Care Med 30:1755-1760, 2004.
73. Bach JR, Alba AS, Bohatiuk G et al: Mouth intermittent positive pressure ventilation in the management of post-polio respiratory insufficiency, Chest 91:859-864, 1987.
74. Vitacca M, Rubini F, Foglio K et al: Noninvasive modalities of positive pressure ventilation improved the outcome of acute exacerbations in COLD patients, Intensive Care Med 19:450-455, 1993.
75. Bach JR: Update and perspective on noninvasive respiratory muscle aids. Part 2: The expiratory aids, Chest 105:1538-1544, 1994.
76. Strumpf DA, Carlisle CC, Millman RP et al: An evaluation of the Respironics BiPAP bi-level CPAP device for delivery of assisted ventilation, Respir Care 35:415-422, 1990.
77. Brochard L, Harf A, Lorino H et al: Inspiratory pressure support prevents diaphragmatic fatigue during weaning from mechanical ventilation, Am Rev Respir Dis 139:513-521, 1989.
78. Schwartz AR, Kacmarek RM, Hess DR: Factors affecting oxygen delivery with bi-level positive airway pressure, Respir Care 49:270-275, 2004.
79. Ferguson GT, Gilmartin M: CO_2 rebreathing during BiPAP ventilatory assistance, Am J Respir Crit Care Med 151(4):1126-1135, 1995.
80. Schettino GPP, Chatmongkolchart S, Hess D et al: Position of exhalation port and mask design affect CO_2 rebreathing during noninvasive positive pressure ventilation, Crit Care Med 31:2178-2182, 2003.
81. Hill NS, Carlisle C, Kramer NR: Effect of a nonrebreathing valve on long-term nasal ventilation using a bilevel device, Chest 122:84-91, 2002.
82. Hill NS: Clinical applications of body ventilators, Chest 90:897-905, 1986.
83. Corrado A, Ginanni R, Villella G et al: Iron lung versus conventional mechanical ventilation in acute exacerbation of COPD, Eur Respir J 23:419-424, 2004.
84. Chervin RD, Guilleminault C: Diaphragm pacing for respiratory insufficiency, J Clin Neurophysiol 14:369-377, 1997.
85. Bach JR, Alba AS, Bodofsky E et al: Glossopharyngeal breathing and noninvasive aids in the management of post-polio respiratory insufficiency, Birth Defects 23:99-113, 1987.
86. Kwok H, McCormack J, Cece R et al: Controlled trial of oronasal versus nasal mask ventilation in the treatment of acute respiratory failure, Crit Care Med 31:468-473, 2003.
87. Maheshwari V, Paioli D, Rothaar R et al: Utilization of noninvasive ventilation in acute care hospitals: a regional survey, Chest 129:1226-1233, 2006.
88. L'Her E, Deye N, Lellouche F et al: Physiologic effects of noninvasive ventilation during acute lung injury, Am J Respir Crit Care Med 172:1112-1118, 2005.
89. Holland AE, Denehy L, Buchan CA et al: Efficacy of a heated passover humidifier during noninvasive ventilation: a bench study, Respir Care 52:38-44, 2007.
90. Devlin J, Bahhady I, Nava S et al: Survey of sedation practices for noninvasive positive pressure ventilation (NPPV) to treat acute respiratory failure, Crit Care Med 35:2298-2302, 2007.
91. Soo Hoo GW, Santiago S, Williams J: Nasal mechanical ventilation for hypercapnic respiratory failure in chronic obstructive pulmonary disease: Determinants of success and failure, Crit Care Med 27:417-434, 1994.
92. Hill NS, Redline S, Carskadon MA et al: Sleep-disordered breathing in patients with Duchenne muscular dystrophy using negative pressure ventilators, Chest 102:1656-1662, 1992.
93. Richards GN, Cistulli PA, Ungar G et al: Mouth leak with nasal continuous positive airway pressure increases nasal airway resistance, Am J Respir Crit Care Med 154:182-186, 1996.
94. Mehta S, McCool FD, Hill NS: Leak compensation in positive pressure ventilators—a lung model study, Eur Respir J 17:259-267, 2001.
95. Meyer TJ, Pressman MR, Benditt J et al: Air leaking through the mouth during nocturnal nasal ventilation: Effect on sleep quality, Sleep 20:561-569, 1997.
96. Nourdine K, Combes P, Carton MJ et al: Does noninvasive ventilation reduce the ICU nosocomial infection risk? A prospective clinical survey, Intensive Care Med 25:567-573, 1999.

CHAPTER

22 Modifications on Conventional Ventilation Techniques

John D. Davies

OUTLINE

OBJECTIVES

- Explain the underlying concepts and application of airway pressure release ventilation.
- Explain the underlying concepts and application of independent lung ventilation.
- Explain the underlying concepts and application of proportional assist ventilation.
- Explain the underlying concepts and application of tracheal gas insufflation.

KEY TERMS

airway pressure release ventilation (APRV)
dual lumen endotracheal tube (DLT)
hyperbaric O_2 (HBO) chamber
independent lung ventilation (ILV)
magnetic resonance imaging (MRI) scanner
proportional assist ventilation (PAV)
selective ventilation distribution circuit (SVDC)
tracheal gas insufflation (TGI)

Conventional positive-pressure ventilation provides respiratory support through periodic lung inflations, often in conjunction with expiratory pressure applications. Additional features usually include patient interactive capabilities (patient breath triggering and patient flow control), various feedback control systems (intermittent mandatory ventilation [IMV], mandatory minute ventilation [MMV], pressure-regulated volume control/volume support [PRVC/VS]), and sophisticated monitoring and alarm systems. In recent years, some variations to this basic strategy have been proposed. One of the most important is discussed in a separate chapter (see high-frequency ventilation in Chapter 23). Several other modifications or variations to conventional strategies, however, also deserve comment and are reviewed in this chapter: airway pressure release ventilation (APRV), independent

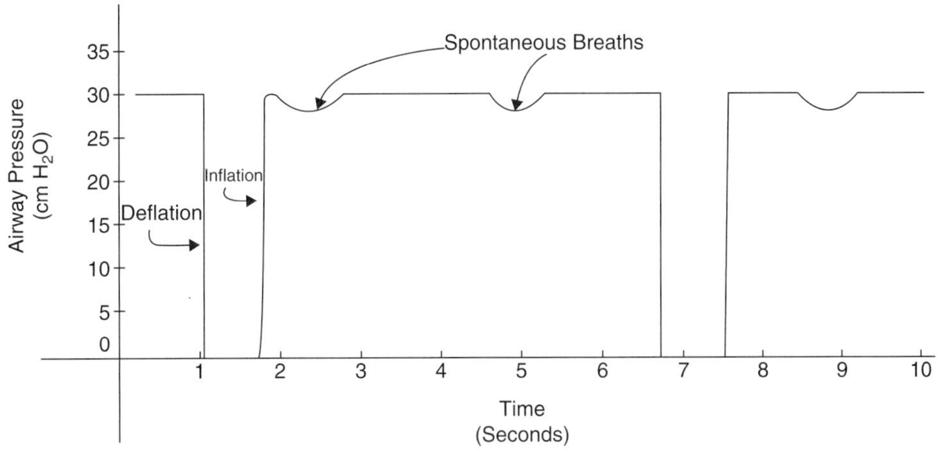

FIGURE 22-1 APRV. Depicted is airway pressure over time with airway pressure release ventilation (APRV). Note the long inspiratory : expiratory time ratio and the fact that spontaneous breaths can be taken from P_{high}. (Modified from Frawley P, Habashi N: Airway pressure release ventilation: Theory and practice. AACN 12(2):234-246, 2001.)

lung ventilation (ILV), proportional assist ventilation (PAV), and tracheal gas insufflation (TGI). Two other technical modifications of conventional ventilation that address the application of positive-pressure ventilation in the magnetic resonance imaging scanner and the hyperbaric environment also are discussed.

AIRWAY PRESSURE RELEASE VENTILATION

Description and Rationale

Airway pressure release ventilation (APRV) was first described in 1987 as continuous positive airway pressure (CPAP) with an intermittent pressure release phase.[1-3] It is a pressure-limited, time-cycled mode of ventilation that permits spontaneous breathing throughout the ventilatory cycle.[2-4]

Although all positive pressure modes have a high (inflation) and a low (deflation) pressure applied, with APRV these are specifically defined as the high pressure setting (P_{high}) and the low pressure setting (P_{low}) during two time periods called time high (T_{high}) and time low (T_{low}). If T_{high} and T_{low} are set in the physiologic range (i.e., an inspiratory time of 0.5 to 1.0 second and an inspiratory : expiratory [I:E] time ratio of 1:2 to 1:4), APRV closely resembles conventional pressure assist-control (A/C) ventilation or pressure-targeted IMV (if spontaneous breaths are taken during the expiratory time). The usual APRV strategy, however, sets T_{high} much longer than traditional inspiratory times, usually between 3 and 5 seconds. Unlike conventional pressure-targeted modes, APRV allows spontaneous breaths during this long inflation period. After P_{high} has timed out, the ventilator releases the pressure down to the P_{low} setting for a short (i.e., less than 1 second) fixed T_{low}. Figure 22-1 illustrates the waveforms associated with APRV. Note the long duration of T_{high} and short duration of T_{low}.

APRV can improve oxygenation because the prolonged period at P_{high} progressively recruits lung units in a "cascade" type manner.[5] That is, throughout T_{high}, the number of lung units steadily increases until T_{low} begins.[5] The ultimate result is that a larger lung surface area gets exposed for gas exchange. Put another way, APRV can increase the mean airway pressure (through the prolonged I:E ratio) without having to use conventional approaches that increase the baseline positive end-expiratory pressure (PEEP) or tidal volume (V_T). It may thus be an attractive strategy in patients in whom end-inspiratory pressures are considered excessive on conventional ventilation (CV).

Another purported advantage to APRV is the ability to have a considerable number of spontaneous breaths. A positive-pressure breath has the tendency to shift ventilation to nondependent areas of the lung as the passive respiratory system accommodates gas delivery.[6] The ability for spontaneous ventilation at P_{high} may lead to dependent regions of the lung being preferentially ventilated.[7] Consequent ventilation-perfusion ($\dot{V}/\dot{Q}$) improvements result in improved oxygenation.[8] Importantly, however, it must be remembered that spontaneous efforts during the APRV inflation period will add to the end-inspiratory transpulmonary pressure. Thus the set

P_{high} is only the maximal mechanical ventilator pressure, not the actual end-inspiratory stretching pressure on the lung. Some ventilators have the ability to augment the spontaneous breaths during APRV with pressure support ventilation (PS). This may further promote patient ventilator synchrony in that the patient's effort is augmented.[7-8] However, clinicians must be careful if using PS above P_{high} because this will further lead to a significant elevation in the end-inspiratory transpulmonary pressure (thus negating a potential benefit to APRV).[7] Also, using PS above P_{high} can sometimes paradoxically increase patient discomfort and reduce $\dot{V}/\dot{Q}$ matching associated with unassisted spontaneous breathing.[7-8]

CO_2 removal occurs both during P_{high} and P_{low}. During P_{high}, if the patient is breathing spontaneously, CO_2 can be released through the spontaneous effort. CO_2 is also released from the lungs through the brief, controlled releases to P_{low} in the same manner as conventional ventilation (elastic recoil of the lungs). The difference between P_{high} and P_{low} determines the tidal volume (V_T). Often P_{low} is set at 0 to achieve a reasonable V_T (e.g., 6 ml/kg ideal body weight [IBW]) while avoiding end-inspiratory overdistention. A concern with a P_{low} so low is that alveolar recruitment may be lost. However, because T_{low} is so short, the development of some intrinsic PEEP may prevent this.

Weaning from APRV may be done in one of two ways. First, the patient can be placed on a more conventional mode and standard ventilator discontinuation strategies employed (see Chapter 18). The second method is somewhat more nontraditional. It is accomplished by a combination of lowering the P_{high} and extending T_{high}. By decreasing the number of releases, the patient will pick up more of the work of breathing through spontaneous ventilation.[7] APRV thus is essentially converted to CPAP.

Clinical Data

There have been various studies performed comparing APRV to other modes of ventilation. Garner showed that patients with mild acute lung injury (ALI) receiving conventional positive-pressure ventilation required higher airway pressures to support oxygenation and ventilation than patients receiving APRV.[11] Kaplan showed that APRV provided similar oxygenation to pressure-controlled inverse ratio ventilation (IRV) with an increase in cardiac function, less pressor use, decreased use of sedation and paralytics, and a decrease in airway pressure in patients with ALI/acute respiratory distress syndrome (ARDS).[12] Sydow compared the use of volume control IRV to APRV and showed similar oxygenation initially. However, after the 8-hour period, the patients on APRV exhibited a continued improvement in oxygenation with lower airway pressures in patients with severe ALI.[5] In the first randomized trial of APRV, Putenson et al[8] demonstrated reduced airway pressures, better oxygenation, and fewer ventilator days with APRV. However, the control group in this study received a mode of support that significantly reduced oxygenation compared with baseline and required paralysis for the first 3 days of the trial. Thus it is difficult to draw conclusions from this study. The most recent trial by Varpula et al[8a] showed no difference in gas exchange, sedation needs, or outcome in patients receiving APRV versus an IMV-PS strategy.

Recommendations

APRV is a physiologically attractive mode of ventilation that may limit lung injury by simultaneously reducing maximal pressures and increasing mean pressures. Crucial questions remain, however, and clinical data are limited. Until a well-designed randomized trial using a "gold standard" conventional strategy, such as the NIH ARDS Network strategy, demonstrates an outcome benefit (not just physiologic improvement), widespread application of APRV cannot be recommended.

INDEPENDENT LUNG VENTILATION

Description and Rationale

Independent lung ventilation (ILV) is a method by which the gas flow to each lung is effectively separated mechanically by either two small endotracheal tubes (ETs) or a single specially designed **dual lumen endotracheal tube (DLT)** (Figure 22-2). The rationale for separation can be either anatomic or physiologic and includes massive hemoptysis, pulmonary alveolar proteinosis, unilateral lung injury, single-lung transplant, and bronchopleural fistula.

Regardless of the indication, the main reason for the use of ILV is to address asymmetric lung pathophysiology in which each lung requires different support strategies. ILV should be considered when the V_T-PEEP combination beneficial for one lung may not be optimal or may even detrimental to the other. For example, whole-lung PEEP application in an emphysematous patient with severe unilateral pneumonia might result in the uninjured lung units

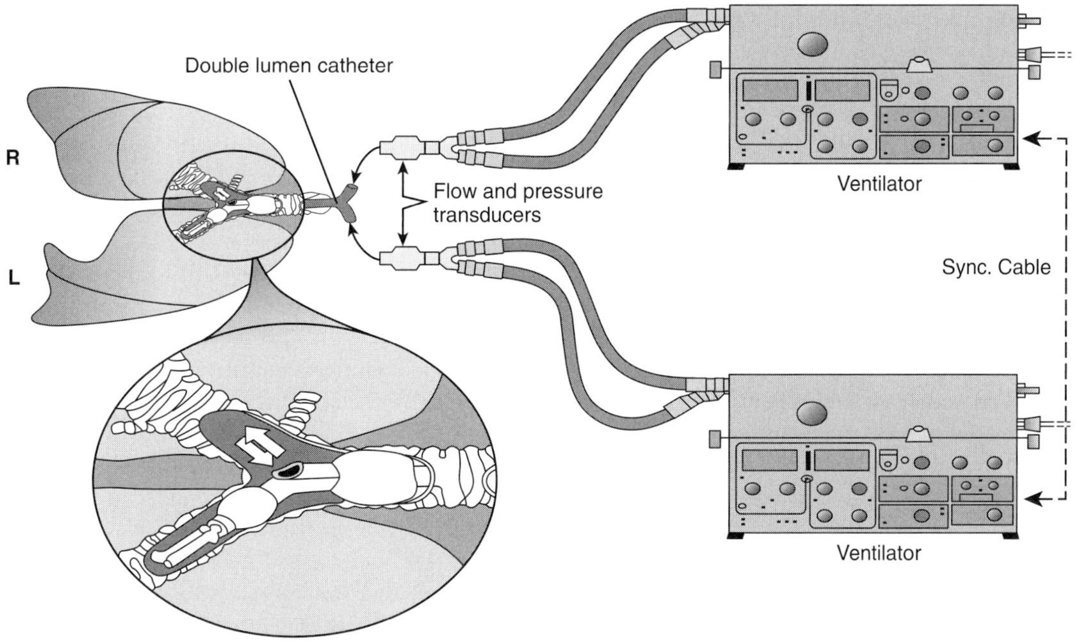

FIGURE 22-2 Setup of an independent lung ventilation system using two synchronized ventilators attached to separate lumens of a double-lumen ET. (Redrawn from Siegel JH, Stoklosa JC, Borg U et al: Quantification of asymmetric lung pathophysiology as a guide to the use of simultaneous independent lung ventilation in posttraumatic and septic adult respiratory distress syndrome, Ann Surg 202:425-439, 1985.)

being overexpanded and underperfused, whereas the injured lung may experience underexpansion and overperfusion. The goal of ILV in this circumstance is to isolate each lung for the purpose of applying aggressive PEEP lung recruitment in the injured lung and lower PEEP application in the emphysematous lung.

With ILV, not only is the ventilation setup different, but specialized airway devices must be employed. The Carlens DLT, introduced in 1949, was the first available device designed to separate the lungs.[12] This tube incorporated a carinal hook, which was intended to help facilitate proper placement and stabilization, but had the unfortunate side effect of tracheal trauma. It was followed with the improved Robertshaw DLT that was designed in both left-sided and right-sided models and did not have a carinal hook.[13] This device eventually fell out of favor due to the fact that it was made of red rubber, which was irritating to the respiratory mucosa. Also, the cuffs were of low volume and high pressure and tended to inflate asymmetrically.

Over the last 3 decades, other devices have been developed to separate the right and left lungs for one of two broad purposes: obstruct one lung (i.e., to control hemoptysis) or provide the capability to ventilate the two lungs differently. When intentional obstruction of an airway is indicated to protect the normal lung from insult by focal processes such as massive hemoptysis, several devices and strategies are available. These include cuffed rubber bronchial blockers, embolectomy balloons, pulmonary artery catheters, and other specially designed plastic tubes.

In some cases, intubation of the mainstem bronchus of the unaffected side is all that is required. The Fogarty embolectomy catheter is the most widely used endobronchial blocker. It usually is passed through a normal ET with the tip of the catheter angled at 30° to help direct it into the correct mainstem bronchus. A fiberoptic bronchoscope can be inserted through the ET with the catheter to assist with positioning. The balloon then is inflated until occlusion of the bronchus occurs.

The disadvantage of using the Fogarty occlusion techniques is that they do not afford access to the affected lung and therefore cannot provide ventilation and pulmonary hygiene. An alternative occlusion strategy is the Univent catheter. This device was first described by Inoue and associates[14] in 1982 and consists of an ET with an extra exterior lumen, 2 mm in internal diameter, in the anterior portion of the tube. Although the lumen is small, it does allow for a special blocking device that passes through the small lumen and can be positioned up to 8 cm beyond the

ET. The Univent has several advantages over the Fogarty catheter. Because the device is attached to the main ET, displacement is less likely. Moreover, suctioning, pulmonary lavage, O_2 insufflation, and even high-frequency ventilation can be provided through the Univent tube to the occluded lung.

If substantial but differential ventilatory support is required for both lungs during ILV, a larger DLT is required. Current versions are made of nontoxic polyvinyl chloride with high-volume, low-pressure cuffs. Generally, one lumen is longer than the other, which allows it to be inserted into a mainstem bronchus (both left and right mainstem designs are available). The more proximal lumen thus opens into the trachea for ventilating the other lung. Because each lumen is less than half the diameter of a regular ET, suctioning and bronchoscopy are difficult.

The challenges in using the DLT involve placement, positioning, and securing the tube. Several authors[15-17] recommend that a DLT should be placed routinely using bronchoscopy. Although a DLT may be placed successfully without direct visualization, the complication rate and procedure time are increased. Once placed, the DLT may have a tendency to migrate. Distal migration potentially could block a mainstem bronchus, creating further collapse or atelectasis. Proximal migration has the potential to compromise the effectiveness of ILV. Because of this, pressures and volumes from each lung should be monitored carefully during ILV.

Ventilator management during ILV depends on the clinical goals for each lung. A single conventional ventilator can be used in circumstances in which one lung needs conventional support while the other is managed with a T tube, a CPAP system, or a high-frequency ventilator. ILV, however, usually involves different PEEP, V_T, F_{IO_2}, pressure targets, and/or flow settings customized for each lung. This generally involves two separate ventilators, each attached to one of the lumens of the DLT.

There also has been successful ILV with a single ventilator when using a specialized **selective ventilation distribution circuit (SVDC).** The SVDC uses a single circuit adapted at the wye with an additional wye that adapts to the two lumens of a DLT. A variable-flow resistance device is used in the inspiratory limb of the uninjured lung. By varying the set resistance, the proportion of the V_T delivered to the injured lung or to the uninjured lung can be varied. Because there are separate expiratory limbs, each with its own PEEP device, PEEP to each lung can be modified individually and according to the severity of injury or need. Yamamura and colleagues[18] have described a one-piece SVDC device for use in anesthesia, but there has been no testing of this device in the critical care setting.

Problems associated with SVDC include (1) limitations of independent ventilation parameters, (2) the additional adapters can be a source for leaks, and (3) rapid changes in the compliance or resistance of either lung alters V_T delivery.

When two ventilators are used, rate synchrony can be achieved by mechanically or electronically linking the two machines.[19] With the increased use of microprocessors, ventilators can be linked electronically in a primary/secondary fashion so that synchronized delivery of two different breaths (each breath specific to a particular lung) should be possible. Two unconnected, noncommunicating (i.e., asynchronous) ventilators also can provide ILV. The concerns with asynchronous independent lung ventilation are the possible compromise of the cardiovascular system and substantial discomfort. However, Hillman and Barber[20] demonstrated no adverse effects with asynchronous ILV compared with standard ventilation and indeed suggested possible benefit to cardiovascular function in the selective reduction in lung volume and consequent decrease in mean airway pressure.

When using ILV, it may not be necessary to have the patient deeply sedated or paralyzed. Assuming the patient has an appropriate respiratory drive, both ventilators could be set in an assist or support mode of ventilation[21] (such as pressure assist, PS, or volume assist). As long as the patient effort is recognized equally for both lungs by appropriate sensitivity settings, both lungs will inflate simultaneously. If, however, there is need for a mandatory respiratory rate, there is evidence to suggest that asynchronous inflation of the individual lung units is not detrimental as long as they are not 180° out of phase.[22]

In setting the V_T for each lung, it is important to remember that each lung represents only a fraction of the total lung capacity and thus the regional V_T should be reduced accordingly. Specifically, if a global 6 ml/kg IBW V_T is desired, each lung should receive 3 ml/kg IBW. A plateau pressure limit of less than 30 cm H_2O on both lungs helps reduce the exposure of both to excessive end-inspiratory stretch. In contrast, PEEP settings in each lung should follow the same guidelines as applying PEEP with a single airway.

Using ILV can create logistical problems as well. First, confusion can arise from having different goals for two separate lung units. For this reason, each ventilator should be labeled clearly as to its control relationship (primary vs. secondary or master vs. slave) and designated right versus left lung clearly on the ventilator. Second, the area required for two ventilators in a patient space can restrict mobility and access to other therapeutic delivery devices and monitors and to the patient.

Clinical Data

Much of the literature available on ILV relates to case studies detailing the accounts of various asymmetric lung processes and how ILV was applied in these particular circumstances. Reports include cases of unilateral pulmonary contusions,[23-25] a bronchopulmonary fistula managed with a variable-resistance valve and a single ventilator,[26] treatment of situations evolving after a single-lung transplant for primary pulmonary hypertension,[27-29] independent lung ventilation using a combination of a conventional ventilator and a high-frequency oscillatory ventilator,[30] and the use of two high-frequency oscillatory ventilators for independent lung ventilation.[31]

Recommendations

ILV provides the opportunity to provide different ventilatory support strategies to the right and left lung in the setting of asymmetric lung disease. The safe use of ILV is dependent on the available resources and the clear establishment of the management goals for each lung. Besides the commitment of equipment, consideration should be given to the level of intensive care required to safely administer ILV. ILV should not be attempted unless there is adequate monitoring, ongoing assessment, and the availability of experienced personnel to respond to management and emergencies.

PROPORTIONAL ASSIST VENTILATION

Description and Rationale

Proportional assist ventilation (PAV) is an innovative mode that is designed to improve synchrony between patient ventilatory demand and the support that the ventilator provides. PAV was first described by Younes in 1992 as an interactive ventilatory mode in which the ventilator provides dynamic inspiratory pressure assistance in linear proportion to patient inspiratory effort (as determined by inspiratory flow measurements).[32,33] If the patient's effort during an inspiration increases, then the ventilator generates an increase in applied pressure and flow. Ventilator assistance in the respiratory cycle stops when the patient's inspiratory effort ends.

In theory, PAV acts by offsetting some percentage of both the elastance (inverse of compliance) and resistance loads of the respiratory system (as measured during test breaths). This percentage is adjustable by the clinician.[34] Figure 22-3 illustrates the differences in applied pressure and flow characteristics of PAV compared with other frequently used ventilator modes.

As can be seen in Figure 22-3, pressure-targeted modes, such as PS and APRV, provide a constant pressure with increasing flow delivery in response to an increasing inspiratory effort. In contrast, in volume-targeted modes such as IMV, A/C, or controlled mandatory ventilation the flow is constant regardless of effort and thus applied pressure during the assisted breaths drops in the face of increasing effort. PAV differs from both of these approaches by increasing the delivered pressure and flow with increased demand. In short, the goal of PAV is to provide: (1) flow to unload a set percentage of the resistive burden and (2) volume to unload a set percentage of the elastic burden.

With PAV being a mode of ventilation that continuously adjusts assistance in an intrabreath fashion (Figure 22-4), a number of advantages potentially exist. Foremost is the concept that the PAV assistance pattern may provide better patient flow synchrony with the ventilator and thus less need for paralysis and/or sedation. PAV is also less affected by pressure artifacts, such as hiccups or heart beats, that cause a premature breath triggering. In PAV, because these false triggers result in very little inspiratory effort, the resulting V_T can be inconsequential, resulting in no increase in ventilation.

There are also potential shortcomings in PAV.

1. There is the dependence on spontaneous effort. If the patient were to become apneic for any reason, the ventilator would not deliver a PAV breath. Therefore, it is of vital importance that any ventilator designed for life support and is equipped with PAV should also be outfitted with backup controlled ventilation.
2. There exists the potential for "runaway" pressure ventilation under circumstances described in more detail below.
3. There is no guaranteed V_T. If the patient tires or fatigues and develops a shallow rapid breathing pattern, PAV will only support the reduced effort and not a target V_T or pressure. The clinician must therefore be skilled in selecting appropriate PAV unloading percentages to assure comfort and avoid fatigue. The clinician must also carefully monitor patients to identify fatigue.

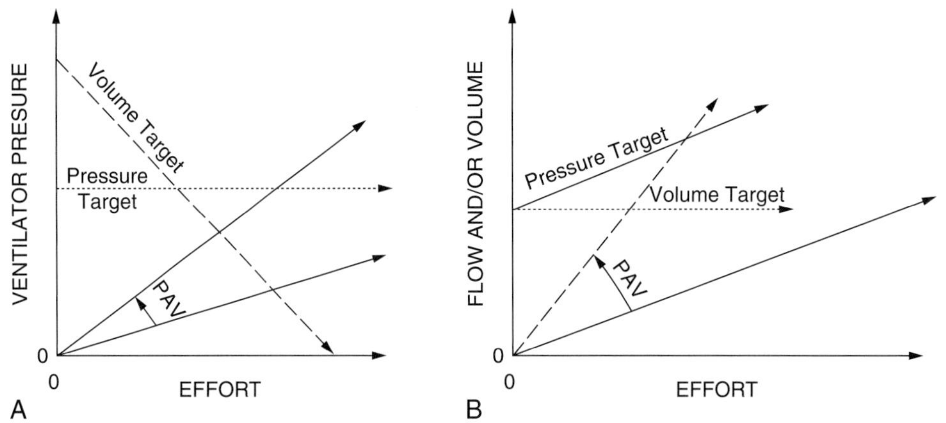

FIGURE 22-3 A, Relationship between patient effort and pressure delivered by the ventilator with different ventilatory support modalities. **B,** Effect of different support modalities on the relation between effort and delivered flow and volume. In panel A, PAV pressure increases with increases in effort, whereas pressure-targeted modes maintain pressure and volume targeted–assisted breaths decrease pressure. In panel B, both PAV and pressure targeting increase flow with increased effort, whereas volume targeting maintains the set flow regardless of effort. (From Younes M: proportional assist ventilation, a new approach to ventilatory support, Am Rev Respir Dis 145:114-120, 1992.)

4. The clinical use of PAV is based on repetitive measurements of respiratory system elastance and resistance. If these are not measured properly or if they change suddenly, proper adjustments in the ventilator may be inaccurate or delayed.
5. PAV is highly susceptible to intrinsic PEEP (PEEPi). If a patient exerts most of his or her inspiratory energy merely to overcome PEEPi and trigger the ventilator, then PAV support may be inadequate due to a lack of energy on the patient's part. Careful attention must be paid to these patients, and it may be necessary to add external PEEP to counterbalance PEEPi so that extensive work is not expended merely to trigger the ventilator.

Clinical Data

Many of the theoretical and early clinical data on PAV have been produced by Younes and colleagues.[33] They developed the concept that PAV was actually providing a "gain" on effort and thus resembled power steering on an automobile. They went on to propose that flow and volume gain settings should be based on providing a percentage unloading of resistance and elastance that would provide comfortable, nonfatiguing patient work. Using their device in patients, this group has demonstrated that PAV is a comfortable form of ventilatory support and that this approach to proportional unloading behaves as predicted. Bigatello and colleagues[35] subsequently used a lung model to study the muscle-unloading effects of PAV. This model produced a sine wave spontaneous flow pattern, and the "ventilatory drive" was varied by adjusting the V_T from 0.2 to 1.2 L. By adjusting the flow and volume gains accordingly, the model illustrated the muscle-unloading effects of PAV.

Navalesi and colleagues[36] studied PAV in eight patients with acute respiratory failure. They also demonstrated that the flow gain provided unloading from resistive loads and that the volume gain provided unloading from the elastance loads. Ranieri and associates[37] compared PAV and PS at two levels of support in 12 mechanically ventilated patients. These patients had stimulation of their ventilatory drive by the addition of dead space into the circuit. They found that, with PS, the compensatory mechanism with induced hypercapnia was an increased patient breathing frequency rather than increased V_Ts. With the same induced hypercapnia in PAV, subjects

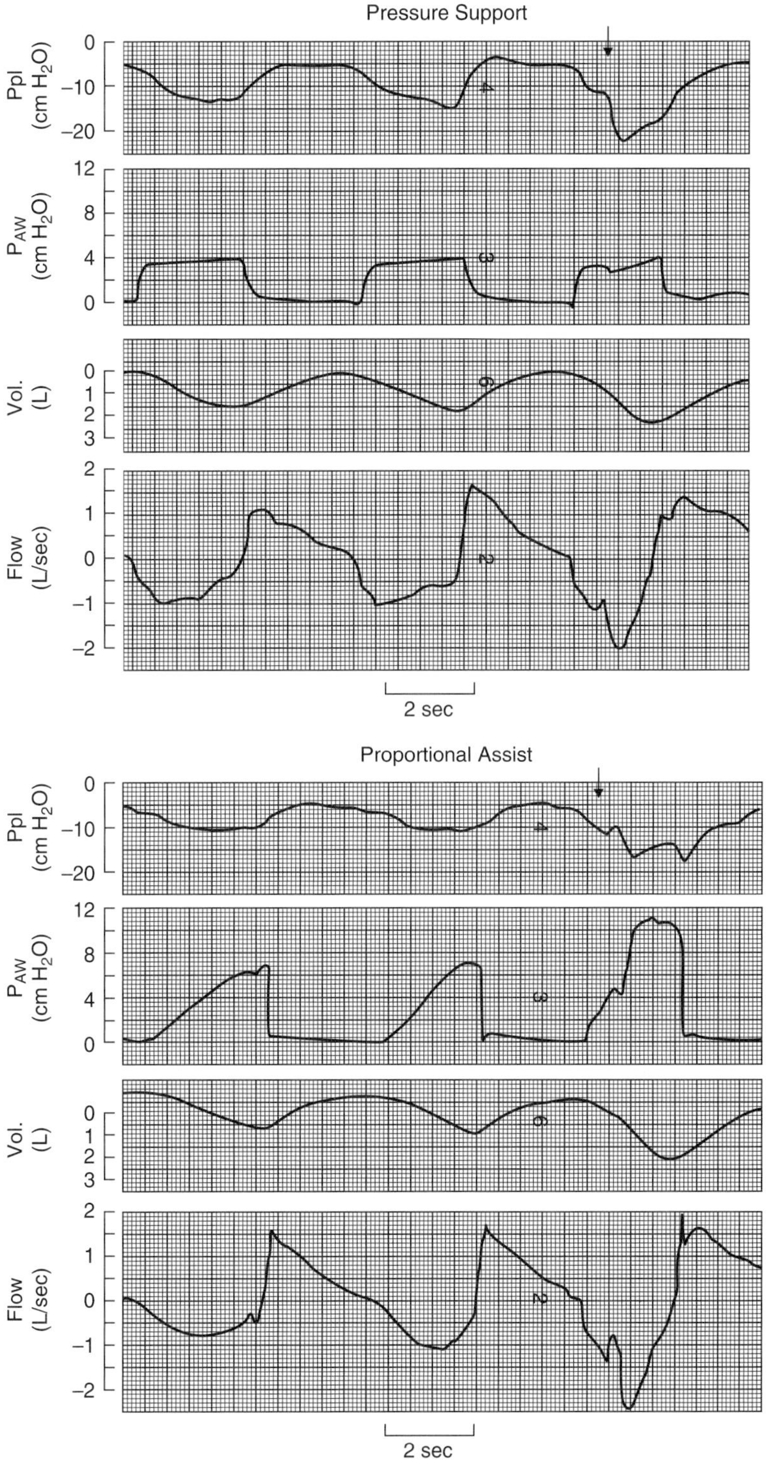

FIGURE 22-4 Effect of increasing patient effort during pressure support (PS) *(upper panel)* and during proportional assist *(lower panel)*. At the arrows, patient pulls with increased effort as reflected by a more negative deflection in the pleural pressure (P_{pl}) tracing. With PS, airway pressure (P_{AW}) remains constant while flow and volume (vol) increase. In contrast, with proportional assist, airway pressure also increases and the delivered flow and volume are even greater. (From Younes M, Puddy A, Roberts D et al: Proportional assist ventilation: results of an initial clinical trial, Am Rev Respir Dis 145:121-129, 1992.)

increased their V_Ts to compensate. They concluded that the compensatory strategy to increase minute ventilation during PS requires more muscle effort and creates more patient discomfort than with PAV. This was also confirmed by a study performed by Grasso et al.[38] They showed that muscle effort in the face of elevated respiratory loads increased with PS as compared with PAV. With PS, although the patients receive mandatory degrees of support, the patients' abilities to alter their ventilatory pattern through changes in motor output were impaired.

Ranieri and associates[39] have also described the "runaway" effect of PAV. This phenomenon can occur under two conditions. First, a leak in the system can result in an apparent excessive flow and volume demand, which elicits even further flow and volume delivery from PAV. Second, flow and volume gains set in excess of those required by passive resistance and elastance of the patient can produce a similar excess delivery of flow and volume by PAV. One way this can occur is if elastance and/or resistance suddenly improves and the ventilator has not yet remeasured these parameters. This runaway potential underscores the need to closely monitor the respiratory mechanics and patient status during PAV. Moreover, ventilators incorporating PAV need to have appropriate safeguards to prevent this from happening.

Recently, PAV has been studied as a mode of noninvasive ventilation. Preliminary results show that PAV may be effective in this manner and may even be superior in terms of respiratory muscle unloading and patient comfort.[40-43]

Recommendations

PAV is a novel ventilatory approach that targets intrabreath synchrony. In small studies, PAV seems to be effective for unloading respiratory muscles in the face of increased ventilatory loads. For general clinical application, however, devices need to be able to accurately and repeatedly assess patient resistance and elastance loads and clinicians need to be able to assess optimal patient muscle loading. More clinical studies are needed to develop management algorithms to comfortably unload patient muscles. Although the idea of amplifying the patient effort has merit, there remains concern about inappropriate adjustments that could lead to fatigue or that do not adequately "train" or challenge the patient. Safety from a "runaway breathing" pattern is a critical component of any PAV system.

TRACHEAL GAS INSUFFLATION

Description and Rationale

Tracheal gas insufflation (TGI) is the process of injecting gas into the trachea with the purpose of clearing CO_2 from the anatomic and mechanical dead space proximal to the catheter tip. This CO_2 represents alveolar gas at the end of expiration in the trachea and/or ET and since this gas volume is the leading edge of the next inspiration, it is essentially rebreathed gas. The idea behind TGI is to flush this gas volume out of the trachea and/or ET during exhalation and thereby reduce functional dead space. TGI was first introduced in 1969 by Stresemann et al[44] and they observed a "proof of concept" by showing a significant reduction in Pa_{CO_2} when 18 L/min (lpm) of TGI gas flow was used.

TGI flow is delivered by a small-diameter catheter usually located at the distal end of the ET. Normal flows are usually in the range of 5 to 10 lpm and can be delivered either continuously or on exhalation only. TGI typically is delivered through either a stand-alone catheter or a catheter imbedded in the ET wall positioned just above the carina. By enhancing CO_2 removal, TGI may lessen the V_T requirement and thus serve to reduce maximal distending pressures in patients at risk for lung stretch injury. TGI also may improve gas mixing because of the turbulent flow created at the tip of the catheter.

There are several limitations and complications associated with the use of TGI. These include altered pressure and volume delivery from the ventilator, PEEPi buildup, assisted breath triggering difficulties, humidification needs, airway trauma, and monitoring interference. Additional flow in the circuit gives rise to altered pressures and/or volumes. This is especially true when TGI is applied in the continuous mode. Because extra flow is added to inspiration, the ventilator must interact properly with the additional flow to ensure that the desired airway pressures and/or volumes are not compromised.

Imanaka and colleagues[45] developed a lung model to look at the effect of TGI on two commonly used modes of support: pressure assist-control ventilation (PACV) and volume assist-control ventilation (VACV). As expected, during PACV, TGI flow during inspiration reduced ventilator flow delivery as the ventilator strove to maintain the inspiratory pressure target. However, the TGI flow added to this reduced ventilator flow resulted in a constant V_T. In contrast, during VACV, TGI flow during inspiration added to the set ventilator flow delivery such that both V_T and peak airway pressure increased.

At higher levels of TGI flow, PEEPi may develop. Although this may have some benefit in reducing atelectasis, it is an unmeasured pressure that could also lead to overdistention. There is also a concern that there may be some interference by TGI on assisted breath triggering. Hoyt and associates[46] showed that this is especially true in patients with weak effort.

Extended use of TGI poses a threat of mucous plug formation unless the fresh gas is humidified. Most of the research has been short term and has not shown issues with plug formation. However, one study did have two different catheter obstructions in a 20-subject ARDS population.[47] There is also a danger of airway trauma with a catheter being introduced into the ventilatory system. If the catheter is malpositioned or inadvertently advanced during the course of treatment, structural damage to the airway mucosa can occur. Careful monitoring of catheter position is vital to prevent this.

Clinical Data

The use of TGI to increase elimination of CO_2 has been well documented in the literature. Kalfon and colleagues[48] showed in mechanically ventilated patients that TGI reduced $Paco_2$ and increased pH. They also showed that TGI can significantly increase tracheal PEEP and mean airway pressure. Adjustments in applied PEEP (preferably with tracheal pressure monitoring) and the use of a pressure relief valve are thus important to maintain desired airway pressures during TGI.[49]

One of the largest clinical studies with TGI comes from Barnett and associates.[50] This was a prospective study spanning a 5-year period in which data were collected on 68 trauma patients suffering from ARDS. The results showed improvement in $Paco_2$ (from 72 ± 5 to 59 ± 5 mm Hg) and pH (from 7.25 ± 0.03 to 7.33 ± 0.03) despite a reduced V_T (from 7.9 ± 0.6 ml/kg to 7.2 ± 0.6 ml/kg) and minute ventilation (from 13 ± 1 to 11 ± 1 L/min) (P less than 0.05). This study was echoed by Oliver in rabbits, where TGI resulted in lower ventilatory requirements (peak inspiratory pressure, V_T, and dead space) and a more favorable histologic trend than that of CV.[51] The importance of this study is that it shows that TGI may be a useful ventilatory adjunct in the neonatal population.

A couple of catheter-related logistical issues have also been studied: (1) catheter position relative to the carina and (2) straight versus inverted style catheter for CO_2 elimination. Nahum and colleagues[52] have shown that the best CO_2 clearance occurs with the catheter placed 1 cm above the carina. Nahum and colleagues[53] also demonstrated that the straight catheter as opposed to an inverted catheter is more effective for CO_2 elimination. However, they also concluded that PEEPi development was less with the inverted catheter.

TGI may also have some benefits in the weaning phase of ventilation. Patients who are difficult to wean from mechanical ventilation may benefit from decreased dead space and work of breathing. Two studies have shown some promising results by reducing ventilatory demand.[54-55]

TGI usage also has been reported in other potential clinical settings. Okamato and colleagues[56] showed that TGI plus APRV was more effective at maintaining normocarbia than APRV alone in a canine restrictive-thorax model with and without pulmonary edema. Miro and associates[57] used TGI in a canine model with methacholine-induced bronchospasm and showed improved CO_2 elimination without any evidence of hyperinflation or hemodynamic instability. In clinical trials of partial liquid ventilation, the elevated $Paco_2$ created by the rapid instillation of perflubron may be decreased with the use of TGI.[58] TGI also has been reported as useful in high-frequency oscillatory ventilation (HFOV) and in reducing intracranial pressure resultant from permissive hypercapnia.[59,60] A study involving helium delivery during TGI also had some promising results. Pizov et al[61] showed that the addition of helium may even be more effective than using O_2 alone during TGI for CO_2 elimination and lower peak pressures in mechanically ventilated patients.

TGI has not been evaluated as extensively in infants as in adults. Animal research suggests that TGI may reduce the risk of ventilation-induced lung disease in the newborn.[51,62] Given the size of the neonatal ET, a TGI catheter could impose a significant increase in airway resistance. In an attempt to address this issue, Danan and colleagues[63] described a technique of TGI in newborns using a specially designed ET with capillaries molded into the wall that produce TGI CO_2 (dead space) washout without the need for a tracheal catheter. Further use of TGI in newborns is contingent on future development of appropriate delivery systems that will not compromise the patient.

Recommendations

Reduction (or elimination) of CO_2-laden dead space has conceptual appeal in a number of circumstances, especially during mechanical ventilatory support when appropriate CO_2 elimination requires unacceptably high ventilation pressures. There are important TGI-ventilator interactions that must be considered before implementation of TGI. Among these are breath triggering issues, monitoring issues with the added flow, peak pressures, and increases in tracheal (intrinsic) PEEP. In addition, optimal catheter positioning and TGI flow rates for different clinical situations are not yet clear. So, despite the appeal of added CO_2 elimination, safety and logistical issues are still present and need to be addressed before TGI can be used on a widespread clinical basis.

MODIFICATIONS FOR NUCLEAR MAGNETIC SCANNERS AND HYPERBARIC CHAMBERS

Many transport versions of mechanical ventilators are available for the purpose of maintaining ventilatory support in various specialized diagnostic or therapeutic areas. However, there exist two areas that can have profound effects on the operation of mechanical ventilators. These areas are the **magnetic resonance imaging (MRI) scanner** and the **hyperbaric O_2 (HBO) chamber.**

The MRI scanner incorporates a large electromagnet that attracts any ferrous material in close proximity. Besides the possibility of equipment involuntarily moving toward the magnet or scanner (or in the case of small metal objects, becoming projectile), components of the mechanical ventilator and accompanying monitors may fail to operate properly in this environment. Additionally, electromagnetic interference from the ventilator may interfere with the MRI process, potentially producing artifact in the finished scans.

The hyperbaric O_2 chamber uses high barometric pressures and high O_2 concentrations. In addition to the possible effect of barometric pressure changes on the accuracy and operation of the mechanical ventilator, the O_2-rich environment is an inherent fire risk.

MRI-Compatible Equipment

Equipment used in the MRI scanner must be free of ferrous materials and electronics. This requires that ventilators operate on either fluidic or pneumatic principles and this does severely limit the choice of ventilators. However, various companies have manufactured MRI-"safe" ventilators, but unfortunately they usually lack the flexibility of the critical care ventilators. This could be an issue with patients who require more extensive ventilatory support. There is a report of a critical care ventilator being modified for use in the MRI scanner.[64] In this case all ferrous material was replaced with MRI-compatible material and the ventilator was shown to be MRI compatible. When modifying or custom building such a ventilator, a disconnect monitoring device or high-low airway pressure detection device must be included. Although manufacturers should have information on compatibility, MRI facilities should test ventilators and monitoring equipment before allowing their use in the scanner.

Hyperbaric Chamber–Compatible Equipment

Hyperbaric O_2 therapy can be provided through either monoplace or multiplace chambers. Mechanical ventilator requirements are different in these two environments.

Monoplace Chamber

In the monoplace chamber, a single patient is exposed to the hyperbaric environment, with most of the support equipment outside. In this type of chamber, there is a minimal fire risk from sparks in a high O_2 environment because all electrical components and mechanically moving parts are outside the hyperbaric environment. Generally, the chamber is compressed with a high level of O_2 (100%), except where mechanical ventilation is used.

Boyle's law should be considered to understand how mechanical ventilators are affected under monoplace hyperbaric conditions. Boyle's law states that an enclosed volume of gas will change in proportion to the pressure exerted on it. For example, if 1 L of gas from an externally controlled ventilator is introduced into a monoplace chamber, the volume will be compressed to 0.5 L at 2 atmospheres absolute (ATA), 0.333 L at 3 ATA, and so forth. In addition, the required airway pressures to drive gas into a thorax with an elevated external pressure will be accordingly higher. Therefore the availability of ventilators for use in monoplace hyperbaric chambers is very limited.

Multiplace Chamber

The other type of hyperbaric chamber is the multiplace chamber, a larger chamber that allows for more than one person's inhabitation, sometimes interconnected to other chambers of similar size. This design can be more efficient and cost-effective, as when treating groups of patients. An additional benefit lies in the ability for physicians, nurses, or respiratory therapists to reside in the chamber with the patient(s) during their treatment, affording hands-on care of patients.

The multiplace chamber usually is not pressurized with 100% O_2. Instead, the ambient level is kept at 21% (room air) while the patient is treated with either a ventilator circuit or a hood containing the appropriate FIO_2. This lower ambient O_2 level in the chamber reduces much of the risk of fire. Any spark is still a potential hazard, and O_2 levels can increase in the chamber under some circumstances. Therefore it is critical to minimize moving parts, electrical components, and anything that may spark.

There are other safety considerations as well; O_2 should not be allowed to flow freely inside the case housing, inside the ventilator, or into the chamber, and all electrical devices used in the chamber should be flushed continuously with nitrogen[49] to lessen the chance that O_2 might come in contact with electrical interfaces. If any device incorporates a battery, a gel cell battery is suggested, when possible, because it is known to be less hazardous under pressurized conditions.

The main concerns when ventilating a patient in a multiplace hyperbaric chamber where the ventilator is physically inside are proper operation, fire hazards, space, and scavenging of expired gases. Therefore the ideal ventilator for the hyperbaric chamber should be one that has multiple ventilatory modes (in case the patient decompensates and needs a different support level), is pneumatically driven (to reduce the possibility of fire from the electrical interface), functions stably in a high-pressure environment (can deliver the desired settings), is compact (space may be an issue), and allows scavenging of expired gases (to prevent the elevation of CO_2 levels).[65] Any ventilator used in the multiplace chamber should therefore be tested for the effect of high ambient pressure on the delivered volume, pressure, or other operating features of the ventilator, such as rate control.

Another consideration is the effect of pressure on electronic controls. In particular, if "touch pad" controls are a feature of the ventilator or any other equipment, make certain that there is not an air interface between the touch pad and the control. Under hyperbaric conditions, any air present might pressurize and inadvertently activate a control.

During all forms of hyperbaric therapy, ET cuffs and tracheostomy tube cuffs must be filled with water.[50] Air in the cuff has the potential for rupturing the cuff, resulting in potential damage to the trachea and loss of a closed system for mechanical ventilation. Sterile water or saline in the cuff, unlike air, does not change volume under pressure. It is also general practice in many hyperbaric chambers to perform a myringotomy to prevent the potential rupture of the ear drum under pressure changes.

In conclusion, these special environments pose serious challenges for both manufacturers and clinicians alike. Because of the limited number of patients who need ventilatory support under these conditions, the available data base on system design and clinical practice is also limited. Considerably more work is needed in these areas as it is likely that these applications will grow.

KEY POINTS

- Conventional mechanical ventilation strategies can still expose the lungs to dangerous stresses and cause unnecessary discomfort during interactive modes.
- APRV offers theoretical advantages in terms of lower applied pressures and encouragement of spontaneous breaths. Important questions about APRV effects on end-inspiratory lung stretch and on ultimate outcome remain.
- PAV offers attractive improvements in patient-ventilator synchrony. Outcome studies are lacking, however, and there are theoretical concerns about both over and under support.
- TGI has physiologic merit but outcome analyses are lacking and concern about the interactions of TGI and ventilator function exist.

ASSESSMENT QUESTIONS

1. True or False. APRV limits the maximal stretching pressure on the lung to the P_{high} setting.
2. True or False. Outcome studies show that APRV reduces ventilator-induced lung injury.
3. True or False. APRV permits spontaneous breathing during P_{high}.
4. True or False. Unlike PS, which adds only flow to patient effort, PAV adds pressure and flow to patient effort.
5. True or False. PAV has a guaranteed minimal V_T.
6. True or False. PAV needs accurate measurements of compliance and resistance to perform properly.

Continued

ASSESSMENT QUESTIONS—cont'd

7. True or False. PAV has been shown to reduce weaning time when compared with daily spontaneous breathing trials.

8. True or False. With ILV, the usual V_T settings are 6 ml/kg IBW in each lung.

9. True or False. With ILV, plateau pressures should ideally be less than 30 cm H_2O in both lungs.

10. True or False. MRI-compatible ventilators cannot have ferrous material.

CASE STUDIES

For additional practice, refer to Case Studies 7 and 8 in the appendix at the back of this book.

REFERENCES

1. Chiang AA, Steinfeld A, Gropper C et al: Demand-flow airway pressure release ventilation as partial ventilatory support mode: comparison with synchronized intermittent mandatory ventilation and pressure support ventilation, Crit Care Med 22:1431-1437, 1994.
2. Stock CS, Downs JB: Airway pressure release ventilation: a new approach to ventilatory support during acute lung injury, Respir Care 32:517-520, 1987.
3. Stock MC, Downs JB: Airway pressure release ventilation, Crit Care Med 15:462-466, 1987.
4. Dart B, Maxwell R, Richart C et al: Preliminary experience with airway pressure release ventilation in a trauma/surgical intensive care unit, J Trauma Infect Crit Care 59(1):71-76, 2005.
5. Sydow M, Bruchardi H, Ephraim E et al: Long-term effects of two different ventilatory modes on oxygenation in acute lung injury, Am J Respir Crit Care Med (149):1550-1556, 1994.
6. Garner W, Downs JB: Airway pressure release ventilation (APRV): a human trial, Chest 94:779-781, 1988.
7. Habashi N: Other approaches to open-lung ventilation: Airway pressure release ventilation: Crit Care Med 33(3) Supplement March 2005: S228-S240.
8. Putensen C, Zech S, Wrigge H et al: Long-term effects of spontaneous breathing during ventilatory support in patients with acute lung injury, Am J Respir Crit Care Med 164:43-49, 2001.
8a. Varpula T, Jousela I, Niemie R et al: Combined effects of prone positioning and airway pressure release ventilation on gas exchange in patients with acute lung injury, Acta Anaesthesiol Scand 47:516-524, 2003.
9. Cane R, Peruzzi W, Shapiro B: Airway pressure release ventilation in severe acute respiratory failure, Chest 100:460-463, 1991.
10. Smith RA, Smith DB: Does airway pressure release ventilation alter lung function after acute lung injury? Chest 107:805-808, 1995.
11. Rasanen J, Cane RD, Downs JB et al: Airway pressure release ventilation during acute lung injury: a prospective multicenter trial, Crit Care Med 19:1234-1241, 1991.
12. Branson R: Independent lung ventilation, Problems Respir Care 2(1):48-60, 1989.
13. Ost D, Corbridge T: Independent lung ventilation, Clin Chest Med 17(3):591-601, 1996.
14. Inoue H, Shotsu H, Ogawa J et al: New device for one lung anesthesia: endotracheal tube with removable blocker, Thorac Cardiovasc Surg 83:940-941, 1991.
15. Charan C, Carvalho C, Hawk P et al: Independent lung ventilation with a single ventilator using a variable resistance valve, Chest 107:256-260, 1995.
16. Benumof J: The position of a double lumen tube should be routinely determined by fiberoptic bronchoscopy, Cardiothoracic Vasc Anesth 7:513-514, 1993.
17. Shinnick J, Freedman A: Bronchofiberscopic placement of a double-lumen endotracheal tube, Crit Care Med 10:544-545, 1982.
18. Yamamura T, Furumido H, Saito Y: A single-unit device for differential lung ventilation with only one anesthesia machine, Anesth Analg 4:1017-1020, 1985.
19. Siegel J, Stoklosa J, Borg U et al: Quantification of asymmetric lung pathophysiology as a guide to the use of simultaneous independent lung ventilation in post-traumatic and septic adult respiratory distress syndrome, Ann Surg 202:425-439, 1985.
20. Hillman K, Barber J: Asynchronous independent lung ventilation (AILV): Crit Care Med 8:390-395, 1980.
21. Schmitt H, Mang H, Kirmse M: Unilateral lung disease treated with patient-triggered independent-lung ventilation: A case report, Respir Care 39:906-911, 1994.
22. Branson R, Hurst J, Davis K: Synchronous independent lung ventilation in the treatment of unilateral pulmonary contusion: A report of two cases, Respir Care 29:361-367, 1984.
23. Branson R, Hurst J, Davis K: Alternative modes of ventilatory support, Problems Respir Care 2:48-60, 1989.
24. Cinnella G, Dambrasio M, Brienza N et al: Independent lung ventilation in patients with unilateral pulmonary contusion. Monitoring with compliance and $EtCO_2$. Intensive Care Med 27:1860-1867, 2001.
25. Miller R, Nelson L, Rutherford E et al: Synchronized independent lung ventilation in the management of a unilateral pulmonary contusion with massive hemoptysis, J Tenn Med Assn 85(8):374-375, 1992.
26. Carvalho P, Thompson W, Riggs R et al: Management of bronchopleural fistula with a variable-resistance valve and a single ventilator, Chest 111:1452-1454, 1997.

27. Badesch D, Zamora M, Jones S et al: Independent ventilation and ECMO for severe unilateral pulmonary edema after SLT for primary pulmonary hypertension, Chest 107:1766-1770, 1995.
28. Officer T, Wheeler D, Frost A et al: Respiratory control during independent lung ventilation, Chest 120:678-681, 2001.
29. Smiley R, Navedo A, Kirby T et al: Postoperative independent lung ventilation in a single-lung transplant recipient, Anesthesiology 74:1144-1148, 1991.
30. Terragni P, Rosboch G, Corno E et al: Independent high-frequency oscillatory ventilation in the management of asymmetric acute lung injury, Anesth Analg 100:1793-1796, 2005.
31. Graciano L, Barton P, Luckett P et al: Feasibility of asynchronous independent lung high-frequency oscillatory ventilation in the management of acute hypoxemic respiratory failure: A case report, Crit Care Med 28:3075-3077, 2000.
32. Younes M, Puddy A, Roberts D et al: Proportional assist ventilation: results of an initial clinical trial, Am Rev Respir Dis 145:121-129, 1992.
33. Younes M: Proportional assist ventilation, a new approach to ventilatory support, Am Rev Respir Dis 145:114-120, 1992.
34. Delaere S, Roeseler J, D'hoore W et al: Respiratory muscle workload in intubated, spontaneously breathing patients without COPD: pressure support vs proportional assist ventilation, Intensive Care Med 29:949-954, 2003.
35. Bigatello L, Nishimura M, Imanaka H et al: Unloading of the work of breathing by proportional assist ventilation in a lung model, Crit Care Med 25:267-272, 1997.
36. Navalesi P, Hernandez P, Wongsa A et al: Proportional assist ventilation in acute respiratory failure: Effects on breathing pattern and inspiratory effort, Am J Respir Crit Care Med 154:1330-1338, 1996.
37. Ranieri VM, Giuliani R, Mascia L et al: Patient-ventilator interaction during acute hypercapnia: pressure support vs. proportional-assist ventilation, J Appl Physiol 81:426-436, 1996.
38. Grasso S, Puntillo F, Mascia L et al: Compensation for increase in respiratory workload during mechanical ventilation, Am J Respir Crit Care Med 161:819-826, 2000.
39. Ranieri VM, Grasso S, Mascia L et al: Effects of proportional assist ventilation on inspiratory muscle effort in patients with chronic obstructive pulmonary disease and acute respiratory failure, Anesthiology 86:79-91, 1997.
40. Dolmage T, Goldstein R: Proportional assist ventilation and exercise tolerance in subjects with COPD, Chest 111:948-954, 1997.
41. Bianchi L, Foglio K, Pagani M et al: Effects of proportional assist ventilation on exercise tolerance in COPD patients with chronic hypercapnia, Eur Respir J 11:422-427, 1998.
42. Ambrosino N, Vitacca M, Polese G et al: Short-term effects of nasal proportional assist ventilation in patients with chronic hypercapneic respiratory insufficiency, Eur Respir J 10:2829-2834, 1997.
43. Wysocki M, Richard JC, Meshaka P: Noninvasive proportional assist ventilation compared with noninvasive pressure support ventilation in hypercapnic acute respiratory failure, Crit Care Med 30:323-329, 2002.
44. Stresemann E, Votteri B, Sattler F: Washout of anatomical dead space for alveolar hypoventilation: preliminary case report, Respiration 26:424-434, 1969.
45. Imanaka H, Kacmarek R, Ritz R et al: Tracheal gas insufflation-pressure control versus volume control ventilation: a lung model study, Am J Respir Crit Care Med 153:1019-1024, 1996.
46. Hoyt J, Marini J, Nahum A: Effect of tracheal gas insufflation on demand valve triggering and total work during continuous positive airway pressure ventilation, Chest 110:775-783, 1996.
47. Kuo P, Wu H, Yu C et al: Efficacy of tracheal gas insufflation in acute respiratory distress syndrome with permissive hypercapnia, Am J Respir Crit Care Med 154:612-616, 1996.
48. Kalfon P, Rao G, Gallart L et al: Permissive hypercapnea with or without expiratory washout in patients with severe acute respiratory distress syndrome, Anesthesiology 87:6-17, 1997.
49. Gowski G, Delgado E, Miro A et al: Tracheal gas insufflation during pressure-control ventilation: effect of using a pressure relief valve, Crit Care Med 25:145-152, 1997.
50. Barnett C, Moore F, Moore E et al: Tracheal gas insufflation is a useful adjunct in permissive hypercapnic management of acute respiratory distress syndrome, Am J Surg 172:518-521, 1996.
51. Oliver R, Rozycki H, Greenspan J et al: Tracheal gas insufflation as a lung-protective strategy: Physiologic, histologic, and biochemical markers, Pediatr Crit Care Med 6:64-69, 2005.
52. Nahum A, Ravenscraft S, Adams A et al: Distal effects of tracheal gas insufflation: changes with catheter position and oleic acid lung injury, J Appl Physiol 81:1121-1127, 1996.
53. Nahum A, Ravenscraft S, Nakos G: Effect of catheter flow direction on CO_2 removal during tracheal gas insufflation in dogs, J Appl Physiol 75:1238-1246, 1993.
54. Nakos G, Lachana A, Prekates A: Respiratory effects of tracheal gas insufflation in spontaneously breathing COPD patients, Intensive Care Med 21:904-912, 1995.
55. Hoffman L, Tasota F, Delgado E et al: Effect of tracheal gas insufflation during weaning from prolonged mechanical ventilation: A preliminary study, Am J Crit Care 12:31-40, 2003.
56. Okamoto K, Kishi H, Choi H et al: Combination of tracheal gas insufflation and airway pressure release ventilation, Chest 111:1366-1374, 1997.
57. Miro A, Hoffman L, Tasota F et al: Tracheal gas insufflation improves ventilatory efficiency during methacholine-induced bronchospasm, J Crit Care 12:13-21, 1997.
58. Meszaros E, Ogawa R: Continuous low-flow tracheal gas insufflation during partial liquid ventilation in rabbits, Acta Anaesthesiol Scand 41:861-867, 1997.

59. Dolan S, Derdak S, Soloman D et al: Tracheal gas insufflation combined with high-frequency oscillatory ventilation, Crit Care Med 24:458-465, 1996.
60. Levy B, Bollaert P, Nace L et al: Intracranial hypertension and adult respiratory distress syndrome: usefulness of tracheal gas insufflation, J Trauma 39:799-801, 1995.
61. Pizov R, Oppenheim A, Eidelman L et al: Helium versus oxygen for tracheal gas insufflation during mechanical ventilation, Crit Care Med 26:290-295, 1998.
62. Bernath M, Henning R: Tracheal gas insufflation reduces requirements for mechanical ventilation in a rabbit model of respiratory distress syndrome, Anaesth Intensive Care 25:15-22, 1997.
63. Danan C, Dassieu G, Janaud J et al: Efficacy of dead-space washout in mechanically ventilated premature newborns, Am J Respir Crit Care Med 153:1571-1576, 1996.
64. Morgan S, Kestner J, Hall J et al: Modification of a critical care ventilator for use during magnetic resonance imaging, Respir Care 47:61-68, 2002.
65. Blanch P, Desautels D, Gallagher T: Deviations in function of mechanical ventilators during hyperbaric compression, Respir Care 36:803-814, 1991.
66. Moon R, Bergquist L, Conklin B et al: Monaghan 225 ventilator use under hyperbaric conditions, Chest 89:846-851, 1986.

CHAPTER

23

High-Frequency Ventilation

Michael A. Gentile; Neil R. MacIntyre

OUTLINE

OBJECTIVES

- Describe nonconvective gas transport.
- List and explain techniques for delivering high-frequency ventilation.
- Recognize the role of various ventilator settings during high-frequency ventilation.
- Assess the outcome data associated with the use of high-frequency ventilation.

KEY TERMS

convective gas transport
high-frequency jet ventilation (HFJV)
high-frequency oscillatory ventilation (HFOV)
high-frequency ventilation (HFV)
jets
lung-protective strategy
nonconvective gas transport
oscillators

Usual approaches to mechanical ventilatory support generally attempt to duplicate the normal bulk flow ventilatory pattern (i.e., tidal volumes (V_Ts) and rates in the physiologic range) in conjunction with elevations in baseline pressures (positive end-expiratory pressure [PEEP]) and inspired O_2 concentration (FIO_2). Despite advances in mechanical ventilation, these strategies may not always provide adequate CO_2 removal and O_2 delivery for diseased lungs. Additionally, conventional mechanical ventilation strategies may damage the lung from excessive lung stretch and/or alveolar collapse/reopening stresses (ventilator induced lung injury or VILI—see Chapter 11).

An alternative approach to ventilatory support that has generated a great deal of interest over the past 2 decades is **high-frequency ventilation (HFV).**[1,2] Generally speaking, HFV is defined as mechanical ventilatory support using higher-than-normal breathing frequencies. For purposes of this discussion, however, only those techniques that use breathing frequencies several fold higher than normal (i.e., greater than 100 breaths/min in the adult and greater than 300 breaths/min in the neonate and/or pediatric patient) are considered. When these frequencies are used, V_Ts are usually much smaller than normal (e.g., less than 1 ml/kg in the alveolar regions) and are often less than anatomic dead space.[1-3]

The major reason for considering HFV is that the smaller tidal pressure swings, coupled with appropriate mean airway pressure applications, create a conceptually ideal **lung-protective strategy.**[1]

Specifically, the combination of a substantial mean airway pressure to maintain recruitment and the limited tidal pressure swings should lead to reductions in both overstretch and repetitive opening-closing stresses in the lung. Put another way, HFV support is applied between the overdistention and the derecruitment points of the injured lung's pressure volume relationship (Figure 23-1), the presumed ideal mechanical range for positive pressure ventilatory support (see Chapters 6 and 15).

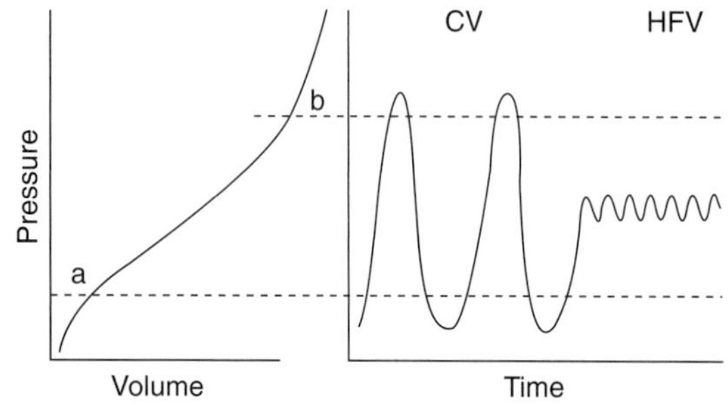

FIGURE 23-1 Conceptual rationale for HFV. Left panel is pressure-volume relationship (plot in a patient with acute lung injury). Points "a" and "b" represent alveolar derecruitment pressure and overdistention pressure, respectively. Right panel illustrates how a high-frequency ventilator with a substantial mean pressure and smaller tidal pressure swings might be expected to ventilate between inflection points more readily than conventional ventilation (CV) with applied PEEP.

DEVICES

Delivery of gas at the frequencies being considered is generally impossible for conventional ventilators with their standard valves and circuits. Different systems therefore must be used, and these usually consist of gas delivery via either **jets (high-frequency jet ventilation [HFJV])** or **oscillators (high-frequency oscillatory ventilation [HFOV])** (Table 23-1).

Jets

High-frequency jets (Figure 23-2) operate on the principle of a nozzle or injector that creates a high velocity "jet" of gas directed into the lung.[4,5] These injectors are usually only 1 to 3 mm in diameter and can be placed in one of several locations in the ventilator circuit and/or patient airway (see Figure 23-2). Generally the further down the airway that the injector is placed, the less is the functional dead space. Jet injectors also can entrain gas from an additional fresh gas source to increase delivered V_T. Because of the inertia of jetted gas, exhalation valves and cuffed airway tubes are unnecessary (although they can be used to manipulate mean and baseline airway pressures). Exhalation with jet ventilation is passive (i.e., due to lung recoil). With a jet ventilator, the clinician usually has control over rate, inspiratory time, jet "drive pressure," and the expiratory pressure. The ultimately delivered jet volume, however, depends on a number of factors (Figure 23-3), including the set drive pressure, the injector diameter, the inspiratory time, the endotracheal tube size (the more narrow the tube, the smaller the volume), the

TABLE 23-1 *High-Frequency Ventilation Devices (Jets and Oscillators) Versus Conventional Ventilation*

	JETS	OSCILLATORS	CONVENTIONAL
Frequencies available	Up to 600 breaths/min	300-3000 breaths/min	2-60 breaths/min
Target delivered volumes	<or> than V_D	$<V_D$	$>>V_D$
Expiration	Passive	Active	Passive
Baseline pressure manipulated by	Extrinsic PEEP valve	Bias flow and extrinsic exhalation valve	Extrinsic PEEP valve
Potential for intrinsic PEEP	+++	++	+
Necessary $f \times V_T$ product for effective VA	>>Conventional	>>Conventional	–
Peak airway pressures	<Conventional	<Conventional	–
Mean airway pressures	<or> Conventional*	<or> Conventional*	–

f, Frequency; *PEEP*, positive end-expiratory pressure; *VA*, alveolar ventilation; V_D, dead-space volume; V_T, tidal volume.

*Standing waves can theoretically create high alveolar/airway pressure relationships near lung resonance frequencies in neonates.

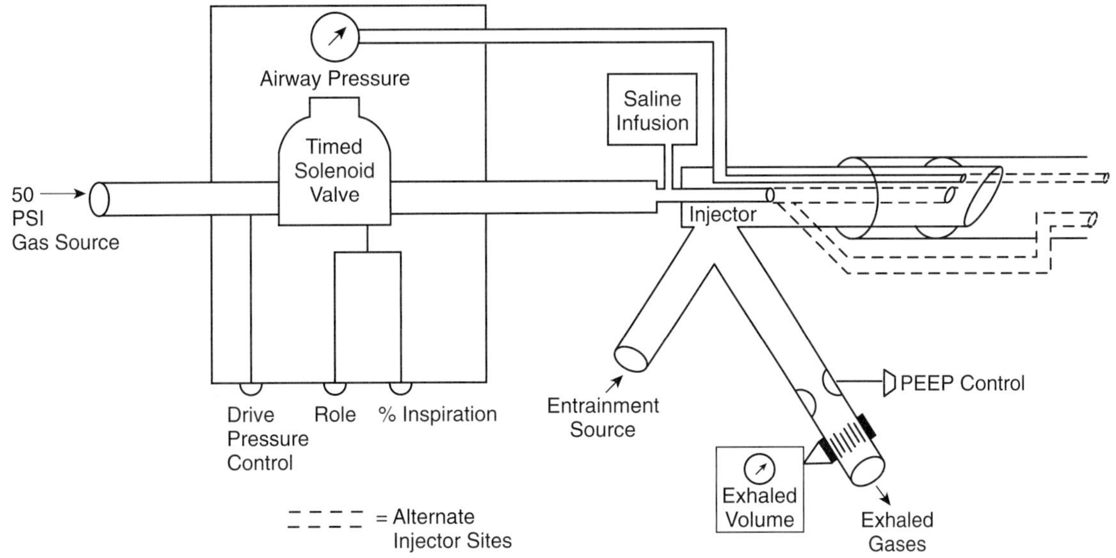

FIGURE 23-2 Schematic diagram of a jet ventilator for delivering HFV. Source gas is supplied to a controlling valve, which then provides jet pulses at the desired pressure, inspiratory duration, and frequency. The delivered pulse may be injected into the distal endotracheal tube or directly into tracheal catheters. In addition, injected pulses can be augmented through entrainment (as shown). Exhalation is passive and does not need an expiratory valve. Positive expiratory pressure can be applied, if desired, in the exhalation circuit. Airway pressure must be measured distal to the jet injector for accuracy. (From Tobin M: Principles and practice of mechanical ventilation, New York, 1994, McGraw-Hill.)

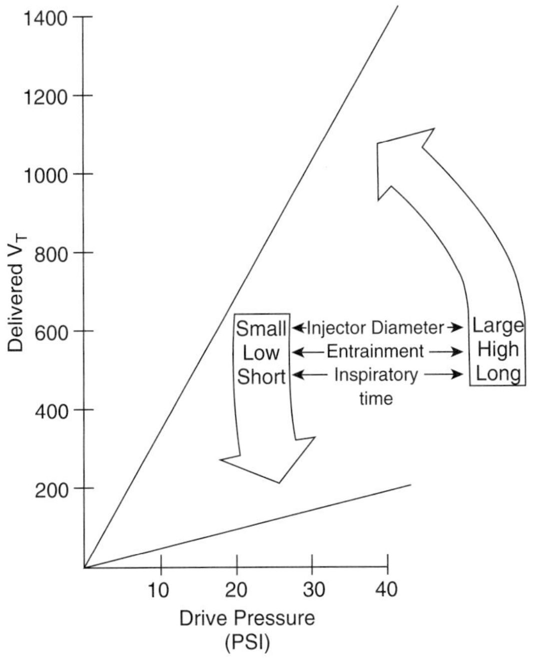

FIGURE 23-3 Relationship between jet drive pressure and ultimately delivered V_T as a function of several system features. (From Tobin M: Principles and practice of mechanical ventilation, New York, 1994, McGraw-Hill.)

presence of an entrainment gas, and the development of air trapping ("intrinsic" PEEP).[1-6]

Monitoring actual volume delivery with flow sensors during HFJV is difficult because the system is often open (see Figure 23-2), and entrainment often is occurring. External chest impedance bands are an alternate approach, but must have appropriate frequency response characteristics to be accurate. Peak and mean airway pressures must be monitored several centimeters distal to the jet nozzle to obtain representative values for the proximal airway.[4,5] In neonates, it is conceivable that at high frequencies (especially near lung resonant frequencies), alveolar pressures can be considerably *higher* than proximal airway pressures because of the development of standing waves.[7] In addition, air trapping from short expiratory times may not be detected in proximal airway sensors.[6] Ventilation parameters with jets usually are set according to pressure monitoring, visual inspection of chest movement, and arterial blood gases. Specific operational considerations are given in Table 23-2. Currently, the only available HFJV devices are for use in neonatal and pediatric patients.

TABLE 23-2 *High-Frequency Ventilation Operational Considerations*

	INFANT JETS	ADULT JETS	INFANT OSCILLATORS	ADULT OSCILLATORS
Initial recommended frequency	7 Hz (IMV background rate of 2)	5 Hz	15 Hz	3-5 Hz
Initial V_T and pressures	Jet drive pressure to produce 90% of CV peak pressure; I time 0.02 sec	Jet drive pressure of 25-35 psi; I:E = 1:2 – 1:1	Amplitude to create chest vibration visually; I:E = 1:1 Mean pressure = CV mean + 5 cm H_2O	Amplitude to create chest vibration visually; I:E = 1:2 – 1:1 Mean pressure = CV mean + 5 cm H_2O
To change effective VA	Alter drive pressure*; alter inspiratory time†; alter frequency‡	Alter drive pressure*; alter inspiratory time†; alter frequency‡	Alter pressure amplitudes*; alter inspiratory time†; alter frequency‡	Alter pressure amplitudes*; alter inspiratory time†; alter frequency‡
To change mean P_{AW} (for $\dot{V}/\dot{Q}$ effects on PaO_2)	Alter applied PEEP; alter inspiratory time†	Alter applied PEEP (if available); alter inspiratory time†	Alter bias flow; alter outflow resistor; alter inspiratory time†	Alter bias flow; alter outflow resistor; alter inspiratory time†

CV, Conventional ventilation; *I*, inspiratory; *I:E*, inspiratory: expiratory; *IMV*, intermittent mandatory ventilation; *PaO_2*, arterial O_2 pressure; *P_{AW}*, airway pressure; *PEEP*, positive end-expiratory pressure; *V_T*, tidal volume; *VA*, alveolar ventilation; $\dot{V}/\dot{Q}$, ventilation-perfusion.

*↑ Pressure = ↑ V_T = ↑ V_A.

†↑ Inspiratory time = ↑ V_T = ↑ V_A *unless* air trapping develops, in which case V_T may ↓.

‡Frequency response may be variable—↑ frequency may increase total ventilation but ↑ frequency can ↓ V_T through shorter inspiratory time and pulse attenuation through narrow endotracheal tubes.

Oscillators

High-frequency oscillators (Figure 23-4) operate with a "to and fro" application of pressure on the airway opening using either pistons or microprocessor gas controllers.[1,2,8] Although simple pistons provide a basic sinusoidal pressure wave form, microprocessor flow controllers can "shape" the inspiratory and expiratory pattern in a variety of ways. Fresh gas is supplied with the ventilator circuit as a "bias flow," and mean airway pressure is adjusted by the relationship between fresh gas inflow and any positive or negative pressure placed on the gas outflow from the bias flow circuit. With oscillators, clinicians usually have the capability to set oscillator frequency, oscillator displacement (volume), inspiratory to expiratory time, and bias flow. A resistor setting on the outflow circuit may also exist and used to interact with bias flow to set mean airway pressure. The actual fresh gas volume delivered to the lung depends on oscillator displacement volume as it interacts with both the magnitude

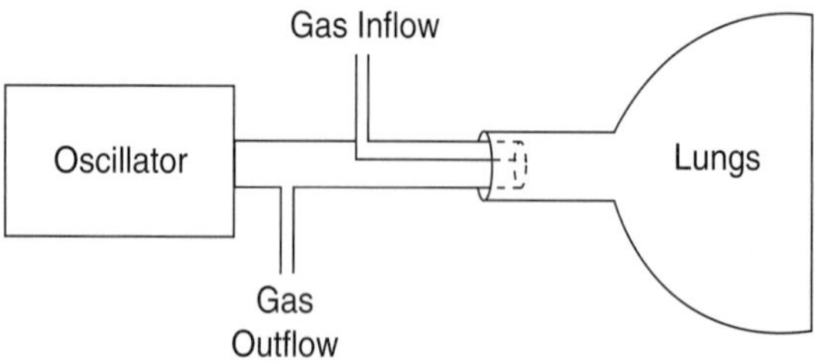

FIGURE 23-4 Schematic diagram of a HFOV for delivering HFV. Airway pressure oscillations are produced by a piston or membrane or microprocessor flow controller at a selected rate and displacement. Fresh gas inflow occurs through a bias flow. Gas outflow and circuit pressure are regulated by adjusting bias flow and/or pressure near the exhalation port. (From Tobin M: Principles and practice of mechanical ventilation, New York, 1994, McGraw-Hill.)

and the location of the bias flow.[8] In general, the magnitude of the bias flow should be adequate to replenish the oscillator displacement volume, and the bias flow location should be as deep as possible in the airways to minimize dead space. Factors such as endotracheal tube size and inspiratory time that affect jetted volumes also affect oscillator delivered volumes.[8]

Similar to HFJV, peak and baseline pressures in the proximal airway may not be reflective of alveolar pressure. Importantly, however, mean airway and alveolar pressures are probably comparable during HFOV.[7,9-11] Intrinsic PEEP also develops with HFOV, but it probably occurs less than with jets because of the active expiratory phase.[6,12]

Because delivered volumes are very difficult to monitor with these systems, ventilation parameters often are set using pressure measurements, visual inspection of chest motion, and arterial blood gases.[13] Specific operational considerations are given in Table 23-2.

MECHANISM OF GAS TRANSPORT

Jet or oscillator tidal breaths are usually small and often are less than anatomic dead space. For effective CO_2 and O_2 transfer to take place between alveoli and the environment under these circumstances, mechanisms other than conventional bulk flow transport (i.e., **nonconvective gas transport**) must be invoked.[14] This is because the traditional relationship between effective alveolar ventilation (VA) and the frequency (f), V_T, and dead-space volume (V_D) (i.e., $VA = f \times [V_T - V_D]$) becomes meaningless when V_T is less than V_D.

At least five different mechanisms exist to explain gas transport under these seemingly "unphysiologic" conditions[2,3,15-20]:

1. Conventional *bulk flow* (i.e., **convective gas transport**) is responsible for gas delivery into the major airways with any high-frequency system. As a consequence, alveoli in close proximity to these airways still can be ventilated principally by this mechanism.[14,17,18]
2. *Coaxial flow* results if the gas-flow profile during one phase of the ventilatory cycle is parabolic and during the other phase is square, a net flow of gas can occur in one direction through the center of the airway and in the other direction via the periphery. Measurements in models of the human tracheobronchial tree have demonstrated such asymmetric flow profiles, but they are quite complex and depend heavily on airway geometry (especially bifurcations) and gas velocity during different phases of the ventilatory cycle.[14,15,17]
3. *Taylor dispersion* is a complex physical concept that describes gas dispersion along the front of a high-velocity gas flow. The dispersion characteristics are different depending on whether flow is turbulent or laminar. Dispersion also is affected by bifurcations in the airway and the development of flow eddies. Net gas transport occurs as a result of this dispersion of gas molecules beyond the bulk flow front.[14,16]
4. *Molecular diffusion* is responsible for gas mixing within alveolar units during conventional ventilation. Molecular diffusion is also likely to serve this role during HFV as well. It is unclear whether augmented molecular diffusion serves any additional role during HFV.
5. *Pendelluft* is the phenomenon of intraunit gas mixing due to impedance differences. This intraunit mixing also can involve airway gas and thus produce effective alveolar ventilation. Pendelluft may be particularly pronounced when HFV is used in a lung with heterogeneous impedances.[14]

The relative importance of each of these mechanisms is not clear. In fact, because these mechanics are not mutually exclusive, all may be operative simultaneously and to varying degrees depending on HFV parameters and the effects of lung disease on regional mechanics.

Predicting gas exchange as a function of ventilator parameters when these nonconvective flow mechanisms are operative during HFV can be difficult. In general, as nonconvective flow mechanisms become more important, alveolar ventilation becomes increasingly a function of frequency times the square of V_T ($f \times V_T^2$). Thus V_T has more effect than f in determining VA. Indeed, increases in frequency, if it produces more air trapping and consequent V_T reduction, can actually reduce effective VA.

The proportionality constant between VA and $f \times V_T^2$ is quite small and thus during nonconvective flow HFV, the $f \times V_T$ product needs to be quite high for effective VA to occur. This is why typical HFV "output" is generally several fold higher than conventional mechanical ventilation (see Table 23-1). Importantly, however, these pressure and volume changes in the major airways are considerably dampened by the time they reach the alveoli and

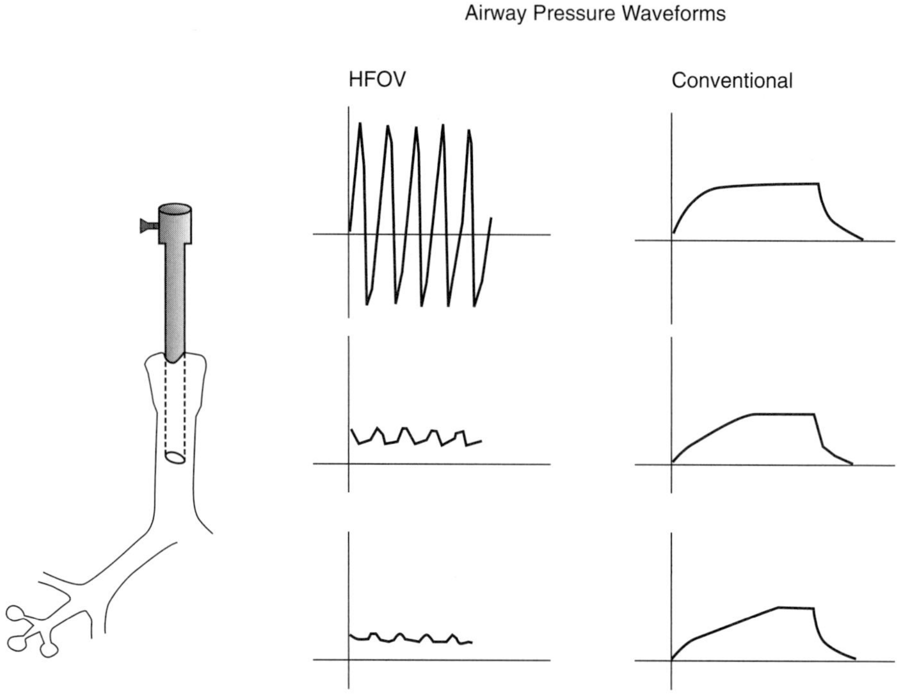

FIGURE 23-5 Airway pressure profiles over time at different sites in the tracheobronchial tree. The left panel reflects HFOV; the right panel reflects conventional ventilation. Note that with HFOV, very large pressure swings in the ventilator circuitry are considerably "dampened" near the alveolar structures. In contrast, with conventional ventilation, circuit pressures equilibrate with alveolar pressures near end inspiration.

thus alveolar pressure and volume changes are small (Figure 23-5). Because of this alveolar pressure profile of small oscillations around a substantial mean during HFOV, some have termed HFOV as being simply "CPAP (continuous positive airway pressure) with a wiggle."

Alveolar capillary gas transport during HFV depends on matching effective ventilation with perfusion ($\dot{V}/\dot{Q}$), just as it does with conventional ventilatory strategies. Thus the alveolar-arterial O_2 difference during HFV remains largely dependent on mean alveolar pressure (and functional residual capacity [FRC]), just as it does with conventional strategies.[1,13,21,22] Interestingly, observational trials with HFV (especially HFOV) described below have often safely used mean pressures higher than conventional ventilation and sometimes higher than what is considered a "safe" maximal pressure during conventional ventilation (i.e., greater than 35 cm H_2O). This may be possible because the tidal pressure swings are so small with HFOV and the application of the higher mean pressure is often a gradual process. Because of this, alveolar epithelial cells may be able to "adapt" to this higher mean stretch.[23]

APPLICATIONS

The strongest clinical data supporting the use of HFV come from studies in neonatal and pediatric populations[13,24-34] (Table 23-3). In these populations, jet breathing frequencies in the range of 250 to 600 breaths/minute or oscillatory frequencies of 500 to 1000 breaths/minute produce adequate gas exchange and often a lower incidence of chronic lung disease in survivors. Several of these studies emphasize the need for HFV to have adequate volume recruitment for successful application. One study even suggests a mortality benefit to HFV in patients with pulmonary interstitial emphysema.[30] As can be seen in Table 23-3, however, not all studies favor HFV although most of the negative trials only showed HFV to be no worse than conventional (i.e., they are equivalent). The one exception to this is the largest randomized trial of HFV ever conducted (the National Institutes of Health [NIH] High Frequency Intervention Trial [HIFI] trial in 673 premature infants),[31] which showed no improvement in respiratory function or outcome but also an increased incidence of intraventricular hemorrhage in the HFV group. The

TABLE 23-3 *Published Randomized Controlled Trials of Neonatal/Pediatric High-Frequency Ventilation*

STUDY	HFV DEVICE	PATIENT POPULATION	MAJOR RESULTS/OUTCOME
Kinsella et al[24]	HFOV	205 PPHN	When combined with inhaled nitric oxide, improved oxygenation with HFOV compared with CV
Gerstman et al[25]	HFOV	125 RDS	When used with a lung-recruitment strategy, HFOV improved PaO_2 and lowered incidence of chronic lung disease compared with CV
Clark et al[26]	HFOV	79 RDS	HFOV had fewer treatment failures than CV
Clark et al[27]	HFOV	83 RDS	HFOV had lower incidence of chronic lung disease than CV
Keszler et al[29]	HFJV	130 RDS	HFJV had lower incidence of chronic lung disease than CV; proper lung recruitment improved oxygenation
Keszler et al[30]	HFJV	144 PIE	HFJV resolved PIE faster than CV; HFJV improved survival when treatment failure cross-over permitted
HIFI[31]	HFOV	673 RDS	No difference between HFOV and CV except for increase IVH in HFOV
Johnson[33]	HFOV	400 RDS	No difference between HFOV and CV
Carlo et al[28]	HFJV	42 RDS	No difference between HFJV and CV
Courtney et al[32]	HFOV	500 RDS	HFOV extubated earlier than CV
Arnold et al[34]	HFOV	75 ARDS	HFOV had lower incidence of chronic lung disease than CV

CV, Conventional ventilation; *HFJV,* high-frequency jet ventilation; *HFOV,* high-frequency oscillatory ventilation; *HIFI,* high-frequency intervention trial; *IVH,* intraventricular hemorrhage; *PaO_2,* partial pressure of O_2; *PIE,* pulmonary interstitial emphysema; *PPHN,* persistent pulmonary hypertension of the newborn; *RDS,* respiratory distress syndrome.

study design of the HIFI trial, however, often has been criticized, especially for its lack of emphasis on alveolar recruitment. Importantly, a recent review of the neonatal-pediatric experience with HFV emphasized that while HFV does provide benefit, the magnitude of that benefit has shrunk over the years as new modalities (e.g., surfactant) and a better appreciation for lung-protective conventional ventilation has emerged.[35]

Adult experience with HFV has been limited because devices with adequate ventilation capabilities for adults are few (Table 23-4). Early jet devices were shown to provide reasonable gas transport with lower peak airway pressures in adult respiratory failure.[36-38] Oscillators with the capabilities to support gas exchange in the adult have been more recently introduced and have shown the capability to support gas exchange safely.[39-41] Our own experience with these devices has been only observational in nature, but has demonstrated that HFOV can supply good gas exchange in patients failing lung-protective conventional ventilation. The largest adult trial to date used an oscillator and demonstrated strong trends in improved mortality in favor of HFV.[40] A concern with this trial was the fact that the control group had a V_T generally considered now to be excessive (see Chapter 10). Larger, better powered trials with appropriate control strategies are thus required.

There do appear to be several potential specific applications for HFV other than support of respiratory failure in the adult. First, the reduced peak pressure and faster rate can alter ventilation distribution and improve gas exchange in patients with very large pulmonary air leaks.[42] However, no data are available demonstrating improved survival in such patients using HFV, and most clinicians would argue that routine bronchopleural fistulas can be ventilated adequately with conventional mechanical ventilation. Second, although cardiac function generally is not affected by HFV compared with conventional ventilation at a given mean airway pressure, synchronizing the HFV pressures with cardiac systole appears to benefit stroke volume in patients with severe cardiac dysfunction.[43] This is an interesting illustration of how intrathoracic pressure swings, if timed to cardiac systole and diastole, can function as a "ventricular assist" device. Third, reduced thoracoabdominal

TABLE 23-4 *Published Adult High-Frequency Ventilation Studies*

STUDY	HFV DEVICE	PATIENT POPULATION	STUDY DESIGN	MAJOR RESULT OUTCOME
Carlon et al[37]	HFJV	300 Respiratory failure	Randomized, controlled	↓Peak P_{AW}; comparable PaO_2, $PaCO_2$, mean P_{AW}, outcome to CV
MacIntyre et al[36]	HFJV	58 Respiratory failure	Crossover	↓Peak P_{AW}; comparable PaO_2, $PaCO_2$, mean P_{AW} to CV
Gluck et al[38]	HFJV	90 ARDS	Crossover	↑ PaO_2/FIO_2, ↓ $PaCO_2$, ↓ Peak P_{AW}, ↓ PEEP need compared with CV; 15% pneumothorax, 15% mucus desiccation in HFJV
Fort et al[39]	HFOV	18 ARDS	Crossover	Comparable PaO_2/FIO_2 compared with CV
Derdak et al[40]	HFOV	148 ARDS	Randomized, controlled	HFOV showed improvement in PaO_2/FIO_2 compared with CV

ARDS, Acute respiratory distress syndrome; *CV,* conventional ventilation; *FIO_2,* inspired O_2 concentration; *HFJV,* high-frequency jet ventilation; *HFOV,* high-frequency oscillatory ventilation; *$PaCO_2$,* alveolar partial pressure of carbon dioxide; *PaO_2,* partial pressure of oxygen; *P_{AW},* airway pressure; *PEEP,* positive end-expiratory pressure.

motion during anesthesia with the use of HFV has been useful in extracorporeal shockwave lithotripsy by minimizing stone motion and, thus procedure time.[44] Finally, the open system provided by the jet ventilator (i.e., a system without a need for an exhalation valve or tight-fitting endotracheal tube) offers additional advantages in two areas: (1) this system allows airway surgical procedures (e.g., bronchoscopy or laryngoscopy) to be performed with adequate ventilatory support and low airway pressures[45]; and (2) transtracheal jet ventilation in emergency situations can be used by trained individuals.[46]

COMPLICATIONS

There are potential problems that are of particular concern when using HFV. Adequate humidification can be difficult to achieve when using high gas flows and delivered minute volumes.[5] Appropriate systems to provide heat and humidity therefore are needed along with frequent assessment of airway function and sputum consistency. The high gas velocity of HFV (especially HFJV) also may cause direct physical airway damage. This, along with inadequate humidification, is thought to be responsible for the necrotizing tracheobronchitis that is observed in some neonates on HFJV.[13] There is also a theoretical concern that the high gas flows of HFV can cause shearing at the interface of different lung regions having different impedances. This may be a cause of barotrauma to both airways and alveoli. Finally, the high mean pressures used with HFV could be an additional source of lung injury and/or reduced cardiac filling.

SUMMARY

HFV is an interesting alternative approach to mechanical ventilatory support that may offer benefits in terms of good gas exchange with a less injurious positive airway pressure pattern. It should be considered when escalating controlled mandatory ventilation support yields little improvement in gas exchange and the required ventilator pattern may be inflicting VILI. Clinical data demonstrating improved outcome exist for neonatal and some forms of pediatric respiratory failure. The data for adults are much less because the devices for such application have only recently been introduced. A randomized controlled trial has yielded a trend toward improved outcomes, but the widespread use of HFV in adults with acute respiratory distress syndrome (ARDS) remains limited. There are important complications that can develop, and an extensive "learning curve" is required for operators to become skilled at delivering proper support in a safe fashion.

KEY POINTS

- HFV provides V_Ts much smaller than anatomic dead space at rates several times faster than normal. It conceptually is an attractive lung-protective strategy since alveolar recruitment can be substantial and tidal pressure/volume changes at the alveolar level are very small.
- Gas transport with HFV involves a number of poorly understood mechanisms that include Taylor dispersion, coaxial flows, augmented diffusion, and pendelluft.
- HFV can be delivered either by jet devices (high-velocity bursts of gas through a nozzle) or by rapidly oscillating a fresh gas bias flow.
- The neonatal/pediatric literature strongly suggests less long-term lung injury when using HFV. The adult literature is much less robust and the one small randomized trial showed only a trend for improved survival. Further studies are clearly needed.

ASSESSMENT QUESTIONS

1. True or False. HFV is defined as breathing frequencies more than 500 breaths per minute.
2. True or False. Conventional ventilators can generally deliver breathing frequencies of 200 to 300 breaths per minute.
3. True or False. Jets and oscillators are the two most common ways to deliver HFV.
4. True or False. An oscillator is essentially a continuous flow CPAP system with oscillations superimposed at the airway.
5. True or False. The traditional alveolar ventilation equation ($VA = f \times [V_T - V_D]$) explains HFV up to breathing frequencies of 1000 breaths per minute.
6. True or False. The largest clinical database supporting the use of HFV comes from studies in neonatal and pediatric populations.
7. True or False. The largest randomized trial of HFV in neonates (the NIH HIFI trial) showed traumatic improvements in outcome with high-frequency ventilation.
8. True or False. One advantage to a high-frequency jet device is that an airway seal is not required and thus the device could be used to support various airway procedures (e.g., bronchoscopy).
9. True or False. There are no high-frequency devices approved for use in adults.
10. True or False. The one randomized controlled trial of HFV in adults showed a trend for improved outcomes with HFV, but this did not reach statistical significance.

CASE STUDIES

For additional practice refer to Case Study 8 in the appendix at the back of this book.

REFERENCES

1. Imai Y, Slutsky AS: High-frequency oscillatory ventilation and ventilator-induced lung injury, Crit Care Med 33(3 Suppl):S129-S134, 2005.
2. Drazen JM, Kamm RD, Slutsky AS: High-frequency ventilation, Physiol Rev 64:505-543, 1984.
3. Slutsky AS, Kamm RD, Rossing TH et al: Effects of frequency, tidal volume, and lung volume on CO_2 elimination in dogs by high frequency (2-30 Hz), low tidal volume ventilation, J Clin Invest 68:1475-1484, 1981.
4. Bunnell JB: High frequency hardware, Med Instrum 19:208-216, 1985.
5. Carlon GC, Miodownik S, Ray C et al: Technical aspects and clinical implications of high frequency jet ventilation with a solenoid valve, Crit Care Med 9:47-50, 1981.
6. Beamer WC, Donald PS, Roger RL et al: High frequency jet ventilation produces auto-PEEP, Crit Care Med 12:734-737, 1984.
7. Spahn DR, Bush EH, Schmid ER et al: Resonant amplification and flow/pressure characteristics in high frequency ventilation, Med Biol Eng Comput 26:355-359, 1988.
8. Fredburg JJ, Glass GM, Boynton BR et al: Factors influencing mechanical performance of neonatal high frequency ventilators, J Appl Physiol 62:2485-2490, 1987.

9. All JL, Frantz ID III, Fredberg JJ: Heterogeneity of mean alveolar pressure during high-frequency oscillations, J Appl Physiol 62:223-228, 1987.
10. Fredberg JJ, Keefe DH, Glass GM et al: Alveolar pressure nonhomogeneity during small amplitude high-frequency oscillation, J Appl Physiol 57:788-800, 1984.
11. Smith DW, Frankel LR, Ariagno RL: Dissociation of mean airway pressure and lung volume during high-frequency oscillatory ventilation, Crit Care Med 16: 531-535, 1988.
12. Bancalari A, Gerhardt T, Bancalari E et al: Gas trapping with high-frequency ventilation: jet versus oscillatory ventilation, J Pediatr 110:617-622, 1987.
13. Coghill CH, Haywood JL, Chatburn RL et al: Neonatal and pediatric high-frequency ventilation: principles and practice, Respir Care 36:596-612, 1991.
14. Chang HK: Mechanisms of gas transport during ventilation by high frequency oscillation, J Appl Physiol Respir Environ Exerc Physiol 56:553-563, 1984.
15. Brusasco V, Knopp TJ, Rehder K: Gas transport during high-frequency ventilation, J Appl Physiol Respir Environ Exerc Physiol 55:472-478, 1983.
16. Fredberg JJ: Augmented diffusion in the airways can support pulmonary gas exchange, J Appl Physiol Respir Environ Exerc Physiol 49:323-338, 1980.
17. Isabey D, Hart A, Chang HK: Alveolar ventilation during high-frequency oscillation: core dead space concept, J Appl Physiol Respir Environ Exerc Physiol 56:700-707, 1984.
18. Sherer PW, Haselton FR: Convective exchange in oscillatory flow through bronchial-tree models, J Appl Physiol Respir Environ Exerc Physiol 53:1023-1033, 1982.
19. Permutt S, Mitzner W, Weinmann G: Model of gas transport during high-frequency ventilation, J Appl Physiol 58:1956-1970, 1985.
20. Vengas JG, Hales CA, Strieder DJ: A general dimensionless equation of gas transport by high-frequency ventilation, J Appl Physiol 60:1025-1030, 1986.
21. Walsh MC, Carlo WA: Sustained inflation during high frequency oscillatory ventilation improves pulmonary mechanics and oxygenation, J Appl Physiol 65:368-372, 1988.
22. Simon BA, Weinmann GC, Mitzner W: Mean airway pressure and alveolar pressure during high-frequency ventilation, J Appl Physiol 57:1069-1078, 1984.
23. Hubmayr RD: Cellular stress failure in ventilator-injured lungs, Am J Respir Crit Care Med 171:1328-1342, 2005.
24. Kinsella JP, Truog WE, Welsh WF et al: Randomized multicenter trial of inhaled nitric oxide and high frequency oscillatory ventilatory in severe PPHN, J Pediatr 131:55-62, 1988.
25. Gerstman DR, Minton SD, Stoddard RA et al: The Provo multicenter early HFOV trial, Pediatrics 98:1044-1057, 1996.
26. Clark RH, Yoder BA, Sells MS: Prospective randomized comparison of HFOV and conventional ventilation in candidates for ECMO, J Pediatr 124:447-454, 1994.
27. Clark RH, Gerstmann DR, Null DM et al: Prospective randomized comparison of HFOV and conventional ventilation in RDS, Pediatrics 89:5-12, 1992.
28. Carlo WA, Siner B, Chatburn RL et al: Early randomized intervention with high-frequency jet ventilation in respiratory distress syndrome, J Pediatr 117:765-770, 1990.
29. Keszler M, Modanlo HD, Brudno DS et al: Multicenter controlled trial of HFJV in a preterm infant with uncomplicated respiratory distress syndrome, Pediatrics 100:593-599, 1997.
30. Keszler M, Donn SM, Bucciarelli RL et al: Multicenter controlled trial comparing HFJV and conventional mechanical ventilation in newborn infants with PIE, J Pediatr 119:85-93, 1991.
31. The HIFI Study Group: High-frequency oscillatory ventilation compared with conventional mechanical ventilation in the treatment of respiratory failure in preterm infants, N Engl J Med 320:88-93, 1989.
32. Courtney SE, Durand DJ, Asselin JM et al: Neonatal Ventilation Study Group. High-frequency oscillatory ventilation versus conventional mechanical ventilation for very-low-birth-weight infants, N Engl J Med 347:643-652, 2002.
33. Johnson AH, Peacock JL, Greenough A et al: High frequency oscillatory ventilation for the prevention of lung disease of prematurity, N Engl J Med 347:633-642, 2002.
34. Arnold JH, Hanson JH, Toro-Figuero LO et al: Prospective, randomized comparison of high-frequency oscillatory ventilation and conventional mechanical ventilation in pediatric respiratory failure, Crit Care Med 22:1530-1539, 1994.
35. Bollen C, Uiterwaal CS, van Vught AJ: Cumulative meta-analysis of high frequency vs. conventional ventilation in premature neonates, Am J Respir Crit Care Med 168:1150-1155, 2003.
36. MacIntyre NR, Follett JV, Deitz JL et al: Jet ventilation at 100 BPM in adult respiratory failure, Am Rev Respir Dis 134:897-901, 1986.
37. Carlon GC, Howland WS, Ray C et al: High-frequency ventilation: a prospective randomized evaluation, Chest 84:551-559, 1983.
38. Gluck E, Heard S, Petel C et al: Use of ultra high frequency ventilator in patients with ARDS, Chest 103:1413-1420, 1993.
39. Fort P, Farmer C, Westerman J et al: HFOV ventilator for ARDS—a pilot study, Crit Care Med 25:937-947, 1997.
40. Derdak S, Metha S, Stewart T et al: High-frequency oscillatory ventilation for acute respiratory distress syndrome in adults: A randomized, controlled trial, Am J Respir Care Med 166:801-808, 2002.
41. Mehta S, Granton J, MacDonald RJ et al: High-frequency oscillatory ventilation in adults: the Toronto experience, Chest 126:518-527, 2004.
42. Carlon GC, Ray C Jr, Klain M et al: High-frequency positive-pressure ventilation in management of a patient with bronchopleural fistula, Anesthesiology 52:160-162, 1980.

43. Pinsky MR, Marquez J, Martin D et al: Ventricular assist by cardiac cycle-specific increases in intrathoracic pressures, Chest 91:709-715, 1987.
44. Carlson CA, Boysen PG, Nabber MJ et al: Conventional vs. high frequency jet ventilation for extracorporeal shock wave lithotripsy, Anesthesiology 63: A530, 1985.
45. MacIntyre NR, Ramage JE, Follett JV: Jet ventilation in support of fiberoptic bronchoscopy, Crit Care Med 15:303-307, 1987.
46. Klain M, Smith RB: High frequency percutaneous transtracheal jet ventilation, Crit Care Med 5:280-285, 1977.

CHAPTER

24

Extracorporeal Techniques for Cardiopulmonary Support

Michael A. Gentile; Ira M. Cheifetz

OUTLINE

OBJECTIVES

- Explain the history of extracorporeal life support (ECLS) and the available technology.
- Identify the populations who might benefit from ECLS, including patient selection criteria.
- List the potential complications of ECLS.
- Describe the outcomes for neonatal, pediatric, cardiac, and adult extracorporeal life support.

KEY TERMS

activated clotting time (ACT)
extracorporeal life support (ECLS)
extracorporeal membrane oxygenation (ECMO)
intravascular oxygenator (IVOX)
partial extracorporeal life support (ECLS)
venoarterial bypass
venovenous bypass

Extracorporeal life support (ECLS) or **extracorporeal membrane oxygenation (ECMO)** is an invasive and complex form of cardiopulmonary bypass for patients with severe reversible cardiac and/or pulmonary failure when maximum conventional therapies are not effective. This technique once was used exclusively in the operating room for short-term support during cardiothoracic surgery. The use of ECLS allows for blood circulation and gas exchange outside the body while theoretically resting the heart and lungs. The major advantage of extracorporeal techniques is to provide adequate gas exchange with less ventilatory support, including a lower inspired O_2 concentration (FIO_2) and reduced airway pressures. Potential complications are significant and include clot formation, extensive bleeding due to systemic anticoagulation, and technical failure.

HISTORY OF EXTRACORPOREAL LIFE SUPPORT

The technology used during ECLS is not new. Extracorporeal circulation first was devised as a tool for

TABLE 24-1 *Neonatal ECLS Diagnoses and Survival Rates to Hospital Discharge or Transfer*

DIAGNOSIS	NO. OF CASES	SURVIVAL RATE (%)
Meconium aspiration syndrome	6867	94
Respiratory distress syndrome	1403	84
Congenital diaphragmatic hernia	4881	52
Sepsis or pneumonia	2444	75
Persistent pulmonary hypertension	3153	78
Air leak syndrome	101	71
Other	1385	63
Total	**20,234**	**76**

Data from ELSO: Neonatal ECLS registry, Ann Arbor, Mich, 2006, Extracorporeal Life Support Organization.

cardiac surgery. As early as 1936, John Gibbon was attempting to research and develop a roller pump that could sustain life during surgical procedures of the heart and great vessels.[1] In 1944, Kolff and Beck reported the oxygenation of venous blood during dialysis.[2] As the technology of open heart surgery was advanced in the 1950s, so was the use of cardiopulmonary bypass. The first membrane oxygenator was developed by Clowes and associates in 1956.[3] This was a substantial technical advancement, but it could not support life for more than a few hours. Common complications of cardiopulmonary bypass at that time were thrombocytopenia, coagulopathy, hemolysis, and renal and pulmonary dysfunction. Soon it was discovered that the silicone rubber used in these initial membrane oxygenators had uncommon gas transfer characteristics and was unreliable.[4]

The 1960s were a time of intensive laboratory research to prolong the time that cardiopulmonary bypass could be performed and to improve the functionality of membrane lungs. An oxygenator constructed of dimethylpolysiloxane similar to the one that currently is commonly used was developed in 1963.[5] With such a device, it was possible to perform extended bypass procedures in animals up to 1 week.[6] Several premature neonates were supported with ECLS, but all died of intraventricular hemorrhage.[7-9] The first successful human ECLS case was reported in 1972, in which a 24-year-old male with multiple trauma injuries was supported for 75 hours.[10]

In 1974, the National Institutes of Health sponsored a multicenter, randomized trial that compared venoarterial ECLS with conventional therapy in adult patients with respiratory failure. The results failed to show an improvement in outcome. Both ECLS and conventional therapies demonstrated a dismal survival rate, with no significant difference (9.5% survival rate in ECLS patients and 8.3% in the conventional therapy group).[11]

Meanwhile, the neonatal population was being treated successfully by Bartlett.[12] Throughout the 1980s, additional centers started to use ECLS technology for neonates with reversible lung disease who were failing conventional support. Over the past 20 years, ECLS has moved into many intensive care units (ICUs) and has become a standard of care for days and even weeks in the support of patients of many age groups with severe cardiopulmonary dysfunction.

PATIENT SELECTION AND CRITERIA FOR EXTRACORPOREAL LIFE SUPPORT

In the ICU, several diagnoses commonly are associated with ECLS. These are detailed in Tables 24-1 through 24-4.[13] Although criteria for ECLS vary from center to center and patient to patient, there are several general recommendations on which most clinicians agree.

The general guidelines for neonatal ECLS include a disease process that is deemed reversible, gestational age older than 32 weeks, weight greater than 2 kg, "significant" mechanical ventilation for no more than 7 to 10 days before ECLS, no significant immunosuppression, absence of intraventricular hemorrhage, no severe neurologic dysfunction, and no significant chromosomal abnormality. However, many centers perform ECLS on patients with trisomy 21.[14] It should be noted that these general criteria do vary among centers.

For all age groups, ECLS usually is considered after failure of other available therapies (e.g., surfactant, high-frequency ventilation, inhaled nitric oxide, and lung protective ventilation often with permissive hypercapnea). Additionally, a persistent significant air leak is a reasonable indication for ECLS. Some centers use an O_2 index (OI) greater than 40 (Figure 24-1) and an alveolar-arterial O_2 difference (A-aDO$_2$) greater than 500 × 4 hours (see Figure 24-1) as ECLS criteria, but other centers use lower cutoffs. These

TABLE 24-2 *Pediatric ECLS Diagnoses and Survival Rates to Hospital Discharge or Transfer*

DIAGNOSIS	NO. OF CASES	SURVIVAL RATE (%)
Bacterial pneumonia	344	56
Viral pneumonia	802	63
Aspiration	174	67
Acute respiratory distress syndrome (ARDS), postoperative/ trauma	80	61
ARDS, not postoperative/trauma	307	52
Acute respiratory failure, non-ARDS	629	48
Pneumocystis pneumonia	24	46
Others	850	53
Total	**3210**	**56**

Data from ELSO: Neonatal ECLS registry, Ann Arbor, Mich, 2006, Extracorporeal Life Support Organization.

TABLE 24-3 *Neonatal (≤30 Days of Age) Cardiac ECLS Diagnoses and Survival Rates to Hospital Discharge or Transfer*

DIAGNOSIS	NO. OF CASES	SURVIVAL RATE (%)
Cardiac surgery	2363	36
Cardiac arrest	28	25
Myocarditis	31	42
Cardiomyopathy	76	64
Cardiogenic shock	29	41
Other	201	43
Total	**2728**	**38**

Data from ELSO: Neonatal ECLS registry, Ann Arbor, Mich, 2006, Extracorporeal Life Support Organization.

TABLE 24-4 *Adult ECLS Diagnoses and Survival Rates to Hospital Discharge or Transfer*

DIAGNOSIS	NO. OF CASES	SURVIVAL RATE (%)
Bacterial pneumonia	216	52
Viral pneumonia	88	63
Aspiration	34	59
Acute respiratory distress syndrome (ARDS), postoperative / trauma	141	52
ARDS, postoperative / trauma	214	50
Acute respiratory failure, non-ARDS	67	64
Others	421	48
Total	**1181**	**52**

Data from ELSO: Neonatal ECLS registry, Ann Arbor, Mich, 2006, Extracorporeal Life Support Organization.

Oxygenation Index

$$OI = \frac{(F_{IO_2})(P_{AW}) \times 100}{Pa_{O_2}}$$

Alveolar–Arterial Oxygen Gradient

$$A - a_{DO_2} = ([P_{IO_2} - \frac{Pa_{CO_2}}{R}]) - Pa_{O_2}$$

P = Atmospheric Pressure

FIGURE 24-1 Alveolar-arterial O_2 difference (A-aDO_2) and O_2 index (OI) calculations.

criteria are based on the mortality risk without ECLS. A pre-ECLS OI of between 25 and 40 has been associated with a 50% mortality rate on conventional therapy. If the OI is greater than 40, the chance of mortality historically has been reported to be as high as 80%.[15]

For cardiac patients, ECLS criteria remain subjective and include severe and reversible cardiac dysfunction for which maximum therapy has failed. Most cardiac ECLS is performed in the postoperative

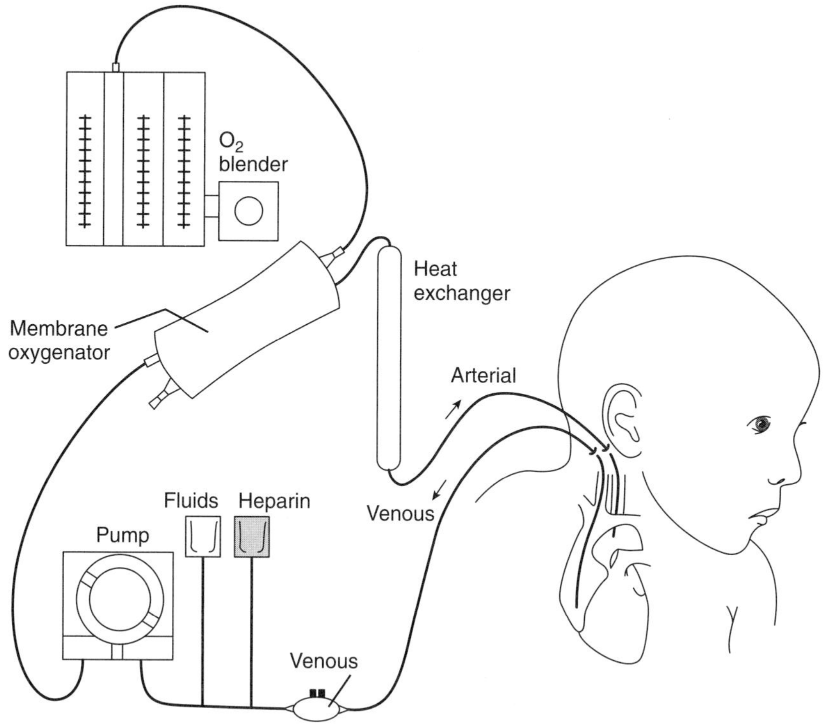

FIGURE 24-2 Venoarterial ECLS. (From MacIntyre NR, Leonard RA: Unconventional support techniques for ventilation and oxygenation. In Dantzker DR, MacIntyre NR, Bakow ED: Comprehensive respiratory care, Philadelphia, 1995, Saunders.)

period, when the patient cannot be weaned from cardiopulmonary bypass or when assistance is needed for poor ventricular performance.[13,16,17] Patients with severe myocarditis may be supported with ECLS until the condition resolves or until transplantation is possible.[17] Additionally, ECLS is an option for patients with complicated post-transplant courses.

The use of ECLS to support patients after surgery for congenital heart disease has been increasing because improvements in myocardial and cerebral protection, surgical techniques, and perioperative care have led to the recommendation of early neonatal repair for most congenital heart lesions, including hypoplastic heart syndrome. Hospital survival is better for those patients who are cannulated for ECLS in the operating room rather than in the ICU.[18] This finding is most likely related to early effective cardiovascular support preventing prolonged periods of hypoperfusion and the avoidance of a catastrophic cardiac arrest. Predictors for adverse outcome for cardiac ECLS includes serious mechanical ECMO complications, need for renal support, residual cardiac lesions, and a prolonged duration of ECLS support.[18]

TYPES OF EXTRACORPOREAL LIFE SUPPORT

Venoarterial Extracorporeal Life Support

Venoarterial bypass ECLS (Figure 24-2) is near complete cardiopulmonary bypass that supports both cardiac and pulmonary functions. The degree of bypass that occurs is primarily a function of the ECLS pump flow rate and the intravascular volume status of the patient. The system consists of six components: an extracorporeal circuit, a blood-circulating pump, a membrane oxygenator, a heat exchanger, monitoring and safety devices, and patient cannulas.[17] The extracorporeal circuit consists of a series of super Tygon tubes and access adapters to circulate venous blood from the patient through the blood-circulating pump and membrane lung back to the patient. The membrane lung can be either a silicone or hollow-fiber oxygenator, which is highly permeable to CO_2 and O_2 gas exchange. The surface area of the membrane lung, selected according to patient size, and the flow of ventilating gases across the membrane determine the rate of gas exchange. The blood pump

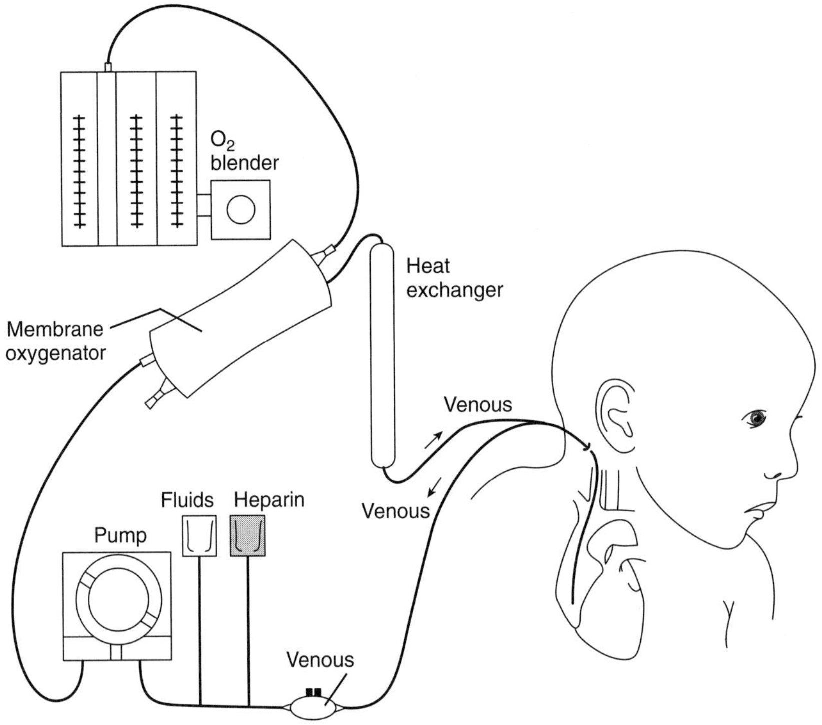

FIGURE 24-3 **Double lumen venovenous ECLS.** (From MacIntyre NR, Leonard RA: Unconventional support techniques for ventilation and oxygenation. In Dantzker DR, MacIntyre NR, Bakow ED: Comprehensive respiratory care, Philadelphia, 1995, Saunders.)

provides the driving pressure from the patient's venous circulation across the membrane lung and back to the arterial circulation.

Two types of extracorporeal pumps commonly are used: the roller head displacement pump and the centrifugal pump.[17] The circuit cardiac output is a function of blood volume and the speed of pump revolutions. A heat exchanger placed proximal to the patient's arterial return warms the circulating blood volume to body temperature to help prevent hypothermia from ambient cooling of extracorporeal blood volumes. Appropriately sized cannulas access the circuit to the patient. Specific monitors within the circuit provide information on circuit safety, function, and performance.

Neonatal and pediatric venoarterial extracorporeal support generally accesses the right atrium for venous return via cannulation of the internal jugular vein. The common carotid artery on both neonatal and pediatric patients is cannulated for blood return to the body. Adult patients typically require alteration of this technique, either by direct transthoracic access to the atrium and aorta or by femoral access.[16] Venoarterial ECLS is almost complete cardiopulmonary bypass, draining venous return from the right atrium, circulating the blood through the extracorporeal circuit, and then returning the blood to the aortic arch. Because it is very effective, the patient can be supported for days to several weeks.[16]

The major advantage of venoarterial ECLS is complete control over the patient's cardiac output and gas exchange. The disadvantages of venoarterial ECLS are that ligation of a major artery is required and there is the possibility of air or clots embolizing to the central nervous system. In larger patients, some centers have successfully started to reconnect the artery after ECLS is discontinued. The major risk to this procedure is again emboli.[19]

Venovenous Extracorporeal Life Support

Venovenous bypass ECLS (Figure 24-3) takes only a portion (e.g., 30% to 60%) of the cardiac output from the venous circulation, passes it through a membrane oxygenator, and returns it to the major veins.[20] Venovenous ECLS is essentially adding another lung to the patient and is generally reserved for patients with adequate cardiac output. If cardiac insufficiency develops, the patient must be supported by inotropic support or surgically converted to venoarterial ECLS.

Venovenous ECLS accesses venous return in neonatal patients and some pediatric patients by placement of a double-lumen cannula into the right atrium through the internal jugular vein (see Figure 24-3). Venous return circulates from the right atrium through the extracorporeal circuit and returns to the right atrium.[21] Cannula outflow is placed proximal to the tricuspid valve to minimize recirculation of the oxygenated blood from the extracorporeal system. Percutaneous cannulation has been successfully used.[22]

In neonatal and pediatric patients, this technique is gaining popularity for patients who previously were considered for venoarterial ECLS. Interest in this technique is increasing because no arterial ligation or repair is needed and all debris, clots, and air are routed to the pulmonary circulation and not to the cerebral or systemic circulation.[16] The major disadvantage to venovenous ECLS is that it does not provide cardiac support.

COMPLICATIONS ASSOCIATED WITH EXTRACORPOREAL LIFE SUPPORT

Complications of ECLS usually are related to anticoagulation, preexisting hypoxic or hypotensive injury to organs, and technical and mechanical complications within the ECLS circuit. Hemorrhage is the most common and potentially disastrous complication of ECLS and occurs in approximately 25% of neonatal cases.[13] Bleeding most commonly occurs in the central nervous system, the gastrointestinal tract, and the lungs, or at operative sites. The most devastating of these occurs in the brain. Proper patient selection (e.g., greater than 2 kg body weight, greater than 32 weeks gestational age, and normal head ultrasound results) and measurements of serum lactate can help minimize the probability of intracranial hemorrhage. Serum lactates greater than 10 mmol/L have been associated with an increased risk of intracranial bleeding.[23] Maintaining **activated clotting times (ACTs)** less than approximately 200 seconds also can decrease the incidence of bleeding complications. It should be noted that the ideal ACT will vary based on the measurement technology used.

Seizures associated with fluid and electrolyte abnormalities can be seen at the time of cannulation and during the early hours of ECLS. Pediatric patients (1 month to 18 years of age) who have a metabolic acidosis, a bicarbonate or inotrope/vasopressor requirement, cardiopulmonary resuscitation, or a left ventricular assist device before initiation of ECLS are at greater risk for the development of central nervous system complications. After initiation of ECLS, pediatric patients who develop renal failure or metabolic acidosis or who undergo venoarterial ECLS should be closely monitored for the development of central nervous system complications.[24]

Other problems applicable to ECLS for all patient populations include renal failure due to the nonpulsatile flow of ECLS, hemolysis, hypotension, hypertension, pneumothorax, infection, and cardiac arrhythmias. Complications should be recognized early to optimize the chance for appropriate treatment.[13,17,25]

Mechanical and technical complications of ECLS are rare but equally potentially hazardous. The most common complication, occurring in as many as 50% of neonatal ECLS cases, is clot formation in the circuit, most commonly in the oxygenator, bridge, or bladder.[13] The incidence of clots increases in linear fashion to the length of time on ECLS. Other mechanical complications commonly reported are oxygenator failure, tubing rupture, pump failure, cannulation kinks, heat exchanger malfunction, air in the circuitry, and cracks in the connectors.[13] Meliones and colleagues found a significant association between a calculated "complication score" and a chance of survival, with nonsurvivors having more complications during ECLS.[26]

PATIENT MANAGEMENT DURING EXTRACORPOREAL LIFE SUPPORT

Ventilator and Respiratory Care

The main intent of ECLS is cardiopulmonary support without the iatrogenic complications known to be associated with high ventilation pressures and O_2 toxicity. With these intentions in mind, ventilatory support may be reduced significantly during ECLS. Maintaining positive end-expiratory pressure (PEEP) levels of approximately 10 cm H_2O and a low tidal volume or peak inspiratory pressure maintains lung expansion while minimizing barotrauma and/or volutrauma. Measurement of dynamic lung compliance may be helpful in the assessment of recovery. A dynamic compliance of 0.8 ml/cm H_2O/kg or greater has predicted successful discontinuation of ECLS.[27]

Successful weaning from ECLS has occurred at lower dynamic compliance values. Chest physiotherapy, endotracheal suctioning, and bronchoscopy may be performed to remove retained pulmonary secretions. Instillation of surfactant also may be beneficial in decreasing the length of ECLS support.

Anticoagulation

Continuous heparin infusion is adjusted to keep the ACTs between approximately 160 and 200 seconds. Again, it must be noted that the ideal ACT range will vary with the measurement technology used. The ACT is influenced by blood product administration and other substances that are injected into the circuit. The ACTs must be adjusted if hemorrhage or clotting (blood coagulation) in the circuit presents problems.

Sedation and Analgesia

A patient receiving ECLS should generally not be treated with neuromuscular blockade with the exception of during the initial catheter placement and other surgical procedures. Maintaining muscle function allows for periodic neurologic examinations, observation for seizures, and the increased potential for mobilizing third-spaced fluids. The more commonly used medications for ECLS sedation are morphine and midazolam. The patients should be sedated only to the point that they are comfortable and not at risk for moving the cannulas or impeding venous return.

Nutrition

Nutritional support for ECLS patients must be tailored to the specific caloric and supplement requirements of each patient. It is common practice to start parenteral nutrition within 24 hours of initiation of ECLS. Total parenteral nutrition may be infused directly into the ECLS circuit, although the administration of intralipids remains controversial. Some centers have reported using enteral feeds via nasogastric tubes without complications, although this practice also remains debatable.[28]

CURRENT STATUS OF EXTRACORPOREAL LIFE SUPPORT AND OUTCOME IN PEDIATRICS

Currently there are more than 100 centers throughout the world that have provided ECLS for almost 32,000 patients since 1986 with an overall ECLS survival rate of 76%.[13] Survival to hospital discharge or transfer is 65%.[13] In recent years, other therapies, including high-frequency ventilation, inhaled nitric oxide, and improved surfactant products, have reduced the number of patients requiring ECLS and the number of centers providing ECLS services.[29-31] It is unclear if this trend will continue, resulting in the need for increased regionalization of ECLS services.

A Cochrane review concludes that mature infants with potentially reversible respiratory failure have improved survival without increased risk of severe disability with ECLS.[32] Neonatal ECLS survivors experience lung injury lasting into childhood; however, many have normal lung function by 15 years of age.[33,34] Lung dysfunction correlates with the extent and duration of barotrauma and O_2 exposure in the peri-ECLS period.[33,34] The cost effectiveness of neonatal ECLS has been supported based on the United Kingdom Collaborative ECMO trial. Over 4 years, neonatal ECMO for mature infants with severe respiratory failure was demonstrated to be cost-effective at reducing known death or severe disability.[35]

Infants and children with congenital heart disease who are supported with ECLS in the postoperative period have survival rates to hospital discharge ranging from 32% to 48%.[13,36-39] Mortality risk for this population has been reported to be increased in males, patients less than 1 month of age, patients with a longer duration of mechanical ventilation before initiation of ECLS, and patients who developed renal or hepatic failure during ECLS. In one report of infants requiring ECLS after cardiac surgery, 75% of survivors to hospital discharge had normal neuromotor outcome but only 50% had normal neurocognitive outcome.[39]

EXTRACORPOREAL LIFE SUPPORT TECHNOLOGY FOR ADULT RESPIRATORY FAILURE

Clinical data supporting outcome benefit to ECLS systems in adult acute respiratory failure are few. As noted above, the original National Institutes of Health trial of ECMO in severe acute respiratory failure in 1979 was clearly negative in that both the treated group and the control group had mortality in excess of 90%. There are many reasons, however, to believe that outcomes from severe adult respiratory failure managed with ECLS might be better today. For example, the technology of ECLS has clearly advanced over the last 25 years and the attendant risks and complications have been dramatically reduced, especially with venovenous systems. Perhaps just as important is that the new appreciation for protecting the lung from ventilator induced lung injury is in marked contrast to the injurious high tidal volume ventilator strategy commonly used in the late 1970s. ECLS for severe ARDS in adults has been gradually increasing over the last 3 decades and has been successful in a subset of those patients who do not respond to conventional mechanical ventilator strategies. Survival rates to hospital discharge today are reported to be as high as 56% (see Table 24-3).[13,38,40,41]

In the United Kingdom, an important randomized controlled trial is underway to hopefully define the role of ECMO in severe acute respiratory failure. Known as the CESAR (**C**onventional Ventilation or **E**CMO for **S**evere **A**cute **R**espiratory Failure) trial (cesar-trial.org), 180 patients were recruited who have: (1) potentially reversible acute respiratory failure, (2) a Murray lung score greater than 3, and (3) been less than 7 days on a ventilator. Sample size calculations are based on an expected mortality of greater than 60%. The trial was begun in April, 2001 at 70 centers and concluded in August, 2006. Interim analyses allowed the trial to continue to its planned conclusion but final results have not yet been released.

In the adult, partial pumpless ECLS systems are the subject of considerable study. **Partial extracorporeal life support (ECLS)** refers to technologies that provide only a portion of the gas exchange function of the lung. Advantages to partial ECLS systems are that they are generally pumpless, maintain substantial flow through the native pulmonary circulation, and would be easier to develop into portable or ambulatory systems.

An early partial ECLS system was the **intravascular oxygenator (IVOX).**[42] This device consisted of thousands of hollow filaments and filled virtually the entire inferior vena cava through a femoral cutdown site. Substantial (30% to 50%) gas exchange support could be provided by a high flow of O_2 through the filaments and subsequent gas transfer with the surrounding blood. Unfortunately, a large trial of 161 patients using the device showed no effect on ultimate outcome. A more recent IVOX system is the Hattler catheter. This can be inserted percutaneously with a 28-31 Fr device and differs from the original IVOX by having a pulsating membrane around the fibers to augment the gas exchange potential. This device is currently being evaluated in clinical trials.

Another novel ECLS technique that does not require a pump is an arteriovenous CO_2 removal ($AVCO_2R$) system.[43] With this technique, an arteriovenous shunt routes approximately 20% of the cardiac output flow through a gas exchange device. Blood flow is driven only by the patient's blood pressure. The current design requires 12-16 Fr percutaneous catheters and can provide nearly total CO_2 removal. Oxygenation cannot be fully supported with this device and thus some level of respiratory system support is required (although apneic oxygenation through high-flow tracheal catheters might be an option).

In sheep studies with 11% to 14% of the cardiac output flowing through an $AVCO_2R$ device, 95% CO_2 removal was noted and mechanical ventilation was reduced from 13 lpm to 5 lpm. Interestingly, there was 100% survival in these injured sheep using this device versus 45% survival in the controls. This device has now gone on to phase 1 clinical trials and the first 10 patients have been recently reported.[44] In these patients, CO_2 clearance was again substantial and the Pa_{CO_2} was reduced from 91 mm Hg to 53 mm Hg. Because of the success and safety of the device, a phase 2 trial in ARDS has begun.

Another potential application of an $AVCO_2R$ device may be to miniaturize it to the point that it could be used for outpatients and ambulatory patients. In concept, an arteriovenous fistula would be established and a small device about the size of a soda can could be strapped to the patient's waist and remove virtually all of the CO_2. A venovenous CO_2 removal device also exists, but its CO_2 removal capabilities are less and thus it could only be used for partial support.

Newer ECLS approaches are attempting to create systems that can provide near total gas exchange support but that last longer and are more portable than current ECMO systems.[44] The short-term goal for these approaches is to create systems that can provide a better "bridge" to transplant or other therapy. The long-term goal might be to develop systems that could provide lifelong support.

In the United States, efforts are being focused on paracorporeal artificial lungs (PALs).[44] These are devices that cannulate either the right atrium or proximal pulmonary artery and route the entire cardiac output through an oxygenator/CO_2 removal device and then back into the distal pulmonary artery. The right ventricle alone can be used to provide flow through the system, although very low resistance devices with compliance chambers appear necessary to prevent right ventricular overload. An alternative is to couple the device with a right ventricular assist device. An additional benefit from this approach is that fully oxygenated blood, a potent vasodilator, is delivered to the entire pulmonary circulation. These approaches have only been studied in animals, but they appear effective and improve outcome through less ventilator induced lung injury.

SUMMARY

The number of neonates being treated with ECLS has decreased over the past several years as techniques such as inhaled nitric oxide, high-frequency ventilation, and surfactant have become commonplace. The number of pediatric and adult ECLS cases has been relatively stable. The largest recent increase in the use of ECLS has been in the postoperative cardiac population. These trends can be expected to continue. Ongoing research and technical advances will continue to make ECLS safer and, hopefully, result in improved survival rates and decreased complication rates. Proper patient selection and early intervention may be the keys to successful treatment of the most critically ill patients with ECLS.

KEY POINTS

- ECLS remains an important life-saving strategy for infants, children, and adults with severe cardiac and/or respiratory failure of various causes.
- The major complications associated with ECLS are bleeding, clotting, and technical problems. Advances in technology are helping to minimize complications and improve outcomes. As the number of ECLS patients decreases, so does the number of ECLS centers. This trend is beginning to promote improved regionalization of care. This regionalization will hopefully result in more standard ECLS criteria and improved data collection.
- Outcomes-based research has become an essential component of ECLS programs. Data from these investigations have been used to further improve ECLS technology and the overall management of the ECLS patient.

ASSESSMENT QUESTIONS

1. True or False. ECLS is a technology that was first developed in the late 1990s.
2. True or False. Extracorporeal pumps are generally either rolled head displacement pumps or centrifugal pumps.
3. True or False. Venovenous bypass ECLS systems generally take only a portion of the cardiac output.
4. True or False. The most serious complication of ECLS is hemorrhage.
5. True or False. Ventilator management in a patient on ECLS should be greatly reduced and focused primarily on reducing atelectasis and minimizing lung expansion.
6. True or False. Anticoagulation during ECLS is generally aimed to keep the ACT between 160 and 200 seconds.
7. True or False. The overall ECLS survival rate since 1986 approaches 76%.
8. True or False. Survival rates in adults receiving ECLS today are reported to be as high as 56%.
9. True or False. A recent randomized controlled trial of ECLS in adult respiratory failure showed statistically better survival.
10. True or False. The intravascular oxygenator is a newer concept in partial ECLS but supportive clinical trials are lacking.

REFERENCES

1. Gibbon JH Jr: Artificial maintenance of circulation during experimental occlusion of the pulmonary artery, Arch Surg 34:1105-1112, 1937.
2. Kolff WJ, Beck HT: Artificial kidney: a dialyzer with a great area, Acta Med Scand 117:121-124, 1944.
3. Clowes GHA Jr, Hopkins AL, Neville WE: An artificial lung dependent upon diffusion of oxygen and carbon dioxide through plastic membranes, J Thorac Surg 32:630-637, 1956.
4. Kammermeyer K: Silicone rubber as a selective barrier, Ind Chem Eng 49:1685, 1957.
5. Kolobow T, Bowman RL: Construction and elimination of an alveolar membrane heart-lung, Trans Am Soc Artif Intern Organs 9:238, 1963.
6. Kolobow T, Zapol WM, Pierce J: High survival and minimal blood damage in lambs exposed to long term venovenous pumping with a polyurethane chamber roller pump with and without a membrane oxygenator, Trans Am Soc Artif Intern Organs 15:172-177, 1969.

7. Dorson WJ, Baker E, Melvin L et al: A perfusion system for infants, Trans Am Soc Artif Intern Organs 15:155-160, 1969.
8. White JJ, Andrews HG, Risemberg H et al: Prolonged respiratory support in newborn infants with a membrane oxygenator, Surg 70:288-296, 1971.
9. Rashkind WJ, Freeman A, Klein D et al: Evaluation of a disposable plastic, low volume, pumpless oxygenator as a lung substitute, J Pediatr 66:94-102, 1965.
10. Hill JD, O'Brien TG, Murray JJ et al: Extracorporeal oxygenation for acute post-traumatic respiratory failure (shock-lung syndrome): use of the Bramson Membrane Lung, N Engl J Med 286:629-634, 1972.
11. Blake LH: Goals and progress of the NHLI collaborative ECMO study. In: Zapol W, Qvist J, editors: Artificial lungs for acute respiratory failure, New York, 1976, Academic Press, pp 513-524.
12. Bartlett RH, Gazzaniga AB: Extracorporeal circulation for cardiopulmonary failure, Curr Problems Surg 15:1-7, 1978.
13. Extracorporeal Life Support Organization: ECLS Registry. Ann Arbor, Mich, 2006, Extracorporeal Life Support Organization.
14. Southgate WM, Annibale DJ, Hulsey TC et al: International experience with trisomy 21 infants placed on extracorporeal membrane oxygenation, Pediatrics 107:549-552, 2001.
15. Ortega M, Ramos A, Atkinson J et al: Oxygenation index can predict outcomes in neonates who are candidates for extracorporeal membrane oxygenation, Pediatr Res 22:462A, 1987.
16. Bartlett RH: Extracorporeal life support for cardiopulmonary failure, Curr Problems Surg 27:621-705, 1990.
17. Kanter KR, Pennington G, Weber TR et al: Extracorporeal membrane oxygenation for postoperative cardiac support in children, J Thorac Cardiovasc Surg 93:27-35, 1987.
18. Chaturvedi RR, Macrae D, Brown KL et al:. Cardiac ECMO for biventricular hearts after paediatric open heart surgery, Heart 90:545-551, 2004.
19. Lupinetti FM, Bove EL, Minich LL et al: Intermediate-term survival and functional results after arterial repair for transposition of the great arteries, J Thorac Cardiovasc Surg 103:421-427, 1992.
20. Ostu T, Merz SI, Holtquist KA et al: Laboratory evaluation of a double lumen catheter for venovenous neonatal ECMO, Trans Am Soc Artif Intern Organs 35:647-650, 1989.
21. Anderson HL, Ostu T, Shapman R et al: Venovenous extracorporeal life support in neonates using a double lumen catheter, Trans Am Soc Artif Intern Organs 35:650-653, 1989.
22. Pranikoff R, Hirschl RB, Remenapp R et al: Venovenous extracorporeal life support via percutaneous cannulation in 94 patients, Chest 115:818-822, 1999.
23. Grayck EN, Meliones JN, Kern FH et al: Elevated serum lactate correlates with intracranial hemorrhage in neonates treated with extracorporeal life support, Pediatrics 96:914-917, 1995.
24. Cengiz P, Seidel K, Rycus PT et al: Central nervous system complications during pediatric extracorporeal life support: Incidence and risk factors, Crit Care Med 33:2817-2824, 2005.
25. Klein MD, Shaheen KW, Whittlesey GC et al: Extracorporeal membrane oxygenation for the support of children after repair of congenital heart disease, J Thorac Cardiovasc Surg 100:498-505, 1990.
26. Meliones JN, Custer JR, Snedecor S et al: Extracorporeal life support for cardiac assist in pediatric patients: review of the ELSO Registry data, Circulation 84:168-172, 1991.
27. Lotze A, Taylor J, Short BL: The use of lung compliance as a parameter for improvement in lung function in newborns with respiratory failure requiring ECMO, Crit Care 15:226-229, 1987.
28. Pettignano R, Heard M, Davis R et al: Total enteral nutrition versus total parenteral nutrition during pediatric extracorporeal membrane oxygenation, Crit Care Med 26:358-363, 1998.
29. Roy BJ, Rycus P, Conrad SA et al: The changing demographics of neonatal extracorporeal membrane oxygenation patients reported to the Extracorporeal Life Support Organization (ELSO) Registry, Pediatrics 106:1334-1338, 2000.
30. Hintz SR, Suttner DM, Sheehan AM et al: Decreased use of neonatal extracorporeal membrane oxygenation (ECMO): How new treatment modalities have affected ECMO utilization, Pediatrics 106:1339-1343, 2000.
31. Wilson JM, Bower LK, Thompson JE et al: ECMO in evolution: the impact of changing patient demographics and alternative therapies on ECMO, J Pediatr Surg 31:1116-1123, 1996.
32. Elbourne D, Field D, Mugford M: Extracorporeal membrane oxygenation for severe respiratory failure in newborn infants, Cochrane Database Syst Rev, 2006.
33. Boykin AR, Quivers ES, Wagenhoffer KL et al: Cardiopulmonary outcome of neonatal extracorporeal membrane oxygenation at ages 10-15 years, Crit Care Med 31:2380-2384, 2003.
34. Hamutcu R, Nield TA, Garg M et al: Long term pulmonary sequelae in children who were treated with ECMO for neonatal respiratory failure, Pediatrics 114:1292-1296, 2004.
35. Petrou S, Edwards L: Cost effectiveness analysis of neonatal extracorporeal membrane oxygenation based on four year results from the UK Collaborative ECMO Trial, Arch Dis Child Fetal Neonatal Ed 89:F263-F268, 2004.
36. Morris MC, Ittenbach RF, Godinez RI et al: Risk factors for mortality in 137 pediatric cardiac intensive care unit patients managed with extracorporeal membrane oxygenation, Crit Care Med 32:1061-1069, 2004.
37. Montgomery VK, Strotman J, Ross MP: Impact of multiple organ system dysfunction and nosocomial infections on survival of children treated with extracorporeal membrane oxygenation after heart surgery, Crit Care Med 28:526-531, 2000.
38. Bartlett RH, Roloff DW, Custer JR et al: Extracorporeal life support: The University of Michigan experience, JAMA 283:904-908, 2000.
39. Hamrick SEG, Cremmels DB, Keet CA et al: Neurodevelopmental outcome of infants supported with

extracorporeal membrane oxygenation after cardiac surgery, Pediatrics 111:e671-e675, 2003.
40. Hemmila MR, Rowe SA, Boules TN et al: Extracorporeal life support for severe acute respiratory distress syndrome in adults, Ann Surg 240:595-607, 2004.
41. Bartlett RH: Extracorporeal life support in the management of severe respiratory failure, Clin Chest Med 21:555-561, 2000.
42. Conrad SA, Bagley A, Bagley B et al: Major findings from clinical trials of the IVOX, Art Organs 18:846-863, 1994.
43. Conrad SA, Zwishenberger JB, Grier LR et al: Total extracorporeal arteriovenous CO_2 removal in acute respiratory failure: a phase I clinical study, Intensive Care Med 27:1340-1351, 2001.
44. Lick SD, Zwischenberger JB: Artificial lung: bench towards bedside, ASAIO J 50:2-5, 2004.

CHAPTER

25

Heliox and Inhaled Nitric Oxide

Dean R. Hess

OUTLINE

OBJECTIVES

- Describe the physical properties that provide the basis for heliox therapy.
- Discuss the role of heliox in the settings of partial upper airway obstruction, croup, bronchiolitis, asthma, and chronic obstructive pulmonary disease.
- Describe the effect of heliox on flowmeters, nebulizers, and mechanical ventilators.
- Explain why inhaled nitric oxide is a selective pulmonary vasodilator.
- Discuss the evidence for clinical use of inhaled nitric oxide.
- Discuss potential toxicities and adverse effects of inhaled nitric oxide.
- Describe the delivery device for inhaled nitric oxide.

KEY TERMS

Bernoulli's principle	inhaled nitric oxide	Reynolds' number (Re)
density	laminar flow	selective pulmonary vasodilation
Graham's law	methemoglobin	turbulent flow
heliox	nitrogen dioxide	

Gas mixtures of air and O_2 are usually administered to produce the desired inspired O_2 concentration (F_{IO_2}). However, there may be clinical circumstances in which it is desirable to substitute helium for air. There is also clinical utility in providing very low concentrations of nitric oxide in the inspired gas of some patients. In this chapter, clinical applications of **heliox** (80% helium/20% O_2) and **inhaled nitric oxide** (iNO) are discussed.

HELIOX

Physics and Physiology

The physical properties of helium are different from those of air or O_2.[1-4] The densities of helium, air, and O_2 are 0.18, 1.29, and 1.43 kg/m^3, respectively. The viscosities of helium, air, and O_2 are 201.8, 188.5, and 211.4 micropoise, respectively. The **density** and viscosity of heliox are 0.43 kg/m^3 and 203.6 micropoise,

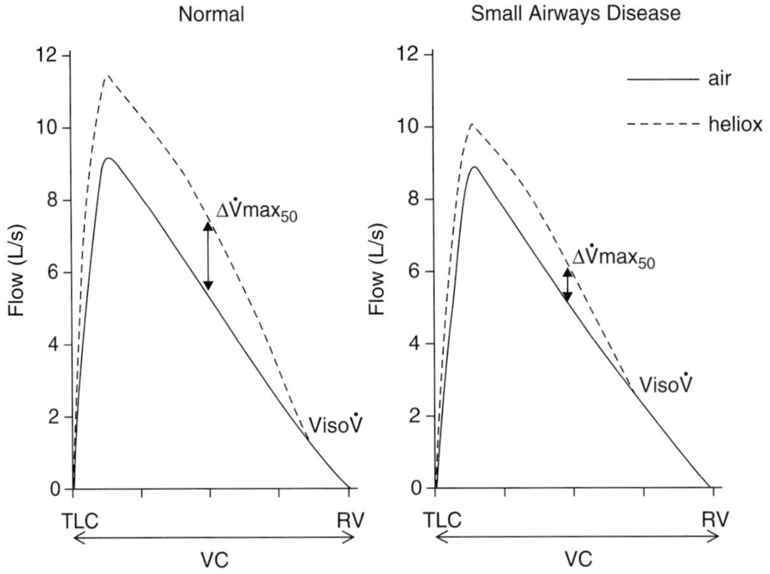

FIGURE 25-1 Expiratory flow-volume loop breathing air and breathing heliox. In the normal case *(left)*, note the greater increase in $\Delta\dot{V}max_{50}$ than in the case of small airways disease. Also note that Viso$\dot{V}$ is larger in the case of small airways disease than normal. With small airways disease, gas flow is laminar in the flow-limiting segment, which is density independent. (From Hess DR: Heliox and noninvasive positive-pressure ventilation: a role for heliox in exacerbations of chronic obstructive pulmonary disease? Respir Care 51:640-650, 2006.)

respectively. Note that the density of helium is lower than that for air or O_2, but its viscosity is higher than air and lower than O_2. Being an inert gas, helium is nonreactive with body tissue. It is also relatively insoluble in body fluids.

According to the Hagen-Poiseuille law, **laminar flow** is affected by the radius of the conducting tube (r), the pressure gradient (ΔP), the viscosity of the gas (η), and the length of the conducting tube (l):

$$\dot{V} \cong (\pi\ r^4\ \Delta P)/(8\ \eta\ l)$$

Turbulent flow is affected by the radius of the conducting tube (r), the pressure gradient (ΔP), the density of the gas (ρ), and the length of the conducting tube (l):

$$\dot{V}^2 \cong (4\ \pi\ r^5\ \Delta P)/(\rho\ l)$$

Note that turbulent flow is density dependent, whereas laminar flow is density independent. In other words, use of heliox would be expected to have a greater effect on turbulent flow. In fact, heliox might adversely affect laminar flow because it has a greater viscosity than air.

Whether flow is laminar or turbulent is determined by the **Reynolds' number (Re):**

$$Re \cong \text{inertial forces/viscous forces} \cong (v\ r\ \rho)/(\eta)$$

where v is velocity of gas movement, r is the radius of the conducting tube, ρ is density, and η is viscosity. A low Reynolds' number causes flow to be laminar. Because of its lower density and higher viscosity, heliox produces a lower Reynolds' number and a greater tendency for laminar flow. Laminar flow is desirable because it is more energy efficient than turbulent flow. According to the Reynolds' number, gas flow tends to be laminar in small peripheral airways of the lungs and turbulent in larger central airways. Therefore heliox might be expected to have limited benefit for diseases affecting small airways (e.g., emphysema), whereas it might be useful for diseases affecting larger airways (e.g., asthma or postextubation stridor) (Figure 25-1).

For gas flow through an orifice (i.e., axial acceleration), flow has only a weak dependence on the Reynolds' number and is affected by density:

$$\dot{V} \cong \Delta P/\rho$$

In other words, flow through an orifice (e.g., constricted airway) increases if the density of the gas decreases (e.g., heliox).

Bernoulli's principle and **Graham's law** are also important relative to heliox therapy. Bernoulli's principle states that the pressure required to produce flow is affected by the mass of the gas:

$$(P_1 - P_2) = (\tfrac{1}{2})(m)(v_2^2 - v_1^2)$$

where $(P_1 - P_2)$ is the pressure required to produce flow, $(v_2^2 - v_1^2)$ is the difference in velocity between P_1 and P_2, and m is the mass of the gas. In other words, less pressure is required to produce flow with heliox than with air or O_2. Graham's law states that the rate of diffusion is inversely related to the square root of gas density. Thus heliox diffuses at a rate 1.8 times greater than O_2. This explains why the flow of heliox through an O_2 flowmeter is 1.8 times greater than the indicated flow.

Clinical Applications

Partial Upper Airway Obstruction

A common use of heliox is to reduce resistance with partial upper airway obstruction.[4-13] An example of this application is postextubation stridor, most of the evidence for which comes from anecdotal reports. In a double-blind, randomized, controlled, crossover trial, Kemper et al[9] assessed the effectiveness of heliox in reducing postextubation stridor in children hospitalized for burns or trauma and reported that stridor was less with heliox than with O_2. In a study of patients with upper airway obstruction from a multitude of causes, Grosz et al[10] evaluated the use of heliox in 42 children treated for severe upper-airway obstruction and observed that a reduced work of breathing was reported in 73% of the children. In a study of 14 consecutive children with severe subglottic edema or injury and severe airway distress, and who met criteria for intubation, Connolly and McGuirt[11] reported that the use of heliox prevented intubation in 71% of the patients. Rodeberg et al[12] evaluated the use of heliox in 8 children with burns and postextubation stridor refractory to racemic epinephrine. Reintubation was avoided in 6 of the 8 children. Jaber et al[13] evaluated heliox immediately postextubation and reported that it significantly improved inspiratory effort (Figure 25-2) and comfort, but had no effect on gas exchange. Although largely anecdotal, the available evidence suggests that heliox therapy for upper-airway obstruction relieves stridor, reduces respiratory distress, and decreases the work of breathing. In some patients, heliox may decrease the need for intubation.[14]

Asthma

There have been a number of reports of the use of heliox for the treatment of acute severe asthma.[15-24] In spontaneously breathing asthmatic patients, heliox has been reported to decrease $Pa{CO_2}$, increase peak flow, and decrease pulsus paradoxus. The reduction in pulsus paradoxus may be particularly important because it reflects a reduction in inspiratory muscle work (Figure 25-3).[18] Kudukis et al[19] conducted a double-blind, randomized, controlled study of the efficacy of heliox in 18 children with status asthmaticus. Heliox was administered through a nonrebreather face mask and supplemental O_2 was supplied via nasal cannula under the mask as needed. Within 15 minutes of the start of administration, heliox was associated with significantly lower pulsus paradoxus and dyspnea, and an increase in peak flow. However, in another double-blind, randomized, controlled trial, Carter et al[21] evaluated the use of heliox on pulmonary function, dyspnea, and clinical symptom score in 11 children hospitalized with status asthmaticus. They reported no difference between the groups in clinical or dyspnea symptom scores or FEV_1.

Gluck et al[20] reported that heliox reduced peak inspiratory pressure and $Pa{CO_2}$ in 7 intubated patients with status asthmaticus. Kass and Castriotta[17] reported similar findings in 12 patients, 5 of whom were mechanically ventilated. Schaeffer et al[22] reported that heliox improved the alveolar-arterial O_2 difference in 11 adult and pediatric mechanically ventilated patients with status asthmaticus. Abd-Allah et al[23] conducted a retrospective review of heliox in 28 mechanically ventilated children with acute severe asthma and reported decreases in peak inspiratory pressure and $Pa{CO_2}$.

The evidence for use of heliox in patients with asthma is conflicting. First line therapy with heliox is not warranted.[14,25,26] Heliox appears to benefit patients with the most severe exacerbations and airflow obstruction. Early use of heliox may decrease work of breathing and dyspnea, improve gas exchange, and prevent intubation in some patients. Heliox is safe when used by clinicians familiar with its use. Its benefits have a rapid onset, allowing discontinuation of heliox in patients who do not respond within minutes of initiation of therapy.

Croup

Duncan[27] reported a case series of seven children with acute airway obstruction; two with croup and five with postextubation edema. Those treated with heliox had a significant decrease in croup score and improvement in gas exchange. In another case series of 14 children, Nelson et al[28] reported an immediate reduction in respiratory distress with the use of heliox, with none requiring intubation. In a randomized, double-blind, controlled trial of 15 pediatric patients with mild croup, Terregino et al[29] reported that

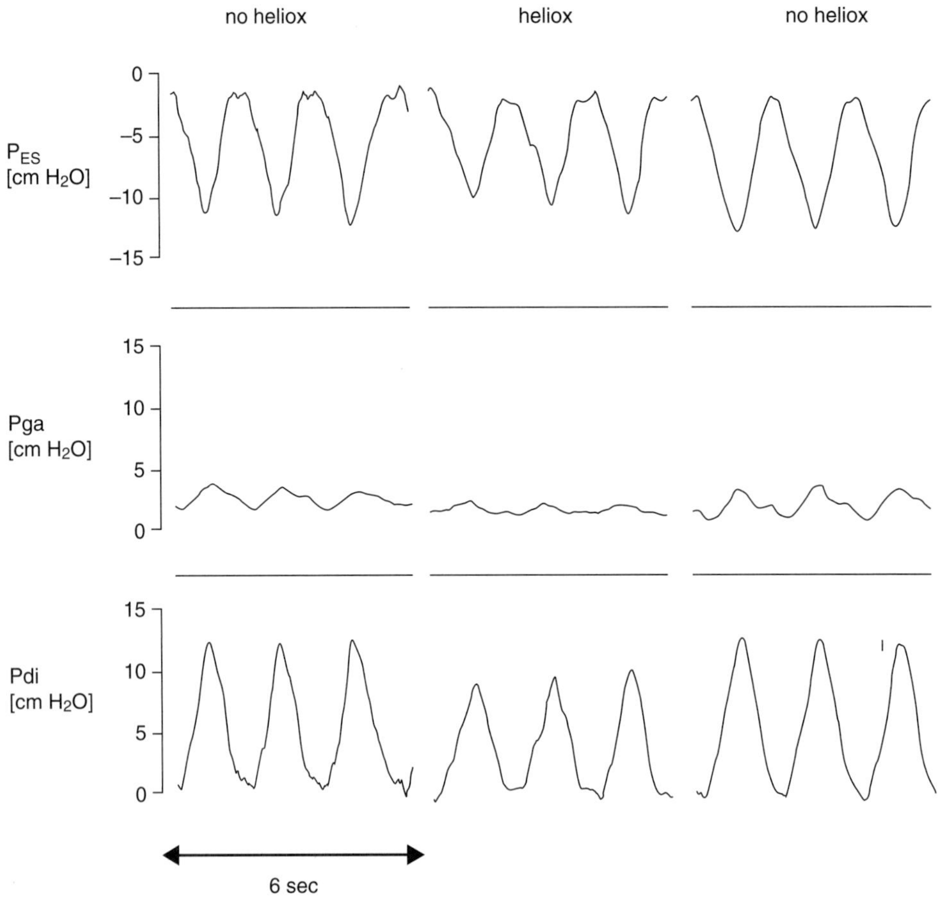

FIGURE 25-2 **Radial artery pressure tracings from a patient with severe asthma before (A), during (B), and after (C) the administration of heliox. Note the reduction in degree of pulsus paradoxus with heliox.** (From Manthous CA, Hall JB, Caputo MA et al: Heliox improves pulsus paradoxus and peak expiratory flow in nonintubated patients with severe asthma, Am J Respir Crit Care Med 151:310-314, 1995, American Lung Association.)

heliox was a safe, well-tolerated, and useful alternative to tracheostomy or tracheal intubation. Weber et al[30] evaluated the additive effect of heliox with racemic epinephrine in 29 children with moderate to severe croup and reported that racemic epinephrine and heliox have equal treatment efficacy in children with croup. These studies suggest that, while heliox improves respiratory distress, it is not superior to other conventional therapies.[14]

Bronchiolitis

Hollman et al[31] evaluated the efficacy of heliox in 13 infants with respiratory syncytial virus bronchiolitis and concluded that heliox provided greater clinical improvement in overall respiratory status. In a multicenter randomized, double-blind, placebo-controlled trial, Liet et al[32] evaluated the use of heliox in 39 infants with severe bronchiolitis. There was no significant difference between the groups in the primary outcomes of the requirement for mechanical ventilation or in secondary outcome measures, such as clinical scores, O_2 requirement, $Paco_2$, or ICU stay. Martinon-Torres et al[33] evaluated heliox in 38 infants with moderate to severe respiratory syncytial virus bronchiolitis. At both 1 hour and at the end of the observation period, the infants who received heliox had a more rapid improvement in clinical score and better clinical improvement, and ICU stay was shorter in the heliox group. Gross et al[34] assessed the response to heliox in a case series involving 10 mechanically ventilated infants with bronchiolitis. Heliox did not improve gas exchange during mechanical ventilation, and there were no significant differences in $Paco_2$ or Pao_2. Though the evidence is limited and inconsistent, heliox may decrease work of breathing and improve gas exchange in nonintu-

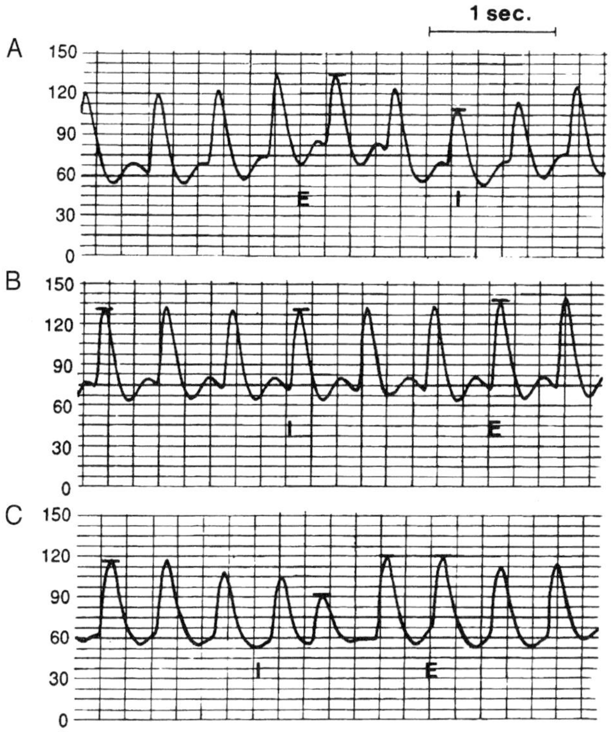

FIGURE 25-3 Tracings of esophageal, gastric, and transdiaphragmatic pressures over time in a patient during the three periods after extubation (no heliox, heliox, and no heliox). These tracings illustrate the reduction in breathing effort obtained with the helium-O_2 mixture. **A,** No heliox. **B,** Heliox. **C,** No heliox.

bated infants with bronchiolitis. However, it may not confer benefit in those who are intubated.[14]

Chronic Obstructive Pulmonary Disease

Johnson et al[35] randomized patients with severe chronic obstructive pulmonary disease (COPD) to air, heliox, or noninvasive positive pressure ventilation (NPPV) during 6 weeks of exercise training. They found no training advantage in the heliox group, compared with the group breathing air without NPPV. Palange et al[36] evaluated the use of heliox in patients with COPD during exercise, and concluded that heliox improved high-intensity exercise endurance. Pecchiari et al[37] explored the effects of heliox on breathing pattern, expiratory flow limitation, and dynamic hyperinflation in 22 patients with COPD and reported that heliox had no effect on dynamic hyperinflation. Swidwa et al[38] evaluated the effect of heliox in 15 patients with severe COPD, and reported that functional residual capacity and Pa_{CO_2} decreased with heliox (Figure 25-4). These short-term physiologic effects support the use of heliox in COPD but provide little insight into the use of heliox during COPD exacerbations.

There have been several impressive case reports of the use of heliox in patients with COPD exacerbation. Polito and Fessler[39] reported a patient with COPD receiving invasive mechanical ventilation who self-extubated. With administration of heliox via face mask, the patient's respiratory rate immediately fell, she became alert, and her Pa_{CO_2} decreased from 90 mm Hg to 50 mm Hg. Gerbeaux et al[40] reported the case of a patient with COPD exacerbation who presented with altered mentation, paradoxical diaphragmatic motion, tachypnea, and hypercarbia. With heliox there was marked improvement in respiratory acidosis and mentation. In a retrospective study, Gerbeaux et al[41] assessed whether 81 patients with COPD treated with heliox have a better prognosis than those treated with standard therapy. The survivors in the heliox group had significantly shorter ICU and hospital stays. However, a Cochrane review[42] concluded that there is insufficient evidence to support the use of heliox to treat COPD exacerbations. Andrews and Lynch[43]

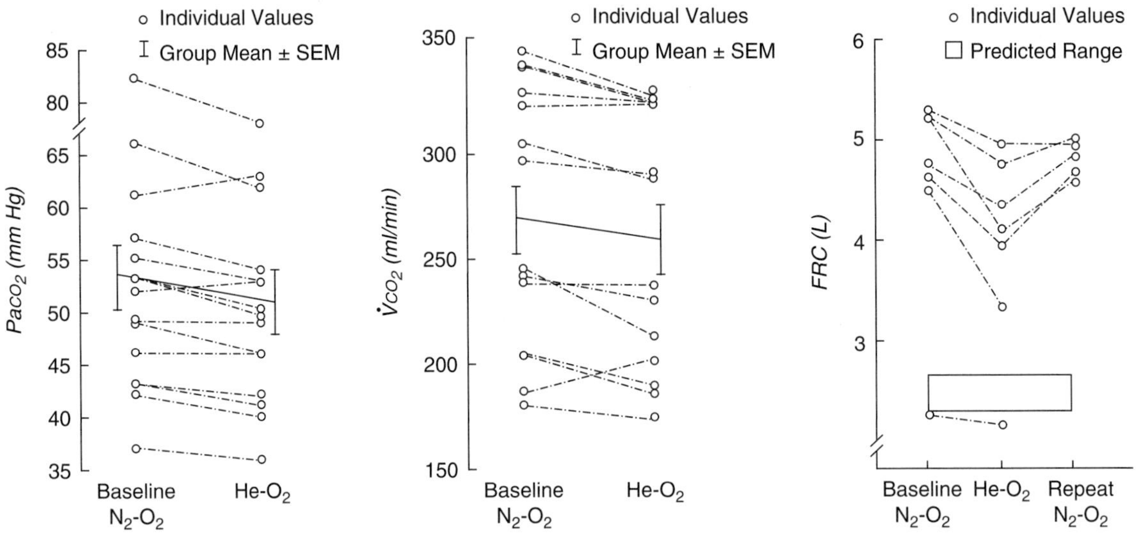

FIGURE 25-4 $PaCO_2$ and functional residual capacity (FRC) in patients with stable COPD breathing air/O_2 (N_2-O_2) and heliox (He-O_2). SEM: standard error of the mean. (From Swidwa DM, Montenegro HD, Goldman MD et al: Helium-oxygen breathing in severe chronic obstructive pulmonary disease. Chest 87:790-795, 1985.)

conducted a meta-analysis to determine if heliox in nonintubated patients with COPD exacerbation reduces $PaCO_2$ or the odds of intubation, and concluded that definitive evidence of a beneficial role of heliox in treatment of severe COPD is lacking.

Several studies have evaluated the combination of heliox with NPPV in patients with COPD. Austan and Polise[44] reported the case of a patient with COPD exacerbation in which there was notable improvement in arterial blood gases, and a reduction in respiratory rate and accessory muscle use with the use of heliox. In a randomized crossover study, Jolliet et al[45] evaluated use of heliox in 19 patients with COPD exacerbation receiving NPPV and reported a reduction in $PaCO_2$ and dyspnea score with heliox. Jaber et al[46] reported a significant decrease in work of breathing and $PaCO_2$ during NPPV with heliox. Jolliet et al[47] conducted a prospective randomized multicenter study to determine whether NPPV with heliox would benefit outcome or cost in 123 patients with COPD exacerbation. Intubation rate and ICU stay were not significantly different, but the post-ICU hospital stay was shorter with heliox. In this study, it is difficult to reconcile the shorter post-ICU hospital stay and lower costs with the fact that the intubation rate and ICU stay were not significantly different. Moreover, the study may have been underpowered.

Heliox has also been evaluated in mechanically ventilated patients with COPD. In a prospective crossover study, Tassaux et al[48] reported that heliox reduced trapped gas volume, auto-PEEP, and peak inspiratory pressure. However, the effect was quite variable between patients. In another prospective crossover study, the same investigators[49] evaluated the impact of heliox on inspiratory effort and work of breathing in 10 intubated patients with COPD. Heliox reduced the number of ineffective triggers, auto-PEEP, the magnitude of negative esophageal pressure swings, and work of breathing. In a prospective randomized crossover study, Gainnier et al[50] reported that heliox reduces inspiratory work of breathing in 23 mechanically ventilated patients with COPD exacerbation. Jolliet et al[51] reported that auto-PEEP and trapped gas volume were comparably reduced by heliox. In 13 mechanically ventilated patients, Diehl et al[52] reported that heliox reduced the work of breathing, but was not consistent among patients. Lee et al[53] evaluated the effect of heliox on cardiac performance in 25 mechanically ventilated patients with severe COPD. Heliox decreased auto-PEEP, trapped gas volume, and respiratory variations in systolic pressure.

The evidence for the use of heliox in patients with COPD exacerbation is not robust or mature. Most of the peer-reviewed literature consists of case reports, case series, and physiologic studies in small samples of carefully selected patients. Even in the physiologic studies, a consistent response in not reported in all patients. It seems that some patients with COPD exacerbation have a favorable physiologic response to heliox therapy, whereas others do not, and it is not clear how to predict who will be a responder and who will not.[54]

TABLE 25-1 *Clinical Studies of Heliox as the Driving Gas for Asthma Medications*

AUTHOR	NUMBER OF SUBJECTS	AGE OF SUBJECTS (Y)	
STUDIES THAT FOUND BENEFIT FROM HELIOX-DRIVEN NEBULIZATION			
Kress (2002)	45	<50	Better improvement in FEV_1 with heliox than with air.
Bag (2002)	31	18-44	Better improvement in FEV_1, FVC, and PEF with heliox.
Sattonnet (2004)	205	Not reported	Significant improvement in PEF at 20, 40, and 60 min with heliox; lower intubation rate with heliox.
Lee (2005)	80	>18	More rapid and greater improvement in PEF with heliox than with O_2. Older patients benefited from heliox.
Kim (2005)	30	2-18	Significantly better clinical scores at 120, 180, and 240 min, and lower rate of hospital admission with heliox.
STUDIES THAT FOUND LITTLE OR NO BENEFIT FROM HELIOX-DRIVEN NEBULIZATION			
Henderson (1999)	205	18-65	No differences in improvement of PEF or FEV_1.
Dorfman (2000)	39	8-55	No difference in PEF. More admissions in heliox group.
Rose (2002)	36	18-55	More improvement in Borg dyspnea score with heliox than with O_2. No improvement in respiratory rate, O_2 saturation, PEF, or FEV_1.
Lanoix (2003)	94	19-55	No difference in PEF, FEV_1, time to best PEF/FEV_1, emergency-department stay, or admission rate.
Rivera (2006)	41	3-16	No difference in clinical scores at 10 and 20 min. Trend toward significant difference at 20 min.

Adapted from Kim IK, Saville AL, Sikes KL et al: Heliox-driven albuterol nebulization for asthma exacerbations: an overview. Respir Care 51:613-618, 2006.
FEV_1, Forced expiratory volume in 1 second; *FVC*, forced vital capacity; *PEF*, peak expiratory flow; *O_2*, oxygen.

Heliox to Improve Aerosol Delivery

Using an inhaled radionuclide deposition study, Anderson et al[55] concluded that heliox was significantly more effective than air in depositing an aerosol in alveolar regions, and this was more pronounced in asthmatic subjects than in healthy subjects. Darquenne and Prisk[56] also used a radionuclide approach to compare upper-respiratory-tract deposition with heliox versus air and concluded that heliox might reduce deposition in the upper respiratory tract and increase deposition in the distal airways and alveoli. In pediatric asthma patients, Piva et al[57] performed a radionuclide study and found better pulmonary aerosol delivery with heliox than with O_2. Heliox has been studied as the driving gas for nebulizing bronchodilators in the treatment of asthma exacerbations in both adult and pediatric patients (Table 25-1).[58-67] These studies have had different results, possibly because of the differences in methods, severity of the asthma exacerbations, aerosol delivery technique, patient characteristics, and duration of therapy. Heliox-driven albuterol nebulization is generating increased interest, but further studies are needed to determine the role of heliox-driven albuterol nebulization in the care of patients with asthma exacerbations.[68]

Delivery Systems for Heliox

For spontaneously breathing patients, heliox is administered by face mask with a reservoir bag (Figure 25-5). A Y-piece is attached to the mask to allow concurrent delivery of aerosolized medications.

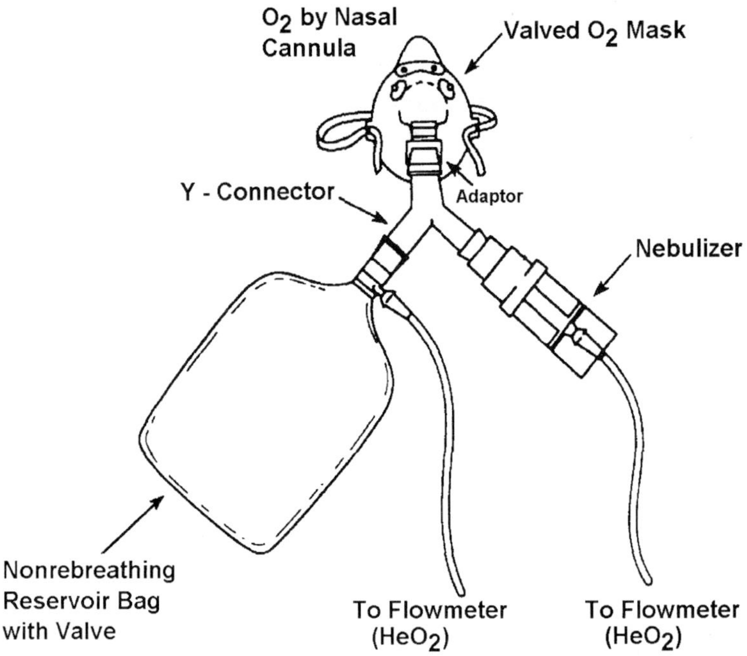

FIGURE 25-5 Schematic illustration of equipment used for heliox administration to spontaneously breathing patients.

Sufficient flow to keep the reservoir bag inflated is required. This is often at least 12 to 15 L/min and requires 3 to 6 cylinders per day.

Heliox administration via mechanical ventilation can be problematic.[69-73] Ventilators are designed to deliver a mixture of air and O_2. The different density and viscosity of helium can affect the delivered tidal volume and the measurement of exhaled tidal volume. For some ventilators (e.g., Puritan Bennett 840, Puritan Bennett, Carlsbad, Calif.), no reliable tidal volume is delivered with heliox. For other ventilators, there may be a much higher delivered tidal volume than desired. This problem can be circumvented partially by using pressure ventilation rather than volume ventilation. Unlike flow sensors, pressure sensors are not affected by a different gas composition.

The effect of heliox on the ability of the ventilator to correctly monitor flow and tidal volume depends on the method that is used for this measurement. Monitoring devices that are density dependent are inaccurate in the presence of heliox. Devices that use the principle of thermal conductivity also are affected. However, devices that are affected by gas viscosity rather than gas density are affected to a lesser degree because the viscosity of helium is only slightly different from that of air or O_2. Screen pneumotachometers, such as those used in the Servo ventilators (Maquet, Bridgewater, N.J.), are affected by viscosity rather than density. Thus the flow sensors in these ventilators are affected to a lesser degree than occurs in other ventilators. The accuracy of commonly used bedside respirometers is also affected by heliox. Regardless of the ventilator, extreme caution must be exercised with the delivery of heliox. This should not be attempted unless the clinicians providing this therapy are familiar with the performance of the ventilator with heliox. Also, many ventilators waste gas as part of the normal pneumatic function of the device, resulting in gas loss and necessitating frequent cylinder changes. It has also been reported that there is a potential for ventilator malfunction in some conditions with heliox use in ventilators designed specifically for NPPV.

The Viasys Avea ventilator is approved by the United States Food and Drug Administration for heliox delivery.[54] Using "smart" connector technology, the Avea can deliver heliox-blended gas instead of air. By changing a connector on the back panel, the ventilator identifies the gas input and adjusts to accommodate the change. All volumes are automatically compensated for the presence of heliox. The Aptaér heliox delivery system (GE Healthcare, Madison, Wis.) is available to administer heliox with NPPV (Figure 25-6).[54] It uses a premixed blend of heliox from a source gas cylinder and delivers it to a

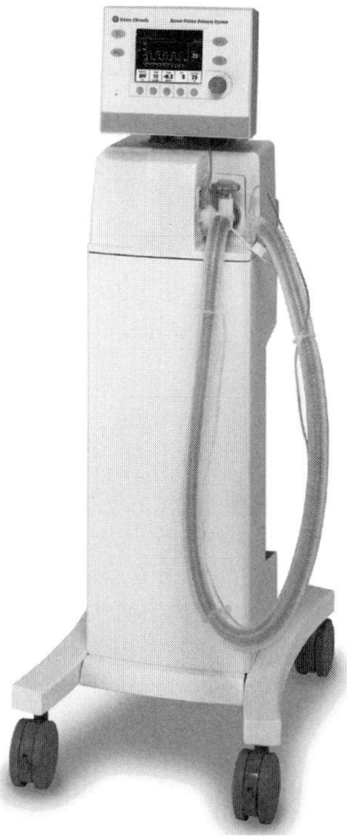

FIGURE 25-6 The Aptaér heliox delivery system. (Courtesy GE Healthcare, Madison, Wis.)

spontaneously breathing patient through a sealed face mask. The Aptaér allows the clinician to adjust the level of pressure support (3 to 20 cm H_2O), trigger sensitivity (−0.1 to −1.5 cm H_2O), rise time, and cycle sensitivity (5% to 75% of peak inspiratory flow). It incorporates a vibrating-mesh nebulizer, but does not include an O_2 blender (so the tank needs to be changed for an FIO_2 change) and the ability to apply PEEP.

The FIO_2 requirement of the patient limits the helium concentration that can be administered. If an FIO_2 greater than 0.40 is required, the limited concentration of helium is unlikely to produce clinical benefit. Heliox can affect nebulizer function,[74-78] resulting in a smaller particle size, reduced output, and longer nebulization time. The effect of heliox on nebulizer function can be circumvented with the use of nebulizers that do not depend on gas flow, such as those that use vibrating mesh technology.[78]

INHALED NITRIC OXIDE

Nitric oxide (NO) is a ubiquitous, highly reactive, gaseous, diatomic radical[79,80] that is important physiologically at very low concentrations (Box 25-1). Atmospheric concentrations of NO usually range between 10 and 100 ppb, and concentrations of 400 to 1000 ppm routinely are inhaled by people who smoke cigarettes.[81] Because it is considered an occupational and environmental pollutant, the Occupational Safety and Health Administration (OSHA) developed exposure limits for NO exposure in the workplace. NO is an important messenger molecule, and many cell types have shown the capacity to produce NO. The action of common nitrosovasodilators (e.g., sodium nitroprusside and nitroglycerin) is a result of their release of NO. NO is present in low concentration in the hospital compressed gas supply.[82-84] Since the mid-1980s, clinical and academic interest in NO moved from environmental and public health to cellular biology and physiology. Because it is a vasodilator, there is much clinical interest in the use of iNO in the treatment of diseases characterized by pulmonary hypertension and hypoxemia.[85]

BOX 25-1 *Concentrations of Nitric Oxide and Nitrogen Dioxide*

NO and NO_2 Usually Are Expressed in Concentrations of Parts per Million (ppm) or Parts per Billion (ppb)
% = $\frac{1}{100}$
ppm = $\frac{1}{1{,}000{,}000}$
10,000 ppm = 1%
1000 ppb = 1 ppm

Biology of Nitric Oxide

L-Arginine is the substrate for NO synthesis in biologic systems (Figure 25-7). NO is produced in the presence of NO synthase (NOS). It is lipophilic and readily diffuses across cell membranes to adjacent cells, thus serving as a local messenger molecule. NO typically diffuses from its cell of origin to a neighboring cell, where it binds with guanylate cyclase. Activation of guanylate cyclase results in the production of cyclic guanosine 3′,5′-monophosphate (cGMP) from guanosine triphosphate (GTP), which produces a biologic effect within the cell (e.g., smooth muscle relaxation). The time between NO production and guanylate cyclase activation is very short because of a half-life of less than 5 seconds for NO in physiologic systems.

NO is metabolized and excreted via a number of pathways. In O_2 mixtures, it is oxidized to NO_2 and converted to nitric and nitrous acids in aqueous

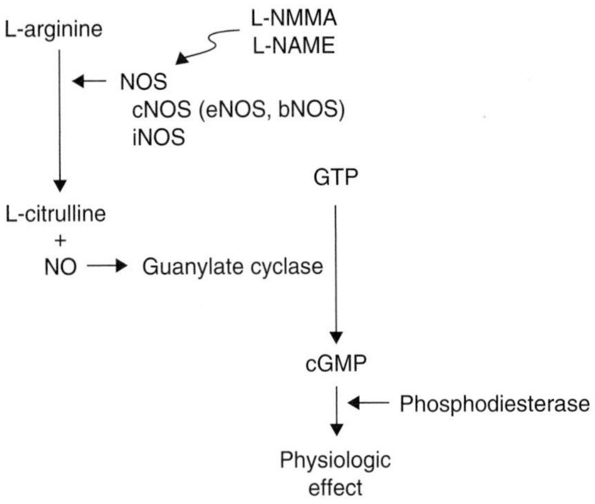

FIGURE 25-7 Biologic pathway for endogenous production of NO. *bNOS,* Neuronal type constitutive nitric oxide synthase; *cGMP,* cyclic guanosine 3′,5′-monophosphate; *cNOS,* constitutive nitric oxide synthase; *eNOS,* endothelial nitric oxide synthase; *GTP,* guanosine triphosphate; *iNOS,* inducible nitric oxide synthase; *L-NAME,* L-NG-arginine methyl ester; *L-NMMA,* L-NG-monomethyl arginine; *NOS,* nitric oxide synthase.

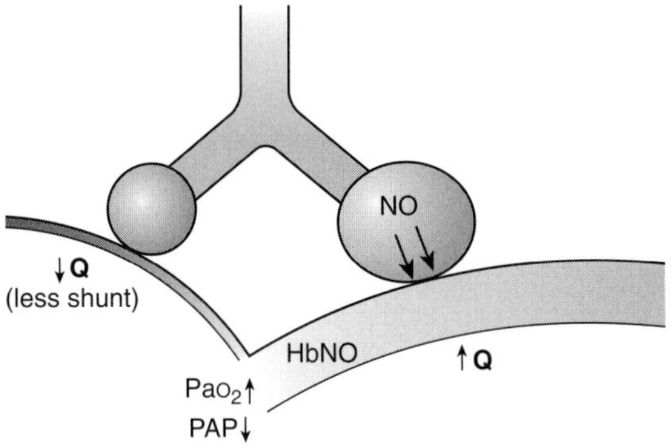

FIGURE 25-8 Because of selective pulmonary vasodilation, iNO redistributes pulmonary blood flow from unventilated lung units to ventilated lung units. iNO does not produce systemic vasodilation because it is rapidly bound to hemoglobin (Hb). *PAP,* Pulmonary artery pressure.

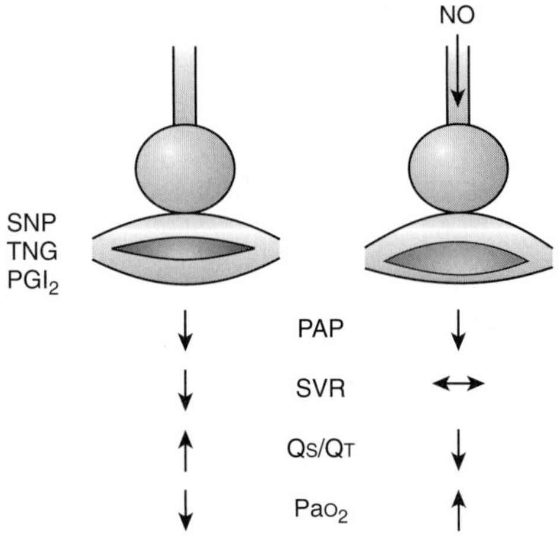

FIGURE 25-9 Physiologic effects of intravenous vasodilators *(left)* compared with the inhaled vasodilator NO *(right)*. *PAP,* Pulmonary artery pressure; *PGI_2,* epoprostenol (prostacyclin); *Q_S/Q_T,* intrapulmonary shunt fraction; *SNP,* sodium nitroprusside; *SVR,* systemic vascular resistance; *TNG,* nitroglycerin.

solutions. In aqueous solutions, NO also reacts rapidly with superoxide (O_2^-) to form peroxynitrite ($OONO^-$), which is a strong oxidant that catalyzes membrane lipid peroxidation. NO forms complexes with transitional metal complexes, including those in metalloproteins such as hemoglobin. In tissues, nitrosation of iron-containing enzymes and iron-sulfur proteins of target cells may be responsible for the cytotoxic action of NO generated by activated macrophages. NO is converted to nitrates and nitrites in plasma and is excreted primarily by the kidney. In the circulation, NO combines extremely rapidly with hemoglobin to form nitrosyl-hemoglobin and then **methemoglobin.**

Selective Pulmonary Vasodilation

The term **selective pulmonary vasodilation** is used to indicate two physiologic phenomena (Figure 25-8). First, selective pulmonary vasodilators reduce pulmonary vascular resistance without affecting systemic vascular resistance. Second, a selective pulmonary vasodilator affects vascular resistance only near ventilated alveoli. Inspired vasodilators are delivered to those lung units that are ventilated. NO is not a selective pulmonary vasodilator per se but becomes one when inhaled. iNO selectively improves blood flow to ventilated alveoli, which produces a reduction in intrapulmonary shunt and improved oxygenation. The selective pulmonary vasodilation demonstrated by iNO is due in large part to high affinity of hemoglobin for NO, which is approximately 10^6 times as great as the affinity of hemoglobin for O_2. In contrast to iNO, intravenous vasodilators (e.g., sodium nitroprusside, nitroglycerin, prostacyclin) are not selective. Although intravenous vasodilators lower pulmonary artery pressure, they also lower systemic blood pressure (Figure 25-9). Moreover, these agents increase blood flow to both ventilated and unventilated lung units, resulting in an increased intrapulmonary shunt and a lower Pao_2.

Clinical Applications

Hypoxemic Respiratory Failure of the Newborn

Since the early 1990s, several case series have reported the use of iNO for hypoxemic respiratory failure of the newborn.[86-102] Randomized double-blinded studies have reported improvement in Pao_2 and a reduced requirement for extracorporeal life support (ECLS) with the use of iNO in this patient population.[86-101] In newborns with congenital diaphragmatic hernia, however, iNO has not been shown to reduce the need for ECMO.[102] A Cochrane review concluded that, based on the evidence presently available, it appears reasonable to use iNO in an initial concentration of 20 ppm for term and near-term infants with hypoxic respiratory failure who do not have a diaphragmatic hernia.[103] iNO is not associated with an increase in neurodevelopmental, behavioral, or medical abnormalities at 2 years of age.[104] The brand name for iNO is INOmax and, currently, the only FDA-approved indication for iNO is in newborns: "INOmax, in conjunction with ventilatory support and other appropriate agents, is indicated for the treatment of term and near-term (more than 34 weeks) neonates with hypoxic respiratory failure associated with clinical or echocardiographic evidence of pulmonary hypertension, where it improves oxygenation and reduces the need for extracorporeal membrane oxygenation." iNO should not be used in the treatment of neonates known to be dependent on right-to-left shunting of blood.

There is also interest in the use of iNO in hypoxemic premature infants.[105-108] However, the evidence for this indication is mixed, and a Cochrane review concluded that the currently published evidence from randomized trials does not support the use of iNO in preterm infants with hypoxemic respiratory failure.[109]

Acute Respiratory Distress Syndrome

There is interest in the use of iNO in patients with the acute respiratory distress syndrome (ARDS) to improve oxygenation and reduce pulmonary hypertension. In many patients with ARDS, there is an increase in Pao_2 and decrease in pulmonary arterial pressure with iNO at doses of 20 ppm or less.[110-113] In a phase II trial, 177 patients with nonseptic ARDS were enrolled in a multicenter placebo-controlled double-blind study.[114] Patients were assigned randomly to receive 0, 1.25, 5, 20, 40, or 80 ppm of iNO. There was a 60% positive response to NO (greater than or equal to 20% increase in Pao_2) compared with 24% with placebo. The intensity of mechanical ventilation was lower for patients breathing NO compared with placebo over the first week of therapy. In a subgroup of patients without organ system failure, iNO at 5 ppm was associated with an increased number of days alive and ventilator free through day 28 after initiation of therapy (62% vs. 44%). However, a subsequent phase III trial comparing 5 ppm of iNO to placebo reported no substantial impact on the duration of ventilatory support or mortality.[115] Similar results have been reported by others.[116-118] That is, although iNO improves Pao_2 in many patients, this effect is not sustained and does not afford a survival benefit. iNO at 5 ppm had no effect on costs and long-term outcomes in ARDS in previously healthy adults.[119] A Cochrane review concluded that iNO did not demonstrate any statistically significant effect on mortality and transiently improved oxygenation in patients with hypoxemic respiratory failure.[120]

Other Applications

iNO is being investigated as treatment for a number of other indications, including sickle cell disease,[121,122] cardiothoracic surgery,[123-126] and lung transplantation.[127-131] Short-term (10 to 30 minute) trials of iNO are also used as a test of pulmonary vascular reactivity. To date, most investigations in these diseases are uncontrolled and anecdotal. iNO cannot be recommended as standard therapy in these settings until appropriately designed studies with relevant endpoints are published.

Toxicity and Complications of Inhaled Nitric Oxide

A number of potential toxicities and complications should be appreciated by those using this treatment modality.[132] In very high concentrations, iNO may have direct toxic effects on the lungs. In a patient who died after iatrogenic poisoning with NO (concentration not specified) from a contaminated NO cylinder, the lungs at autopsy were edematous and solid.[133] To date, however, no toxic effects have been reported in patients receiving therapeutic doses of iNO.

Nitrogen dioxide (NO_2) is produced spontaneously from NO and O_2. The conversion rate of NO to NO_2 is determined by the O_2 concentration, the square of the NO concentration, and the residence time of NO with O_2.[134] OSHA has set safety limits for NO_2 at 5 ppm, but airway reactivity and parenchymal lung injury have been reported with inhalation of 2 ppm NO_2 or less.[135-140] Thus it is prudent to keep the iNO_2 concentration as low as possible because its effects in an injured lung are unknown.

Methemoglobin (metHb) results when the iron in heme is oxidized from Fe^{-2} to Fe^{-3}. In the oxidized form, iron cannot bind to O_2 and the affinity of the other heme groups for O_2 increases (i.e., shifts the oxyhemoglobin dissociation curve to the left). Normal methemoglobin is less than 2%, and levels of less than 5% do not require treatment. The normal methemoglobin blood level may be due, in part, to metabolism of endogenous NO. Methemoglobin reductase within erythrocytes converts endogenously produced methemoglobin to normal hemoglobin. Methemoglobinemia is uncommon at the NO doses used for therapeutic inhalation (= 20 ppm). There have been a few cases of methemoglobinemia reported in association with iNO therapy, generally with high doses of iNO (e.g., 80 ppm).[141-143] In patients with decreased methemoglobin reductase (e.g., newborns and those with a hereditary deficiency), methemoglobinemia may be more likely. The usual treatment of methemoglobinemia is infusion of methylene blue, which increases NADH methemoglobin reductase. Methemoglobinemia also can be treated with ascorbic acid (vitamin C). The production of methemoglobin in patients treated with iNO is dose-dependent; methemoglobinemia is rare at usual therapeutic doses of less than 20 ppm.

Some patients fail to respond to iNO, although this is not necessarily seen as an adverse effect. In patients with ARDS, approximately 40% do not have an initial improvement in PaO_2/FIO_2 or pulmonary vascular resistance of at least 20%. A paradoxical response to iNO in a newborn infant has been reported, in whom there was a worsening of arterial oxygenation and arterial blood pressure with NO doses of 7 and 15 ppm.[144] Worsening of hypoxemia in patients with COPD who received iNO also has been reported[145,146] and has been attributed to impaired ventilation-perfusion ($\dot{V}/\dot{Q}$) matching. This suggests that iNO should be used cautiously in patients in whom hypoxemia is due to $\dot{V}/\dot{Q}$ imbalance rather than shunt.[147]

Inhibition of platelet adhesion, aggregation, and agglutination has been reported with iNO. When healthy volunteers were exposed to 30 ppm iNO for 15 minutes, bleeding time increased by 33%.[148] In patients with ARDS, platelet aggregation and agglutination were decreased significantly with iNO.[149] However, the antithrombotic effect was not associated with a change in bleeding time. Although it is prudent to consider coagulopathy when deciding to use iNO, the clinical importance of this effect remains unclear. An increased incidence of bleeding diathesis has not been noted in prospective randomized trials of NO inhalation.

Several studies have examined the effects of iNO in patients with left ventricular dysfunction.[150-152] At high doses (40 to 80 ppm), iNO has been reported to decrease pulmonary vascular resistance and increase pulmonary capillary wedge pressure in some patients with severe left ventricular dysfunction. Presumably, the acute reduction of right ventricular afterload may produce an increase in pulmonary venous return to the left heart. This would increase left ventricular filling pressure and might worsen pulmonary edema. Although this effect may be dose related, iNO should be avoided in patients with severe left ventricular dysfunction (pulmonary capillary wedge pressure = 25 mm Hg).

Withdrawal of iNO has been found to be problematic for some patients. In some cases, the degree of hypoxemia and pulmonary hypertension is greater after discontinuation of NO than at baseline, leading to hemodynamic instability. The reasons for this rebound effect are not entirely known, but they may relate to feedback inhibition of nitric oxide synthase activity. The following guidelines may help avoid the deleterious effects of rebound during withdrawal of iNO. First, use the lowest effective NO dose (5 ppm or less). Second, do not withdraw iNO until the patient's clinical status has improved sufficiently. Third, increase the FIO_2 to 0.60 to 0.70 before withdrawal of iNO,[153,154] and prepare to support the patient's hemodynamics if necessary. Discontinuation of iNO has been well tolerated under these conditions. Case studies and case series have reported benefit for use of phosphodiesterase inhibitors to attenuate rebound when iNO is discontinued.[155-162]

Delivery Systems for Inhaled Nitric Oxide

Various delivery systems have been constructed for investigational use in patients.[158,159] Because investigators have used different delivery systems and analysis methods, it is difficult to compare the actual dose administered in various studies. The following are important considerations when building a system for delivery of iNO:[163-165]

- Dependable and safe system: Complex systems will more likely permit errors that could compromise ventilation, oxygenation, or delivery of the correct NO dose. The function of NO delivery systems must be thoroughly evaluated in the laboratory before patient use.

- Precise and stable NO dose delivery: A precise and stable dose must be delivered to prevent complications associated with iNO. The dose should not vary with changes in ventilatory pattern or F_{IO_2}.
- Limit NO_2 production: The level of iNO_2 must be kept as low as possible.
- NO and NO_2 monitoring: Inhaled NO must be monitored to ensure that the correct dose is delivered, and inhaled NO_2 must be monitored because of its potentially injurious effects.
- Maintain proper ventilator function: Care must be taken to ensure that adapting the ventilator to deliver NO does not affect its function. The alarm systems should not be affected. The addition of NO lowers the F_{IO_2}, and for that reason, it should be monitored after the site of NO titration into the system (note that it is impossible to deliver 100% O_2 during iNO therapy). There is concern regarding the effect of NO on the internal components of ventilators, blenders, and flowmeters that are exposed to NO. However, damage or malfunction of equipment related to NO exposure has not been reported.
- The system should allow emergency administration of iNO (e.g., during manual ventilation).

The INOvent delivery system (INO Therapeutics, Clinton, N.J.) is a universal NO delivery system designed for use with most conventional critical care ventilators.[166,167] It can be used with either phasic-flow ventilators (e.g., adults) or continuous-flow ventilators (e.g., neonates). It can also be used with a face mask during spontaneous breathing. In its typical configuration, the delivery system is mounted on a transport cart that holds two NO therapy gas cylinders (Figure 25-10). The system is configured for 0 to 80 ppm using an 800-ppm cylinder. An integral battery provides 30 minutes of uninterrupted NO delivery in the absence of an external power source. An injection module is inserted into the inspiratory circuit at the outlet of the ventilator. The injection module consists of a hot film flow sensor and a gas injection tube. Flow in the ventilator circuit is measured precisely, and NO is injected proportional to that flow to provide the desired NO dose. This design allows a precise and constant NO concentration in the inspired gas for any ventilatory pattern. NO flows through either a high- or a low-flow controller. The high- and low-flow controllers ensure that the delivered NO concentration is accurate over a wide range of ventilator flows and desired NO concentrations. Further, residence time is short and thus NO_2 generation is minimal.

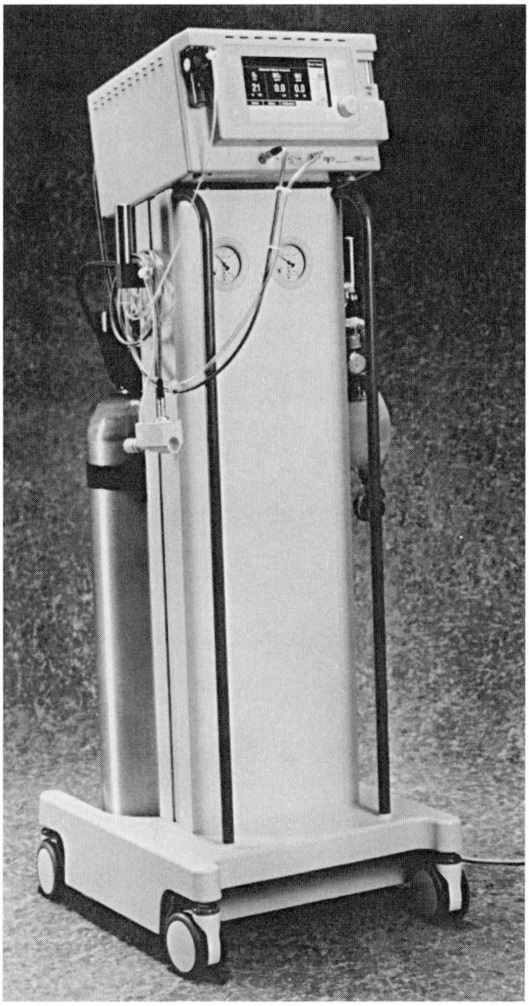

FIGURE 25-10 Ohmeda INOvent nitric oxide delivery system. (Courtesy INO Therapeutics, Clinton, N.J.)

The INOvent includes gas monitoring of O_2, NO, and NO_2. Gas is sampled downstream from the point of injection near the Y-piece in the inspiratory circuit. Gas concentrations are measured using electrochemical cells that can be calibrated at regular intervals by the user. A number of gas delivery alarms can be set by the user: high NO, low NO, high NO_2, high O_2, and low O_2. Additional alarms include those for loss of source gas pressure, weak or failed electrochemical cells, calibration required, delivery system

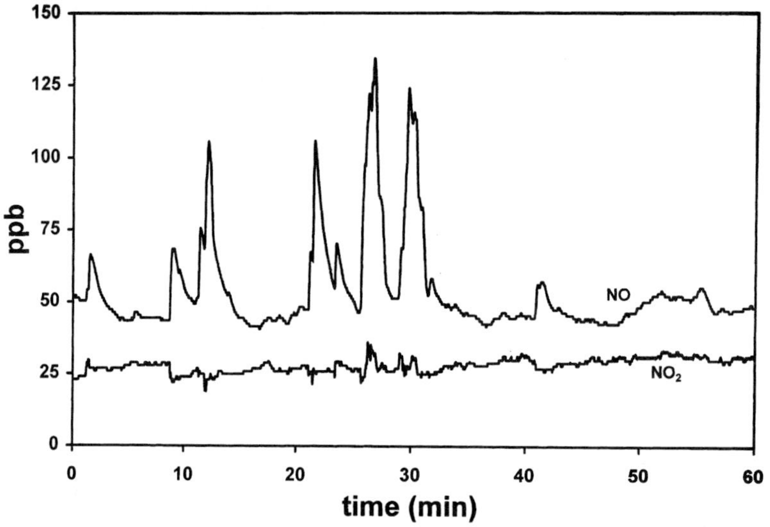

FIGURE 25-11 Ambient NO levels with 100 ppm delivered into a patient room at a flow of 8 L/min. Note that the ambient levels remain very low.

failures, and monitoring failures. The INOvent delivery system uses a dual-channel design. One channel controls NO delivery, and the other controls monitoring. This design permits NO delivery independent of monitoring, which is an important safety feature. Further, the monitoring system can be calibrated without interruption of NO delivery. A manual NO delivery system is provided by the INOvent delivery system. With an O_2 flow to the manual ventilator set at 15 L/min, INOvent injects gas to provide an NO concentration of 20 ppm. As with any manual ventilator system for NO, the bag should be squeezed three to five times to clear residual NO_2 before it is attached to the patient.

There are concerns regarding contamination of the environment with NO and NO_2, and the potential for adverse effects on health care providers. The OSHA exposure limit for NO (a time-weighted average of 25 ppm for 8 hours in the workplace) is higher than the typical NO dose (less than or equal to 20 ppm). In ICU environments that have more than six air exchanges/hour, ambient NO levels should remain very low. Ambient NO levels are very low during NO administration (less than 0.25 ppm), with or without scavenging (Figure 28-11). Available evidence suggests that scavenging is not necessary during iNO therapy.[168-170]

KEY POINTS

- The clinical benefits of heliox relate to its low density.
- Heliox has been used in the settings of partial upper airway obstruction, acute severe asthma, croup, bronchiolitis, and COPD.
- Bronchodilator delivery may be improved if it is delivered with heliox.
- Heliox affects the performance of many types of respiratory care equipment, including flowmeters, nebulizers, and ventilators.
- iNO is a selective pulmonary vasodilator.
- iNO is approved by the FDA for hypoxemic respiratory failure of the newborn.
- The role of iNO in settings other than that approved by the FDA is unclear.
- The toxicity of iNO is presumably low when the dose is less than 20 ppm.
- iNO is administered using the INOvent.
- Environmental contamination is minimal when iNO is used and thus scavenging is not necessary.

ASSESSMENT QUESTIONS

1. Which of the following statements are true regarding helium:
  I. The density of helium is less than that of O_2.
  II. The viscosity of helium is greater than that of air.
  III. It is an inert gas.
    A. I only
    B. III only
    C. I and II only
    D. II and III only
    E. I, II, and III

2. True or False. Laminar flow is density independent.

3. True or False. Turbulent flow is density independent.

4. What variables are components of the Hagen-Poiseuille law?
  I. Density
  II. Viscosity
  III. Radius
  IV. Length of the tube
    A. I and II only
    B. I, II, and III only
    C. III and IV only
    D. I, III, and IV only
    E. I, II, III, and IV

5. True or False. Reynolds' number determines if gas flow is turbulent or laminar.

6. The components of Reynolds' number include:
  I. Density
  II. Viscosity
  III. Radius of the tube
  IV. Velocity of the gas flow
    A. I, II, and III only
    B. I, II, and IV only
    C. II, III, and IV only
    D. I, II, III, and IV

7. Heliox may benefit patients with asthma during aerosol therapy by
  I. improving nebulizer performance.
  II. increasing the work of breathing.
  III. reducing auto-PEEP.
  IV. increasing gas density.
    A. I, II, and IV only
    B. I, III, and IV only
    C. III and IV only
    D. I and IV only

8. True or False. Caution should be used during delivery of heliox during mechanical ventilation because the presence of helium may alter ventilator function.

9. What is the minimum helium concentration, below which it is unlikely that a change in gas density will provide clinical benefit?
  A. 20%
  B. 40%
  C. 60%
  D. 80%

10. Which of the following are properties of NO?
  I. Highly reactive
  II. Short half-life
  III. High affinity for hemoglobin
    A. I only
    B. II only
    C. III only
    D. I and III only
    E. I, II, and III

11. NO and O_2 combine to form the toxic gas NO_2. The production of NO_2 is accelerated by
  I. High FIO_2
  II. High NO
  III. High pressure
  IV. Time
    A. I and II only
    B. I, II, and III only
    C. II and IV only
    D. I, II, III, and IV

12. iNO is approved by the FDA for use in
  A. adults with ARDS and pulmonary hypertension.
  B. premature infants with hypoxic respiratory failure.
  C. term infants with congenital heart disease.
  D. infants with bronchiolitis.
  E. term or near term infants with hypoxemia and pulmonary hypertension.

Continued

ASSESSMENT QUESTIONS—cont'd

13. Complications of iNO include:
I. Carboxyhemoglobinemia
II. Pulmonary edema
III. Methemoglobinemia
IV. Rebound hypoxemia during discontinuation of NO
A. I and II only
B. III and IV only
C. II and III only
D. I, III, and IV only
E. I, II, III, and IV

14. iNO improves oxygenation owing to its ability to improve
A. $\dot{V}/\dot{Q}$ matching by alveolar recruitment.
B. $\dot{V}/\dot{Q}$ matching by reducing pulmonary artery pressure.
C. $\dot{V}/\dot{Q}$ matching by selective pulmonary vasodilation.
D. $\dot{V}/\dot{Q}$ matching by increasing cardiac output.

15. True or False. Exposure of caregivers during NO delivery has been shown to result in adverse clinical effects.

REFERENCES

1. Manthous CA, Morgan S, Pohlman A et al: Heliox in the treatment of airflow obstruction: a critical review of the literature, Respir Care 42:1034-1042, 1997.
2. Eisenkraft JB, Barker SJ: Helium and gas flow, Anesth Analg 76:452-453, 1993.
3. Papamoschou D: Theoretical validation of the respiratory benefits of helium-oxygen mixtures, Respir Physiol 99:183-190, 1995.
4. Hess DR, Fink JB, Venkataraman ST et al: The history and physics of heliox, Respir Care 51:608-661, 2002.
5. Skrinskas GJ, Hyland RH, Hutcheon MA: Using helium-oxygen mixtures in the management of acute upper airway obstruction, Can Med Assoc J 128:555-558, 1983.
6. Lu TS, Ohmura A, Wong KC et al: Helium-oxygen in treatment of upper airway obstruction, Anesthesiology 45:678-680, 1976.
7. Curtis JL, Mahlmeister M, Fink JB et al: Helium-oxygen gas therapy: use and availability for the emergency treatment of inoperable airway obstruction, Chest 90:455-457, 1986.
8. Boorstein JM, Boorstein SM, Humphries GN et al: Using helium-oxygen mixtures in the emergency management of acute upper airway obstruction, Ann Emerg Med 18:688-690, 1989.
9. Kemper KJ, Ritz RH, Benson MS et al: Helium-oxygen mixture in the treatment of postextubation stridor in pediatric trauma patients, Crit Care Med 19:356-359, 1991.
10. Grosz AH, Jacobs IN, Cho C et al: Use of helium-oxygen mixtures to relieve upper airway obstruction in a pediatric population, Laryngoscope 111:1512-1514, 2001.
11. Connolly KM, McGuirt WF Jr: Avoiding intubation in the injured subglottis: the role of heliox therapy, Ann Otol Rhinol Laryngol 110:713-717, 2001.
12. Rodeberg DA, Easter AJ, Washam MA et al: Use of a helium-oxygen mixture in the treatment of postextubation stridor in pediatric patients with burns, J Burn Care Rehabil 16(5):476-480, 1995.
13. Jaber S, Carlucci A, Boussarsar M et al: Helium-oxygen in the postextubation period decreases inspiratory effort, Am J Respir Crit Care Med 164:633-637, 2001.
14. Myers TR: Use of heliox in children, Respir Care 51:619-631, 2006.
15. Martin-Barbaz F, Barnoud D, Carpendier F et al: Use of helium and oxygen mixtures in status asthmaticus, Rev Pneumol Clin 43:186-189, 1987.
16. Shiue ST, Gluck EH: The use of helium-oxygen mixtures in the support of patients with status asthmaticus and respiratory acidosis, J Asthma 26:177-180, 1989.
17. Kass JE, Castriotta RJ: Heliox therapy in acute severe asthma, Chest 107:757-760, 1995.
18. Manthous CA, Hall JB, Caputo MA et al: Heliox improves pulsus paradoxus and peak expiratory flow in nonintubated patients with severe asthma, Am J Respir Crit Care Med 151:310-314, 1995.
19. Kudukis TM, Manthous CA, Schmidt GA et al: Inhaled helium-oxygen revisited: effect of helium-oxygen during the treatment of status asthmaticus in children, J Pediatr 130:217-224, 1997.
20. Gluck EH, Onorato DJ, Castriotta R: Helium-oxygen mixtures in intubated patients with status asthmaticus and respiratory acidosis, Chest 98:693-698, 1990.
21. Carter ER, Webb CR, Moffitt DR: Evaluation of heliox in children hospitalized with acute severe asthma: a randomized crossover trial, Chest 109:1256-1261, 1996.
22. Schaeffer EM, Pohlman A, Morgan S et al: Oxygenation in status asthmaticus improves during ventilation with helium-oxygen, Crit Care Med 27:2666-2670, 1999.
23. Abd-Allah SA, Rogers MS, Terry M et al: Helium oxygen therapy for pediatric acute severe asthma requiring mechanical ventilation, Pediatr Crit Care Med 4:353-357, 2003.
24. Austan F: Heliox inhalation in status asthmaticus and respiratory acidemia: a brief report, Heart Lung 25:155-157, 1996.

25. Rodrigo GJ, Rodrigo C, Pollack CV et al: Use of helium-oxygen mixtures in the treatment of acute asthma: a systematic review, Chest 123:891-896, 2003.
26. Ho AM, Lee A, Karmakar MK et al: Heliox vs air-oxygen mixtures for the treatment of patients with acute asthma: a systematic overview, Chest 123:882-890, 2003.
27. Duncan PG: Efficacy of helium-oxygen mixtures in the management of severe viral and post-intubation croup, Can Anaesth Soc J 26:206-212, 1979.
28. Terregino CA, Nairn SJ, Chansky ME et al: The effect of heliox on croup: a pilot study, Acad Emerg Med 5:1130-1133, 1998.
29. Nelson DS, McClellan L: Helium-oxygen mixtures as adjunctive support for refractory viral croup, Ohio State Med J 78:729-730, 1982.
30. Weber JE, Chudnofsky CR, Younger JG et al: A randomized comparison of helium-oxygen mixture (heliox) and racemic epinephrine for the treatment of moderate to severe croup, Pediatrics 107:E96, 2001.
31. Hollman G, Shen G, Zeng L et al: Helium-oxygen improves clinical asthma scores in children with acute bronchiolitis, Crit Care Med 26:1731-1736, 1998.
32. Liet JM, Millotte B, Tucci M et al: Noninvasive therapy with helium-oxygen for severe bronchiolitis, J Pediatr 147:812-817, 2005.
33. Martinon-Torres F, Rodriguez-Nunez A, Martinon-Sanchez JM: Heliox therapy in infants with acute bronchiolitis, Pediatrics 109:68-73, 2002.
34. Gross MF, Spear RM, Peterson BM: Helium-oxygen mixture does not improve gas exchange in mechanically ventilated children with bronchiolitis, Crit Care 4:188-192, 2002.
35. Johnson JE, Gavin DJ, Adams-Dramiga S: Effects of training with heliox and noninvasive positive pressure ventilation on exercise ability in patients with severe COPD, Chest 122:464-472, 2002.
36. Palange P, Valli G, Onorati P et al: Effect of heliox on lung dynamic hyperinflation, dyspnea, and exercise endurance capacity in COPD patients, J Appl Physiol 97:1637-1642, 2004.
37. Pecchiari M, Pelucchi A, D'Angelo E et al: Effect of heliox breathing on dynamic hyperinflation in COPD patients, Chest 125:2075-2082, 2004.
38. Swidwa DM, Montenegro HD, Goldman MD et al: Helium-oxygen breathing in severe chronic obstructive pulmonary disease, Chest 87:790-795, 1985.
39. Polito A, Fessler H: Heliox in respiratory failure from obstructive lung disease, N Engl J Med 332:192-193, 1995.
40. Gerbeaux P, Boussuges A, Torro D et al: Heliox in the treatment of obstructive hypoventilation, Am J Emerg Med 16:215-216, 1998.
41. Gerbeaux P, Gainnier M, Boussuges A et al: Use of heliox in patients with severe exacerbation of chronic obstructive pulmonary disease, Crit Care Med 29:2322-2324, 2001.
42. Rodrigo G, Pollack C, Rodrigo C et al: Heliox for treatment of exacerbations of chronic obstructive pulmonary disease, Cochrane Database Syst Rev CD003571, 2002.
43. Andrews R, Lynch M: Heliox in the treatment of chronic obstructive pulmonary disease, Emerg Med J 21:670-675, 2004.
44. Austan F, Polise M: Management of respiratory failure with noninvasive positive pressure ventilation and heliox adjunct, Heart Lung 31:214-218, 2002.
45. Jolliet P, Tassaux D, Thouret JM et al: Beneficial effects of helium : oxygen versus air : oxygen noninvasive pressure support in patients with decompensated chronic obstructive pulmonary disease, Crit Care Med 27:2422-2429, 1999.
46. Jaber S, Fodil R, Carlucci A et al: Noninvasive ventilation with helium-oxygen in acute exacerbations of chronic obstructive pulmonary disease, Am J Respir Crit Care Med 161:1191-1200, 2000.
47. Jolliet P, Tassaux D, Roeseler J et al: Helium-oxygen versus air-oxygen noninvasive pressure support in decompensated chronic obstructive disease: A prospective, multicenter study, Crit Care Med 31:878-884, 2003.
48. Tassaux D, Jolliet P, Roeseler J et al: Effects of helium-oxygen on intrinsic positive end-expiratory pressure in intubated and mechanically ventilated patients with severe chronic obstructive pulmonary disease, Crit Care Med 28:2721-2728, 2000.
49. Tassaux D, Gainnier M, Battisti A et al: Helium-oxygen decreases inspiratory effort and work of breathing during pressure support in intubated patients with chronic obstructive pulmonary disease, Intensive Care Med 31:1501-1507, 2005.
50. Gainnier M, Arnal JM, Gerbeaux P et al: Helium-oxygen reduces work of breathing in mechanically ventilated patients with chronic obstructive pulmonary disease, Intensive Care Med 29:1666-1670, 2003.
51. Jolliet P, Watremez C, Roeseler J et al: Comparative effects of helium-oxygen and external positive end-expiratory pressure on respiratory mechanics, gas exchange, and ventilation-perfusion relationships in mechanically ventilated patients with chronic obstructive pulmonary disease, Intensive Care Med 29:1442-1450, 2003.
52. Diehl JL, Mercat A, Guerot E et al: Helium/oxygen mixture reduces the work of breathing at the end of the weaning process in patients with severe chronic obstructive pulmonary disease, Crit Care Med 31:1415-1420, 2003.
53. Lee DL, Lee H, Chang HW et al: Heliox improves hemodynamics in mechanically ventilated patients with chronic obstructive pulmonary disease with systolic pressure variations, Crit Care Med 33:968-973, 2005.
54. Hess DR: Heliox and noninvasive positive-pressure ventilation: a role for heliox in exacerbations of chronic obstructive pulmonary disease? Respir Care 51:640-650, 2006.
55. Anderson M, Svartengren M, Bylin G et al: Deposition in asthmatics of particles inhaled in air or in helium-oxygen, Am Rev Respir Dis 147:524-528, 1993.
56. Darquenne C, Prisk GK: Aerosol deposition in the human respiratory tract breathing air and 80:20 heliox, J Aerosol Med 17:278-285, 2004.

57. Piva JP, Menna Barreto SS, Zelmanovitz F et al: Heliox versus oxygen for nebulized aerosol therapy in children with lower airway obstruction, Pediatr Crit Care Med 3:6-10, 2002.
58. Kress JP, Noth I, Gehlbach BK et al: The utility of albuterol nebulized with heliox during acute asthma exacerbations, Am J Respir Crit Care Med 165:1317-1321, 2002.
59. Bag R, Bandi V, Fromm RE Jr et al: The effect of heliox driven bronchodilator aerosol therapy on pulmonary function tests in patients with asthma, J Asthma 39:659-665, 2002.
60. Sattonnet P, Plaisance P, Lecourt L et al: The efficacy of helium-oxygen mixture (65%-35%) in acute asthma exacerbations, Eur Respir J 24:Suppl 48:540s, 2004.
61. Lee DL, Hsu CW, Lee H et al: Beneficial effects of albuterol therapy driven by heliox versus by oxygen in severe asthma exacerbation, Acad Emerg Med 12:820-827, 2005.
62. Kim IK, Phrampus E, Venkataraman S et al: Helium/oxygen-driven albuterol nebulization in the treatment of children with moderate to severe asthma exacerbations: a randomized, controlled trial, Pediatrics 116:1127-1133, 2005.
63. Henderson SO, Acharya P, Kilaghbian T et al: Use of heliox-driven nebulizer therapy in the treatment of acute asthma, Ann Emerg Med 33:141-146, 1999.
64. Dorfman TA, Shipley ER, Burton JH et al: Inhaled heliox does not benefit ED patients with moderate to severe asthma, Am J Emerg Med 18:495-497, 2000.
65. Rose JS, Panacek EA, Miller P: Prospective randomized trial of heliox-driven continuous nebulizers in the treatment of asthma in the emergency department, J Emerg Med 22:133-137, 2002.
66. Lanoix R, Lanigan MD, Radeo MS et al: A prospective, randomized trial to evaluate heliox as a delivery vehicle to nebulize albuterol in acute asthma exacerbations in the emergency department (abstract), Acad Emerg Med 10:507, 2003.
67. Rivera ML, Kim TY, Stewart GM et al: Albuterol nebulized in heliox in the initial ED treatment of pediatric asthma: a blinded, randomized controlled trial, Am J Emerg Med 24:38-42, 2006.
68. Kim IK, Saville AL, Sikes KL et al: Heliox-driven albuterol nebulization for asthma exacerbations: an overview, Respir Care 51:613-618, 2006.
69. Brown MK, Willms DC: A laboratory evaluation of 2 mechanical ventilators in the presence of helium-oxygen mixtures, Respir Care 50:354-360, 2005.
70. Oppenheim-Eden A, Cohen Y, Weissman C et al: The effect of helium on ventilator performance: study of five ventilators and a bedside Pitot tube spirometer, Chest 120:582-588, 2001.
71. Tassaux D, Jolliet P, Thouret JM et al: Calibration of seven ICU ventilators for mechanical ventilation with helium-oxygen mixtures, Am J Respir Crit Care Med 160:22-32, 1999.
72. Chatmongkolchart S, Kacmarek RM, Hess DR: Heliox delivery with noninvasive positive pressure ventilation: a laboratory study, Respir Care 46:248-254, 2001.
73. Venkataraman ST: Heliox during mechanical ventilation, Respir Care 51:632-639, 2006.
74. Hess DR, Acosta FL, Ritz RH et al: Effect of heliox on nebulizer function, Chest 115:184-189, 1999.
75. Goode ML, Fink JB, Dhand R et al: Improvement in aerosol delivery with helium-oxygen mixtures during mechanical ventilation, Am J Respir Crit Care Med 163:109-114, 2001.
76. deBoisblanc BP, DeBleiux P, Resweber S et al: Randomized trial of the use of heliox as a driving gas for updraft nebulization of bronchodilators in the emergent treatment of acute exacerbations of chronic obstructive pulmonary disease, Crit Care Med 28:3177-3180, 2000.
77. Corcoran TE, Gamard S: Development of aerosol drug delivery with helium oxygen gas mixtures, J Aerosol Med 17:299-309, 2004.
78. Fink JB: Opportunities and risks of using heliox in your clinical practice, Respir Care 51:651-660, 2006.
79. Hurford WE: The biological basis for inhaled nitric oxide, Respir Care Clin North Am 3:357-369, 1997.
80. Steudel W, Hurford WE, Zapol WM: Inhaled nitric oxide: basic biology and clinical applications, Anesthesiology 91:1090-1121, 1999.
81. Dupuy PM, Lancon JP, Francoise M et al: Inhaled cigarette smoke selectively reverses human hypoxic vasoconstriction, Intensive Care Med 21:941-944, 1995.
82. Pinsky MR, Genc F, Lee KH et al: Contamination of hospital compressed air with nitric oxide: unwitting replacement therapy, Chest 111:1759-1763, 1997.
83. Tan PS, Genc F, Delgado E et al: Nitric oxide contamination of hospital compressed air improves gas exchange in patients with acute lung injury, Intensive Care Med 28:1064-1072, 2002.
84. Mourgeon E, Levesque E, Duveau C et al: Factors influencing indoor concentrations of nitric oxide in a Parisian intensive care unit, Am J Respir Crit Care Med 156:1692-1695, 1997.
85. Griffiths MJ, Evans TW: Inhaled nitric oxide therapy in adults, N Engl J Med 353:2683-2695, 2005.
86. Roberts JD, Polaner DM, Lang P et al: Inhaled nitric oxide in persistent pulmonary hypertension of the newborn, Lancet 340:818-819, 1992.
87. Kinsella JP, Neish SR, Shaffer E et al: Low-dose inhalational nitric oxide in persistent pulmonary hypertension of the newborn, Lancet 340:818-820, 1992.
88. Goldman AP, Tasker RC, Haworth HG et al: Four patterns of response to inhaled nitric oxide for persistent pulmonary hypertension of the newborn, Pediatrics 98:706-713, 1996.
89. Biban P, Trevisanuto D, Pettenazzo A et al: Inhaled nitric oxide in hypoxaemic newborns who are candidates for extracorporeal life support, Eur Respir J 11:371-376, 1998.
90. Mercier JC, Lacaze T, Storme L et al: Disease-related response to inhaled nitric oxide in newborns with

severe hypoxemic respiratory failure, French Paediatric Study Group of Inhaled NO, Eur J Pediatr 157:747-752, 1998.
91. Gupta A, Rastogi S, Sahni R et al: Inhaled nitric oxide and gentle ventilation in the treatment of pulmonary hypertension of the newborn—a single-center, 5-year experience, J Perinatol 22:435-441, 2004.
92. Day RW, Lynch JM, White KS et al: Acute response to inhaled nitric oxide in newborns with respiratory failure and pulmonary hypertension, Pediatrics 98:698-705, 1996.
93. Hoffman GM, Ross GA, Day SE et al: Inhaled nitric oxide reduces utilization of extracorporeal membrane oxygenation in persistent pulmonary hypertension of the newborn, Crit Care Med 25:352-359, 1997.
94. Wessel DL, Adatia I, Van Marter LJ et al: Improved oxygenation in a randomized trial of inhaled nitric oxide for persistent pulmonary hypertension of the newborn, Pediatrics 100:e7-e13, 1997.
95. The Neonatal Inhaled Nitric Oxide Study Group: Inhaled nitric oxide in full-term and nearly full-term infants with hypoxic respiratory failure, N Engl J Med 336:597-604, 1997.
96. Roberts JD Jr, Fineman J, Morin FC III et al: Inhaled nitric oxide and persistent pulmonary hypertension of the newborn, N Engl J Med 336:605-610, 1997.
97. Kinsella JP, Truog WE, Walsh WF et al: Randomized, multicenter trial of inhaled nitric oxide and high frequency oscillatory ventilation in severe, persistent pulmonary hypertension of the newborn, J Pediatr 131:55-62, 1997.
98. Davidson D, Barefield ES, Kattwinkel J et al: Inhaled nitric oxide for the early treatment of persistent pulmonary hypertension of the term newborn: a randomized, double-masked, placebo-controlled, dose-response, multicenter study, Pediatrics 101:325-334, 1998.
99. Clark RH, Kueser TJ, Walker MW et al: Low-dose nitric oxide therapy for persistent pulmonary hypertension of the newborn, N Engl J Med 342:469-474, 2000.
100. Sadiq HF, Mantych G, Benawra RS et al: Inhaled nitric oxide in the treatment of moderate persistent pulmonary hypertension of the newborn: a randomized controlled, multicenter trial, J Perinatol 23:98-103, 2003.
101. Konduri GG, Solimano A, Sokol GM et al: A randomized trial of early versus standard inhaled nitric oxide therapy in term and near-term newborn infants with hypoxic respiratory failure, Pediatrics 113:559-564, 2004.
102. The Neonatal Inhaled Nitric Oxide Study Group (NINOS): Inhaled nitric oxide and hypoxic respiratory failure in infants with congenital diaphragmatic hernia, Pediatrics 99:838-845, 1997.
103. Finer NN, Barrington KJ: Nitric oxide for respiratory failure in infants born at or near term, Cochrane Database Syst Rev CD000399, 2006.
104. The Neonatal Inhaled Nitric Oxide Study Group (NINOS): Inhaled nitric oxide in term and near-term infants: neurodevelopmental follow-up of the neonatal inhaled nitric oxide study group (NINOS), J Pediatr 136:611-617, 2000.
105. Kinsella JP, Cutter GR, Walsh WF et al: Early inhaled nitric oxide therapy in premature newborns with respiratory failure, N Engl J Med 355:354-364, 2006.
106. Ballard RA, Truog WE, Cnaan A et al: Inhaled nitric oxide in preterm infants undergoing mechanical ventilation, N Engl J Med 355:343-353, 2006.
107. Schreiber MD, Gin-Mestan K, Marks JD et al: Inhaled nitric oxide in premature infants with the respiratory distress syndrome, N Engl J Med 349:2099-2107, 2003.
108. Van Meurs KP, Wright LL, Ehrenkranz RA et al: Inhaled nitric oxide for premature infants with severe respiratory failure, N Engl J Med 353:13-22, 2005.
109. Barrington KJ, Finer NN: Inhaled nitric oxide for respiratory failure in preterm infants, Cochrane Database Syst Rev CD000509, 2006.
110. Rossaint R, Falke KJ, Lopez F et al: Inhaled nitric oxide for the adult respiratory distress syndrome, N Engl J Med 328:399-405, 1993.
111. Bigatello LM, Hurford WE, Kacmarek RM et al: Prolonged inhalation of low concentrations of nitric oxide in patients with severe adult respiratory distress syndrome: effects on pulmonary hemodynamics and oxygenation, Anesthesiology 80:761-770, 1994.
112. Manktelow C, Bigatello LM, Hess D et al: Physiologic determinants of the response to inhaled nitric oxide in patients with acute respiratory distress syndrome, Anesthesiology 87:297-307, 1997.
113. Bigatello LM, Hurford WE, Hess D: Use of inhaled nitric oxide for ARDS, Respir Care Clin North Am 3:437-458, 1997.
114. Dellinger RP, Zimmerman JL, Taylor RW et al: Inhaled nitric oxide in patients with acute respiratory distress syndrome: results of a randomized phase II trial, Crit Care Med 26:15-23, 1998.
115. Taylor RW, Zimmerman JL, Dellinger RP et al: Low-dose inhaled nitric oxide in patients with acute lung injury: a randomized controlled trial, JAMA 291:1603-1609, 2004.
116. Lundin S, Mang H, Smithies M et al: Inhalation of nitric oxide in acute lung injury: results of a European multicentre study. The European Study Group of Inhaled Nitric Oxide, Intensive Care Med 25:911-919, 1999.
117. Troncy E, Collet JP, Shapiro S et al: Inhaled nitric oxide in acute respiratory distress syndrome: a pilot randomized controlled study, Am J Respir Crit Care Med 157:1483-1488, 1998.
118. Michael JR, Barton RG, Saffle JR et al: Inhaled nitric oxide versus conventional therapy: effect on oxygenation in ARDS, Am J Respir Crit Care Med 157:1372-1380, 1998.
119. Angus DC, Clermont G, Linde-Zwirble WT et al: Healthcare costs and long-term outcomes after acute respiratory distress syndrome: A phase III trial of inhaled nitric oxide, Crit Care Med 34:2883-2890, 2006.
120. Sokol J, Jacobs SE, Bohn D: Inhaled nitric oxide for acute hypoxemic respiratory failure in children and

adults, Cochrane Database Syst Rev CD002787, 2003.

121. Head CA, Brugnara C, Martinez-Ruiz R et al: Low concentrations of nitric oxide increase oxygen affinity of sickle erythrocytes in vitro and in vivo, J Clin Invest 100:1193-1198, 1997.
122. Weiner DL, Hibberd PL, Betit P et al: Preliminary assessment of inhaled nitric oxide for acute vaso-occlusive crisis in pediatric patients with sickle cell disease, JAMA 289:1136-1142, 2003.
123. George I, Xydas S, Topkara VK et al: Clinical indication for use and outcomes after inhaled nitric oxide therapy, Ann Thorac Surg 82:2161-2169, 2006.
124. Fattouch K, Sbraga F, Sampognaro R et al: Treatment of pulmonary hypertension in patients undergoing cardiac surgery with cardiopulmonary bypass: a randomized, prospective, double-blind study, J Cardiovasc Med (Hagerstown) 7:119-123, 2006.
125. Maxey TS, Smith CD, Kern JA et al: Beneficial effects of inhaled nitric oxide in adult cardiac surgical patients, Ann Thorac Surg 73:529-533, 2002.
126. Fattouch K, Sbraga F, Bianco G et al: Inhaled prostacyclin, nitric oxide, and nitroprusside in pulmonary hypertension after mitral valve replacement, J Card Surg 20:171-176, 2005.
127. Adatia I, Lillehei C, Arnold JH et al: Inhaled nitric oxide in the treatment of postoperative graft dysfunction after lung transplantation, Ann Thorac Surg 57:1311-1318, 1994.
128. Date H, Triantafillou AN, Trulock EP et al: Inhaled nitric oxide reduces human lung allograft dysfunction, J Thorac Cardiovasc Surg 111:913-919, 1996.
129. Bacha EA, Sellak H, Murakami S et al: Inhaled nitric oxide attenuates reperfusion injury in non-heart beating-donor lung transplantation, Transplantation 63:1380-1386, 1997.
130. Ardehali A, Laks H, Levine M et al: A prospective trial of inhaled nitric oxide in clinical lung transplantation, Transplantation 72:112-115, 2001.
131. Meade MO, Granton JT, Matte-Martyn A et al: A randomized trial of inhaled nitric oxide to prevent ischemia-reperfusion injury after lung transplantation, Am J Respir Crit Care Med 167:1483-1489, 2003.
132. Hess DR: Adverse effects and toxicity of inhaled nitric oxide, Respir Care 44:315-330, 1999.
133. Clutton-Brock J: Two cases of poisoning by contamination of nitrous oxide with higher oxides of nitrogen during anaesthesia, Br J Anaesth 39:388-392, 1967.
134. Nishimura M, Hess D, Kacmarek RM et al: Nitrogen dioxide production during mechanical ventilation with nitric oxide in adults: effects of ventilator internal volume, air versus nitrogen dilution, minute ventilation, and inspired oxygen fraction, Anesthesiology 82:1246-1254, 1995.
135. Bauer MA, Utell MJ, Morrow PE et al: Inhalation of 0.30 ppm nitrogen dioxide potentiates exercise-induced bronchospasm in asthmatics, Am Rev Respir Dis 134:1203-1208, 1986.
136. Frampton MW, Morrow PE, Cos C et al: Effects of nitrogen dioxide exposure on pulmonary function and airway reactivity in normal humans, Am Rev Respir Dis 143:522-527, 1991.
137. Hazucha MJ, Folinsbee LJ, Seal E et al: Lung function responses of healthy women after sequential exposures to NO_2 and O_3, Am J Respir Crit Care Med 150:642-647, 1994.
138. Kleinman MT, Bailey RM, Linn WS et al: Effect of 0.2 ppm nitrogen dioxide on pulmonary function and response to bronchoprovocation in asthmatics, J Toxicol Environ Health 12:815-826, 1983.
139. Orehek J, Massari JP, Gayard P et al: Effects of short-term, low level nitrogen dioxide exposure on bronchial sensitivity of asthmatic patients, J Clin Invest 74:301-307, 1976.
140. Blomberg A, Krishna MT, Bocchino V et al: The inflammatory effects of 2 ppm NO_2 on the airways of healthy subjects, Am J Respir Crit Care Med 156:418-424, 1997.
141. Taylor MB, Christian KG, Patel N et al: Methemoglobinemia: Toxicity of inhaled nitric oxide therapy, Pediatr Crit Care Med 2:99-101, 2001.
142. Wessel DL, Adatia I, Thompson JE et al: Delivery and monitoring of inhaled nitric oxide in patients with pulmonary hypertension, Crit Care Med 22:930-938, 1994.
143. Hovenga S, Koenders ME, van der Werf TS et al: Methaemoglobinaemia after inhalation of nitric oxide for treatment of hydrochlorothiazide-induced pulmonary edema, Lancet 348:1035-1036, 1996.
144. Oriot D, Boussemart T, Berthier M et al: Paradoxical effect of inhaled nitric oxide in a newborn with pulmonary hypertension, Lancet 342:364-365, 1993.
145. Barbera JA, Roger N, Roca J et al: Worsening of pulmonary gas exchange with nitric oxide inhalation in chronic obstructive pulmonary disease, Lancet 347:436-440, 1996.
146. Katayama Y, Higenbottam TW, Diaz DA et al: Inhaled nitric oxide and arterial oxygen tension in patients with chronic obstructive pulmonary disease and severe pulmonary hypertension, Thorax 52:120-124, 1997.
147. Hopkins SR, Johnson EC, Richardson RS et al: Effects of inhaled nitric oxide on gas exchange in lungs with shunt or poorly ventilated areas, Am J Respir Crit Care Med 156:484-491, 1997.
148. Hogman M, Frostell C, Arnberg H et al: Bleeding time prolongation and NO inhalation, Lancet 341:1664-1665, 1993.
149. Samama CM, Diaby M, Fellahi JL et al: Inhibition of platelet aggregation by inhaled nitric oxide in patients with acute respiratory distress syndrome, Anesthesiology 83:56-65, 1995.
150. Bocchi EA, Bacal F, Auler JO Jr et al: Inhaled nitric oxide leading to pulmonary edema in stable severe heart failure, Am J Cardiol 74:70-72, 1994.
151. Loh E, Stamler JS, Hare JM et al: Cardiovascular effects of inhaled nitric oxide in patients with left ventricular dysfunction, Circulation 90:2780-2785, 1994.
152. Semigran MJ, Cockrill BA, Kacmarek R et al: Hemodynamic effects of inhaled nitric oxide in heart failure, J Am Coll Cardiol 24:982-988, 1994.
153. Davidson D, Barefield ES, Kattwinkel J et al: Safety of withdrawing inhaled nitric oxide therapy in persistent pulmonary hypertension of the newborn, Pediatrics 104:231-236, 1999.

154. Aly H, Sahni R, Wung JT: Weaning strategy with inhaled nitric oxide treatment in persistent pulmonary hypertension of the newborn, Arch Dis Child Fetal Neonatal Ed 76:F118-122, 1997.
155. Behrends M, Beiderlinden M, Peters J: Combination of sildenafil and bosentan for nitric oxide withdrawal, Eur J Anaesthesiol 22:155-157, 2005.
156. Keller RL, Hamrick SE, Kitterman JA et al: Treatment of rebound and chronic pulmonary hypertension with oral sildenafil in an infant with congenital diaphragmatic hernia, Pediatric Crit Care Med 5:184-187, 2004.
157. Saiki Y, Nitta Y, Tsuru Y et al: Successful weaning from inhaled nitric oxide using dipyridamole, Eur J Cardiothorac Surg 24:837, 2003.
158. Buysse C, Fonteyne C, Dessy H et al: The use of dipyridamole to wean from inhaled nitric oxide in congenital diaphragmatic hernia, J Pediatr Surg 36:1864-1865, 2001.
159. Ivy DD, Kinsella JP, Ziegler JW et al: Dipyridamole attenuates rebound pulmonary hypertension after inhaled nitric oxide withdrawal in postoperative congenital heart disease, J Thorac Cardiovasc Surg 115:875-882, 1998.
160. Atz AM, Adatia I, Wessel DL: Rebound pulmonary hypertension after inhalation of nitric oxide, Ann Thorac Surg 62:1759-1764, 1996.
161. Namachivayam P, Theilen U, Butt WW et al: Sildenafil prevents rebound pulmonary hypertension after withdrawal of nitric oxide in children, Am J Respir Crit Care Med 174:1042-1047, 2006.
162. al-Alaiyan S, al-Omran A, Dyer D: The use of phosphodiesterase inhibitor (dipyridamole) to wean from inhaled nitric oxide, Intensive Care Med 22:1093-1095, 1996.
163. Hess D, Kacmarek RM, Ritz R et al: Inhaled nitric oxide delivery systems: a role for respiratory therapists, Respir Care 40:702-705, 1995.
164. Branson RD, Hess DR, Campbell RS et al: Inhaled nitric oxide: delivery systems and monitoring, Respir Care 44:281-306, 1999.
165. Hess D, Ritz R, Branson RD: Delivery systems for inhaled nitric oxide, Respir Care Clin North Am 3:371-410, 1997.
166. Young JD, Roberts M, Gale LB: Laboratory evaluation of the INOvent nitric oxide delivery device, Br J Anaesth 79:398-401, 1997.
167. Kirme M, Hess D: Delivery of inhaled nitric oxide using the Ohmeda INOvent delivery system, Chest 113:1650-1657, 1998.
168. Phillips ML, Hall TA, Sekar K et al: Assessment of medical personnel exposure to nitrogen oxides during inhaled nitric oxide treatment of neonatal and pediatric patients, Pediatrics 104:1095-1100, 1999.
169. Qureshi MA, Shah NJ, Hemmen CW et al: Exposure of intensive care unit nurses to nitric oxide and nitrogen dioxide during therapeutic use of inhaled nitric oxide in adults with acute respiratory distress syndrome, Am J Crit Care 12:147-153, 2003.
170. Markhorst DG, Leenhoven T, Uiterwijk JW et al: Occupational exposure during nitric oxide inhalational therapy in a pediatric intensive care setting, Intensive Care Med 22:954-958, 1996.

APPENDIX 1

Mechanical Ventilation Case Studies

NEIL MACINTYRE

CASE STUDY 1
PARENCHYMAL LUNG INJURY

(See Chapter 15 for further information.)

MJ, a 46-year-old man without a prior history of cardiopulmonary disease, is brought to the hospital after a massive exposure to chlorine gas in a workplace accident. He is intubated in the emergency department and comes into the intensive care unit unresponsive and on a mechanical ventilator. His chest x-ray shows bilateral infiltrates and his arterial blood gases with an FIO_2 of 0.6 are PO_2 51, PCO_2 42, and pH 7.35.

QUESTIONS

Refer to MJ's ventilator graphics in Figure 1-1 to answer the following questions.

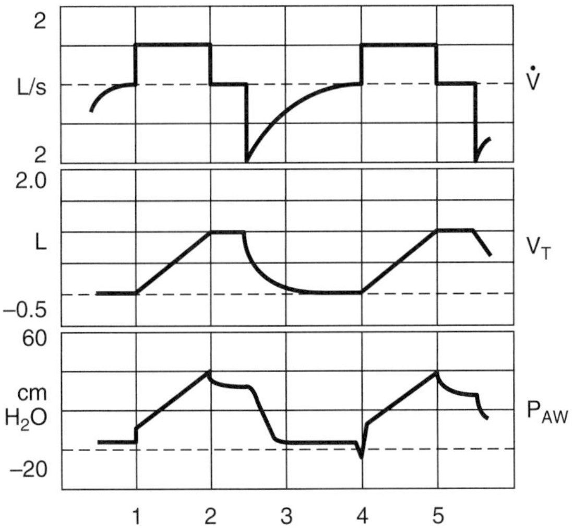

FIGURE 1-1

1. What mode of support is he receiving?
2. What is the peak airway pressure (P_{PEAK})?
3. What is the plateau airway pressure (P_{PLAT})?
4. What is the baseline airway pressure (PEEP)?
5. What is the inspiratory flow ($\dot{V}$)?
6. What is the delivered tidal volume (V_T)?
7. Calculate static compliance (V_T/P_{PLAT} − PEEP).
8. Calculate inspiratory airway resistance $P_{PEAK} - P_{PLAT}/\dot{V}$).

In Figure 1-2, PEEP has been increased and the PO_2 has improved to 81. Refer to this figure to answer the following questions.

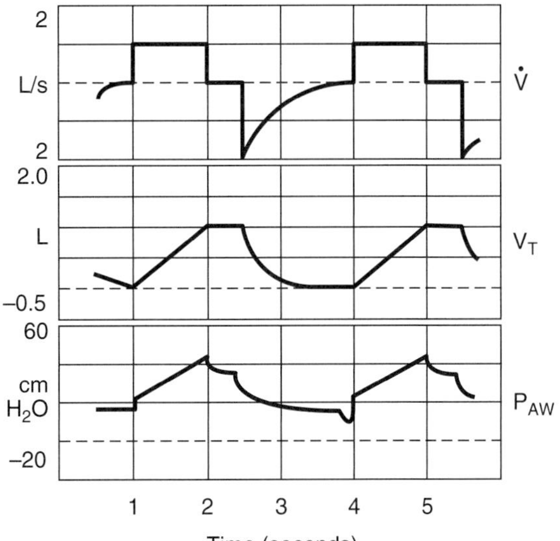

FIGURE 1-2

9. What is the PEEP setting now?
10. What is the P_{PLAT} now?
11. What is the compliance now?
12. Does this represent alveolar recruitment?

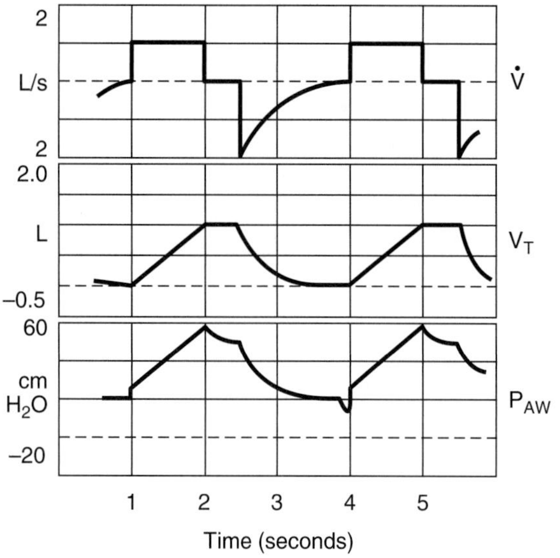

FIGURE 1-3

13. Why or why not does this represent alveolar recruitment?

In Figure 1-3, PEEP has been further increased and the Po_2 has gone to 71. Refer to this figure to answer the following questions.

14. What is the PEEP setting now?
15. What is the P_{PLAT} now?
16. What is the compliance now?
17. Does this represent alveolar recruitment?
18. Why or why not does this represent alveolar recruitment?

The PEEP is returned to the levels in Figure 1-2 and the Po_2 to 85. Pco_2 remains 42 and pH remains 7.35.

19. Should anything else be done at this time? Why or why not?

CASE STUDY 2
PARENCHYMAL LUNG INJURY

(See Chapter 15 for further information.)

PD is a 65-year-old woman with febrile neutropenia and progressive bilateral pulmonary infiltrates on chest x-ray. She is on a ventilator with an Fio_2 of 1.0. The Po_2 is 54, the Pco_2 is 62, and the pH is 7.17.

QUESTIONS

Refer to PD's ventilator graphics in Figure 2-1 to answer the following questions.

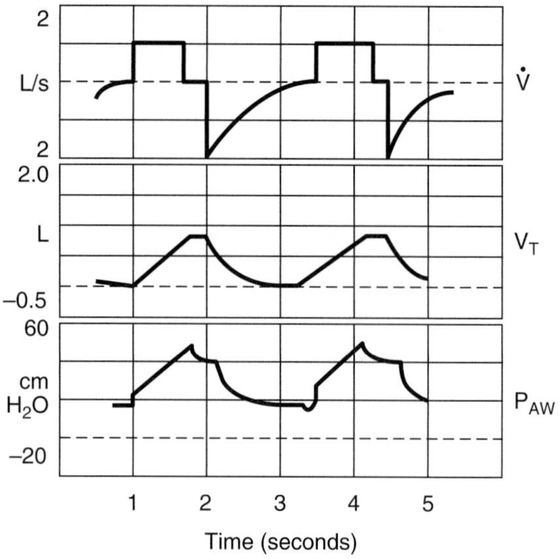

FIGURE 2-1

1. What is the mode?
2. What is the peak airway pressure (P_{PEAK})?
3. What is the plateau airway pressure (P_{PLAT})?
4. What is the baseline airway pressure (PEEP)?
5. What is the inspiratory flow ($\dot{V}$)?
6. What is the delivered tidal volume (V_T)?
7. What is the static compliance (V_T/P_{PLAT} – PEEP)?

Refer to Figure 2-2 to answer the following questions.

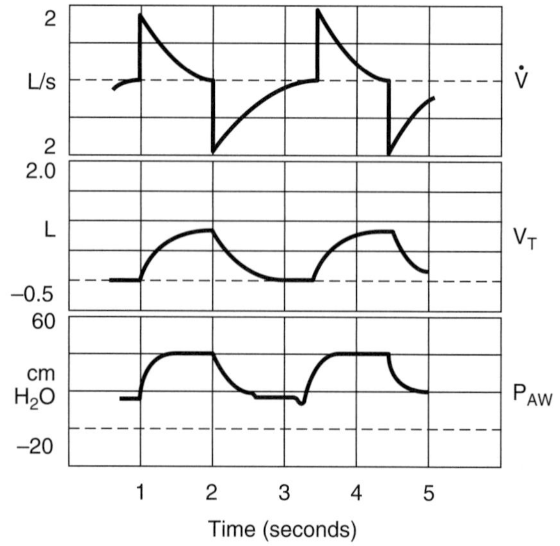

FIGURE 2-2

8. What change has been made between Figures 2-1 and 2-2?
9. How was the inspiratory pressure set to give the same V_T as that in Figure 2-1?

10. What considerations were made in setting the inspiratory time to match ventilation of Figure 2-1?
11. What is the static compliance now?
12. Is the static compliance different from what is shown in Figure 2-1?
13. Would you have expected the static compliance to be different?

In Figure 2-3, the blood gases remain essentially unchanged. Refer to this figure to answer the following questions.

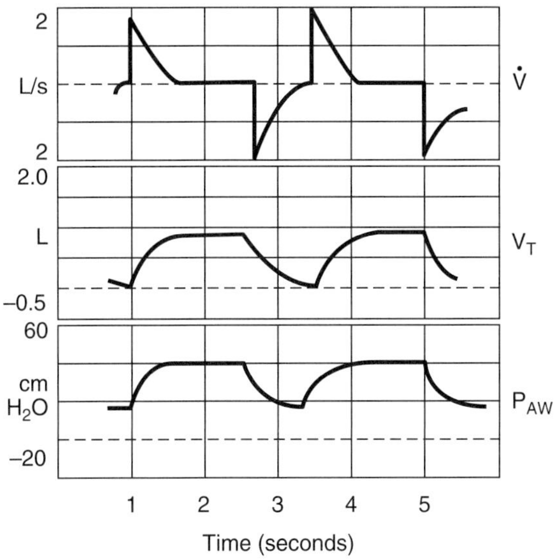

FIGURE 2-3

14. What change has been made between Figures 2-2 and 2-3?
15. Did mean airway pressure change?
16. Why or why not did mean airway pressure change?
17. Did air trapping develop?
18. Give two graphical signs why or why not air trapping developed.
19. If you performed an expiratory hold maneuver, what would you observe?

Figure 2-4 shows some improvement in blood gases. Refer to this figure to answer the following questions.

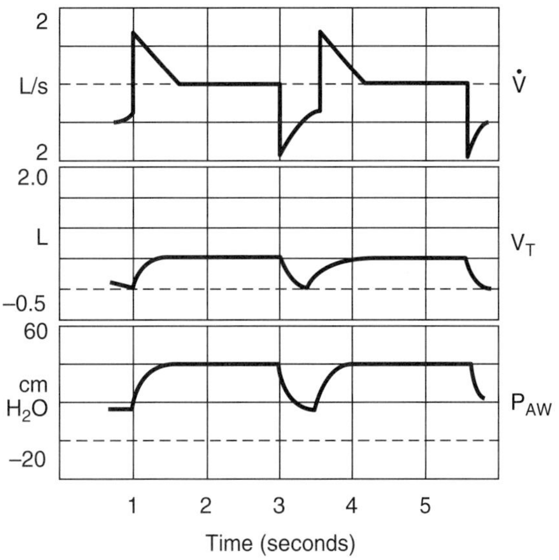

FIGURE 2-4

20. What change has been made between Figures 2-3 and 2-4?
21. Did mean airway pressure change?
22. Did air trapping develop?
23. Give two graphical signs why or why not.
24. What is the calculated static compliance now?
25. Why is this different from that in Figure 2-3?
26. If you assume that true static compliance did not change between Figures 2-3 and 2-4, can you calculate the intrinsic PEEP that developed?
27. If you performed an expiratory hold maneuver, what would you observe?

You return to the settings of Figure 2-3 and arterial blood gases improve. Two hours later, the patient becomes hypotensive and develops the graphics shown in Figure 2-5.

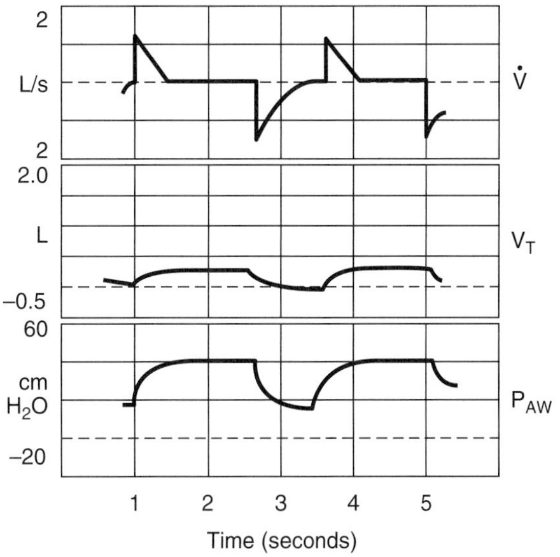

FIGURE 2-5

28. What ventilator parameter has been most affected?
29. What is the compliance now?
30. What are the most important diagnoses to consider?
31. Had this been volume-targeted ventilation and assuming that alarms were not activated, what would have happened to P_{PLAT}?
32. What would have happened to V_T?

CASE STUDY 3
ACUTE AIRFLOW OBSTRUCTION

(See Chapter 16 for further information.)

BF is a 39-year-old woman with severe asthma who cones to the emergency room with respiratory arrest. She is resuscitated, intubated, and placed on a mechanical ventilator. Her initial blood gases on 100% O_2 are Po_2 102, Pco_2 38, and pH 7.42.

QUESTIONS

BF's initial ventilator graphics are displayed in Figure 3-1. Refer to this figure to answer the following questions.

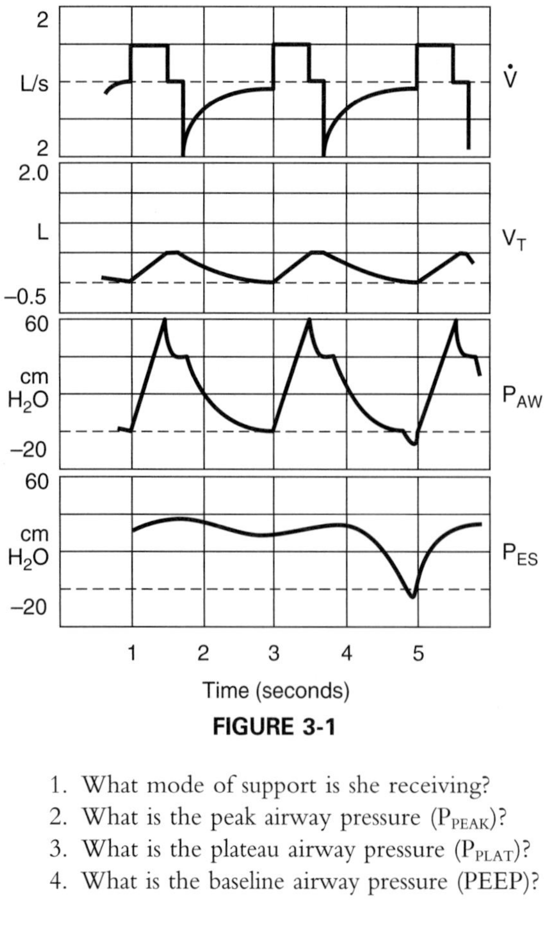

FIGURE 3-1

1. What mode of support is she receiving?
2. What is the peak airway pressure (P_{PEAK})?
3. What is the plateau airway pressure (P_{PLAT})?
4. What is the baseline airway pressure (PEEP)?
5. What is the inspiratory flow ($\dot{V}$)?
6. What is the delivered tidal volume (V_T)?
7. Calculate static compliance (V_T/ P_{PLAT} – PEEP).
8. Calculate inspiratory airway resistance (P_{PEAK} – $P_{PLAT}/\dot{V}$).
9. Is air trapping present?
10. Why or why not is air trapping present?
11. Using the esophageal pressure tracing during the assisted breath, what level of intrinsic PEEP is present?
12. Is this air trapping/intrinsic PEEP contributing to the increased P_{PLAT}?
13. If this pressure is taken into account, what is the true inspiratory change in intra-alveolar (plateau-PEEP) pressure?
14. What is true respiratory system compliance?
15. Name four actions that could be taken to reduce air trapping/intrinsic PEEP in this patient.
16. What additional step could be taken to improve triggering of the assisted breath?

CASE STUDY 4
ACUTE EXACERBATION OF CHRONIC AIRWAY OBSTRUCTION

(See Chapter 16 for further information.)

LT is a 66-year-old man with COPD who is intubated in the emergency room for respiratory failure. His initial blood gases on an F_{IO_2} of 0.5 are Po_2 98, Pco_2 78, and pH 7.08.

QUESTIONS

Figure 4-1 shows LT's ventilator graphics. Refer to this figure to answer the following questions.

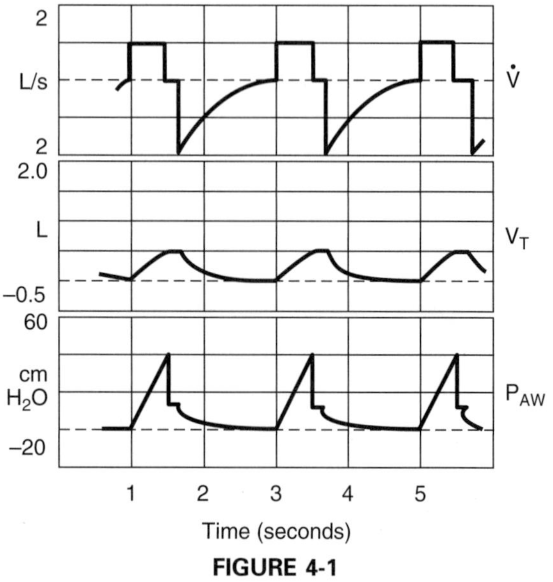

FIGURE 4-1

1. Is air trapping present?
2. Why or why not is air trapping present?
3. What would happen with an expiratory hold maneuver?
4. What would happen to this expiratory hold maneuver if the patient made inspiratory/expiratory efforts?
5. Calculate static compliance ($V_T/P_{PLAT} - PEEP$).
6. Calculate inspiratory airway resistance ($P_{PEAK} - P_{PLAT}/\dot{V}$).
7. What change would you make at this time?
8. What two parameters would you monitor as you did this?

The next day, blood gases have improved and you have returned to the settings of Figure 4-1. However, later that day, the patient becomes hypotensive and the graphics in Figure 4-2 appear.

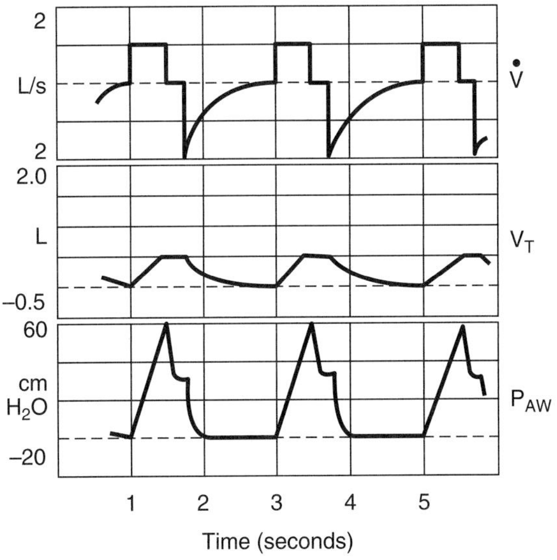

FIGURE 4-2

9. What is the static compliance?
10. What diagnoses must be considered immediately?
11. Had this been pressure-targeted ventilation and assuming that no alarms were activated, what would have happened to P_{PLAT}?
12. What would have happened to V_T?

CASE STUDY 5

RECOVERING RESPIRATORY FAILURE/ WEANING AND PARTIAL SUPPORT

(See Chapters 8 and 18 for further information.)

JR is a 54-year-old man with mild COPD who is intubated for respiratory failure following bilateral pneumonia. After 4 days of antibiotics and mechanical ventilatory support, his chest x-ray is clearing, PEEP has been reduced to 5, and F_{IO_2} is 0.4. He is awake and making efforts to breathe.

QUESTIONS

1. What assessments are most likely to determine his potential for ventilator discontinuation?
2. How often should these assessments be performed if he is deemed unfit for discontinuation today?

After appropriate assessment, it is decided that he is not ready for ventilator discontinuation. He is then placed on a substantial level of volume-targeted ventilation as displayed in Figure 5-1.

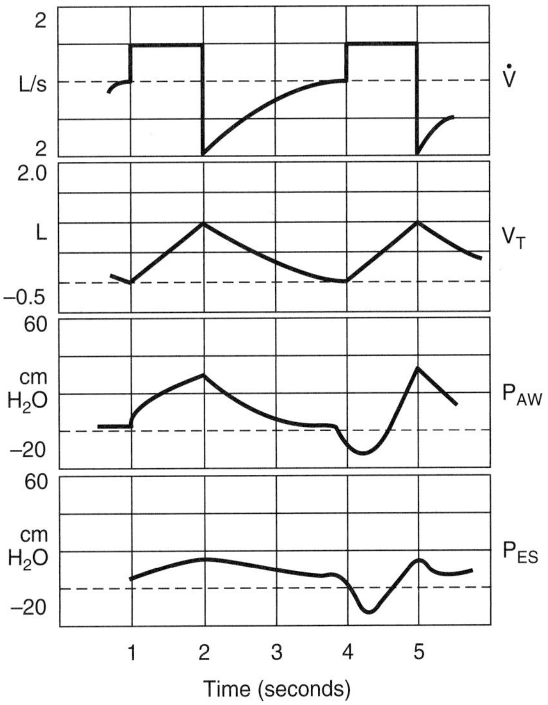

FIGURE 5-1

3. What are two obvious sources of imposed loading in Figure 5-1?
4. List two things that can be done.

You choose another mode of assisted ventilation for this patient (Figure 5-2).

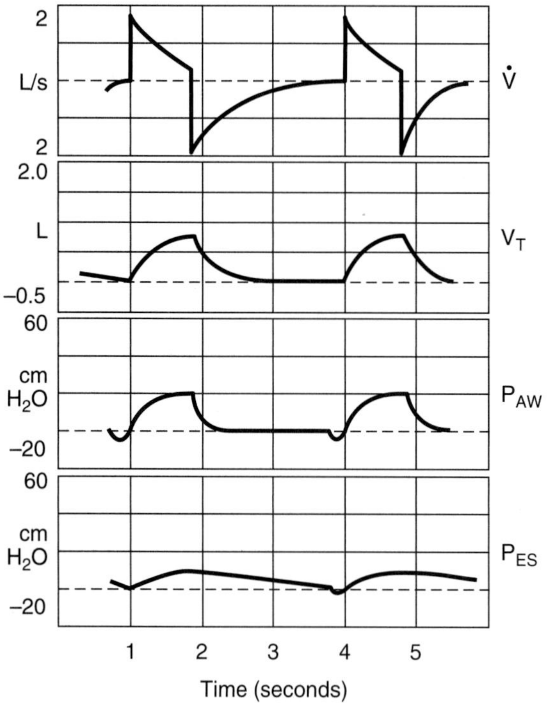

FIGURE 5-2

5. What is this mode?
6. How does pressure support differ from pressure assist?
7. Does this mode appear synchronous with ventilatory efforts?
8. Why is it or why is it not better than the volume-targeted breaths of Figure 5-1?
9. What new mode has been introduced that may be helpful under these circumstances?

In an effort to improve flow synchrony, you adjust the pressure rate of rise setting in Figure 5-3.

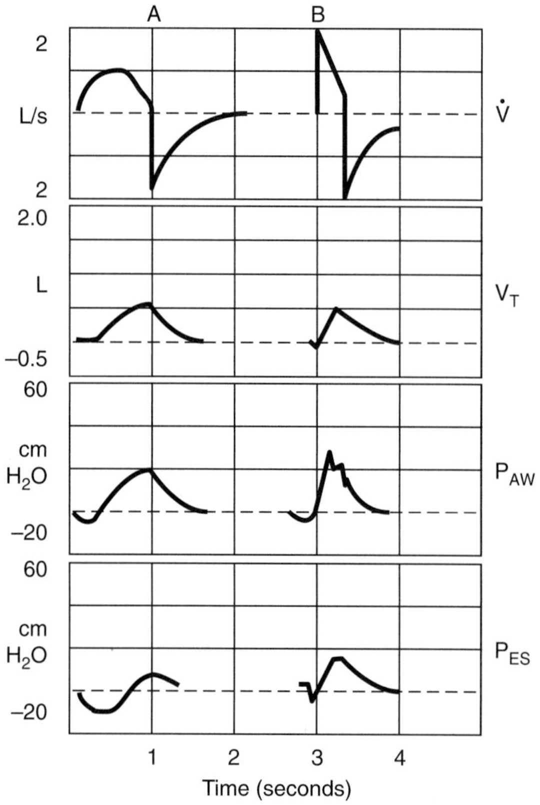

FIGURE 5-3

10. Did you make the rise time faster or slower in breath A?
11. Did you make the rise time faster or slower in breath B?
12. Which rate of rise (Figure 5-2; Figure 5-3, *A* or *B*) seems most synchronous with the patient?

You set the optimal pressure rate of rise settings and maintain support until the next morning. The patient, however, again is deemed not ready for discontinuation and you return him to pressure support. Later that morning the patient seems to have difficulty synchronizing breath termination. You switch to pressure assist in an effort to control inspiratory time and improve cycle synchrony. In Figure 5-4 are three different inspiratory time settings.

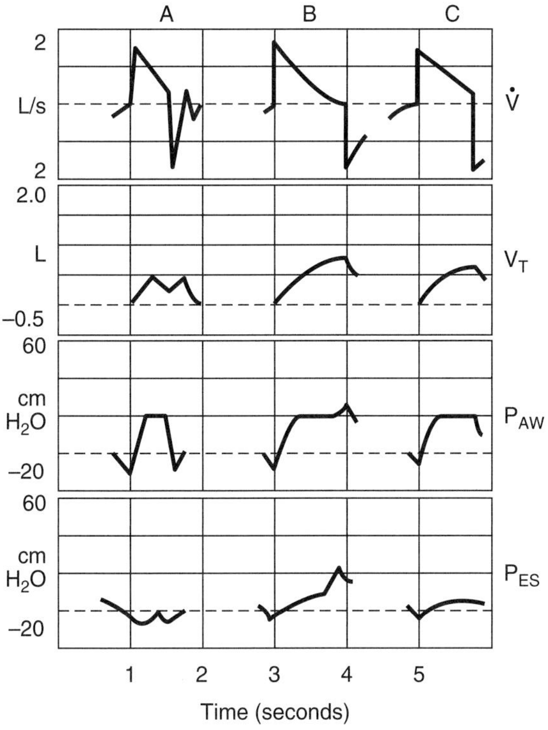

FIGURE 5-4

13. Which setting is too long and forces the patient to actively force the breath off?
14. Which setting is too short and leaves the patient demanding more gas at end inspiration?
15. Which breath has the proper inspiratory time?

CASE STUDY 6

PARTIAL VENTILATORY SUPPORT AND LOAD SHARING

(See Chapter 8 for further information.)

PH, a 42-year-old alcoholic man, is recovering from respiratory failure caused by aspiration pneumonia. You insert an esophageal balloon to assess load distribution between patient and ventilator. As you adjust the level of pressure support, you see three different patterns displayed on the pressure-time graphics as ventilatory loads are borne entirely by the ventilator, as ventilatory loads are shared between ventilator and patient, and as ventilatory loads are borne entirely by the patient (Figure 6-1). In these displays, load is characterized as a shaded pressure-time product (PTP).

QUESTIONS

1. Which shaded PTP represents ventilator load during total ventilatory support?

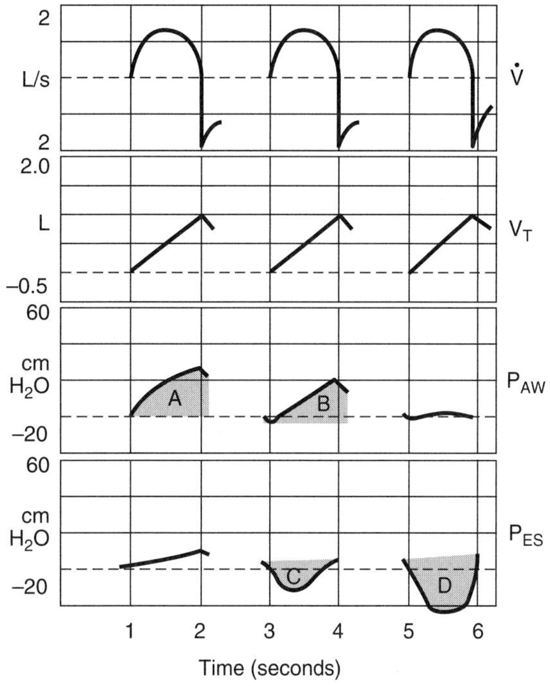

FIGURE 6-1

2. Which shaded PTP represents ventilator load during partial (shared) support?
3. Which shaded PTP represents patient load during an unassisted and unsupported breath?
4. Which shaded PTP represents patient load during partial (shared) support?
5. If flow and volume are equal during the three breaths in Figure 6-1, should PTP in *A* be equal to PTP in *D*?
6. Why or why not should PTP in *A* be equal to PTP in *D*?
7. Should the sum of PTP in *B* plus PTP in *C* = PTP in *A* or *D*?

CASE STUDY 7

NEW MODES FOR ACUTE RESPIRATORY FAILURE

(See Chapters 2, 7, 15, 22, and 23 for further information.)

EW, a patient with acute respiratory distress syndrome (ARDS), is being ventilated with the mode depicted in Figure 7-1.

QUESTIONS

Refer to Figure 7-1 to answer the following questions.

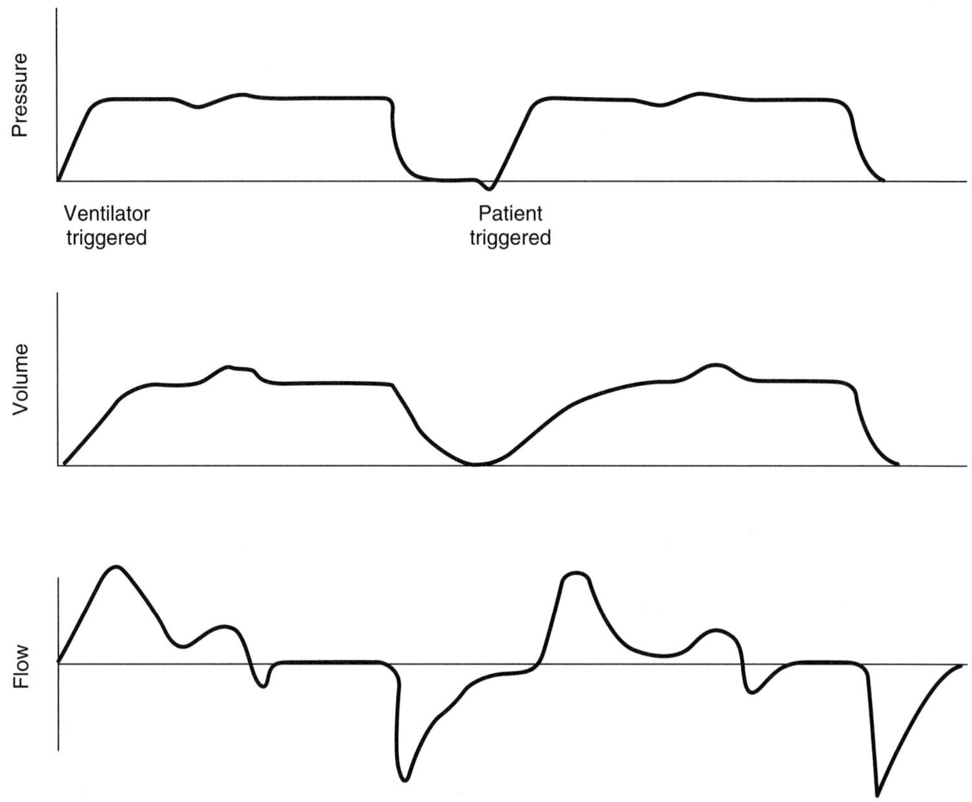

FIGURE 7-1

1. What description best fits this mode?
2. What are the triggers, target, and cycle criteria for this mode?
3. Is air trapping present?
4. What are the two purported benefits to this mode?
5. Is the maximal stretching pressure on the lung equal to the inflation (high pressure) setting?
6. How does this mode differ from pressure controlled inverse ratio ventilation (PCIRV)?

CASE STUDY 8
NEW MODES FOR ACUTE RESPIRATORY FAILURE

(See Chapters 2, 7, 15, 22, and 23 for further information.)

CS, a patient with acute respiratory distress syndrome (ARDS), is receiving high-frequency oscillatory ventilation.

QUESTIONS

Refer to Figure 8-1 to answer the following questions.

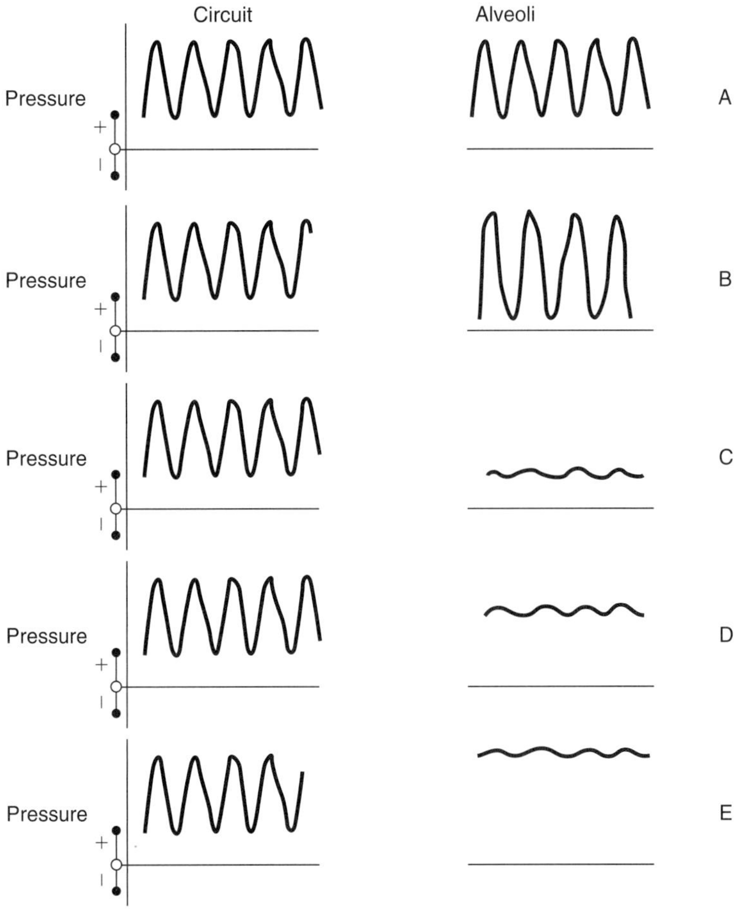

FIGURE 8-1

1. The relationship of pressures in the ventilator circuitry and pressures at the alveolar level is best represented by which panel in Figure 8-1?
2. Why are the other panels wrong?
3. What two changes could be made with this device to improve oxygenation?

CASE STUDY 9
CHANGING RESPIRATORY SYSTEM MECHANICS

(See Chapters 2, 6, and 8 for further information.)

MH, a patient with acute respiratory distress syndrome (ARDS), is being ventilated with volume assist-control ventilation. Her graphical pattern is depicted in Panel A of Figure 9-1.

QUESTIONS

Refer to Figure 9-1 to answer the following questions.

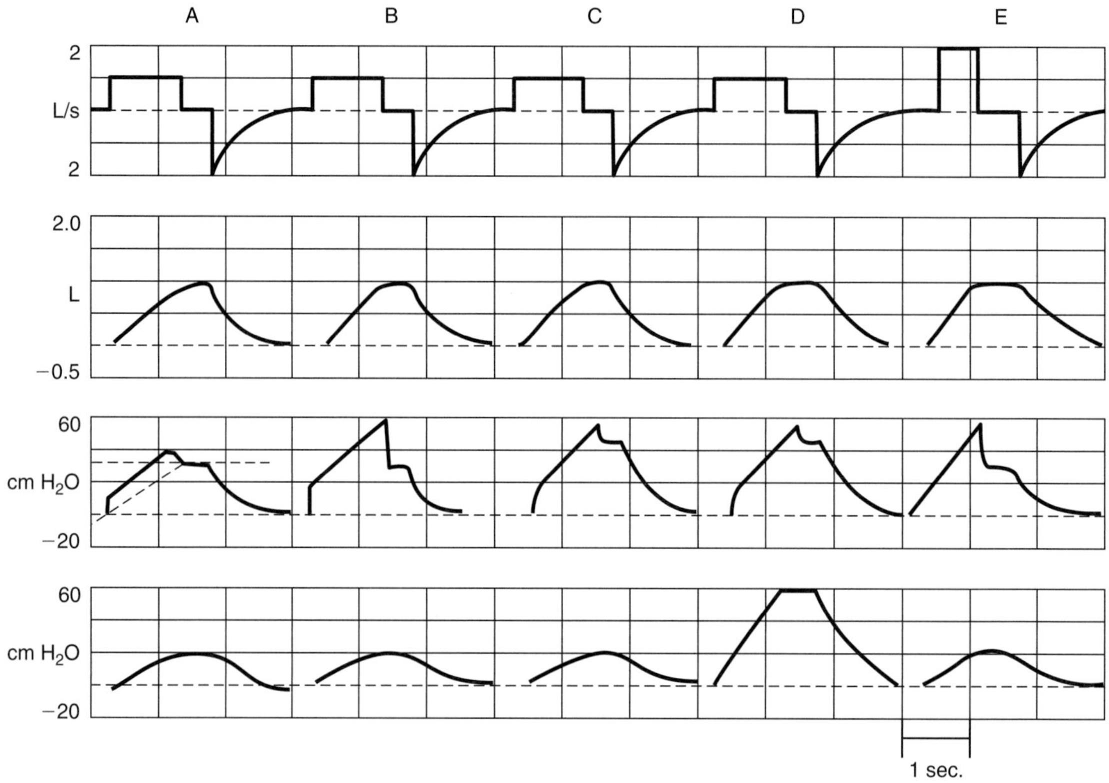

FIGURE 9-1

1. What changes would explain panel B?
2. What changes would explain panel C?
3. What changes would explain panel D?
4. What changes would explain panel E?

This same patient is being ventilated with pressure assist-control, with her graphics depicted in panel A of Figure 9-2.

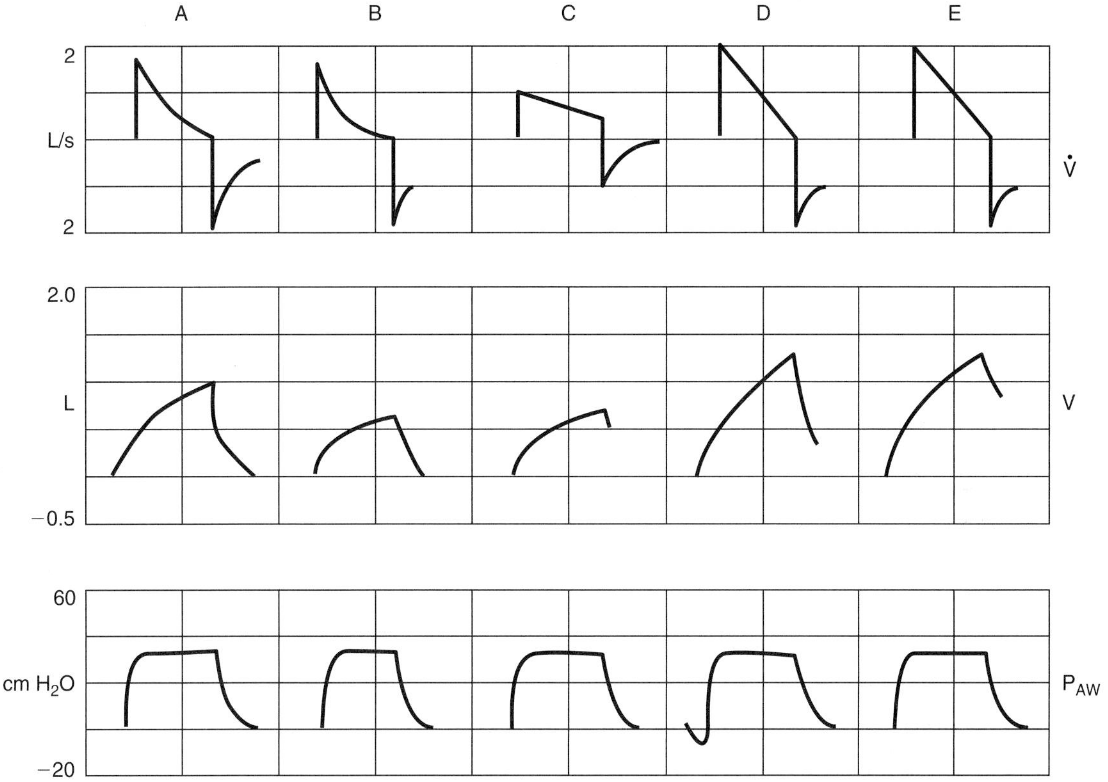

FIGURE 9-2

5. What changes would explain the graphics in Panel B?
6. What changes would explain the graphics in Panel C?
7. What changes would explain the graphics in Panel D?
8. What changes would explain the graphics in Panel E?

CASE STUDY 10
LUNG PROTECTION

(See Chapters 10 and 15 for additional information.)

CJ, a 37-year-old man with a seizure disorder, experiences a grand mal seizure and has a massive witnessed aspiration. He is intubated in the emergency department for severe hypoxemia and sent to the ICU. His chest x-ray shows diffuse bilateral infiltrates. His initial blood gases on 100% O_2, a volume control mode (rate of 20, a V_T of 420 ml [ideal body weight is 70 kg]), and a PEEP of 5 cm H_2O shows a Po_2 of 50 mm Hg, Pco_2 48 mm Hg, and pH of 7.36. His inspiratory plateau pressure (P_{plat}) is 29 cm H_2O and his flow graphic indicates an adequate expiratory time.

QUESTION

1. What three things should be done and why?

CASE STUDY 11
FEEDBACK CONTROL

(See Chapter 2 for additional information.)

JL is a 67-year-old alcoholic with severe pancreatitis, who has severe acute respiratory distress syndrome (ARDS) requiring mechanical ventilation. Figure 11-1 shows airway flow ($\dot{V}$), volume (V_T), and pressure (P_{AW}) over time at baseline (left panel). A mucus plug acutely develops and his ventilator graphics change to the right panel.

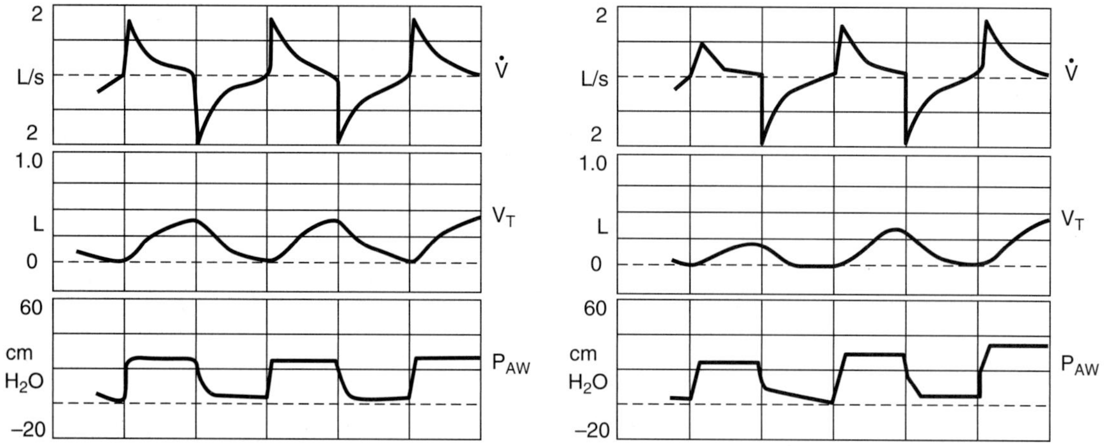

FIGURE 11-1

QUESTIONS

1. What ventilator mode would behave like this?
2. What is the name of the patient-triggered, flow-cycled version of this mode?
3. What happens to the pressure applied to the airway if effort increases? If it decreases?
4. What happens to the volume delivered if the effort increases?

CASE STUDY 12
EFFECTS OF PARALYSIS ON PRESSURE-TARGETED MODES

(See Chapters 2 and 12 for additional information.)

SC, a patient recovering from acute respiratory distress syndrome (ARDS), is receiving pressure assist-control ventilation and is triggering virtually all of the ventilator breaths (Figure 12-1 [left panel]). An upper endoscopy is required to evaluate new upper GI bleeding and a neuromuscular blocker (NMB) is administered to facilitate this. The ventilator graphics abruptly change to Figure 12-1 (right panel).

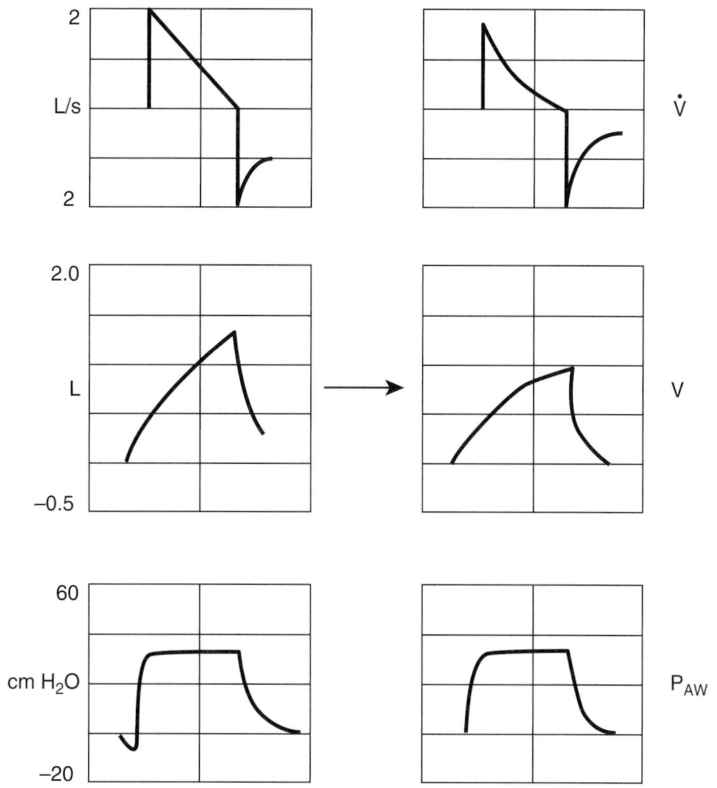

FIGURE 12-1

QUESTIONS

1. What is the best explanation for this?
2. What are four other possible causes for this change?

CASE STUDY 13
A NEW APPROACH TO SYNCHRONY

(See Chapters 2 and 8 for additional information.)

CJ, a patient recovering from acute respiratory failure and capable of spontaneous breathing, is being ventilated with the mode depicted in Figure 13-1. The thick arrow indicates a vigorous patient effort as reflected by a large change in esophageal pressure (P_{ES}); the thin arrow indicates a less vigorous patient effort as reflected by a much smaller change in P_{ES}.

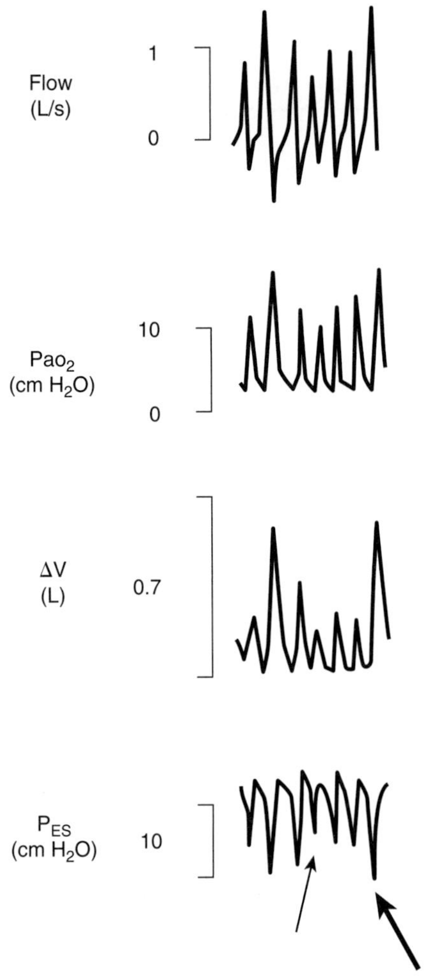

FIGURE 13-1

QUESTIONS

1. What is this mode of mechanical ventilation?
2. How does the response to increased effort differ from a pressure support breath?
3. How does the response to decreased effort differ from pressure support?
4. How does the response to increased effort differ from a volume assist breath?
5. How does the response to decreased effort differ from volume assist?

ANSWERS

Case Study 1

1. VACV
2. 40
3. 30
4. 5
5. 1 L/sec
6. 1000 ml
7. 1000/25 = 40
8. 10/1 = 10
9. 15
10. 35
11. 1000/20 = 50
12. Yes
13. Improved compliance
14. 20
15. 50
16. 1000/30 = 33 (rounded)
17. No
18. Worsening compliance and increased P_{PLAT} suggest overdistention
19. P_{PLAT} of 35 is still excessive; reduce V_T, accept higher CO_2

Case Study 2

1. VACV
2. 50
3. 40
4. 15
5. 1 L/sec
6. 750 ml
7. 750/25 = 30
8. Change to PACV
9. Match P_{PLAT}
10. Adequate to match V_T during VACV, short pause, adequate T_e
11. 750/25 = 30
12. No
13. No; same lung disease; same V_T; same PEEP
14. Longer T_i with I:E reversal
15. Yes
16. Longer time of inspiratory pressure
17. No
18. No change V_T; Adequate T_e
19. No change in baseline pressure
20. Longer T_i
21. Yes
22. Yes
23. V_T decreased; inadequate T_e with flow not returning to zero
24. 500/25 = 20
25. Intrinsic PEEP not included in the calculation of P_{PLAT} − PEEP
26. Yes; Static compliance = V_T/P_{PLAT} − total PEEP (applied plus intrinsic). Thus with a V_T of 500, a static compliance of 30 (Figure 2-3), and a P_{PLAT} of 40, total PEEP must be 24 (compliance = V_T/P_{PLAT} − total PEEP; 30 = 500/40 − 24) and intrinsic PEEP (total − applied) is 24 − 15 = 9.

27. Increase in baseline pressure
28. V_T
29. 250/25 = 10
30. Pneumothorax, airway obstruction
31. Increased
32. Not changed

Case Study 3

1. VACV
2. 60
3. 40
4. 0
5. 1 L/sec
6. 500
7. 500/40 = 12.5
8. 20/1 = 20
9. Yes
10. Inadequate expiratory time such that flow does not return to zero
11. 30
12. Yes
13. 40 − 30 = 10
14. 500/10 = 50
15. Reduce V_T; reduce T_i; reduce frequency; and use a low-density gas (heliox)
16. Apply PEEP to equilibrate circuit PEEP with intrinsic PEEP

Case Study 4

1. No
2. Expiratory flow returns to zero
3. No change in baseline pressure
4. Baseline pressure would be falsely reduced or elevated
5. 500/10 = 50
6. 30/1 = 30
7. Increase frequency
8. P_{PLAT}; keep below 30-35; expiratory flow tracing to assess adequacy of T_e
9. 500/30 = 17 (rounded)
10. Pneumothorax, airway obstruction
11. Nothing
12. Decreased

Case Study 5

1. Breathing pattern, hemodynamics, mental status, discomfort after 1- to 2-hour discontinuation assessment (SBT)
2. Daily
3. Insensitive trigger; inadequate flow delivery
4. Increase sensitivity or change to flow trigger; increase set flow or change to pressure-targeted mode
5. PSV
6. Pressure support terminates on flow reduction (T_i can vary), whereas pressure assist has a clinician-set T_i
7. Yes
8. Adjustable flow responds to patient effort
9. Proportional assist ventilation (PAV); it also adjusts to patient effort
10. Slower
11. Faster
12. Figure 5-2
13. B
14. A
15. C

Case Study 6

1. A
2. B
3. D
4. C
5. Yes
6. Same respiratory system mechanical properties and ventilatory pattern
7. Yes

Case Study 7

1. Airway pressure release ventilation
2. Patient or machine triggered, pressure targeted, time cycled
3. Yes, expiratory flow has not reached zero before next breath given
4. Higher mean pressure without an increase in V_T or PEEP, spontaneous breaths permitted
5. No, spontaneous efforts during the higher pressure period further increase transpulmonary (lung stretching) pressure
6. APRV permits spontaneous breaths during the high pressure inflation period, PCIRV does not

Case Study 8

1. D
2. HFO has similar means but dampened peak and PEEP values. A has equal peaks and PEEPs, B has excessive peaks and PEEPs in alveoli, C has mean too low in alveoli, E has mean too high in alveoli
3. Increase mean pressure or increase FIO_2

Case Study 9

1. Increased airway resistance reflected by an increased peak to plateau pressure difference

2. Decreased lung compliance with increased P_{PLAT} and unchanged esophageal pressure (increased transpulmonary pressure)
3. Decreased chest wall compliance with increased plateau and increased esophageal pressure (unchanged transpulmonary pressure)
4. Increased set flow producing increased peak to plateau pressure difference
5. Decreased respiratory system compliance (cannot distinguish lung from chest wall effect without esophageal pressure)
6. Increased airway resistance characterized by low initial flow compared with the decreased compliance effects in Question 5
7. Active patient effort increased flow and volume
8. Improved mechanics (i.e., increased compliance or decreased resistance)

Case Study 10

1. *First*, given the severe hypoxemia, PEEP is needed to better recruit alveoli and reduce FIO_2. In this patient, however, applied PEEP will further increase inspiratory plateau pressure (P_{PLAT}), which is already approaching an overdistention range (i.e., with a PEEP increase of 5 cm H_2O, P_{PLAT} could be expected to rise as much as 5 to a total of 34 cm H_2O). Thus the *second* thing that should be done is that V_T should be reduced at the same time. A consequence of this, however, is that the reduced minute ventilation will worsen the hypercapnia. The fact that there is adequate expiratory time to prevent air trapping means that the *third* thing that could be done to address this is to provide some additional breaths.

Case Study 11

1. Pressure regulated volume control (PRVC)
2. Volume support
3. Pressure decreases, pressure increases
4. There is no change in volume

Case Study 12

1. Loss of effort reduced patient contribution to the breath and thus there was a loss of flow and volume with an unchanged set pressure
2. Idiosyncratic reaction to the NMB agent causing flash pulmonary edema; bronchospasm; mucus plugging; tension pneumothorax

Case Study 13

1. Proportional assist ventilation (PAV)
2. More flow and pressure with PAV, more flow but no change in pressure with pressure support
3. Less flow and less pressure with PAV, less flow but same pressure with pressure support
4. More flow and pressure with PAV, no change in flow and less pressure with volume assist
5. Less flow and less pressure with PAV, same flow and more pressure with volume assist

APPENDIX 2

Answers to Assessment Questions

CHAPTER 1

1. B
2. D
3. True
4. False
5. C
6. D
7. D
8. False
9. D
10. False
11. A
12. B
13. A
14. D
15. B
16. C
17. B
18. C

CHAPTER 2

1. A
2. C
3. True
4. False
5. C
6. D
7. A
8. False
9. D
10. True
11. A
12. B
13. A
14. B
15. A
16. C
17. B
18. D
19. A
20. D

CHAPTER 3

1. C
2. D
3. True
4. False
5. A
6. B
7. B
8. True
9. D
10. False
11. A
12. D
13. D
14. B
15. A
16. C
17. B

CHAPTER 4

1. D
2. B
3. A
4. C
5. B
6. A
7. False
8. True
9. B
10. D
11. D
12. D
13. True

14. False
15. C
16. False
17. False
18. D
19. True
20. A
21. False
22. A

CHAPTER 5

1. True
2. True
3. False
4. False
5. False
6. True
7. False
8. True
9. True
10. True

CHAPTER 6

1. True
2. True
3. False
4. False
5. True
6. False
7. False
8. True
9. True
10. True

CHAPTER 7

1. False
2. True
3. True
4. True
5. False
6. True
7. False
8. False
9. True
10. True

CHAPTER 8

1. The administration of sedation has been associated with a longer duration of mechanical ventilation, weaning time, and ICU stay.
2. The three feedback signals are: (1) chemoreceptor-mediated (chemical), (2) mechanoreceptor-mediated (mechanical), and (3) cortical-mediated (behavioral) feedback.
3. Hypocapnia and the resulting respiratory alkalosis are expected to suppress the respiratory controller. However, at high assist levels with ACV or PSV, despite hypocapnia, the subject continues to trigger the ventilator.
4. Increasing ventilator flow rate exhibits an excitatory response, manifests as increased respiratory rate.
5. Compared with flow triggering, the flow-waveform triggering is more sensitive to patient effort and results in fewer ineffective efforts.
6. Auto-triggering is automatic delivery of mechanical breaths without inspiratory efforts. Ineffective triggering is the inability of patient-generated effort to trigger the ventilator-derived breath; essentially the ventilator is insensitive to patient effort. Applicable methods to decrease the frequency of ineffective triggering are: (1) setting PEEPe at 75% of PEEPi, and (2) increasing the ventilator inspiratory flow (i.e., decrease inspiratory time).
7. With ACV, there is an inverse relationship between P_{AW} and Pmus. With PSV, there is no relationship between P_{AW} and Pmus. With PAV, there is a proportional relationship between P_{AW} and Pmus.
8. Expiratory dys-synchrony is defined by the cessation of ventilator flow before or after the end of T_{IN}. It increases both the inspiratory and expiratory work of breathing, and a delay in ventilator triggering.
9. An expiratory trigger set at equal to or greater than 50% of peak flow improves PEEPi and decreases the frequency of ineffective triggering.
10. The feedback signals are diaphragmatic electrical activity for both NAVA and targeted-neural drive pressure support; and transdiaphragmatic pressure for transdiaphragmatic pressure-driven servo-ventilator.

CHAPTER 9

1. Mean systemic pressure is the weighed average of all the pressures in the systemic circulation, and the pressure to which the circulation will equilibrate if the heart stops. It is not mean arterial pressure, and averages only about 7 mm Hg in humans and many other species. It is the functional upstream pressure driving venous return back to the heart.
2. Sudden increases in venous return will distend the right heart. This can limit filling of the left

ventricle, especially when the pericardium is thickened or effusion is present.

3. Lung inflation increases right ventricular afterload.
4. Positive pressure inspiration increases P_{pl}, which lowers left ventricular afterload. Spontaneous inspiration has the opposite effect.
5. The most important circulatory stress during spontaneous breathing is the effect of changing P_{pl} on venous return. Systolic arterial pressure normally falls, by less than 10 mm Hg, during inspiration. This is the reflection of the lower systemic venous return during the preceding expiratory phase, delayed because of the transit time through the lungs. When the fall in pressure exceeds 10 to 15 mm Hg, this is termed pulsus paradoxicus. (It was originally so-named because the radial pulse would disappear while the apical pulse was still palpable.)
6. A common cause of hypotension after intubation in a patient with obstructive disease is breath-stacking and the worsening of intrinsic PEEP. Once intubated, V_T and respiratory rate are often greater than while the exhausted patient was breathing spontaneously. In addition, the negative P_{pl} during spontaneous inspiratory efforts may have been helping to sustain venous return. This assist is lost after the patient is placed on positive pressure ventilation. Of course, a misplaced endotracheal tube, tension pneumothorax, sedative side effects, or other causes of hypotension must be considered.
7. "Alveolar vessels" behave as if surrounded by alveolar pressure, and decrease capacitance with lung inflation. "Extra-alveolar vessels" behave as if surrounded by P_{pl}. They expand (increase capacitance) with lung inflation. These changes occur regardless of whether lung inflation is on positive pressure ventilation or during spontaneous breathing.
8. Pulmonary vascular resistance decreases during expiration, regardless of the form of ventilation. If subjects continue to exhale below functional residual capacity, resistance starts to rise again as vessels become more tortuous at very low lung volumes.
9. Although the rise in P_{pl} is commonly invoked, increased venous resistance appears to be equally or more important.
10. A large (>10%) change in pulse pressure with the respiratory cycle predicts a large cardiac output response to a fluid bolus.
11. Straining on the toilet is like a Valsalva maneuver. Patients with heart failure have better preservation of arterial pressure during a Valsalva, and therefore would be less likely to faint.

CHAPTER 10

1. Although high airway pressure was originally believed to be the cause of extra-alveolar air, several experiments have suggested that it is alveolar overdistention with excessive alveolar volume that leads to alveolar rupture and air dissection. Patients with underlying obstructive lung diseases like COPD and asthma and those with ALI/ARDS are at high risk of developing extra-alveolar air during mechanical ventilation.
2. Although extra-alveolar air (particularly tension pneumothorax) can be very dangerous, barotrauma is generally not associated with increased mortality. Patients who have more severe lung injury and multiple organ failure are more likely to develop barotrauma and to die, but it is rare for barotrauma to directly contribute to death.
3. Mechanical ventilation–induced alveolar rupture and extra-alveolar air probably usually occur near the alveolar base where it contacts the vascular sheath. Dissection of air likely occurs along vascular sheaths, with the air then passing to the mediastinum, subcutaneous tissue, and retroperitoneum.
4. During mechanical ventilation, air is preferentially forced into more normal and compliant areas of the acutely injured lung. Thus these normal areas are inflated more than the injured, less compliant areas. When high V_Ts are delivered, the normal areas become even more overdistended, which is thought to contribute to VILI.
5. Ventilating with high volumes is thought to contribute most to VILI. In the ARDS Network low V_T trial, ventilating with 6 ml/kg versus 12 ml/kg predicted body weight resulted in a decrease in mortality from 40% to 31%.
6. Biotrauma is the hypothesis that release of inflammatory mediators in the lungs from VILI might perpetuate or worsen lung injury. These inflammatory mediators might also contribute to the development of MODS by "spilling over" into the systemic circulation and causing other organ injury.
7. The only intervention that has ever been convincingly shown to decrease mortality in ALI in a large randomized trial is using a low V_T

ventilation strategy, which means ventilating at 6 ml/kg predicted body weight to keep the P_{PLAT} at or below 30 cm H_2O (please also see answer to question No. 8 for further details).

8. The initial V_T should be 6 ml/kg predicted body weight, and the goal P_{PLAT} is 30 cm H_2O or less. If the P_{PLAT} exceeds 30 cm H_2O, the V_T should be decreased to as low as 4 ml/kg predicted body weight to achieve a P_{PLAT} of 30 cm H_2O or less.
9. In the ARDS Network trial of higher versus lower PEEP, survival was not different between the two groups. This study suggests that, when ALI patients receive low V_T ventilation, there does not appear to be a mortality benefit with the use of higher levels of PEEP.
10. There are preliminary data suggesting that low V_T ventilation may be beneficial in patients at risk for ALI. This hypothesis is currently unproven, however, and a large randomized controlled trial would be needed to provide strong evidence. While this therapy may provide additional benefit, it should not be recommended for general use until strong evidence exists.

CHAPTER 11

1. A
2. False
3. D
4. A
5. E
6. C
7. C
8. D

CHAPTER 12

1. True
2. True
3. False
4. True
5. False
6. True
7. False
8. True
9. True
10. False

CHAPTER 13

1. False
2. True
3. True
4. True
5. False
6. True
7. True
8. True
9. False
10. True

CHAPTER 14

1. C
2. A
3. A
4. A
5. C
6. B
7. A
8. C
9. B
10. A

CHAPTER 15

1. False
2. False
3. True
4. True
5. False
6. True
7. False
8. False
9. False
10. False

CHAPTER 16

1. True
2. True
3. False
4. False
5. True
6. False
7. False
8. False
9. False
10. True

CHAPTER 17

1. True
2. False
3. True
4. False
5. True
6. False
7. True
8. True

9. True
10. True

CHAPTER 18

1. True
2. True
3. False
4. False
5. True
6. False
7. False
8. False
9. False
10. False

CHAPTER 19

1. True
2. True
3. False
4. False
5. True
6. False
7. False
8. False
9. False
10. False

CHAPTER 20

1. B
2. B
3. True
4. A
5. D
6. B
7. C
8. D
9. B
10. C
11. D
12. B
13. D
14. C
15. False

CHAPTER 21

1. F
2. C
3. True
4. D
5. C
6. D
7. D
8. B
9. B
10. False
11. D
12. A
13. C
14. D
15. A
16. True
17. E
18. C

CHAPTER 22

1. False
2. False
3. True
4. True
5. False
6. True
7. False
8. False
9. True
10. True

CHAPTER 23

1. False
2. False
3. True
4. True
5. False
6. True
7. False
8. True
9. False
10. True

CHAPTER 24

1. False
2. True
3. True
4. True
5. True
6. True
7. True
8. True
9. False
10. True

CHAPTER 25

1. B
2. True
3. False
4. D
5. True

6. D
7. D
8. True
9. D
10. F
11. A
12. F
13. B
14. C
15. False

Glossary

100,000 Lives Campaign An initiative to engage US hospitals in a commitment to implement changes in healthcare proven to improve patient care and prevent avoidable deaths.

A

abdominal pressure Pressure within the abdominal space. This is often used as a reference to intrathoracic pressures to calculate transdiaphragmatic pressures. This pressure is commonly measured in either the gastric space or the urinary bladder.

absolute humidity The amount of water vapor present in a gas mixture. Typically expressed in mg H_2O/L.

active heat and moisture exchanger A device that combines a passive humidifier and a heated humidifier to reduce water usage and increase moisture output.

activated clotting times (ACT) The time it takes whole blood to clot after the addition of particulate activators.

acute lung injury (ALI) A condition characterized by alveolar inflammation caused by an acute insult (for example, sepsis). According to the American-European Consensus Conference, ALI is distinguished from ARDS by the PaO_2/FIO_2 ratio: ALI is 200-300, ARDS is <200.

Acute Physiologic and Chronic Health Evaluation Score (APACHE) A method for classifying the severity of illnesses in patients. It represents a simple scoring system used to predict outcome.

acute respiratory distress syndrome (ARDS) A severe pulmonary inflammatory response to a variety of insults, resulting in capillary leak, interstitial edema, intra-alveolar hemorrhage and exudate, decreased pulmonary compliance, decreased ventilation-perfusion matching, and progressive hypoxemic respiratory failure. It is defined by the American European Consensus Conference clinically as an acute lung injury characterized by bilateral chest radiograph abnormalities and abnormal oxygenation ($PaO_2/FIO_2 < 200$) not explained by cardiogenic edema.

adaptive support ventilation A mode of ventilatory support in which the ventilator can choose ventilator settings following the input of patient weight and percent minute volume and is based upon a "minimal work" concept. The ventilator operates in the pressure control and pressure support modes and can change I:E during mandatory breaths.

afterload The impedence that the ventricles must overcome to eject blood. In the left ventricle it is the impedance of the great vessels, in the right ventricle it is the pulmonary vasculature.

agitation Excessive motor activity associated with internal tension.

air trapping See *Intrinsic PEEP*. This is sometimes also called "occult" PEEP.

airway pressure Pressure in the airways of the lung, often assumed to be identical to ventilator circuit pressure.

airway pressure release ventilation (APRV) A pressure-targeted time-cycled ventilator mode often described as two levels of continuous positive airway pressure (CPAP) applied for set periods of time, allowing spontaneous breathing to occur at both levels.

alarm A visual and/or auditory signal that occurs when a monitored parameter has exceeded a set limit.

alarm event Any condition or occurrence that triggers an alarm and requires clinician awareness or action.

American Heart Association device classification system The system by which devices used during cardiopulmonary resuscitation are classified based on usefulness and possibility of doing harm. This system includes the following: *Class I*—A therapeutic option that is usually indicated, is always acceptable, and is considered useful and effective. *Class II*—A therapeutic option that is acceptable, is of uncertain efficacy, and may be controversial. *Class IIa*—A therapeutic option for which the weight of evidence is in favor of its usefulness and efficacy. *Class IIb*—A therapeutic option that is not well established by evidence but may be helpful and probably is not harmful. *Class III*—A therapeutic option that is inappropriate, is without scientific supporting data, and may be harmful.

analgesic A drug that relieves pain.

anticholinergic Of or pertaining to a blockade of acetylcholine receptors that results in the inhibition of the transmission of parasympathetic nerve impulses.

anxiety A sustained state of apprehension in response to new or perceived threats.

ARDS Network Clinical network initiated by the National Heart, Lung, and Blood Institute and the National Institutes of Health to carry out multicenter clinical trials of acute respiratory distress syndrome (ARDS) treatments. The goal of the network is to efficiently test promising agents, devices, or management strategies to hasten the development of effective therapy and improve the care of patients with ARDS.

aspiration Describes the introduction of oral, nasal, pharyngeal, or gastric contents into the lung.

assist-control (A-C) ventilation Mode of ventilator operation in which assisted breaths are provided along with backup mandatory breaths delivered at a set frequency, pressure or volume, and inspiratory flow.

assisted mechanical ventilation (AMV) A proposed version of A-C ventilation in which all breaths are patient triggered and delivered at the ventilator's set tidal volume or pressure; all breaths are assisted breaths.

asynchrony Pertaining to ventilatory support, a situation in which interaction between the patient and machine is poorly coordinated, causing extra patient effort and discomfort.

atelectrauma Lung injury caused by repetitive opening-closing of alveolar units.

automatic tube compensation A technique of ventilator operation that uses the known resistive characteristics of artificial airways to overcome the imposed work of breathing caused by those airways with pressure support.

autoPEEP See *Intrinsic PEEP.*

auto-triggering Delivery of assisted mechanical breaths without inspiratory efforts.

B

bag-valve resuscitator Consists of a self-inflating bag, oxygen reservoir, and nonrebreathing valve. The operator ventilates the patient by squeezing the self-inflating bag, which forces air into the nonrebreathing valve and to the patient. The self-inflating bag is typically made of a resilient material, such as rubber, silicone, or polyvinylchloride. Most self-inflating bags have a volume of around 2.0 L for adults.

barotrauma Injury to the lung due to excessive pressure in the lung.

barrier device A flexible sheet that typically contains a valve and/or filter separating the rescuer from the patient.

benzodiazepine Psychotropic agent; most commonly used drugs in the ICU for sedation therapy.

Bernoulli's principle The physical principle of a lowered pressure around a moving fluid or gas.

biotrauma A systemic inflammatory response resulting from alveolar overdistention and/or repetitive recruitment-derecruitment.

bradycardia An abnormally slow heart rate—in the adult, a heart rate less than 60 beats/min.

bronchoalveolar lavage (BAL) The procedure whereby distal regions of the lung are washed with fluid for the purpose of obtaining samples for diagnosis.

bronchodilator A drug that expands the lumina of the air passages of the lungs.

bronchoscope A medical device that allows examination of the airways; used for irrigating distal airways, suctioning, and passing brushes and biopsy forceps. Often a flexible fiberoptic device but can be a rigid system, it is used mainly for diagnosis but can be therapeutic when used to remove mucus plugs or foreign bodies or when placing stents.

bronchoscopy The procedure in which the patient's airways are examined with a bronchoscope.

bubble humidifier A humidifier that imparts heat and moisture to gas as it is released under the surface of the water and "bubbles" to the surface.

bundles Group of effective evidence-based interventions applied at the same time.

C

calcium chloride A hygroscopic chemical substance that enhances the heat- and moisture-exchanging capabilities of the passive humidifier.

cascade humidifier A type of bubble humidifier that uses an underwater grid to increase the gas-liquid interface and increase humidity.

cerebral perfusion pressure (CPP) A parameter that is related to the amount of blood flow to the brain. It is the difference between the mean arterial pressure (MAP) and the intracranial pressure (ICP).

clinical pneumonia infection score (CPIS) An algorithm used to diagnose ventilator associated pneumonia that relies on easily available clinical, radiographic, and microbiologic criteria.

closed circuit suction catheter A suction catheter designed to be used in-line with the ventilator circuit so that the ventilator does not need to be disconnected. Closed circuit suctioning has been associated with fewer complications than traditional suctioning techniques.

closed-loop control A control scheme in which the actual output of a system is measured and compared with the desired output. If there is a difference caused by external disturbances, the actual output is modified to bring it closer to the desired output.

colorimetric CO_2 detector A device that detects the presence of carbon dioxide (CO_2) in expired gas and indicates the presence of CO_2 by changing color (usually yellow to purple).

compliance The relative ease with which a body or tissue stretches or deforms. In the respiratory system it is quantified as the volume delivered divided by the pressure applied.

compressible volume The volume of gas that distends the ventilator circuit during delivery of a positive pressure breath. This volume is considered "lost," as it is not delivered to the patient.

compressor A device that is designed to compress a gas (usually air).

condensation Water that collects in the ventilator circuit as gas cools when the amount of water vapor present exceeds the carrying capacity of the gas.

continuous mandatory ventilation (CMV) Mode of ventilator operation in which all breaths are mandatory and are delivered by the ventilator at a preset frequency (f), volume or pressure, and inspiratory time.

continuous positive airway pressure (CPAP) A therapeutic modality that maintains a constant transrespiratory pressure. CPAP is not a ventilatory mode because it does not generate a tidal volume.

control circuit The ventilator subsystem responsible for controlling the drive mechanism and/or the output control valves.

control variable The variable (either pressure, volume, flow, or time) that the ventilator manipulates to cause inspiration. This variable is identified by the fact that its behavior remains consistent despite changes in ventilatory load.

convective gas transport Gas transport that moves O_2 and CO_2 in discrete volumes ("bulk flow").

cricoid pressure Pushing down on the cricoid membrane, thereby collapsing the esophagus against the cervical vertebrae. Cricoid pressure has been shown to prevent gastric insufflation during mask ventilation.

critical care ventilators Positive pressure ventilators designed mainly for invasive ventilation (i.e., through an artificial airway) in the acute setting.

cuff pressure The pressure exerted by the tracheal tube cuff on the airway mucosa.

cycle time The duration of the delivery of gas under positive pressure during inspiration until a cycle criterion is met.

cycle variable The variable used by the ventilator control circuit to end inspiration.

D

dead space Respired gas volume that does not participate in gas exchange; may be anatomic, alveolar, or mechanical.

dead volume Volume of medication in a nebulizer that cannot be aerosolized due to device construction.

deep sulcus sign A radiographic sign indicative of the presence of pneumothorax.

de-escalation Therapeutic approach that reduces the level of an intervention as the patient's condition becomes more focused or improves. For example, in treating ventilator-associated pneumonia physicians initially prescribe broad-spectrum agents that are active against likely pathogens. When culture results become available the antibiotic selection is narrowed to target the known cause of the infection.

delirium An acute, potentially reversible impairment of consciousness and cognitive function resulting in inappropriate behavior that may wax and wane.

dexmedetomidine An α_{-2} adrenoceptor agonist sedative; it exhibits sedative, analgesic, and sympatholytic properties.

diaphragm pacers Ventilatory method used in selected patients with impaired neuromuscular function to enhance independence from mechanical ventilation; consists of a radiofrequency transmitter and antenna that signal a surgically implanted receiver and electrode to stimulate the phrenic nerve.

disease management programs Approach to patient care that emphasizes coordinated, comprehensive care along the continuum of disease and across health care delivery systems.

dual control Modes of ventilation whereby two or more variables may control breath delivery depending upon certain circumstances.

dry powder inhaler (DPI) Creates an aerosol by drawing air through a powder that contains micronized particles; commonly used for drug delivery in ambulatory patients.

dynamic hyperinflation (DH) An increase in functional residual capacity (FRC) above the elastic equilibrium volume of the respiratory system. Causes include increased flow resistance, short expiratory time, and increased postinspiratory muscle activity (see also *intrinsic PEEP*).

dys-synchrony See *Patient-ventilator dys-synchrony*.

E

elastance Tendency of a structure to return to its original form after being stretched or acted on by an outside force. Elastance is the inverse of compliance.

electromechanical transducer A mechanical device that is capable of converting one form of energy into another. Commonly used to convert pressure into an electrical current.

end-expiratory pressure (EEP) The baseline transrespiratory pressure that exists at the end of the expiratory time. This pressure is often positive (PEEP).

end-expiratory valve A mechanical valve that regulates pressure during the expiratory phase.

end points Measurements used to determine safety and efficacy.

endotracheal tube An artificial airway passed through the nose or mouth past the vocal cords and into the trachea.

esophageal detector device (EDD) A device such as a syringe or squeeze bulb connected to an endotracheal tube that determines proper tube placement through the use of negative pressure applied to the airway—if a negative pressure is applied to the lungs the bulb re-inflates easily, if it is in the esophagus it will not reinflate.

esophageal pressure Pressure measured in the midesophagus and taken to represent pleural pressure.

event Any condition or occurrence that requires clinician awareness or action.

expiratory flow time The time during which expiratory flow occurs.

expiratory pause time The time during the expiratory phase when no flow is occurring. At this point, airway and alveolar pressures are equal.

expiratory phase The part of the ventilatory cycle from the beginning of expiratory flow to the beginning of inspiratory flow.

expiratory time The duration of the expiratory phase.

expired air resuscitation (EAR) Rescue breathing during cardiopulmonary resuscitation in which the rescuer's exhaled gas provides ventilation for the victim. Types of expired air resuscitation include mouth-to-mouth and mouth-to-mask ventilation.

external compressor A device external to the ventilator used to supply a pneumatic source power.

extracorporeal life support (ECLS) Life support provided from outside the body, e.g., extracorporeal membrane oxygenation.

extracorporeal membrane oxygenation (ECMO) A technique whereby blood is taken from a vein, passed through a device that adds O_2 and removes CO_2, and then returned to the patient into either one of the great veins or the arterial circuit.

F

flow Rate of gas delivery in and out of the lung.

flow triggering Inspiratory flow from the ventilator that begins when a set drop of a continuous flow through the patient circuit is detected.

flow-waveform triggering Requires patient effort to generate flow until 6 ml of volume accumulates above the baseline flow (volume method), or when patient effort distorts the expiratory flow waveform to a certain extent, whichever occurs first (shape-signal method).

functional residual capacity (FRC) The volume of gas remaining in the lungs at the end of exhalation.

G

gas consumption Gas consumed by a ventilator that does not participate in ventilation of the patient. The gas is used to control ventilator function and is wasted.

gastric insufflation Forcing air into the stomach during positive pressure ventilation.

Glasgow Coma Scale A quick, standardized system for assessing the degree of conscious impairment in the critically ill and for predicting the duration and ultimate outcome of coma, primarily in patients with head injuries.

glossopharyngeal (frog) breathing Uses intermittent gulping motions of the tongue and pharyngeal muscles to force air into the trachea; can be used to provide freedom from mechanical ventilation for periods of up to several hours.

gravitational sedimentation Deposition of aerosol due to weight of the particle in a stagnant air stream.

H

heat and moisture exchanger (HME) A passive humidifier that uses only physical means of heat and moisture exchange.

heat and moisture exchanging filter (HMEF) A passive humidifier that uses physical means of heat and moisture exchange and includes a breathing circuit filter.

heated wire circuit A ventilator circuit that contains electric wires that heat the gas as it travels down the circuit. These devices help eliminate or minimize condensate.

heliox Gas mixture of helium and O_2; used clinically because of its low density.

high flow humidifier A humidification device used to add moisture to inspired gases and flows used during mechanical ventilation.

high-frequency jet ventilation (HFJV) Operate on the principle of a nozzle or injector that creates a high velocity "jet" of gas directed into the lung.

high-frequency oscillatory ventilation (HFOV) Operate with a "to and fro" application of pressure on a fresh gas bias flow at the airway opening using either pistons or microprocessor gas controllers.

high-frequency ventilation (HFV) Ventilatory support characterized by breathing frequencies greater than physiologic breathing rates.

HME booster A device that adds moisture to inspired gas between the passive humidifier and the patient.

hygroscopic heat and moisture exchanger (HHME) A passive humidifier in which both physical and chemical means of heat and moisture exchange are used.

hygroscopic heat and moisture exchanging filter (HHMEF) A passive humidifier in which both physical and chemical means of heat and moisture exchange are used; it incorporates a breathing circuit filter.

hyperbaric oxygen (HBO) therapy The administration of O_2 at levels of pressure greater than atmospheric. During hyperbaric exposure, plasma-dissolved O_2 increases approximately 2 vol % for every atmosphere increase in inspired O_2. Typical applications of HBO include decompression sickness, gas gangrene, CO poisoning, cyanide poisoning, and circulatory disorders.

hypercapnia Excess CO_2 in the blood; may be caused by hypoventilation, increased dead space, and increased CO_2 production.

hyperventilation Ventilation in excess of that necessary to meet metabolic needs; signified by a P_{CO_2} less than 35 mm Hg.

hypotension Abnormal condition in which the blood pressure is not adequate for normal perfusion and oxygenation of the tissues.

hypoventilation Respiratory condition resulting in elevated blood CO_2 and generalized reduction in respiratory function; signified by P_{CO_2} greater than 45-50 mm Hg.

hysteresis The difference in a respiratory system mechanical property during inflation versus deflation.

I

idiopathic pulmonary fibrosis (IPF) The formation of scar tissue in the connective tissue of the lungs without known cause.

impedance threshold device (ITD) A spring-loaded valve that limits air entry into the lungs during recoil of the chest wall following cardiac compressions.

independent lung ventilation (ILV) A method by which the gas flow to each lung is effectively separated mechanically by either two small endotracheal tubes or one specifically designed double-lumen endotracheal tube for the purpose of differential ventilation of each lung, with different ventilation parameters.

indirect calorimetry A technique that measures O_2 consumption and CO_2 production to predict nutritional needs and to quantify metabolic activity.

ineffective triggering Delivery of mechanical breaths with the ventilator is impaired because the ventilator is insensitive to patient effort.

inertial impaction Aerosol deposition because of particles striking circuit/airway structures during flow. Baffles in a nebulizer system use inertial impaction to eliminate large particles from the delivered aerosol.

isothermic saturation boundary (ISB) The point at which gases reach alveolar conditions (37° C and 100% relative humidity).

inspiratory : expiratory ratio The ratio of inspiratory time to expiratory time (I : E ratio).

inspiratory flow time The time during the inspiratory phase when flow is being delivered.

inspiratory pause time The time between the end of inspiratory flow and the beginning of expiration. During this period, pressure is held constant and flow is zero. Under those conditions, airway pressure is equal to end-inspiratory alveolar pressure. The pause may also improve gas mixing.

inspiratory phase The part of the ventilatory cycle from the beginning of inspiratory flow to the beginning of expiratory flow. Any inspiratory pause is included in the inspiratory phase.

inspiratory time Inspiratory time (expressed in seconds) is the duration of the inspiratory phase. As inspiratory time increases, mean airway pressure increases and the I : E ratio becomes higher.

inspired gas concentrations The partial pressures of O_2, nitrogen, and other therapeutic gases, such as helium or nitric oxide, that may be in the inspired gas mixture.

intermittent mandatory ventilation (IMV) Mode of ventilator operation in which mandatory (machine) breaths are delivered at a set frequency and volume or pressure; the patient can breathe spontaneously from either a continuous flow of gas or a demand system between machine breaths.

internal compressor A device inside the ventilator used to convert either pneumatic or electric source power into inspiratory pressure.

intravascular oxygenation A technique whereby blood oxygenation devices are inserted into the vasculature.

intrinsic PEEP (PEEPi) End-expiratory pressure in the lung as a consequence of excessive minute ventilation, an inadequately set expiratory time, or airway obstruction preventing lung emptying. Intrinsic PEEP is sometimes referred to as air trapping, autoPEEP, and occult PEEP.

inverse ratio ventilation (IRV) Ventilation in which inspiratory time exceeds expiratory time.

isothermic saturation boundary The point at which gases reach alveolar conditions of 37° C and 100% relative humidity.

J

jets Ventilatory devices used in a technique to deliver high-frequency ventilation.

L

laminar flow Flow through a tube that flows parallel to the tube walls in concentric layers with linear velocities that increase toward the center of the tube.

lateral decubitus Position in which the patient is lying on one side.

lithium chloride A hygroscopic chemical substance that enhances the heat- and moisture-exchanging capabilities of the passive humidifier.

limit To set a maximum value for pressure, volume, or flow during mechanically supported inspiration (or expiration); the preset maximum value for pressure, volume, or flow during an assisted inspiration (or expiration). Inspiration (or expiration) does not necessarily terminate because the limit value has been met.

lung protective strategy Mechanical ventilation strategies designed to limit and/or reduce overdistention and repetitive opening-closing of alveolar units so as to minimize ventilator induced lung injury.

M

mandatory breath A mechanical breath that is initiated and terminated by the ventilator rather than by the patient's ventilatory drive.

mandatory minute ventilation (MMV) Mode of ventilator operation that allows the patient to breathe spontaneously yet ensures that a minimum level of minute ventilation, set by the clinician, always is achieved.

manometer An expandable chamber that responds to pressure changes by changing its volume and moving a gear that rotates a needle around a calibrated dial.

mass median aerodynamic diameter (MMAD) The particle diameter around which the mass of particle diameters is equally distributed.

mean airway pressure (P_{AW}) The average pressure that exists at the airway opening over the ventilatory period. It is usually measured as gauge pressure. Mean airway pressure is mathematically equivalent to the area under the time-pressure curve (from the beginning of one breath to the beginning of the next breath) divided by the ventilatory period.

metered dose inhaler (MDI) A device in which a pressurized canister is used to deliver a precise dose of aerosolized medication.

methemoglobin A form of hemoglobin that is produced when the iron in heme is oxidized from Fe^{+2} to Fe^{+3}.

minimal leak technique Technique for maintaining the endotracheal tube cuff in which cuff inflation volume is adjusted so that at end-inspiration there is a small leak of air around the cuff.

minimal occlusive technique See *Minimal seal technique.*

minimal seal technique The technique for maintaining the endotracheal tube cuff in which the clinician adds volume to the endotracheal tube cuff sufficient to prevent a leak at end-inspiration. Also known as the minimal occlusive technique.

minute ventilation (MV) The total amount of gas moving in or out of the lungs during 1 minute.

monitor A routine repetitive or continuous measurement of a parameter.

moisture output The amount of moisture delivered to the patient from a passive humidifier expressed in mg H_2O/L.

multiple organ dysfunction syndrome (MODS) A condition in which dysfunction of many different organs occurs, often accompanying acute lung injury.

muscle fatigue A condition of muscle dysfunction that is recoverable by rest.

muscle overload A condition in which the load on the muscles is excessive and may cause fatigue.

myasthenia gravis A condition characterized by chronic fatigue and muscle weakness, especially in the face and throat.

myopathy Any disease of muscle.

N

nasal pillows Small rubber cones that are inserted directly into the nostrils; can be used to apply positive air pressure.

neuromuscular blockade (NMB) The pharmacologic inhibition of a muscular contraction activated by the nervous system.

nitric oxide (NO) Colorless gas that is naturally synthesized in human tissue and plays an important role in vascular smooth muscle relaxation, inhibition of platelet aggregation, neurotransmission, and immune regulation.

nitrogen dioxide (NO_2) Irritating brownish gas that can be produced spontaneously from NO and O_2.

nonconvective gas transport Movement of O_2 and CO_2 by mechanisms other than bulk flow movement of discrete tidal volumes.

noninvasive positive pressure ventilation (NPPV) Mechanical ventilation provided noninvasively (by mask or similar interface) rather than through an endotracheal tube or tracheostomy.

noninvasive ventilation (NIV) Techniques of assisting or controlling ventilation using devices that do not require artificial airway placement. This includes NPPV as well as external negative pressure systems.

nonsteroidal antiinflammatory drug (NSAID) A group of drugs with antipyretic, analgesic, and antiinflammatory effects to counteract or reduce inflammation that do not involve corticosteroids.

nosocomial infection An infection acquired at least 72 hours after hospitalization.

O

obesity hypoventilation syndrome (OHS) Combination of hypercapnia and obesity (BMI >30) in the absence of other causes for hypoventilation, such as hypothyroidism or neuromuscular disease.

obstructive lung disease Disease characterized by airway narrowing.

open-loop control A control scheme in which the output of a system is determined by the initial setting of the controller with no corrections made to accommodate disturbances in the output caused by external factors.

opioid Natural and synthetic chemicals that have opium-like effects.

oropharyngeal and nasopharyngeal airways Devices inserted into the mouth or the nose to help maintain airway patency.

orthopnea Breathlessness, especially when reclined.

oscillators A technique to deliver high-frequency ventilation using an oscillating piston or membrane.

overdistention The process of providing excessive volume to lung regions, thereby causing a "stretch" injury.

oxygen delivery system A device used to deliver O_2 concentrations above ambient air to the lungs through the upper airway.

oxygen-powered breathing device (OPD) A device that consists of a demand valve that can be manually or patient triggered. The OPD is connected to a 50-psig source of gas and connects to the patient via a standard 15/22 mm connector. During manual activation of the demand valve, the operator depresses the actuator, allowing flow to travel to the patient.

P

parenchymal lung injury Lung injury resulting from processes affecting the alveolar capillary interface, and the interstitium.

partial extracorporeal life support (ECLS) Technologies that provide only a portion of the gas exchange function of the lung.

partial support Mechanical ventilatory support in which the patient and the ventilator share the ventilatory load.

passover humidifier A humidifier that imparts heat and moisture to gas flowing over the surface of the water.

patient-ventilator dys-synchrony A situation in which the patient breathing pattern and ventilator breathing pattern are not harmonious.

peak inspiratory pressure (PIP) The highest pressure achieved during inspiration on positive pressure ventilation; also called peak pressure and peak airway pressure.

percutaneous dilatational tracheostomy (PDT) An invasive procedure in which the placement of a tracheostomy tube is achieved after establishing a tracheal stoma through percutaneous dilation, rather than surgical creation of a stoma.

permissive hypercapnia Ventilatory support strategy that accepts hypercapnia as a trade-off to excessive lung distention.

phase variable A variable (such as pressure, volume, flow, or time) that is measured and used to initiate some phase of the ventilatory cycle. Phases represent one of four significant events that occur during a ventilatory cycle: (1) the change from expiratory time to inspiratory time, (2) inspiratory time, (3) the change from inspiratory time to expiratory time, and (4) expiratory time.

phase variable value The magnitude of a phase variable.

pleural pressure (P_{pl}) Pressure inside the pleural space (between the lungs and chest wall) often reflected as esophageal pressure.

pneumonia Infection in lung parenchyma.

pneumothorax The presence of air or gas in the pleural space of the thorax; if this air or gas is trapped under pressure, a tension pneumothorax exists.

polyneuropathy A condition in which many peripheral nerves are afflicted with a disorder.

positive pressure ventilation (PPV) Use of positive airway pressure to support ventilation.

positive end-expiratory pressure (PEEP) Pressure above atmospheric, applied to the airway during exhalation; elevated baseline pressure during mechanical ventilation.

preload The filling pressure of the ventricle at the end of ventricular diastole.

pressure assist control ventilation An assist-control mode of ventilation that is pressure targeted/limited and time cycled.

pressure control inverse ratio ventilation (PCIRV) Particular version of pressure assist control in which inspiration is longer than expiration.

pressure gradient The difference in pressure across a resistance or a compliance structure.

pressure-regulated volume control (PRVC) Pressure assist control ventilation that adjusts the pressure target to a set tidal volume.

pressure support ventilation (PSV) Patient-triggered, pressure-targeted, flow-cycled mechanical ventilation mode.

pressure-time product A quantification of ventilation load that is obtained by integrating pressure over time. (See *Work* for an alternative load expression.)

pressure triggering When a change in pressure starts gas flow from the ventilator to deliver inspiration.

prone Position in which the patient is lying face downward.

propofol Intravenous anesthetic agent that is useful for sedation when titrated at lower doses; it can provide anterograde amnesia.

proportional assist ventilation (PAV) An interactive ventilatory support mode that provides patient-triggered breaths in which flow and volume delivery are controlled by clinician-set "gains" placed on sensed patient effort. With PAV, increases in patient effort result in increased flow, volume, and airway pressure.

protected specimen brush (PSB) A small brush at the end of a long catheter designed to sample distal airways for microorganisms. It has an outer sheath to "protect" it from contamination from upper airway microorganisms.

pulmonary artery wedge pressure (PAWP) Measure that provides an estimate of left atrial (LA) and left ventricular end-diastolic or filling pressure (LVDEP).

pulmonary edema Accumulation of excess fluid in the interstitial and alveolar spaces in the lung.

pulmonary vascular resistance (PVR) Resistance in the pulmonary vascular bed against which the right ventricle must eject blood.

pulse oximeter A device that assesses oxygen-hemoglobin saturation through the skin by using infrared light absorption technology.

pulse pressure The difference between systolic and diastolic arterial pressure.

pulsus paradoxus Abnormal decrease in systolic pressure and pulse wave amplitude during inspiration.

R

rainout See *Condensation.*

recruitment maneuver Sustained inflation at high airway pressure that has been advocated as an adjunct to mechanical ventilation in patients with ARDS; the result of a recruitment maneuver is decreased atelectasis.

relative humidity The amount of water vapor in a gas compared with the maximum amount of water that gas can carry. Relative humidity is expressed as a percent.

resistance Impedance to flow in a tube or conduit; quantified as ratio of the difference in pressure between the two points along a tube length divided by the volumetric flow of the fluid per unit of time.

respiratory quotient (RQ) Ratio of CO_2 production to O_2 consumption.

resting energy expenditure (REE) The caloric consumption of a patient.

Reynolds' number A dimensionless number that predicts whether flow will be laminar or turbulent based on gas velocity, viscosity, density, and tube diameter. A Reynolds' number <2000 indicates laminar flow and >2000 indicates turbulent flow.

S

saturated The state of gas that is carrying the maximum possible amount of water vapor. Saturated gas is at 100% relative humidity.

sedation The allaying of irritability or excitement, especially by administration of a sedative drug.

selective pulmonary vasodilation Reducing pulmonary vascular resistance without affecting systemic vascular resistance.

Sellick maneuver Technique of providing cricoid pressure named for its inventor.

shunting Pulmonary capillary blood completely bypassing ventilated alveoli.

silver-coated/silver-impregnated tube Endotracheal tubes used in the ICU may have a silver chloride coating. Silver is known for its bacteriostatic properties. Other medically useful properties include prevention of biofilm formation, a reduction in bacterial burden, and reduction in inflammation.

small-volume nebulizer An aerosol generator that requires a gas source to nebulize liquid medications.

spacer A device used to improve aerosol delivery by stabilizing particle size reducing velocity and reducing the need for breath/actuation coordination. Can be used in ambulatory and mechanically ventilated patients.

spontaneous breathing trial (SBT) Integrated patient assessment during spontaneous breathing with little or no ventilator assistance to assess ventilator discontinuation potential; respiratory pattern, hemodynamic status, gas exchange, and patient comfort should all be assessed.

spontaneous breath/ventilation Breath that is both patient triggered and patient cycled.

stroke volume Volume of blood ejected by the left ventricle during each contraction.

subglottic suction tube Special endotracheal tube used to remove secretions above the endotracheal tube cuff (subglottic secretion drainage [SSD]); it has a second lumen embedded in the body of the tube that opens just above the cuff on the posterior aspect.

suction catheter A thin, hollow plastic tube containing several distal holes used for removal of airway secretions by application of negative pressure.

supine Position in which the patient is lying face up on their back.

synchronous intermittent mandatory ventilation (SIMV) Mode for breath delivery or ventilatory support using pressure or flow/volume assist control breaths interspersed with spontaneous or pressure supported breaths.

T

tidal volume The volume of air that is inhaled or exhaled from the lungs during a breath.

time cycling When the ventilator ends inspiration after measuring a specific time that has elapsed. Time is commonly based on rate or frequency control setting.

titration Method of estimating the amount of solute in a solution.

torsades de pointes Type of ventricular tachycardia that is precipitated by a long Q-T interval, which often is induced by drugs but may also be the result of hypokalemia or profound bradycardia.

tracheal gas insufflation (TGI) A technique whereby a low flow of fresh gas is delivered to the distal end of the endotracheal tube through a small-diameter catheter. This flow can be either continuous (i.e., throughout the ventilatory cycle) or delivered only during exhalation. The primary purpose of TGI is to flush the upper airway with fresh gas during exhalation and thereby to reduce functional dead space.

tracheostomy An opening in the trachea in which sutures are used to provide a connection from the trachea to the skin and secure an opening for a tracheostomy tube.

train-of-four A method of monitoring neuromuscular blockade in patients. A sequence of four electrical stimuli is delivered to electrodes placed over a nerve (usually the temporal or radial nerve) and the twitch of the involved muscle group is measured to gauge neuromuscular blockade. If four stimuli are provided and no twitches are present, blockade is deep. If two of four stimuli result in twitches, blockade is usually sufficient.

transducer A device capable of converting one form of energy into another and commonly used for measurement of physical events; for example, a pressure transducer may convert the physical phenomenon of force per unit area into an analog electrical signal.

transrespiratory pressure The pressure difference between airway and body surface.

traumatic brain injury (TBI) Characterized by primary irreversible injury from the initial insult, and potentially secondary injury related to physiologic abnormalities and nosocomial complications.

trigger variable To initiate the inspiratory phase of a breath.

turbulent flow Flow characterized by formation of currents and eddies resulting in chaotic movement of gas molecules and a Reynolds' number > 2000.

V

Valsalva maneuver Any forced expiratory effort against a closed glottis.

venoarterial bypass Technique for cardiopulmonary bypass (see *Extracorporeal oxygenation*).

venovenous bypass Technique for cardiopulmonary bypass (see *Extracorporeal oxygenation*).

venous return Filling of the heart with blood from the venous circulation

ventilator associated pneumonia (VAP) Pneumonia that develops in the hospital in a patient receiving mechanical ventilation.

ventilator circuit The plastic nondisposable or disposable tubing (22 mm OD for adults) that connects the mechanical ventilator to the artificial airway or mask.

ventilation distribution The description of how the tidal volume is distributed to the millions of alveolar units.

ventilation/perfusion ($\dot{V}/\dot{Q}$) relationships Quantification of the relationship of ventilation to perfusion in alveolar capillary units. This is normally 1. Very high $\dot{V}/\dot{Q}$ units are effectively dead space. $\dot{V}/\dot{Q}$ units of 0 are shunts.

ventilator dependence Need for mechanical ventilation.

ventilator discontinuation Discontinuation of mechanical ventilation support from a patient.

vibrating mesh nebulizer Uses a vibrating mesh or plate with multiple apertures to create an aerosol; does not require a gas source for power and eliminates problems associated with the addition of a continuous flow to the ventilator circuit.

volume Space occupied by matter measured in milliliters or liters.

volume assist control ventilation An assist-control mode of ventilation that is floor targeted/limited and volume cycled.

volume-assured pressure support Pressure support ventilation that provides automated adjustment of inspiratory pressure (pressure support) based upon tidal volume.

volume control Variable in the equation of motion that the ventilator is maintaining constant during breath delivery; breaths are volume constant and pressure variable.

volume cycling Inspiration ends when a preset volume is delivered to the patient.

volume triggering The beginning of inspiration initiated by a ventilator when it detects a small drop in volume in the patient circuit.

volutrauma Injury to the lung due to excessive volume in the lung.

W

weaning Gradual reduction in partial ventilatory support.

weaning techniques Ventilator strategies that accomplish weaning.

wean screen Assessment of lung injury, gas exchange, hemodynamics, and spontaneous breathing as indications for readiness for a formal ventilatory discontinuation assessment (e.g., spontaneous breathing trial or SBT).

wick humidifier A modified passover humidifier that directs gas into a cylinder lined with a wick of blotter paper; as the wick absorbs water and the gas contacts the heated wick, the relative humidity of the gas increases.

work A quantification of ventilation load that is obtained by integrating pressure over volume. (See *Pressure-time product* for an alternative load expression.)

Index

Note: Page numbers followed by "f" refer to illustrations; page numbers followed by "t" refer to tables; page numbers followed by "b" refer to boxes.

J

K

L

N

O

Q

R

S

U

V

W